Handbook of Research on Disease Prediction Through Data Analytics and Machine Learning

Geeta Rani
Manipal University Jaipur, India

Pradeep Kumar Tiwari
Manipal University Jaipur, India

A volume in the Advances in Medical Diagnosis, Treatment, and Care (AMDTC) Book Series

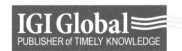

Published in the United States of America by
    IGI Global
    Medical Information Science Reference (an imprint of IGI Global)
    701 E. Chocolate Avenue
    Hershey PA, USA 17033
    Tel: 717-533-8845
    Fax: 717-533-8661
    E-mail: cust@igi-global.com
    Web site: http://www.igi-global.com

Library of Congress Cataloging-in-Publication Data

Names: Rani, Geeta, 1980- editor. | Tiwari, Pradeep Kumar, 1982- editor.
Title: Handbook of research on disease prediction through data analytics
  and machine learning / Geeta Rani and Pradeep Kumar Tiwari, editors.
Description: Hershey, PA : Medical Information Science Reference, [2020] |
  Includes bibliographical references and index. | Summary: "This book
  explores the use of data analytics algorithms and machine learning
  techniques for disease prediction"-- Provided by publisher.
Identifiers: LCCN 2019043256 (print) | LCCN 2019043257 (ebook) | ISBN
  9781799827429 (hardcover) | ISBN 9781799827436 (ebook)
Subjects: MESH: Machine Learning | Diagnosis, Computer-Assisted | Fuzzy
  Logic | Data Interpretation, Statistical | Sampling Studies
Classification: LCC R853.S7 (print) | LCC R853.S7 (ebook) | NLM W
  26.55.A7 | DDC 616.0072/7--dc23
LC record available at https://lccn.loc.gov/2019043256
LC ebook record available at https://lccn.loc.gov/2019043257

This book is published in the IGI Global book series Advances in Medical Diagnosis, Treatment, and Care (AMDTC) (ISSN: 2475-6628; eISSN: 2475-6636)

British Cataloguing in Publication Data
A Cataloguing in Publication record for this book is available from the British Library.

All work contributed to this book is new, previously-unpublished material. The views expressed in this book are those of the authors, but not necessarily of the publisher.

For electronic access to this publication, please contact: eresources@igi-global.com.

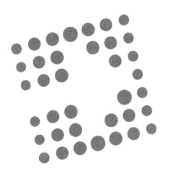

Advances in Medical Diagnosis, Treatment, and Care (AMDTC) Book Series

ISSN:2475-6628
EISSN:2475-6636

MISSION

Advancements in medicine have prolonged the life expectancy of individuals all over the world. Once life-threatening conditions have become significantly easier to treat and even cure in many cases. Continued research in the medical field will further improve the quality of life, longevity, and wellbeing of individuals.

The **Advances in Medical Diagnosis, Treatment, and Care (AMDTC)** book series seeks to highlight publications on innovative treatment methodologies, diagnosis tools and techniques, and best practices for patient care. Comprised of comprehensive resources aimed to assist professionals in the medical field apply the latest innovations in the identification and management of medical conditions as well as patient care and interaction, the books within the AMDTC series are relevant to the research and practical needs of medical practitioners, researchers, students, and hospital administrators.

COVERAGE

- Disease Management
- Patient-Centered Care
- Medical Testing
- Chronic Conditions
- Medical Procedures
- Disease Prevention
- Experimental Medicine
- Critical Care
- Internal Medicine
- Alternative Medicine

IGI Global is currently accepting manuscripts for publication within this series. To submit a proposal for a volume in this series, please contact our Acquisition Editors at Acquisitions@igi-global.com or visit: http://www.igi-global.com/publish/.

Titles in this Series

For a list of additional titles in this series, please visit:
https://www.igi-global.com/book-series/advances-medical-diagnosis-treatment-care/129618

Handbook of Research on Evidence-Based Perspectives on the Psychophysiology of Yoga and Its Appliations
Shirley Telles (Patanjali Research Foundation, India) and Ram Kumar Gupta (Patanjali Research Foundation, India)
Medical Information Science Reference • © 2021 • 577pp • H/C (ISBN: 9781799832546) • US $345.00

New Developments in Diagnosing, Assessing, and Treating ADHD
Rejani Thudalikunnil Gopalan (Mahatma Gandhi Medical College and Hospital, India)
Medical Information Science Reference • © 2021 • 419pp • H/C (ISBN: 9781799854951) • US $265.00

Handbook of Research on Oncological and Endoscopical Dilemmas in Modern Gynecological Clinical Practice
Konstantinos Dinas (2nd Department of Obstetrics and Gynaecology, Aristotle University of Thessaloniki, Greece)
Stamatios Petousis (2nd Department of Obstetrics and Gynaecology, Aristotle University of Thessaloniki, Greece)
Matthias Kalder (Department of Obstetrics and Gynaecology, Philipps-University of Marburg, Germany) and George
Mavromatidis (2nd Department of Obstetrics and Gynaecology, Aristotle University of Thessaloniki, Greece)
Medical Information Science Reference • © 2021 • 460pp • H/C (ISBN: 9781799842132) • US $385.00

Diagnostic Techniques and Therapeutic Strategies for Parotid Gland Disorders
Mahmoud Sakr (Alexandria University, Egypt)
Medical Information Science Reference • © 2021 • 362pp • H/C (ISBN: 9781799856030) • US $295.00

Evaluation and Management of High-Risk Pregnancies Emerging Research and Opportunities
Sapna Nanda (Panjab University, India)
Medical Information Science Reference • © 2021 • 216pp • H/C (ISBN: 9781799843573) • US $195.00

Noninvasive Ventilation Technologies and Healthcare for Geriatric Patients
César Fonseca (Universidade de Évora, Portugal) Manuel José Lopes (Universidade de Évora, Portugal) David
Mendes (Universidade de Évora, Portugal) Jose Garcia-Alonso (University of Extremadura, Spain) and Felismina
Mendes (Universidade de Évora, Portugal)
Medical Information Science Reference • © 2020 • 252pp • H/C (ISBN: 9781799835318) • US $245.00

Diagnostic and Treatment Methods for Ulcerative Colitis and Colitis-Associated Cancer
Ashok Kumar Pandurangan (B.S. Abdur Rahman Crescent Institute of Science and Technology, India)
Medical Information Science Reference • © 2020 • 300pp • H/C (ISBN: 9781799835806) • US $295.00

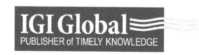

701 East Chocolate Avenue, Hershey, PA 17033, USA
Tel: 717-533-8845 x100 • Fax: 717-533-8661
E-Mail: cust@igi-global.com • www.igi-global.com

Editorial Advisory Board

List of Contributors

Table of Contents

Detailed Table of Contents

Chapter 1

    Meet Ganpatlal Oza, Manipal University, Jaipur, India
    Geeta Rani, Manipal University Jaipur, India
    Vijaypal Singh Dhaka, Manipal University Jaipur, India

The increase in use of ICT tools and decrease in physical activities has increased the risk of disorders such as diabetes, hypertension, myopia, hypermetropia, etc. These disorders make the person more prone to eye disease such as glaucoma. The actual causes of glaucoma are still unknown. But the study of medical literature reveals that the factors such as intraocular pressure, thyroid, diabetics, eye injuries, eye surgeries, ethnic background, and myopia makes the person more prone to glaucoma. The difficulty in early detection make it an invisible thief of sight. Therefore, it is the demand of the day to design a system for its early detection. The aim of this chapter is to develop a convolutional neural network model "GlaucomaDetector" for detection of glaucoma at an early stage. The evaluation of the model on the publicly available dataset reports the accuracy of 99% for prediction of glaucoma from the input images of retina. This may prove a useful tool for doctors for quick prediction of glaucoma at an early stage. Thus, it can minimize the risk of blindness in patients.

Chapter 2

    Shivani Batra, KIET Group of Institutions, Delhi-NCR, India
    Shelly Sachdeva, National Institute of Technology, Delhi, India

EHRs aid in maintaining longitudinal (lifelong) health records constituting a multitude of representations in order to make health related information accessible. However, storing EHRs data is non-trivial due to the issues of semantic interoperability, sparseness, and frequent evolution. Standard-based EHRs are recommended to attain semantic interoperability. However, standard-based EHRs possess challenges (in terms of sparseness and frequent evolution) that need to be handled through a suitable data model. The traditional RDBMS is not well-suited for standardized EHRs (due to sparseness and frequent evolution).

Thus, modifications to the existing relational model is required. One such widely adopted data model for EHRs is entity attribute value (EAV) model. However, EAV representation is not compatible with mining tools available in the market. To style the representation of EAV, as per the requirement of mining tools, pivoting is required. The chapter explains the architecture to organize EAV for the purpose of preparing the dataset for use by existing mining tools.

The image processing task, aimed at interpreting and classifying the contents of the images, has attracted the attention of researchers since the early days of computers. With the advancement of computing system technology, image categorization has found increasingly broader applications, covering new generation disciplines such as image analysis, object recognition, and computer vision, with applications quite general both in scientific and humanistic fields. The automatic recognition, description, and classification of the structures contained in the images are of fundamental importance in a vast set of scientific and engineering fields that require the acquisition, processing, and transmission of information in visual form. Classification tasks also include those related to the categorization of images, such as the construction of a recognition system, the representation of patterns, the selection and extraction of features, and the definition of automatic recognition methods. Image analysis is of collective interest and it is a hot topics of current research.

Having/living convenient life through smart devices, people are more interested or more dependent on to predict something for future (i.e., with respect to their health, business, etc.). For that, many prediction models by several researchers are being used in many applications. Due to a vast (rapid) change in lifestyle, people are more prone to a number of life-threatening diseases when it comes to their well-being. Many of these diseases start developing their symptoms in their early stages. But, still many of these diseases like cancer, kidney damages remain unidentified in their developing stages. The earlier a disease is predicted, the easier it becomes to cure it and even prevent it. Predictive modeling provides a huge step forward in medical science in preventing the risk among patients. Prediction modeling is the process of analyzing current conditions to predict future results.

Healthcare is always a sensitive issue for all of us, and it will always remain. Predicting various types of health issues in advance can lead us to a better life. Various types of health problems are there like cancer, heart diseases, diabetes, arthritis, pneumonia, lungs disease, liver disease, and brain disease, which all are at high risk. To reduce the risk of health issues, some suitable models are needed for prediction.

Thus, it became as a motivational factor for the authors to survey the existing literature on this topic thoroughly and have consequently to identify suitable machine learning techniques so that improvement can be possible while selecting a prediction model. In this chapter, concept of survey is used to provide the prediction models for healthcare issues along with the challenges associated with each model. This chapter will broadly cover the following: machine learning algorithms used in health industry, study various prediction models for Cancer, Heart diseases, Diabetes and Brain diseases, comparative study of various machine learning algorithms used for prediction.

Chapter 6

Devesh Kumar Srivastava, Manipal University Jaipur, India
Pradeep Kumar Tiwari, Manipal University Jaipur, India

In today's contemporary world, it is important to know about the odds of having a disease because of changing living standards of the population overall in the continent. The disease on which the authors are working is chronic kidney disease. Once the person gets chronic kidney disease (CKD), his working capability decreases along with other adverse effects. It is possible to get rid of diseases like CKD with new methodologies that will help us to predict the stage of kidney disease at an early stage. Under big data analytics, data may be structured, unstructured, quasi- or semi-structured. The CKD detected and predicted by applying classification models: support vector machine (SVM), K-nearest neighbor (KNN), and logistic regression algorithm. It helps in predicting the likelihood of occurrence of disease on various different features. The two algorithms KNN and SVM are compared to find the algorithm that gives better accuracy. Further regression technique has been used to detect the disease based on, which the stages are classified by using GFR (glomerular filtration rate) formula.

Chapter 7

Ahan Chatterjee, The Neotia University, India
Swagatam Roy, The Neotia University, India
Rupali Shrivastava, The Neotia University, India

One of the most talked about diseases of the 21st century is none other than cancer. In this chapter, the authors take a closer look to prevent cancer through machine learning approach. At first, they ran their classifier models (e.g., decision tree, K-mean, SVM, etc.) to check which algorithm gives the best result in terms of choosing right features for further treatment. The classified results are compared, and then various feature reduction algorithm is being used to identify exactly which features affects the most. Various data mining algorithms are being used, namely rough-based theory, graph-based clustering, to extract the most important features which influence the results. In the next section they take a look in the cancer analytics part. A simulation model has been designed that can easily manage the patient flow in OPDs and a bed rotation model also have been designed to give patients an insight that how much time they will spend in the queue. Further they analyzed a risk analysis model for chemotherapy treatment, and finally, an econometric discussion has been drawn in how it affects the treatment.

Chapter 8

Aman Sharma, IT Department, Jaypee University of Information Technology, Solan, India
Rinkle Rani, Computer Science and Engineering Department, Thapar Institute of Engineering and Technology, Patiala, India

Advancement in genome sequencing technology has empowered researchers to think beyond their imagination. Researchers are trying their hard to fight against various genetic diseases like cancer. Artificial intelligence has empowered research in the healthcare sector. Moreover, the availability of opensource healthcare datasets has motivated the researchers to develop applications which can help in early diagnosis and prognosis of diseases. Further, next-generation sequencing (NGS) has helped to look into detailed intricacies of biological systems. It has provided an efficient and cost-effective approach with higher accuracy. The advent of microRNAs also known as small noncoding genes has begun the paradigm shift in oncological research. We are now able to profile expression profiles of RNAs using RNA-seq data. microRNA profiling has helped in uncovering their relationship in various genetic and biological processes. Here in this chapter, the authors present a review of the machine learning perspective in cancer research.

Chapter 9

This chapter is devoted to the study of mathematical modelling part of infectious diseases, especially the nipah virus. In the past few decades, one cannot deny that enormous new unanticipated diseases have been the cause of serious concern among the human community and that so many viruses have begun emerging and re-emerging though people are trying all means to get rid of diseases. It can even be said that diseases of all sorts are ruling the world. Early prediction of diseases that spread in humans plays a vital role to protect living beings. Most of such diseases are highly infectious, get transmitted from human to human or through some other vectors. Several research and developments take place in the pharma industry notably after the Second World War. Hence, the predictions are not just for theoretical purposes as quite a number of pharma industries use mathematical models for their findings in new medicines and even to decide the quantity of medicine production. This chapter gives an overview of the different researches conducted in mathematical modelling of nipah virus.

Chapter 10

Early detection and proper treatment of brain tumors are imperative to prevent permanent damage to the brain even patient death. The present study proposed an AI-based computer-aided diagnosis (CAD) system that refers to the process of automated contrast enhancement followed by identifying the region of interest (ROI) and then classify ROI into benign/malignant classes using significant morphological feature selection. This tool automates the detection procedure and also reduces the manual efforts required in widespread screening of brain MRI. Simple power law transformation technique based on different performance metrics is used to automate the contrast enhancement procedure. Finally, benignancy/malignancy of brain tumor is examined by neural network classifier and its performance is assessed by well-known receiver operating characteristic method. The result of the proposed method is enterprising with very low computational time and accuracy of 87.8%. Hence, the proposed method of CAD procedure may encourage the medical practitioners to get alternative opinion.

Upendra Kumar, Institute of Engineering and Technology, Lucknow, India
Shashank Yadav, Institute of Engineering and Technology, Lucknow, India

Interest in research involving health-medical information analysis based on artificial intelligence has recently been increasing. Most of the research in this field has been focused on searching for new knowledge for predicting and diagnosing disease by revealing the relation between disease and various information features of data. However, still needed are more research and interest in applying the latest advanced artificial intelligence-based data analysis techniques to bio-signal data, which are continuous physiological records, such as EEG (electroencephalography) and ECG (electrocardiogram). This study presents a survey of ECG classification into arrhythmia types. Early and accurate detection of arrhythmia types is important in detecting heart diseases and choosing appropriate treatment for a patient.

M. Nandhini, Department of Computer Science, Government Arts College, Udumalpet, India
S. N. Sivanandam, Department of Computer Science and Engineering, Karpagam College of Engineering, Coimbatore, India
S. Renugadevi, Department of Computer Science and Engineering, PSG College of Technology, Coimbatore, India

Data mining is likely to explore hidden patterns from the huge quantity of data and provides a way of analyzing and categorizing the data. Associative classification (AC) is an integration of two data mining tasks, association rule mining, and classification which is used to classify the unknown data. Though association rule mining techniques are successfully utilized to construct classifiers, it lacks in generating a small set of significant class association rules (CARs) to build an accurate associative classifier. In this work, an attempt is made to generate significant CARs using Artificial Bee Colony (ABC) algorithm, an optimization technique to construct an efficient associative classifier. Associative classifier, thus built using ABC discovered CARs achieve high prognostic accurateness and interestingness value. Promising results were provided by the ABC based AC when experiments were conducted using health care datasets from the UCI machine learning repository.

Abhranil Gupta, Auctus Solutions, India

This chapter gives a brief overview of the state of the art of machine learning approaches in detection of the neurodegenerative disease from medical records (brain scans, etc.). It starts with an understanding of the sub-field of artificial intelligence, machine learning, then goes to understand neurodegenerative disease, with a focus on four major diseases and then goes on to giving an overview of how such diseases are detected using machine learning. In the end, it discusses the future areas of research that needs to be done in order to improve the field of research.

Clinical data is increasing day-by-day mainly in hospitals by an ageing of the human population. Patients discharged from hospitals are readmitted due to health issues. As the number of patients increases, there are a smaller number of hospitals and an increase in healthcare costs. This results in ineffective decision making that minimizes the healthcare. Machine learning techniques score better for solving this kind of problem. The proposed work, minimum entropy feature selection with logistic regression (MELR), is performing better for the readmission rates. Decision cannot be based on the clinical knowledge and personal data about the patient. It must be precise in choosing the future patient outcomes. This chapter produces promising results for clinical data.

Acquisition of the standard plane is the prerequisite of biometric measurement and diagnosis during the ultrasound (US) examination. Based upon the analysis of existing algorithms for the automatic fetal development measurement, a new algorithm known as neuro-fuzzy based on genetic algorithm is developed. Firstly, the fetal ultrasound benchmark image is auto-pre-processed using normal shrink homomorphic technique. Secondly, the features are extracted using gray level co-occurrence matrix (GLCM), grey level run length matrix (GLRLM), intensity histogram (IH), and rotation invariant moments (IM). Thirdly, neuro-fuzzy using genetic approach is used to distinguish among the fetus growth as abnormal or normal. Experimental results using benchmark and live dataset demonstrate that the developed method achieves an accuracy of 97% as compared to the state-of-the-art methods in terms of parameters such as sensitivity, specificity, recall, f-measure, and precision rate.

Chapter 16

Cardiovascular diseases are a major cause of death worldwide. Cardiologists detect arrhythmias (i.e., abnormal heart beat) with the help of an ECG graph, which serves as an important tool to recognize and detect any erratic heart activity along with important insights like skipping a beat, a flutter in a wave, and a fast beat. The proposed methodology does ECG arrhythmias classification by CNN, trained on grayscale images of R-R interval of ECG signals. Outputs are strictly in the terms of a label that classify the beat as normal or abnormal with which abnormality. For training purpose, around one lakh ECG signals are plotted for different categories, and out of these signal images, noisy signal images are removed, then deep learning model is trained. An image-based classification is done which makes the ECG arrhythmia system independent of recording device types and sampling frequency. A novel idea is proposed that helps cardiologists worldwide, although a lot of improvements can be done which would foster a "wearable ECG Arrhythmia Detection device" and can be used by a common man.

Genome-wide association studies (GWAS) or genetic data analysis is used to discover common genetic factors which influence the health of human beings and become a part of a disease. The concept of using genomics has increased in recent years, especially in e-healthcare. Today there is huge improvement required in this field or genomics. Note that the terms genomics and genetics are not similar terms here. Basically, the human genome is made up of DNA, which consists of four different chemical building blocks (called bases and abbreviated A, T, C, and G). Based on this, we differentiate each and every human being living on earth. The term 'genetics' originated from the Greek word 'genetikos'. It means 'origin'. In simple terms, genetics can be defined as a branch of biology, which deals with the study of the functionalities and composition of a single gene in an organism. There are mainly three branches of genetics, which include classical genetics, molecular genetics, and population genetics.

Chapter 18

Heart disease is one of the most common and serious health issues in all the age groups. The food habits, mental stress, smoking, etc. are a few reasons for heart diseases. Diagnosing heart issues at an early stage is very much important to take proper treatment. The treatment of heart disease at the later stage is very expensive and risky. In this chapter, the authors discuss machine learning approaches to predict heart disease from a set of health parameters collected from a person. The heart disease dataset from the UCI machine learning repository is used for the study. This chapter discusses the heart disease prediction capability of four well-known machine learning approaches: naive Bayes classifier, KNN classifier, decision tree classifier, random forest classifier.

This chapter aimed to evaluate heuristic approach performances for artificial neural networks (ANN) training. For this purpose, software that can perform ANN training application was developed using four different algorithms. First of all, training system was developed via back propagation (BP) algorithm, which is the most commonly used method for ANN training in the literature. Then, in order to compare the performance of this method with the heuristic methods, software that performs ANN training with genetic algorithm (GA), particle swarm optimization (PSO), and artificial immunity (AI) methods were designed. These designed software programs were tested on the breast cancer dataset taken from UCI (University of California, Irvine) database. When the test results were evaluated, it was seen that the most important difference between heuristic algorithms and BP algorithm occurred during the training period. When the training-test durations and performance rates were examined, the optimal algorithm for ANN training was determined as GA.

Many apps and analyzers based on machine learning have been designed to help and cure the stress issue. This chapter is based on an experiment that the authors performed at Research Labs and Scientific Spirituality Centers of Dev Sanskriti VishwaVidyalaya, Haridwar and Patanjali Research Foundations, Uttarakhand. In the research work, the correctness and accuracy have been studied and compared for two biofeedback devices named as electromyography (EMG) and galvanic skin response (GSR), which can operate in three modes: audio, visual and audio-visual with the help of data set of tension type headache (TTH) patients. The authors used some data visualization techniques that EMG (electromyography) in audio mode is best among all other modes, and in this experiment, they have used a data set of SF-36 and successfully clustered them into three clusters (i.e., low, medium, and high) using K-means algorithm. After clustering, they used classification algorithm to classify a user (depending upon the sum of all the weights of questions he had answered) into one of these three class. They have also implemented various algorithms for classifications and compared their accuracy out of which decision tree algorithm has given the best accuracy.

Chapter 21

This chapter presents a comparative study of the proposed approaches (i.e., extended dark block extraction [EDBE], extended cluster count extraction [ECCE], and extended co-VAT approaches). This chapter evaluates pre-clustering and post-clustering algorithms on real-time data and synthetic datasets. Unlike traditional clustering algorithms, pre-clustering algorithms provide a prior clustering on different datasets. Simulation studies are carried out using datasets having both class-labeled and unlabeled information. Comparative studies are performed between results of existing pre-clustering and proposed pre-clustering approaches. A simulated RDI-based preprocessing method is also applied for data diversification. Extensive simulation on real and synthetic datasets shows that pre-clustering algorithms with simulated RDI-based pre-processing performs better compared to conventional post-clustering algorithms.

Liver diseases avert the normal activity of the liver. Discovering the presence of liver disorder at an early stage is a complex task for the doctors. Predictive analysis of liver disease using classification algorithms is an efficacious task that can help the doctors to diagnose the disease within a short duration of time. The main motive of this study is to analyze the parameters of various classification algorithms and compare their predictive accuracies so as to find the best classifier for determining the liver disease. This chapter focuses on the related works of various authors on liver disease such that algorithms were implemented using Weka tool that is a machine learning software written in Java. Also, orange tool is utilized to compare several classification algorithms in terms of accuracy. In this chapter, random forest, logistic regression, and support vector machine were estimated with an aim to identify the best classifier. Based on this study, random forest with the highest accuracy outperformed the other algorithms.

Chapter 23

Ashwani Kumar Yadav, Amity University Rajasthan, Jaipur, India
Vaishali, Manipal University, Jaipur, India
Raj Kumar, Shri Vishwakarma Skill University, Palwal, India
Archek Praveen Kumar, Malla Reddy College of Engineering for Women, Hyderabad, India

Texture analysis is one of the basic aspects of human visual system by which one can differentiate the objects and homogenous areas in an image. Manual diagnosis is not possible for huge database of images. Automatic diagnosis is required for greater accuracy in a shorter time. Texture analysis is required for effective diagnosis of medical images like functional MRI (magnetic resonance image) and diffusion tensor MRI, where only visualization is not sufficient to get the pathological information. This chapter explains the basic concepts of texture analysis and features available for analysis of medical images. Specifically, the intense review of texture segmentation and texture feature extraction and entropy measures of medical images have been done. The chapter also explores the available techniques for it. Common findings, comparative analysis, and gaps identified have also been mentioned on both issues.

Chapter 24

Nilamadhab Mishra, School of Computing Science and Engineering, VIT Bhopal University,
     India
Johny Melese Samuel, Debre Berhan University, Ethiopia

The eye is the most important sensory organ of vision function. But some eye diseases can lead to vision loss, so it is important to identify and treat eye disease as early as possible. Eye care professionals can help protect their patients from vision loss or blindness by recognizing common eye diseases and recommending for an eye exam. Eye diseases with early detection, treatment, and appropriate follow-up care, vision loss, and blindness from eye disease can be prevented or delayed. In this study, rule-based eye disease identification and advising the knowledge-based system are projected. The projected system is targeting using hidden knowledge extracted by employing the extraction algorithm of data mining. To identify the best prediction model for the diagnosis of eye disease, four experiments for four classification algorithms were performed. Finally, the researchers decided to use the rules of the J48 pruned classification algorithm for further use in the development of a knowledge base of KBS because it exhibited better performance with a 98.5% evaluation result.

Chapter 25

Rohit Rastogi, ABES Engineering College, India
Devendra Kumar Chaturvedi, Dayalbagh Educational Institute, Agra, India
Mayank Gupta, Tata Consultancy Services, India

This chapter applied the random sampling in selection of the subjects suffering with headache, and care was taken that they ensure to fulfill the International Headache Society criteria. Subjects under consideration were assigned the two groups of GSR-integrated audio-visual feedback, GSR (audio-visual)- and EMG (audio-visual)-integrated feedback groups. In 10 sessions, the subjects experienced the GSR and EMG BF therapy for 15 minutes. Twenty subjects were subjected to EEG therapy. The variables for stress (pain) and SF-36 (quality of life) scores were recorded at starting point, 30 days, and 90 days after the starting of GSR and EMG-BF therapy. To reduce the anxiety and depression in day-to-day routine, the present research work is shown as evidence in favor of the mindful meditation. The physical, mental, and total scores increased over the time duration of SF-36 scores after 30- and 90-days recordings ($p<0.05$). Intergroup analysis has demonstrated the improvement. EMG-audio visual biofeedback group also showed highest improvement in SF-36 scores at first and third month follow up. EEG measures the Alpha waves for the subjects after meditation. GSR, EMG, and EEG-integrated auditory-visual biofeedback are efficient in solution of stress due to TTH with most advantage seen.

Chapter 26

Amit Kumar, Sanaka Educational Trust's Group of Institutions, India
Manish Kumar, Vellore Institute of Technology, Chennai, India
Nidhya R., Madanapalle Institute of Technology & Science, India

In recent years, a huge increase in the demand of medically related data is reported. Due to this, research in medical disease diagnosis has emerged as one of the most demanding research domains. The research reported in this chapter is based on developing an ACO (ant colony optimization)-based Bayesian hybrid prediction model for medical disease diagnosis. The proposed model is presented in two phases. In the first phase, the authors deal with feature selection by using the application of a nature-inspired algorithm known as ACO. In the second phase, they use the obtained feature subset as input for the naïve Bayes (NB) classifier for enhancing the classification performances over medical domain data sets. They have considered 12 datasets from different organizations for experimental purpose. The experimental analysis advocates the superiority of the presented model in dealing with medical data for disease prediction and diagnosis.

Foreword

This is my pleasure to write the forward for the book titled *Handbook of Research on Disease Prediction Through Data Analytics and Machine Learning*. The book covers the pre-processing techniques for the sparse data, image classification algorithms and a rigorous review of machine learning and deep learning techniques employed for prediction of diseases.

The book provides a window for the technologies involved for detection and classification of diseases such as glaucoma, cancer, heart disease, brain tumour, chronic kidney diseases, neuro-generative diseases and liver diseases.

The book gives good insights about the use of Internet of Things (IoT), bio-medical signals, bio-medical feedback for medical data analysis and disease prediction. This book covers the modelling techniques involved for detecting the behavior of Nipah Virus. The book gives the detailed description of the techniques involved in diagnosis and prognosis of fetal growth by analyzing the ultrasound images of fetus.

The book *Handbook of Research on Disease Prediction Through Data Analytics and Machine Learning* gives a clear idea about the deep learning techniques employed for analysis and classification of ECG images. The book covers the roles of Artificial Neural Networks (ANNs) in diagnosis of diseases by medical data analysis. The data mining algorithms for knowledge extraction and the texture segmentation and feature extraction techniques attract the readers working in the field of medical image analysis. The book provides the mechanisms involved in designing and developing the clinical decision support systems.

Handbook of Research on Disease Prediction Through Data Analytics and Machine Learning is a must-read book for the academicians, researchers and students working in the field of applications of machine learning and deep learning for disease diagnosis and prognosis. The book is important to read for the clinical experts who are keen to adopt the techno-tools as assistants for diagnosis and prognosis of diseases.

I would like to congratulate the Editor in Chief, Dr. Geeta Rani and Associate Editor, Dr. Pradeep Kumar Tiwari for bringing the ideas of academicians and research community together at a single platform. I strongly believe that their expertise in the field of machine learning, cloud computing and medical image analysis will be effective in attracting the readers in the field.

Anurag Singh
Department of Computer Science and Engineering, National Institute of Technology, Delhi, India

Preface

In recent era, use of data analytics and machine learning algorithms has been observed in the arena of medical filed. Literature shows the successful application of data analytics and machine learning techniques for making predictions using real time data collected from medical fields. The efficacy of machine learning models in image processing, big data analytics, object detection, automatic extraction and tailoring of features is a great motivation for employing these models in the medical field. A boom in the use of machine learning and deep learning models is observed since the last decade. The machine learning or deep learning models automatically extracts the features from the medical images, identify the most prominent features and predict the disease. For example, the lung disorders and diseases such as pneumonia, COVID-19, emphysema, lung tuberculosis, tumour etc. can predicted by training the deep learning model with the chest radiographs and CT scans. These models not only predict the disease but also useful in visualizing the infection in the organs. For reliable prediction, there is a need to design the custom architecture of the model. The architecture designer must focus on the size of dataset, versatility and quality of dataset, types and number of predictions to be provided. The architecture is also dependent on the type of analysis required for the disease prediction.

Literature reveals a lot of information about the designing of architectures for disease prediction.

But, poor availability of systematic information at one source becomes challenging for the students, academicians as well as researchers working in this field. Researchers face problems in identifying suitable algorithms for pre-processing, transformations and integration of clinical data. They also seek for different ways to build models, prepare data sets for training and evaluating the models. Moreover, it becomes significant for them, to observe the impact of decision making strategies on accuracy and precision of the predictive models designed on the basis of techniques such as Logistic Regression, Neural Networks, Decision Trees and Nearest Neighbors etc. Thus, there is a strong need of providing well organized study material with practical aspect and validation. The book smartly fills the gaps.

This book invited the ideas, proposals, review articles and experimental works from the researchers working in the field. The systematic organization of the research works in the field of applying machine learning for disease prediction will be fruitful in providing the insights to readers about the existing works and the gaps available in the field. This book is a significant contribution towards providing, the detailed study about data analytics algorithms and machine learning techniques for disease prediction. The book includes rigorous review of related literature, methodology for data set preparation, model building, training and testing the model. It contains comparative analysis of versatile algorithms applied for making predictions in the challenging arena of medical science and disease prediction. The provides a good insight about the topics such as Data Analytics, Machine Learning, Information Retrieval from medical data, Data Integration, Prediction Models, Genetic Data Analysis, Medical Data Analysis, Smart ICT and Universal Health Care.

The book is written as a companion and as a must-read, for academicians, people from industries, graduate and post graduate students, researchers, physicians and for everyone who is involved in the fields of medical, data analytics or machine learning directly or indirectly. The book is compiled in such a way that each chapter is suffice to give a complete study set from problem formulation to its solutions. All chapters are independent of each other and can be studied individually without consulting other chapters.

Each chapter starts with important key terms and introduction of the topic. It is followed by model building, training, testing and result analysis. The chapter ends with the concluding remarks and future directions.

This book welcomes the chapters from industry experts, researchers, and physicians. Topics of interest include but not limited to:

- Review in the fields of Data Analytics, Machine Learning and Medical Data Analysis.
- Applications and Practical Systems for Healthcare
- Information Retrieval from medical data
- Data Integration
- Prediction Models
- Mathematical methods for analysis of data collected using ECG, EEG, MRI, X-Ray and CT Scan
- Biomedical Image Analysis
- Sensor Data Analysis in Medical Science
- Analysis of Biomedical Signals such as EEG and ECG
- Genetic Data Analysis
- Role of Text Mining in Disease Prediction
- Advanced Data Analytics for Healthcare.
- Data Analytics for Pharmaceutical Discoveries
- Clinical Decision Support Systems
- Computer-Aided Diagnosis
- Mobile Imaging for Biomedical Applications
- Smart ICT and Universal Health Care

The brief summary of chapters is presented as follows.

Chapter 1: Glaucoma Detection Using Convolutional Neural Networks

The aim of this chapter is to develop a convolutional neural network model "GlaucomaDetector" for detection of glaucoma at an early stage. The evaluation of the model on the publicly available dataset reports the accuracy of 99% for prediction of Glaucoma from the input images of retina. This may prove a useful tool for doctors for quick prediction of glaucoma at an early stage. Thus, it can minimize the risk of blindness in patients.

Chapter 2: Pre-Processing Highly Sparse and Frequently Evolving Standardized Electronic Health Records for Mining

This chapter presents the strategies involved in maintaining the Electronic Health Records (EHRs) to provide a digital support to the healthcare industry. The authors claim that a database of EHRs assembles health data of a patient from various departments of a healthcare organization including administration, pharmacy, clinical, radiology, laboratory and nursing. The gathered data is stored within EHRs in structured, semi-structured, unstructured, or a hybridization of these storage architectures.

Chapter 3: Image Classification Techniques

This chapter presents a discussion on computers, machine learning and artificial intelligence in the field of image classification. The chapter gives details of different classification techniques proficient in categorizing images.

Chapter 4: Prediction Models

This chapter presents the prediction analytics and prediction modeling using the techniques such as Logistic Regression, Random Forest, Ridge Regression, K-nearest Neighbor and XGBoost for forecasting/prediction purpose. The authors in this chapter also discuss about the differences among popular terms like data analytics, predictive analytics, and prediction modeling.

Chapter 5: Predictions Models for Healthcare Using Machine Learning – A Review

In this chapter, the authors present different types of machine learning algorithms and their implementation on various diseases. The diseases selected to fulfil this purpose are general, so as to bolster the reader's understanding of the disease. The algorithms emphasized in this chapter are K-Nearest Neighbor, Classification and Regression Trees, Support Vector Machine (SVM), Naive Bayes, Gradient Boosted Regression Tree, Perceptron Back-Propagation, Random Forest in Supervised learning. Linear Regression and Logistic Regression in Semi Supervised learning. K-Means Clustering and Classification in Unsupervised Learning.

Chapter 6: Chronic Kidney Disease Prediction Using Data Mining Algorithms

This chapter presents a discussion based on the set of experiments conducted using Machine Learning algorithms for disease diagnosis. A sample Chronic disease dataset available publicly is used for the experimentation. Different Models are created using various machine learning algorithms like Linear Regression, Generalized Regression, Discriminant Analysis, Classification Tree, regression Tree, Support Vector Machine, K-Nearest Neighbours and Ensemble methods.

Chapter 7: A Machine Learning Approach to Prevent Cancer

In this chapter, the authors aim to find a performance comparison between various algorithms namely, Support Vector Machine (SVM), Decision Tree, Naïve Bayes (NB) and K-Nearest Neighbor (KNN). All the algorithms are applied on Wisconsin Breast Cancer (Original) Dataset.

Chapter 8: Machine Learning Perspective in Cancer Research

This chapter presents a comprehensive review of the machine learning perspective in cancer research. The chapter give a discussion about the techniques and algorithms employed for diagnosis of cancer from the medical data available online or collected from the hospitals.

Chapter 9: A Pathway to Differential Modelling of Nipah Virus

This chapter presents a discussion on spreading mechanism of Nipah Virus. It identifies the challenges such as finding the illness dynamics in non-human proximal types of species, intensifying the model for cross-species, detection of adaption and human-animal interface to map the transmission, incorporation of analyzation methods like stochasticity after pathogen introduction leads to observation errors etc and suggest the ways to deal with these challenges.

Chapter 10: Application of AI for Computer-Aided Diagnosis System to Detect Brain Tumors

The main objective of this chapter is to present a new AI based CAD system to analyze the brain MRI to detect the lesion characteristics in early stage. For improving that poor visibility, brain MRI requires the automated and efficient enhancement technique. This chapter focuses on approaches for exploiting very simple power-law transformation techniques based on some quantitative parameter measurement in an iterative manner to achieve the best enhancement results.

Chapter 11: Application of Machine Learning to Analyse Biomedical Signals for Medical Diagnosis

The main purpose of this chapter is to present a detailed overview of the computational techniques that have been utilized in analysing biomedical signals, especially ECG for detecting the heart diseases. Some common methods in biomedical signal analysis include some additional steps like pre-processing, biomedical signal wave characterization, feature extraction and classification. The chapter addressed different types of machine learning techniques that are used for ECG analysis to classify different heart diseases. These techniques are fuzzy logic, neural networks, rough set theory and hidden markov model, genetic algorithm, and support vector machines, etc.

Chapter 12: Artificial Bee Colony-Based Associative Classifier for Healthcare Data Diagnosis

This chapter presents the Data mining techniques employed to explore hidden patterns from the huge quantity of data. It specifically focuses on the Associative Classification (AC), an integration of two data mining tasks, association rule mining and classification used to classify the unknown data. The authors made an attempt to generate significant CARs using Artificial Bee Colony algorithm, an optimization technique to construct an efficient associative classifier.

Chapter 13: Artificial Intelligence Approaches to Detect Neurodegenerative Disease From Medical Records – A Perspective

The aim of this chapter is to give common platform for the medical professionals, diagnostic centers, machine learning algorithm professionals and the most importantly the patients. It presents a discussion about the neurodegenerative diseases, factors responsible for these disease and affects caused by these diseases.

Chapter 14: Clinical Decision Support Systems – Decision-Making System for Clinical Data

In this chapter, the authors present an efficient pyspark model EBHTLR implemented for readmission prediction. They also present a comparison of various classifiers. The chapter also gives insights about the feature selection techniques for high volume data.

Chapter 15: Diagnostic and Prognosis of Ultrasound Fetal Growth Analysis Using Neuro-Fuzzy Based on Genetic Algorithm

The objective of this chapter is to perform Image enhancement using application of Ultrasound Fetus Development through the study of various Denoising Filtering, Feature Extraction and Machine Learning techniques. It also evaluates the quantitative denoising filtering techniques on the basis of Peak Signal-to-Noise Ratio (PSNR), Signal-to-Noise Ratio (SNR), Edge Preservation Index (EPI) and Coefficient-of-Correlation (CoC) measures.

Chapter 16: ECG Image Classification Using Deep Learning Approach

The study presented in this chapter aims to help the cardiologists worldwide with the developments of AI in the health care sector. This chapter presents the techniques involved in refining the vast clinical data and to find patterns. The authors claim that the technique proposed in this chapter outperforms the existing techniques.

Chapter 17: Genetic Data Analysis

In this chapter, the authors present the study of massive amount of genetic data. The authors discussed that the analysis of genetic data can revolutionize the field of healthcare, pharmaceutical and agricultural industries. The techniques of Genome sequencing and re-sequencing are useful to develop modern plant breeding techniques. There are new methods that enable DNA to be modified more precisely.

Chapter 18: Heart Disease Prediction Using Machine Learning

This chapter presents the techniques for the early detection of heart diseases. The authors focused on four well-known machine learning techniques namely naive Bayes classifier, KNN classifier, decision tree classifier and random forest classier for heart disease prediction.

Chapter 19: Heuristic Approach Performances for Artificial Neural Networks Training

This chapter focuses on the information about artificial neural cells and Artificial Neural Network (ANN) algorithms. The chapter also highlights the visual design tool, experiments conducted for comparing the performance of different ANN techniques.

Chapter 20: Mental Health Through Biofeedback Is Important to Analyze – An App and Analysis

The work presented in this chapter is based on an experiment performed at Research Labs and Scientific Spirituality Centers of Dev Sanskriti VishwaVidyalaya, Haridwar and Patanjali Research Foundations, Uttarakhand. The authors compared the feedback of two biofeedback devices named as Electromyography(EMG) and Galvanic Skin Response (GSR) which can operate in three modes: audio, visual and audio-visual with the help of data set of Tension Type Headache (TTH) patients.

Chapter 21: Pre-Clustering Techniques for Healthcare System – Evaluation Measures, Evaluation Metrics, Comparative Study of Existing vs. Proposed Approaches

This chapter presents a comparative study of the proposed approaches viz., Extended Dark Block Extraction (EDBE), Extended Cluster Count Extraction (ECCE), and Extended Co-VAT approaches. This chapter evaluates Pre-Clustering and Post-Clustering algorithms on real-time data and synthetic datasets. Unlike traditional clustering algorithms, Pre-Clustering algorithms provide a prior clustering on different datasets. Simulation studies are carried out using datasets having both class-labeled and unlabeled information. Comparative studies are performed between results of existing Pre-Clustering and proposed Pre-Clustering approaches. A simulated RDI based preprocessing method is also applied for data diversification. Extensive simulation on real and synthetic datasets shows that Pre-Clustering algorithms with simulated RDI based pre-processing performs better compared to conventional Post-Clustering algorithms.

Chapter 22: Strategic Analysis in Prediction of Liver Disease Using Different Classification Algorithms

This chapter provides an overview of different classification algorithms popular in the field of data driven prediction of liver disease. The authors analyzed various classification algorithms that can help doctors to predict the liver disease at an early stage. They found that the Random forest algorithms outperforms the Support Vector Machine and Logistic Regression.

Chapter 23: Texture Segmentation and Features of Medical Images

This chapter presents the comparison of the texture segmentation techniques. The authors have presented the research gaps and the challenges identified in the existing techniques. The authors claimed that the watershed transformation algorithm could extract shape and form related information from images precisely. They claimed that the Vajda entropy measures is very much faster than the Kapur's entropy measure.

Chapter 24: Towards Integrating Data Mining With Knowledge-Based System for Diagnosis of Human Eye Diseases – The Case of an African Hospital

This chapter focuses on developing the system using hidden knowledge extraction. The system employs the extraction algorithms of data mining. This chapter also focus on identifying the best prediction model for the diagnosis of eye disease. The authors conducted four experiments for classification. They claimed that employing the rules of the J48 pruned classification algorithm for extracting information from a knowledge base of KBS achieves the good performance with a 98.5% accuracy.

Chapter 25: Use of IoT and Different Biofeedback to Measure TTH – An Approach for Healthcare 4.0

The authors in this chapter covers all possible aspects of TTH, IOT and big data and their applications to field of medical study. The authors presented the causes, effects, cures, biofeedback therapies of TTH. The study provides good insights about the work done and the future scope in this direction of research.

Chapter 26: ACO_NB-Based Hybrid Prediction Model for Medical Disease Diagnosis

In this chapter, the authors present a comparative analysis of most of the standard data set related to medical disease diagnosis. On the basis of the results claimed in the literature, they claim that their proposed model outperforms the models namely GA_NB and PSO_NB for diagnosis of distinct diseases.

Acknowledgment

With great pleasure, I would like to avail this opportunity to thank all the people who have supported me in the successful completion of this book. First and foremost, I wish to express my sincere gratitude to my collogue Dr. Pradeep Kumar Tiwari, Assistant Professor, Manipal University Jaipur for working tirelessly to reach this milestone.

I forward my sincere thanks to my Head of the Department Prof. Vijaypal Singh Dhaka for motivating me, and for providing the constant guidance and encouragement in executing each aspect of this book.

I would like to thank all the authors who have contributed to this book by submitting their ideas and experimental conclusions. I would like to thank my colleagues and friends who always motivated me to take and complete the challenges we encountered during this book. I convey my special thanks to my seniors and juniors who were always there for me to input their valuable suggestions and motivation.

My family deserves special mention for their inseparable support and prayers. I wish to take myself of this opportunity to express a sense of gratitude and love to my husband Satyawrat and kids Sonam and Archit. I am also grateful to my mother-in-law for providing me their mental support, strength and help every time I needed it. I owe my deep gratitude to my father 'Late Shri Jaibir and mother 'Indrawati' who taught me the first step of learning. Their blessings always inspired me to go ahead on this path.

Last but not least, I express my regard and love to all those who directly or indirectly contributed in the completion of the book *Handbook of Research on Disease Prediction Through Data Analytics and Machine Learning*.

Chapter 1
Glaucoma Detection Using Convolutional Neural Networks

Meet Ganpatlal Oza
Manipal University, Jaipur, India

Geeta Rani
Manipal University Jaipur, India

Vijaypal Singh Dhaka
Manipal University Jaipur, India

ABSTRACT

The increase in use of ICT tools and decrease in physical activities has increased the risk of disorders such as diabetes, hypertension, myopia, hypermetropia, etc. These disorders make the person more prone to eye disease such as glaucoma. The actual causes of glaucoma are still unknown. But the study of medical literature reveals that the factors such as intraocular pressure, thyroid, diabetics, eye injuries, eye surgeries, ethnic background, and myopia makes the person more prone to glaucoma. The difficulty in early detection make it an invisible thief of sight. Therefore, it is the demand of the day to design a system for its early detection. The aim of this chapter is to develop a convolutional neural network model "GlaucomaDetector" for detection of glaucoma at an early stage. The evaluation of the model on the publicly available dataset reports the accuracy of 99% for prediction of glaucoma from the input images of retina. This may prove a useful tool for doctors for quick prediction of glaucoma at an early stage. Thus, it can minimize the risk of blindness in patients.

INTRODUCTION

In modern era, the change in life style and increase in use of computer and mobile devices has increased the sensitivity of eyes towards defects and diseases. The diseases such as glaucoma can lead to loss of vision. This disease can cause the damage to the optic nerves which carry signals from the eyes to brain and vice-versa (National Eye Institute, n.d.).

DOI: 10.4018/978-1-7998-2742-9.ch001

At the initial stage, the Glaucoma may remain unnoticeable for the person. Even, it is difficult for the ophthalmologist to detect the Glaucoma at an early stage. At moderate stage the symptoms such as poor vision, loss of peripheral vision and eye pain appears. At severe stage, this disease can lead to blindness.

The factors such as intraocular pressure, thyroid, diabetics, eye injuries, eye surgeries, ethnic background, and myopia makes the person prone to Glaucoma (McMonnies, 2017). The difficulty in early detection make it invisible thief of sight. The regular eye check-up is important to minimize the risk of severe stage of Glaucoma. The glaucoma is categorized into four categories.

(i) **Open- angle glaucoma**: This is the primary stage of glaucoma. It is difficult to diagnose, therefore the person remains unaware to take the precautions. This may cause severe impacts at later stage.

(ii) **Angle- closure glaucoma**: In this type, the person feels pain in the eyes. It leads to a rapid loss in vision.

(iii) **Normal tension glaucoma**: This is the rarely observed type of glaucoma. The medical experts are still struggling to delve into the depth of this category. It is difficult to diagnose because it is observed under normal nerve pressure in the eyes. But, the blood supply in the eyes becomes low in the patients of this category.

(iv) **Congenital glaucoma**: This is hereditary disorder. It is generally observed in the babies of one year age (Medical News Today, n.d.).

As per reports presented in (Glaucoma Today, n.d.; National Health Portal, n.d.), about 11.2 billion people in India are suffering from glaucoma. Among these cases about 90% cases remain undetected. Thus, there is a potential risk of increase in severity of glaucoma with increase in age (Glaucoma Today, n.d.). The report published by World Health Organization (WHO) (National Health Portal, n.d.), shows that approximately 4.5 million people lose their vision due to glaucoma. Therefore, it is the demand of the time to provide an automatic tool for the early stage detection of this disease. The effectiveness of Artificial Intelligence (AI) in object detection, image classification, feature extraction, trend analysis and learning gives good insights for employing the AI techniques for early diagnosis of Glaucoma.

In this chapter, the authors propose a Convolutional Neural Network (CNN) model for early diagnosis of glaucoma.

ARCHITECTURE AND WORKING

Convolutional Neural Networks (CNNs) are a type of deep learning networks. These are effective used for image classification (Albawi et al., 2017; Chen et al., 2015). These networks replaced the manual feature extraction with the automatic feature extraction. These are efficient in the tailoring of most prominent features from the image datasets. These are effective in finding the differences in features of images, hence precise in making image classification.

In this chapter, the authors designed a shallow CNN **"GlaucoDetector"** for detection of **glaucoma**. The architecture of the model consists of four Convolution and four Max Pooling layers. These layers are defined at alternate positions as shown in Figure 1. The architecture employs the ReLu activation function between the convolution and max pooling layers. The kernel size for the first convolution layer is set as (3x3). The remaining three convolution layers use the kernal size of (2x2). The size of pool for each max pooling layer is set as (2x2).

The convolution layer of the model performs the convolution operation for extraction of low level and high level **features** from the image. The initial layers extract the low level features such as pixel intensity while the later layers work on high level features such as edge and shape detection. The later layers are actually involved in classification of images based on the high level features extracted from images. The pooling layers work to reduce the spatial size of the convolved features. The **Max Pooling operation** returns the **maximum value** from the feature map bounded in the kernel size. On the other hand, the **Average Pooling operation** returns the **average of all the values** from the feature map included in the Kernel. The pooling operation is important to fetch the most prominent and dominant features from the complete feature map. These layers also reduce the computation time and cost of the network. and also decreases the computational time required for processing. Now, the fully connected (FC) layers connects to all activations of the previous layer. The drop out layers are embedded in the architecture to inactivate the outputs of some randomly selected neurons. This is useful in avoiding the computations which may have minimum importance in classification. The dense layers actually involved in the analysis of feature maps for the detection and classification.

Figure 1. Architecture of **"GlaucoDetector"**

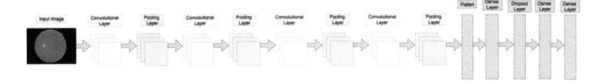

DATASET

For this research, the authors used the dataset of Fundus images available online at (Kaggle, n.d.).

Fundus imaging produces 2-Dimensional images of the 3-Dimensional retina by the reflection of light. The authors used the dataset of 1022 retinal fundus images for training the model. The authors used 511 images of the retina with glaucoma disease and 511 images of the healthy retina or non-glaucoma. The sample input image is shown in Figure 2. Before initiating the training of CNN, the authors divided the dataset into the training, testing and validation sets. By conducting a set of experiments, the authors put 80% dataset into the training set, 20% in the testing set. The training set is further divided into the 10% validation dataset. The optimum ratio selection of these sets is important to minimize the impacts of underfitting and/or overfitting.

Now, they applied the pre-processing techniques to yield the useful insights from our dataset. The pre-processing functions are shown in Table 1. The first column of Table 1 contain the function applied, column 2 shows the description of the function applied and the last column shows the output generated by the pre-processing function. After applying the pre-processing functions, a sequence of steps is followed to detect the glaucoma in the retina of human eye. The steps are given in Algorithm 1.

Figure 2. Sample Input Image

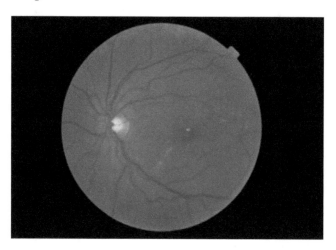

Table 1. Pre-Processing Techniques

Function	Description	Output
Global Thresholding (v=110)	This function segments the optic disc from the complete image. Its output can be used as a mask for the disc segmentation	
Adaptive Mean Thresholding	This function is used to extract the nerves from the images. The structure of the neurons become visible in its output.	
Adaptive Gaussian Thresholding	This function is similar to the mean thresholding. But the less structural view of neurons is visible in its output.	

Algorithm 1: Steps for Glaucoma Detection

```
Input: 2-D image of eye retina.
Output: Detected Class: Glaucoma or Non-Glaucoma.
(i) Convert the input image into an array.
(ii) Resize the input image to a uniform size to fit the model.
(iii) Pass the input image into GlaucomaDetector.
(iv) Employ the ReLu activation function. It returns positive values without
any change and returns zero for the negative values.
(v) Connect the dense layers with dropout layers in series to minimize over-
fitting. Set the dropout value as 0.5.
(vi) Receive the output.
```

EXPERIMENTAL RESULTS

The model was trained for 20 epochs on the dataset available at (Kaggle, n.d.). The model predicts the presence of glaucoma from the input images. The confusion matrix of the model is given in table 2. The authors evaluated the performance of the model in terms of the evaluation metrics precision, recall, F1 score and Support. The definitions of evaluation metrics are given below.

(i)   Precision: It is the ratio of the number of correct predictions in a particular class to that of the total number of correct predictions made in all the classes. The model 'GlaucomaDetector' achieves the average precision of 99% on the test dataset as shown in column 2 of table 3. The high values of precision prove that the model is effective in extracting the relevant instances of each class label from the total number of extracted instances.

(ii) Recall: It is the ratio of the number of correct predictions to a particular class to that of the total number of predictions made in that class. The proposed model gives an average recall of 99% as shown in column 3 of table 3. The high value of recall proves that the model extracts all the relevant instances from the given instances. It makes the correct predictions for the glaucoma.

(iii) F1 Score: This is the harmonic mean of precision and recall. The proposed model yields an average F1 score of 99% as shown in column 4, table 3. The high values of the F1 score prove its efficacy in classifying the test images correctly into their actual classes viz. glaucoma and non-glaucoma.

The experimental results are demonstrated in Table 3. The first column shows the class predicted for the input image, column 2 gives the precision, column 3 shows the recall, and column 4 gives the F1 score achieved by the "GlaucomaDetector". The authors also calculated the accuracy of the model. The accuracy for the training, validation and testing datasets is shown in Table 4. The accuracy of model may increase or decrease with increase in the number of epochs. The trends achieved by the training and validation accuracy are shown in Figure 3.

The loss function of the model changes dynamically for better training the model The trends of the values of the loss function are demonstrated in Figure 4. On conducting the experiments at multiple epochs, the model achieved the testing accuracy of 99.02%. The high value of accuracy shows that the model is effective in classifying the input images into glaucoma and non-glaucoma classes.

Table 2. Confusion Matrix

	Glaucoma	**Non- Glaucoma**
Glaucoma	(TP) 97	(FP) 1
Non- Glaucoma	(FN) 1	(TN) 106

Table 3. Experimental Results

Class	**Precision**	**Recall**	**F1-Score**
Glaucoma	0.990	0.990	0.990
Non-Glaucoma	0.991	0.991	0.991

Table 4. Accuracy of GlaucomaDetector

Split	**Train**	**Test**	**Validation**
Accuracy	99.05%	99.02%	99.00%

Figure 3. Accuracy of GlaucomaDetector

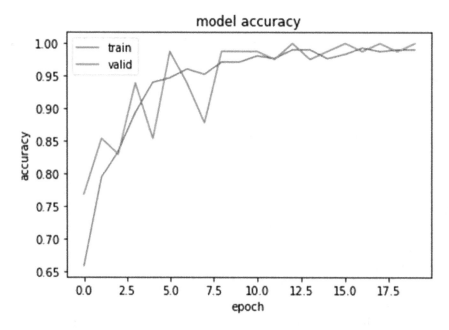

CONCLUSION

In this chapter, the authors applied the shallow CNN model "GlaucomaDetector" for detecting the glaucoma in the retina of human eye. The shallow CNN gave the accuracy of 99.02% on the test dataset. The authors designed the architecture of the model using shallow CNN because the dataset used for training and testing the model is small. The performance of the model proves that it is effective in dealing with the problem of overfitting or underfitting. This model may prove useful for doctors in detection of glaucoma at an early stage. This can minimize the risk of blindness. The functionality of this model can be enhanced to find the severity of glaucoma in patients. This will be useful in determining the type of treatment for the patients.

Figure 4. Loss values of GlaucomaDetector

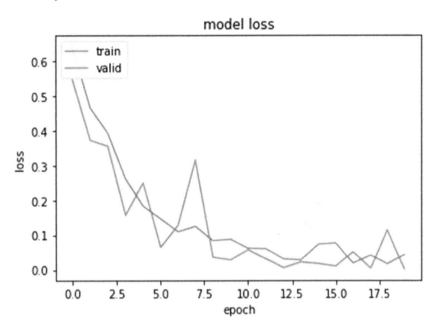

REFERENCES

Albawi, S., Mohammed, T. A., & Al-Zawi, S. (2017). Understanding of a convolutional neural network. *2017 International Conference on Engineering and Technology (ICET)*, 1-6. doi: 10.1109/ICEngTechnol.2017.8308186

Chen, X., Xu, Y., Kee Wong, D. W., Wong, T. Y., & Liu, J. (2015). Glaucoma detection based on deep convolutional neural network. *2015 37th Annual International Conference of the IEEE Engineering in Medicine and Biology Society (EMBC)*, 715-718. 10.1109/EMBC.2015.7318462

Glaucoma Today. (n.d.). https://glaucomatoday.com/articles/2013-jan-feb/glaucoma-care-in-india

Kaggle. (n.d.). Available at https://www.kaggle.com/himanshuagarwal1998/glaucomadataset

McMonnies, C. W. (2017). Glaucoma history and risk factors. *Journal of Optometry, 10*(2), 71-78. doi:. doi:10.1016/j.optom.2016.02.003

Medical News Today. (n.d.). https://www.medicalnewstoday.com/articles/9710

National Eye Institute. (n.d.). https://www.nei.nih.gov/learn-about-eye-health/eye-conditions-and-diseases/glaucoma

National Health Portal. (n.d.). https://www.nhp.gov.in/world-glaucoma-week_pg

Phan, S., Satoh, S., Yoda, Y., Kashiwagi, K., & Oshika, T. (2019). Evaluation of deep convolutional neural networks for glaucoma detection. *Japanese Journal of Ophthalmology, 63*(3), 276–283. doi:10.100710384-019-00659-6 PMID:30798379

Chapter 2
Pre–Processing Highly Sparse and Frequently Evolving Standardized Electronic Health Records for Mining

Shivani Batra
KIET Group of Institutions, Delhi-NCR, India

Shelly Sachdeva
 https://orcid.org/0000-0003-4088-1271
National Institute of Technology, Delhi, India

ABSTRACT

EHRs aid in maintaining longitudinal (lifelong) health records constituting a multitude of representations in order to make health related information accessible. However, storing EHRs data is non-trivial due to the issues of semantic interoperability, sparseness, and frequent evolution. Standard-based EHRs are recommended to attain semantic interoperability. However, standard-based EHRs possess challenges (in terms of sparseness and frequent evolution) that need to be handled through a suitable data model. The traditional RDBMS is not well-suited for standardized EHRs (due to sparseness and frequent evolution). Thus, modifications to the existing relational model is required. One such widely adopted data model for EHRs is entity attribute value (EAV) model. However, EAV representation is not compatible with mining tools available in the market. To style the representation of EAV, as per the requirement of mining tools, pivoting is required. The chapter explains the architecture to organize EAV for the purpose of preparing the dataset for use by existing mining tools.

DOI: 10.4018/978-1-7998-2742-9.ch002

INTRODUCTION

Electronic Health Records (EHRs) provide a digital support to the healthcare industry. A database of EHRs assembles health data of a patient from various departments of a healthcare organization including administration, pharmacy, clinical, radiology, laboratory and nursing. Contents within EHRs can be structured, semi-structured, unstructured, or a hybridization of these. For example, the contents of EHRs can be in the form of plain text, basic types (such as state variable and Boolean), time, date, date-time (including partial date/time), paragraphs, coded text, encapsulated data (such as parsable and multimedia content), measured quantities (providing units with values), uniform resource identifiers (URI) and container types (such as set and list) (Sachdeva S. & Bhalla S., 2012). EHRs aid in exchanging patients' health information electronically from one hospital to another. This electronic exchange of EHRs diminishes the burden of patients to carry reports printed on papers and other health related documents. However, exchange of EHRs needs to be semantic interoperable i.e. communicating parties must depict the same meaning of the exchanged EHRs data without any ambiguity.

Semantic Interoperability

To attain semantic interoperability, distinguished standard organizations, such as ISO (ISO 13606-1. 2008. Health informatics -- Electronic health record communication -- Part 1: Reference Model,.; ISO/DIS 13606-2 - Health informatics -- Electronic health record communication -- Part 2: Archetype interchange specification), openEHR (Beale T., Heard S., Kalra D., & Lloyd D., OpenEHR architecture overview, 2006), and HL7 (Health Level Seven International - Homepage) suggest adopting a dual model approach for the management of EHRs in an information system. Dual model approach segregates the information regarding the structure of various medical concepts (such as blood pressure, thyroid, and body mass index) from the knowledge about constraints on different attributes (that belong to an underlying medical concept). The first layer of the dual model approach, i.e., Reference Model (RM) (Beale T., Heard S., Kalra D., & Lloyd D., The OpenEHR Reference Model, 2007) is defined by various IT experts in the form of numerous classes that describe all possible data type and data structures that an EHR can use. RM aids in capturing the complex structure of EHRs. The second layer of the dual model approach, i.e., Archetype Model (AM) (Beale T., The openEHR archetype model-archetype object model, 2008) enables various clinical experts to portray their knowledge regarding various medical concepts in terms of participating attributes, their data types, and any other constraints such as, ranges and cardinality. AM delivers the maximal definition of a medical concept in form of an artefact known as archetype. Archetypes are released on a standard online library after a rigorous review process. Further, any revision in the definition of an existing archetype is released as a new version. Thus, adoption of archetypes enables semantic interoperability and capturing any future evolution. However, evolution within the medical concept also needs to be reflected to the database level. Moreover, EHRs are characterized by highly sparse behavior. Thus, there is a need of database that can efficiently store standardized EHRs data considering sparseness and frequent evolution. Moreover, database used for storing EHRs must possess the compatibility with mining tools for successful implementation of analytics.

Database Approaches

Two widely adopted data modeling approaches are schema-based (such as, relational database (Codd E. F., 1970)) and schema-less (such as, Not Only SQL (NoSQL) (NoSQL - Wikipedia,; Exploring the different types of nosql databases part ii)). A well-known schema-based approach is relational database that stores data with a predefined schema. However, definition of schema abolishes the elimination of NULL values. Thus, the presence of sparseness (NULL values) results as wastage of the storage space. Moreover, frequent evolution of schema incurs an extra cost such as re-paying schema designer, shutting down a running application and cost of shifting data from existing table to the newly structured table. Thus, frequent evolution is not appreciated in relational model. On the other side, schema-less database approach is trending nowadays to provide a solution to the issues of sparseness and frequent evolution. NoSQL introduced a schema-less organization of data to facilitate the flexibility for storing any possible structure of data (more formally, unstructured data). However, the well-established mining tools available in market seek for schema definition. Thus, NoSQL requires an external SQL support (i.e., needs to define a schema) for utilizing the existing mining tools. Also, NoSQL compromises on consistency to improve the data availability. Authors favour the relational database over NoSQL, since Relational Database Management System (RDBMS) provides capabilities, such as transactional support, read-write concurrency control, statistics gathering, storage-integrated access-control, and cost-based query optimization.

RELATED WORK

Relational model is assumed to be the first choice of user, as it is very easy to use and a variety of RDBMS are available in market. Further, RDBMS provide transactional support. Relational model simplicity is a result of the fact that relational tables are schema-based database. However, technology swing stresses to have a flexible data model that exterminates the need of reserving space for null values and possess the ability to hold any future add-ons in the existing list of attributes.

Although existing RDBMS allows making modifications in schema of existing table but it incurs cost. Whole dataset (in existing schema) needs to be moved to the newly designed schema. Moreover, many RDBMS impose an upper limit on the number of columns that a table can contain to avoid disk-overflow.

Various modifications are proposed at the logical layer of RDBMS to eradicate sparseness and to capture evolving attributes. Entity Attribute Value (EAV) (Agrawal R., Somani A., & Xu Y., 2001), Dynamic Tables (DT) (Corwin J., Silberschatz A., Miller P. L., & Marenco L., 2007), Optimized Entity Attribute Value (OEAV) (Paul R. & Hoque A. S. M. L., Optimized entity attribute value model: a search efficient representation of high dimensional and sparse data, 2009) and Optimized Column Oriented Model (OCOM) (Paul R. & Hoque A. S. M. L., Optimized column-oriented model: a storage and search efficient representation of medical data, 2010) are the popular logical modifications of relational model to handle frequent schema evolution and sparseness in healthcare domain. EAV, DT, OEAV and OCOM define a generic structure that capture only non-null values and can accommodate any future schema evolution.

EAV defines data in form of triplets constituting entity, attribute and value. It is the most widely adopted model in healthcare domain. EAV was first exercised in the TMR (The Medical Record) system and the HELP Clinical Data Repository (CDR) (Pryor T. A., 1988; Warner H. R., Olmsted C. M., &

Rutherford B. D., 1972). EAV can be easily implemented in an existing RDBMS environment. Utilization of RDBMS for employing the EAV system has been advocated by a group at the Columbia-Presbyterian Medical Center (Johnson, 1996).

DT resolves the issue of sparseness and frequent evolution by constructing binary tables for each attribute of the data. Each binary table stores the pairs of primary key and corresponding non-null value of the underlying attribute. On the arrival of any new attribute, a corresponding binary table is added to the existing set of binary tables.

OEAV and OCOM extend EAV and DT respectively through a well-defined coding mechanism. Coding algorithm of OEAV/OCOM considers attribute code (numeric) /position number (attribute code is used in OEAV and position number is used in OCOM) and corresponding data value as input. The coded value received as output replaces the attribute/position and value pair as one column.

EAV, DT, OEAV and OCOM store only non-null values. Information regarding null values can be attained from metadata. Thus, sparseness issue is resolved in EAV, DT, OEAV and OCOM. Moreover, any new knowledge (attribute) can be accommodated by simply placing the name in attribute column (EAV and OEAV), adding new attribute table (DT and OCOM), and constructing new code for attribute (OEAV and OCOM). Thus, EAV, DT, OEAV and OCOM structures are assumed to be generic in terms of capturing any future schema amendments without changing underlying definitions.

Storing Highly Sparse and Frequently Evolving Data

Issues of sparseness and handling frequent evolution arise due to restriction of defining schema in RDBMS. Thus, a generic data model is required that can efficiently deal with sparseness and frequent evolution. The most widely adopted generic data model for EHRs is Entity Attribute Value (EAV) model. Data in EAV is represented vertically in form of entity-attribute-value triplets. The vertical representation breaks non-null entry into a single tuple of EAV as depicted in Figure 1. The entity column stores the unique identifier of equivalent relational table. The attribute and corresponding value column defines each non-null entry as attribute-value pair.

Figure 1. Entity Attribute Value Model

Relational Model

Entity	Attribute1	Attribute2
Entity_id1	1	2
Entity_id2	3	NULL
Entity_id3	NULL	4

EAV Model

Entity	Attribute	Value
Entity_id1	Attribute1	1
Entity_id1	Attribute2	2
Entity_id2	Attribute1	3
Entity_id3	Attribute2	4

EAV model abolishes the need of reserving space for null entries. Moreover, any new attribute can be accommodated without making any amendments to the existing schema. The newly evolved attribute can be appended as a new tuple by designating name of attribute in the attribute column of EAV table as presented in Figure 2.

Figure 2. Capturing Newly Entity Attribute Value Model

Relational Model

Entity	Attribute1	Attribute2	Attribute3
Entity_id1	1	2	NULL
Entity_id2	3	NULL	NULL
Entity_id3	NULL	4	NULL
Entity_id4	NULL	NULL	5

EAV Model

Entity	Attribute	Value
Entity_id1	Attribute1	1
Entity_id1	Attribute2	2
Entity_id2	Attribute1	3
Entity_id3	Attribute2	4
Entity_id4	Attribute3	5

EAV model aids in handling highly sparse and frequently evolving data but, this representation is not compatible with mining tools available in the market. To discover relationship among various parameters of data, mining tools seeks data to be horizontally represented i.e., row depicts complete data related to one entity and one column captures whole data corresponding to one attribute. On the other hand, row in EAV depicts only one non-null data entry and three fixed column depicts entity identifier, attribute name and corresponding non-null values.

To style the representation of EAV as per the requirement (i.e., relational table) of mining tools, pivoting is required. The next section explains the architecture to organize EAV for the purpose of preparing the dataset for use by existing mining tools.

The need for a horizontal representation (i.e., relational table) to perform mining makes the adoption of EAV based storage questionable. To maintain compatibility with existing mining tools, data must be stored as relational table initially. However, this approach will not resolve the issues of sparseness and frequent evolution in standardized EHRs. Thus, the huge amount of EHRs data is maintained as per EAV storage to handle sparseness, frequent evolution to save associated cost. Further, the small portion of EHRs data that need to undergo mining must be reorganized (whenever required). For example, a sample EHRs data constitutes five patients' instances that can store data corresponding to three medical concepts (i.e., Blood Pressure, Body Mass Index and Heart Rate) as listed below.

- **For patient 1**, details of three medical concepts i.e., *Blood Pressure, Body Mass Index and Heart Rate* are recorded.
- **For patient 2**, details of one medical concepts i.e., *Body Mass Index* are recorded.
- **For patient 3**, details of two medical concepts i.e., *Body Mass Index and Heart Rate* are recorded.
- **For patient 4**, details of two medical concepts i.e., *Blood Pressure and Heart Rate* are recorded.
- **For patient 5**, details of three medical concepts i.e., *Blood Pressure, Body Mass Index and Heart Rate* are recorded.

If the above-described data is stored as per relational table, space will be wasted for storing null values corresponding to absent entries. The example quoted above presents only five patients and three medical concepts, however, in a real scenario the database is huge and highly sparse that results in consumption of massive storage space. Also, any evolution in knowledge will seek for corresponding changes in the schema design. Thus, at the database level, data is stored as per EAV storage approach.

Assuming that a data analyst desires to mine the Blood Pressure records (i.e., blood pressure details of patient 1, patient 4 and patient 5). Thus, Blood Pressure records (stored as EAV to resolve sparseness and frequent evolution issues) need to be extracted and transformed as per relational table. This raises a demand for an architecture that can transform the EAV based dataset in accordance to relational table.

PRELIMINARIES

This section provides details of preliminaries of architecture proposed for organizing an EAV based dataset for the purpose of mining.

Extending EAV Table

The architecture proposed in the next section considers an extended EAV table as shown in Figure 3. However, the proposed architecture will also work for basic EAV table (without any extension). The basic three column EAV structure can be extended to capture columns such as ID (unique identifier of EAV row), Archetype_Name (name of the archetype to which attribute belong), and Attribute_Path (a unique hierarchical path defined by openEHR for each attribute). The extension is done to account for following.

1) A patient is uniquely identified in the system through his Patient_ID. However, the value of ID will help in identifying the particular episode of patient admittance.
2) Archetype_Name and Attribute_Path columns are introduced to track the hierarchical path (as defined by openEHR) of every element.

Figure 3. Extended EAV table

ID	Patient_ID	Archetype_Name	Attribute_Path	Attribute_Name	Value

Extension of the EAV table is an optional step for pre-processing that is solely dependent upon the requirements of the end user. If the user wishes to extract details, such as ID, Archetype_Name and Attribute_Path, then basic EAV structure is extended accordingly.

Single Value Column

In addition to the above-specified extension, the Value column is defined to follow 'String' data type. 'String' datatype allows capturing any type of information. This eliminates the need for having multiple Value column or multiple EAV tables (one corresponding to each data type) for storing heterogeneous data. However, using 'String' data type for numeric data can lead to errors. For example, comparing '25' with '221' (when string data type is used) will produce a result that '25' is greater than '221'. This happens because strings are compared character-wise. As soon as a character is found greater (according to ASCII value) in a string, the corresponding string is declared larger. However, the architecture proposed for pre-processing the EAV based dataset, takes into consideration this issue of 'String' data type and organizes data accordingly.

Metadata

In addition to extending EAV table, the metadata database is also defined to be associated with EAV based dataset to aid in the organization of data. The metadata database defines one table for one archetype to store its related attributes and corresponding data types as presented in Figure 4. Each table in the metadata database is named as the name of the underlying archetype (which is uniquely defined by openEHR).

Defining one table for each archetype in the metadata database provides the following advantages.

1) Metadata is free from sparseness. Various tables will record the details of attributes which can't be null.
2) Metadata is search efficient since, one table captures only one archetype details. Thus, details of attributes related to one archetype can be extracted in constant time (i.e., time complexity is $O(1)$). Further, extracting details of more than one archetype will require a simple UNION operation among the corresponding metadata tables. Since all tables of metadata database follow the same schema, they are union-compatible.

No schema changes are required in the metadata database on knowledge evolution. Any changes in the list of attributes participating in an archetype can be reflected by changing a corresponding tuple in the table designated for the underlying archetype. This implementation of metadata can also be replaced with a link to archetype repository and thus, accessing the underlying archetype dynamically to gain information regarding attributes participating in the archetype.

Architecture to Organize EAV Dataset Into Mining Compatible Format

To cater the need for pre-processing, an architecture to organize EAV based dataset for the purpose of mining (as shown in Figure 5) is proposed.

The procedure for organizing EAV based data is divided into six steps, i.e., extracting the list of entities and attributes, building a new query, executing the query, storing results in a temporary table, pivoting, and extracting attribute data types. For a better understanding of the working of the proposed architecture, an example query is considered as "*apply mining to data of patients suffering high blood pressure to predict the effect of thyroid disease on high blood pressure patients*".

Figure 4. Metadata for organizing EAV based dataset for mining

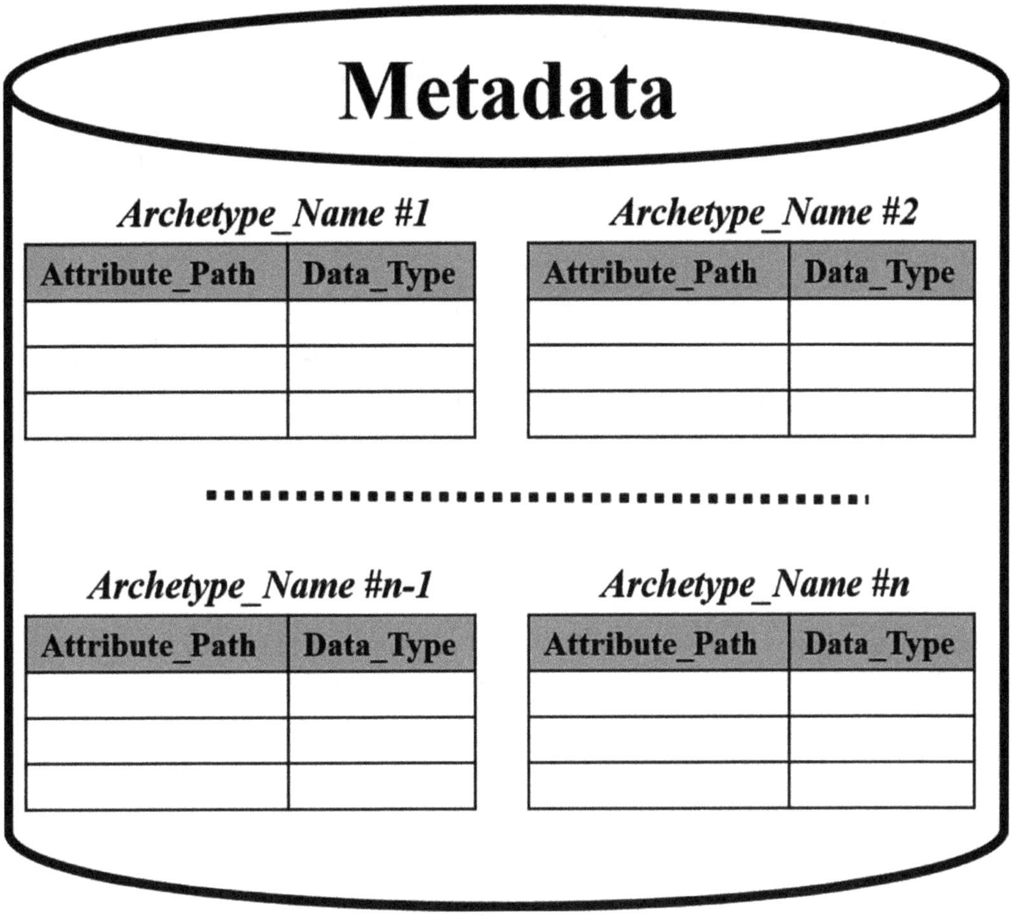

1. **Extracting list of entities and attributes:** Desired set of entities (from EAV table) and attributes (from metadata) is identified in two following sub-steps.
   a. An exhaustive set of entities is identified whose elements can be a potential member of the entity set desired for mining. For example, to identify patients suffering from blood pressure and thyroid, all patients suffering from high blood pressure are identified first. The Patient_ID of entities that fulfil the desired criteria (high blood pressure in this case) is stored in a temporary table. It is assumed that two entities (say, having Patient_ID as E1 and E2) are suffering from high blood pressure. Thus, E1 and E2 are stored in a temporary table.
   b. Metadata is enquired to extract the list of Attribute_Path corresponding to the desired medical concept (thyroid in this case). Thus, the table named as thyroid (in metadata database) is accessed for the identification of desired attributes. It is assumed that three attributes (say, having Attribute_Path as at1, at2, and at3) belong to thyroid archetype.

Figure 5. Architecture to organize standardized EHRs for the purpose of data mining (Batra S., 2016)

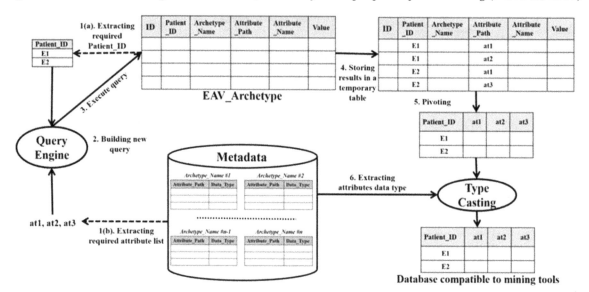

2. **Building a new query:** After the identification of a potential list of entities and desired set of attributes, the query builder composes a query to scrutinize the tuple set required for mining. Structure of the query formulated is as follows.

Select * from EAV_table_name

where Patient_ID IN (*extracted list of Patient_ID*) and

Attribute_Path IN (*extracted list of Attribute_Path*) and

Archetype_Name IS name_of_desired_archetype;

Attribute_Path needs to be tested along with Archetype_Name for scrutiny of EAV records, since Attribute_Path can overlap in two archetypes. However, within an archetype, Attribute_Path is unique. Thus, the query composed by the query builder inspects the records of EAV table based on the desired Patient_IDs (identified in step 1(a)), extracted Attribute_Paths (identified in step 1(b)) and Archetype_Name (i.e., thyroid in this case).

3. **Executing the query:** The query composed by the query builder is executed on the EAV table. An exhaustive scan of EAV table is performed to extract the records based on the conditions specified (in terms of Patient_IDs, Attribute_Paths and Archetype_Name) in the query composed in step 2.

4. **Storing results in a temporary table:** Shortlisted records are stored in a temporary table. However, records extracted are still in the EAV format which needs to be converted to NSM format to make it compatible with mining tools.

5. **Pivoting:** The process of converting EAV format to relational table format involves multiple self JOINS and is known as Pivoting (Dinu V., Nadkarni P., & Brandt C., Pivoting approaches for bulk extraction of Entity–Attribute–Value data, 2006; Luo G. & Frey L. J., 2016). Application of pivoting change the representation of extracted records from EAV to relational table. Three well known techniques for pivoting are following (Dinu V., Nadkarni P., & Brandt C., Pivoting approaches for bulk extraction of Entity–Attribute–Value data, 2006).

a. **Using full outer joins:** Each attribute is segregated from other attributes. An inner join operation is performed to construct a tuple corresponding to an underlying entity. Further, records corresponding to various entities are conjoined using a full outer join operation.

b. **Using left outer joins:** List of entities is extracted based on the condition imposed. Further, each attribute is segregated from other attributes. An inner join operation is performed to construct a tuple corresponding to an underlying entity. Finally, records corresponding to various entities are conjoined using a left outer join operation.

c. **Using hash tables and memory to perform the equivalent of multiple joins:** SQL imposes a limit of 256 join operations per query. However, the number of join operation in pivoting can range beyond the specified limit (i.e., 256). Thus, the following algorithm is used:

   i.   Hash table is designed to arrange attributes in the desired sequence. Hash table provides indexing that assists in faster access to data.

   ii. Unique identifiers (i.e., Patient_ID) corresponding to the desired entities are extracted.

   iii. A string type two-dimensional array is constructed with rows equal to the number of entities (patients) and columns equal to the number of attributes.

   iv. The two dimensional array is filled with the values retrieved from the EAV table at the position specified by the order of Patient_ID and Attribute_ID

The proposed architecture exploits the left outer joins mechanism for pivoting since, it is simple to adopt in contrast to hash tables, and it provides a faster turnaround time in contrast to full outer join.

6. **Extracting attribute data types:** The data stored in the pivoted table follows 'String' data type. Thus, to retain the semantics of the extracted data, type casting is done on the pivoted table. Information regarding various data types belonging to different attributes is extracted from the metadata. As type casting is done, resultant database is compatible with the existing mining tools available in market.

RESULTS

Performance of the proposed architecture is evaluated considering the time taken by it to organize the EAV based dataset.

Experimental Setup

The processor of the machine on which the experiment is performed is quad-core Intel processors. RAM available in the machine is 4 GB RAM. The operating system used is Windows 8.1. The implementation is done using JDK 1.8 and PostgreSQL 9.5.

Dataset Collection

The datasets (on which experiment is performed) are collected using three different methodologies listed below.

1.   From two private clinics,
2.   From the UCI machine learning repository (Liver Disorder and Thyroid) (UCI Machine Learning Repository: Liver Disorders Data Set) (UCI Machine Learning Repository: Thyroid Disease Data Set), and
3.   Fabricated using the knowledge (about blood pressure and heart pulse) available from reliable resources and the internet (such as, if range of systolic pressure systolic pressure lies between 120 to 139 and 80 to 89 respectively, then the patient is suffering from prehypertension (The Facts about High Blood Pressure—American Heart Association)). Since, ethical and legal issues are associated with EHRs, no clerical data is collected. Thus, to simulate a real-life scenario, clerical data is also fabricated.

Dataset collected corresponds to a total of 12.9 million records of an EAV table.

Performance

To measure the performance of the proposed architecture, the number of instances participating in the experiment is varied. The time taken by the proposed architecture to organize the EAV based data (considering the varying size of the dataset) is presented in Table 1 and Figure 6.

Table 1. Performance results of architecture proposed for the organization of EAV based data

S.No.	Number of Instances Prepared for Mining	Time Taken (seconds)
1	100	0.194
2	300	0.284
3	600	0.293
4	1000	0.381
5	1500	0.364
6	3000	0.54
7	5000	0.618
8	10000	0.885
9	20000	1.221
10	50000	2.882
11	80000	4.8
12	120000	7.1
13	160000	10
14	190000	11.2
15	210000	13
16	213664	13.6

Figure 6. Graphical representation of results presented in Table 1

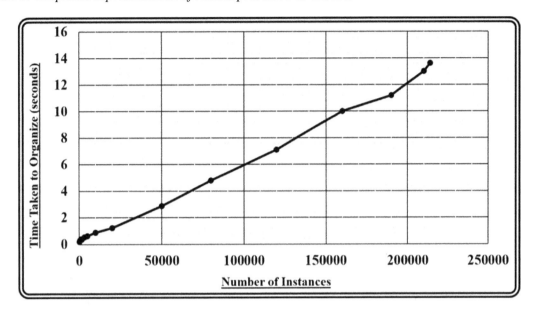

It is witnessed that to organize 100 records, 194 milliseconds are sufficient and to pre-process approximately 2.1 million records, 13.6 seconds are required by the proposed architecture. Data extraction corresponding to a patient (i.e., a patient-centric query) is always desired to be answered in real time. However, analytical queries can be delayed (Dinu V. & Nadkarni P., Guidelines for the effective use of entity–attribute–value modeling for biomedical databases, 2007). However, the proposed architecture organizes EAV based data within a few seconds. Thus, the time taken to organize EAV based data for mining is considered to be acceptable.

CONCLUSION

Standard based EHRs possess challenges (in terms of sparseness, frequent evolution and query efficiency) that need to be handled through a suitable data model. In addition, medical practitioners recommend visualizing EHRs as a set of attribute-value pairs. However, any changes to the data model (for handling issues of sparseness, frequent evolution and query efficiency) or attribute-value representation are not compatible with mining tools available in the market.

Mining reveals the hidden information that can lead to useful discoveries. Thus, in order to utilize existing mining tools for standard based EHRs (stored as EAV), organization of EHRs data is required. This chapter introduces an architecture to organize the standard based EHRs that are modeled as EAV representation for handling issues of sparseness, frequent evolution and query efficiency. Experiments are conducted to observe the time taken for the organization of EAV based dataset. The number of instances in the dataset is varied to notice the effect of dataset size on the performance of the proposed architecture. It is witnessed that the proposed architecture organizes EAV based data within a few seconds. Moreover, analytical queries need not to be answered in real time. Thus, the time taken by the proposed architecture is acceptable.

REFERENCES

Agrawal, R., Somani, A., & Xu, Y. (2001). Storage and querying of e-commerce data. *VLDB*, *1*, 149–158.

Batra, S. S. S., & Sachdeva, S. (2016). Organizing standardized electronic healthcare records data for mining. *Health Policy and Technology*, *5*(3), 226–242. doi:10.1016/j.hlpt.2016.03.006

Beale T. (2008). The openEHR archetype model-archetype object model. *The openEHR Release, 1*(2).

Beale T., Heard S., Kalra D., & Lloyd D. (2006). *OpenEHR architecture overview.* The OpenEHR Foundation.

Beale, T., Heard, S., Kalra, D., & Lloyd, D. (2007). *The OpenEHR Reference Model.* EHR Information Model.

Codd, E. F. (1970). A relational model of data for large shared data banks. *Communications of the ACM*, *13*(6), 377–387. doi:10.1145/362384.362685

Corwin, J., Silberschatz, A., Miller, P. L., & Marenco, L. (2007). Dynamic tables: An architecture for managing evolving, heterogeneous biomedical data in relational database management systems. *Journal of the American Medical Informatics Association*, *14*(1), 86–93. doi:10.1197/jamia.M2189 PMID:17068350

Dinu, V., & Nadkarni, P. (2007). Guidelines for the effective use of entity–attribute–value modeling for biomedical databases. *International Journal of Medical Informatics*, *76*(11-12), 769–779. doi:10.1016/j.ijmedinf.2006.09.023 PMID:17098467

Dinu, V., Nadkarni, P., & Brandt, C. (2006). Pivoting approaches for bulk extraction of Entity–Attribute–Value data. *Computer Methods and Programs in Biomedicine*, *82*(1), 38–43. doi:10.1016/j.cmpb.2006.02.001 PMID:16556470

Exploring the different types of nosql databases part ii. (n.d.). Retrieved June 22, 2017, from https://www.3pillarglobal.com/insights/exploring-the-different-types-of-nosql-databases

Health Level Seven International - Homepage. (n.d.). Retrieved June 22, 2017, from http://www.hl7.org/

ISO 13606-1. 2008. Health informatics -- Electronic health record communication -- Part 1: Reference Model. Retrieved June 22, 2017, from https://www.iso.org/standard/40784.html

ISO/DIS 13606-2 - Health informatics -- Electronic health record communication -- Part 2: Archetype interchange specification. Retrieved June 22, 2017, from https://www.iso.org/standard/62305.html

Johnson, S. B. (1996). Generic data modeling for clinical repositories. *Journal of the American Medical Informatics Association*, *3*(5), 328–339. doi:10.1136/jamia.1996.97035024 PMID:8880680

Luo, G., & Frey, L. J. (2016). Efficient execution methods of pivoting for bulk extraction of entity-attribute-value-modeled data. *IEEE Journal of Biomedical and Health Informatics*, *20*(2), 644–665. doi:10.1109/JBHI.2015.2392553 PMID:25608318

NoSQL - Wikipedia. (n.d.). Retrieved June 22, 2017, from https://en.wikipedia.org/wiki/NoSQL

Paul, R., & Hoque, A. S. M. L. (2009). Optimized entity attribute value model: A search efficient representation of high dimensional and sparse data. *IBC, 3*, 1–6. doi:10.1109/ICCIT.2009.5407131

Paul, R., & Hoque, A. S. M. L. (2010). Optimized column-oriented model: A storage and search efficient representation of medical data. *Information Technology in Bio-and Medical Informatics, ITBAM, 2010*, 118–127. doi:10.1007/978-3-642-15020-3_12

Pryor, T. A. (1988). The HELP medical record system. *MD Computing: Computers in Medical Practice, 5*(5), 22.

Sachdeva, S., & Bhalla, S. (2012). Semantic Interoperability in Standardized Electronic Health Record Databases. *ACM Journal of Data and Information Quality, 3*(1), 1–37. doi:10.1145/2166788.2166789

The Facts about High Blood Pressure—American Heart Association. (n.d.). Retrieved June 22, 2017, from http://www.heart.org/HEARTORG/Conditions/HighBloodPressure/GettheFactsAboutHighBlood-Pressure/The-Facts-About-High-Blood-Pressure_UCM_002050_Article.jsp

UCI Machine Learning Repository: Liver Disorders Data Set. (n.d.). Retrieved June 22, 2017, from https://archive.ics.uci.edu/ml/datasets/Liver+Disorders

UCI Machine Learning Repository: Thyroid Disease Data Set. (n.d.). Retrieved June 22, 2017, from https:// archive.ics.uci.edu/ml/datasets/Thyroid+Disease

Warner, H. R., Olmsted, C. M., & Rutherford, B. D. (1972). HELP—A program for medical decision-making. *Computers and Biomedical Research, an International Journal, 5*(1), 65–74. doi:10.1016/0010-4809(72)90007-9 PMID:4553324

Chapter 3
Image Classification Techniques

Eugenio Vocaturo
 https://orcid.org/0000-0001-7457-7118
Università della Calabria, Italy

ABSTRACT

The image processing task, aimed at interpreting and classifying the contents of the images, has attracted the attention of researchers since the early days of computers. With the advancement of computing system technology, image categorization has found increasingly broader applications, covering new generation disciplines such as image analysis, object recognition, and computer vision, with applications quite general both in scientific and humanistic fields. The automatic recognition, description, and classification of the structures contained in the images are of fundamental importance in a vast set of scientific and engineering fields that require the acquisition, processing, and transmission of information in visual form. Classification tasks also include those related to the categorization of images, such as the construction of a recognition system, the representation of patterns, the selection and extraction of features, and the definition of automatic recognition methods. Image analysis is of collective interest and it is a hot topics of current research.

INTRODUCTION

The image processing task, aimed at interpreting and classifying the contents of the images, has attracted the attention of researchers since the early days of computers. With the advancement of computing system technology, image categorization has found increasingly broader applications, covering new generation disciplines such as image and scene analysis, image understanding, object recognition and Computer Vision, with applications quite general both in scientific and humanistic fields.

The objective of this chapter is to provide an overview of some of the main techniques used for image classifications by introducing the general issue of interest for this research topic.

DOI: 10.4018/978-1-7998-2742-9.ch003

BACKGROUND

Discussions on computers, machine learning and artificial intelligence seem, nowadays, entirely smooth. However the road that has taken us here has been very complex and difficult due to the skepticism surrounding such field of research.

MACHINE LEARNING

The term "Machine Learning (ML)" refers to techniques and approaches used for automatic detection of relevant patterns from data collections. The growing availability of digital data makes the ML approaches widely used for information extraction. We are surrounded by machine learning based technology: search engines learn how to deliver results in the most efficient way, anti-spam software learns to filter our email messages, and credit card transactions are secured by software solutions that learn how to detect frauds. Smartphones are now equipped with advanced digital cameras through which they are able to detect faces interacting with voice commands. In sectors such as bioinformatics and medicine, ML approaches are increasingly adopted to address specific challenges.

The growing digitalization of our world and the following proliferation of data allow the proposal of algorithms for large-scale machine learning (Big Data), giving rise to a wide spectrum of different learning techniques. Machine Learning aims at teaching computers and robots to perform actions and activities in a natural way like humans: learning from experience.

Summing up, machine learning algorithms exploit mathematical - computational methods to obtain learning information directly from data. Machine Learning algorithms may improve their performance in an "adaptive" way, as the examples with which they work increase without having been explicitly programmed.

Machine Learning allows computers to learn from experience; there exists "learning" whenever the performance of the program improves after the performance of a task or the completion of a possibly wrong action. Instead of writing the programming code through which, step by step, the machine is "told" what to do, the computer is only provided with data sets inserted in a generic algorithm that develops its own logic to perform the function, the activity, the task required. The evolution of the concept of "intelligence" in "artificial intelligence" follows (Russell, S. J., & Norvig, P., 2016).

How Machine Learning Works

In principle, machine learning works on the basis of two distinct approaches, which were originally identified by Arthur Samuel at the end of the 1950s. These approaches make possible to differentiate machine learning in two general sub-categories depending on whether the computer is given examples on how to perform the required task (supervised learning) or let the software work without any "help" (unsupervised learning).

Indeed, a more rich taxonomy is available which allows us to make a further and even more detailed classification of the Machine Learning techniques based on its modus operandi (Figure 1). All these techniques are used to classify data.

Figure 1. Fundamental approaches of Machine Learning

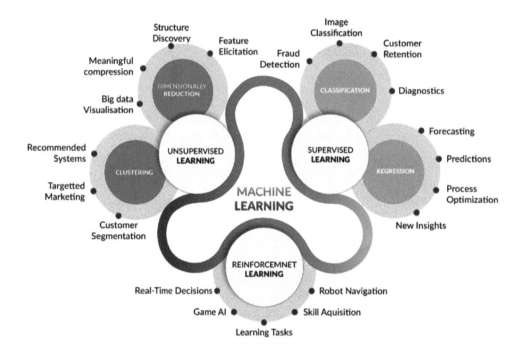

A- Machine Learning with Supervised Learning

In this area of machine learning, both the data sets used as inputs and the information on the desired results "feed" the system with the aim of identifying general rules that link incoming data with outgoing data. The so identified rules can then be reused for other similar tasks.

Interesting examples of Machine Learning with supervised learning come from scientific research in medical field where algorithms learn to make increasingly accurate predictions to prevent outbreaks of epidemics or to accurately and promptly diagnose tumors or rare diseases. Typical applications of Supervised Learning include Classification and Regression task.

B- Machine Learning with Unsupervised Learning

In this second Machine Learning area, only data sets are supplied to the system with- out any indication of the desired result. The purpose of this second learning method is to "go back" to hidden patterns and models, i.e. to identify the logical structures which have not been previously labeled. Two of the main methods used in unsupervised learning are "principal component" and "cluster analysis".

C- Machine Learning with Reinforcement Learning

In this case, the system must interact with a dynamic environment and achieve a goal also by learning from errors. The behavior of the system is determined by a learning routine based on reward and punishment. With such a model, the computer learns, for example, to beat an opponent in a game by concentrating its efforts on performing a certain task, aiming to reach the maximum value of the reward; in other words, the system learns by playing and by the mistakes made improving performance precisely in relation to the results previously achieved. Systems based on reinforcement learning are the foundation for the development of self-driving cars which, through Machine Learning, learn to recognize the surrounding environment (with data collected by sensors, GPS, etc.) and to adapt their "behavior" to specific situations they encounter.

D- Machine Learning with Semi-supervised Learning

In this area, the computer is supplied, through "hybrid" model, with a set of incomplete training / learning data; some of these inputs are "endowed" with examples of output (as in supervised learning), others lack them (as in unsupervised learning). The basic objective is always the same: to identify rules and functions for solving problems, as well as models and data structures useful for achieving certain objectives.

E- Other Approaches to Machine Learning: from probabilistic models to Deep Learning

There are other ways for classifying Machine Learning approaches which suggest the adoption of sub-categories functional to a "practical" classification of Machine Learning algorithms.

In machine learning a decision tree is a predictive model, where each internal node represents a variable, an arc towards a child node represents a possible value for a certain property and a leaf node represents the predicted value for the target variable. A decision tree is a graph representing possible decisions and their implications, used to create actions aimed at a specific purpose.

Then there is the sub-category of "probabilistic models" where the system's learning process is based on the calculation of probabilities; the best known is the "Bayes network", a probabilistic model that represents the set of random variables in a graph and its conditional dependencies.

Finally, we mention the artificial neural networks (ANN) that use algorithms inspired by the structure, functioning and connections of biological neural networks (i.e.those of the human being) for learning, (Vocaturo, E., & Veltri, P., 2017). More advanced models, such as the so-called multilayer neural networks, lead to Deep Learning (Figure 2).

Classification and Machine Learning

Before considering pattern recognition and image analysis themes, it is appropriate to recall some basic concepts of machine learning. The definition of learning for computational models will be functional for the three fundamental approaches of machine learning: supervised unsupervised and reinforcement.

Machine Learning tasks are often described in terms of how the system deals with a collection of features evaluated on the referred data. Typically, the input is represented by a vector $x \in \mathbb{R}^n$ where each x_i represents a descriptive characteristic (feature) of the input data. To evaluate the abilities of a machine learning algorithm, a quantitative measure P must be estimated indicating its performance. Often the measure of P is specific to a certain task T which the system must perform. For tasks such as classification, P is evaluated by measuring the accuracy of the model, evaluating percentage of examples for which the model provides a correct output. Another reference parameter may be the error rate, defined instead as the proportion of examples for which the system provides a wrong output.

Figure 2. Relations between diverse areas of Data Mining

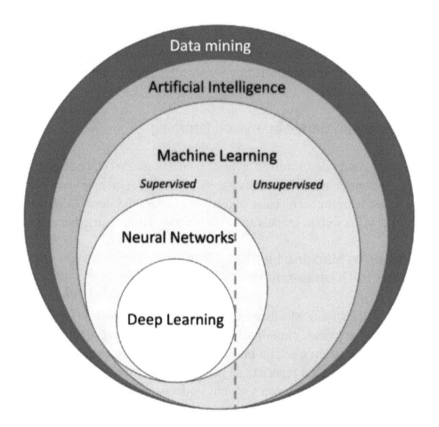

It is important to check how the algorithms are able to evaluate unseen data, enhancing performance indices on testing set, and on training sets, in order to evaluate the performance on independent assessments.

Machine Learning approaches are typically classified depending on the nature of the "signal" used for learning or the "feedback" available to the learning system. As mentioned earlier, in literature, we find three general categories of machine learning: supervised, unsupervised and reinforced learning. Halfway between supervised and unsupervised learning is the semi-supervised learning in which the teacher provides an incomplete training data set, that is, a set of training data among which there are data without the respective desired output (Zhu, X. J., 2005). Another categorization of machine learning approaches considers the output of the machine learning system (Harrington, P., 2012).

- In classification, the outputs are divided into two or more classes and the learning system must produce a model that assigns the inputs not yet seen to one or more of the classes. This is usually dealt with in a supervised manner. Anti-spam filtering is an example of classification, where the inputs are emails and the classes are "spam" and "not spam".
- In regression, which is a problem usually solved using supervised approach, the output and model used are continuous. An example is the prediction of the value of the exchange rate of a currency in the future, given its values in recent times.
- In clustering an input set is divided into groups. Unlike the case of classification, groups are not known before, typically making it an unsupervised task.

Image Processing

The image processing task, aimed at interpreting and classifying the contents of the images, has attracted the attention of researchers since the early days of computers (Figure 3). With the advancement of computing system technology, image categorization has found increasingly broader applications, covering new generation disciplines such as image and scene analysis, image understanding, object recognition and Computer Vision, with applications quite general both in scientific and humanistic fields. On a more general level, the problem is part of Pattern Recognition, the discipline that deals with the automatic recognition and classification of the entity of interest of a phenomenon under observation.

Classification tasks also include those related to the categorization of images, such as the construction of a recognition system, the representation of patterns, the selection and extraction of features and the definition of automatic recognition methods.

Figure 3. Major Supervised and Unsupervised learning methods

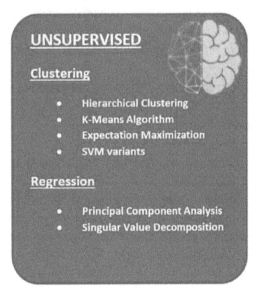

The automatic recognition, description and classification of the structures contained in the images are of fundamental importance in a vast set of scientific and engineering fields that require the acquisition, processing and transmission of information in visual form. Digital imaging techniques are constantly evolving not only in terms of technological refinement, but also from a conceptual view point. The images obtained, thanks to the intervention of electronic processing, lose much of their purely "iconographic" character, in order to acquire an ever greater functional meaning, with an information content to be correctly interpreted. Examples of applications in this sense are:

- Text recognition;
- Medical Imaging;
- Industrial automation;
- Robotics;
- Cartography;
- Remote sensing;
- Environmental modeling;
- Simulation and mobility control in transport;
- Biometrics;
- Conservation of cultural assets;
- Radar Images Recognition in the military sphere.

Pattern Recognition and Image Analysis

Pattern recognition (PR) has its origins in engineering and it is popular in the context of computer vision. Through the Machine Learning approach, interest is focused on maximizing the recognition rates, while in pattern recognition there is a greater interest in detecting significant patterns. A useful definition of pattern recognition is:

The field of pattern recognition is concerned with the automatic discovery of regularities in data through the use of computer algorithms and with the use of these regularities to take actions such as classifying the data into different categories (Bishop, C. M., 2006).

The construction of a PR system essentially requires the development of three aspects:

- data acquisition and pre-processing;
- patterns representation;
- the definition and improvement of a decision function for patterns recognition.

When the data are images, the process of developing a PR system is generally instantiated with specific operations concerning the acquisition and processing of the images, the extraction of the structures to be recognized or classified and their representation, operations that fall within the framework of Image Processing and Analysis.

In particular, this process can be schematized as shown in Figure 4, which also shows the operations performed for each phase and the corresponding results.

The first two phases are related to image processing, or rather to the digitization of analog data and optimization of the obtained images; the two subsequent phases belong to the image analysis characterized by the extraction of the features of interest, through the segmentation process: such features are used for the representation of the patterns.

Finally, the last phase consists in defining a classification method translating the quantitative analysis into qualitative information. Furthermore, it is possible to design post-processing phases to improve the entire classification process (Lampinen, J., Laaksonen, J., & Oja, E. 1997).

Figure 4. Steps of an Image Classification System

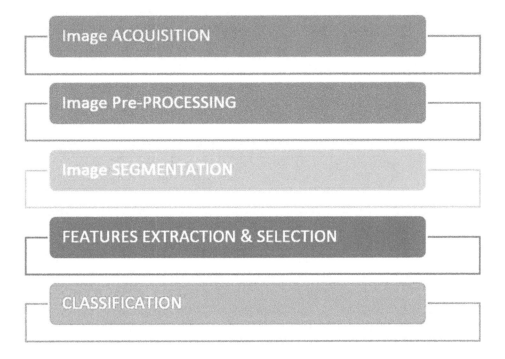

Useful Types of Classifiers for Image Analysis

The classification methods are quite numerous, also due to the fact that several classifiers can be combined together. In general, we can identify two main types of approaches: the statistical and the syntactic ones.

Statistical approach generally seeks to maximize the posterior probability (i.e. the probability that a sample belongs to a given class), starting from the estimates (obtained from the training set) of the a priori probabilities of the classes.

Syntactic approach focuses on the analysis of distinctive features of the objects to be classified: the classification involves the comparison between the structural features of the examples to be tested and those ones of the training set, by using supervised, unsupervised e semi-supervised algorithms.

Apart from the Bayesian classifiers (Friedman, N., Geiger, D., & Goldszmidt, M., 1997), which minimize the probability of misclassifying based on the Bayes theorem, in the following we list the classifiers used in image analysis, highlighting the advantages and disadvantages of their adoption.

Support Vector Machine

Given two classes of data, the Support Vector Machine (SVM) is a well-known supervised machine learning technique (Vapnik, V., 2013), aiming at separating the two classes, with the maximum margin, by means of a hyperplane. When dealing with linearly separable classes, no particular problems arise; if, on the other hand, we are dealing with classes that are not linearly separable we need to use a sort of trick, modifying the SVM algorithm so that it looks for the hyperplane in spaces of higher dimensionality.

In fact, if two classes are not linearly separable in a certain multidimensional space, it is probable that they will be if we increase space dimensionality. Although, the SVM operates generally with two classes, there are also some variants that allow us to obtain good results even in case of n classes. Interesting surveys of SVM can be found in (Burges, C. J., 1998; Cristianini, N., & Shawe-Taylor, J., 2000).

The aim of the algorithm is to determine a hyperplane that separates examples with positive labels from examples with negative labels. Support Vector Machine requires the trans- formation of labels into numbers, so the positive label, for example with the numeric value of $+1$, may represent the class of "sick patients" instead the negative label, with the numeric value of -1, may represent the class of "healthy patients". The equation of the hyperplane is given by two parameters: a real-valued vector w with the same dimensionality as input feature vector x, and a real number b. The equation that defines the hyperplane is:

$$w^T x + b = 0$$

where the expression $w^T x$ is the inner product between vectors $w, x \in \mathbb{R}^d$. The predicted label for an input feature vector x is given by:

$$y = sign(w^T x + b)$$

where sign is a mathematical operator that takes any value as input and returns $+1$ if the input is a positive number or -1 if the input is a negative number.

The goal of SVM learning algorithm is to find the optimal values w^* and b^* for parameters w and b. Once the learning algorithm identifies these optimal values, the model $f(x)$ is then defined as:

$$f(x) = sign(w^{*T} x + b^*)$$

For the determination of w^* and b^*, it is necessary to solve an optimization problem under constraints. As a first step, the model has to correctly predict the labels of the considered examples (*training phase*): each example i is given by a pair (x_i, y_i), where x_i is the feature vector representing the example i and y_i is its label equal to -1 or $+1$. So the constraints are:

$$w^T x_i + b \geq +1 \;\; if \;\; y_i = +1$$

$$w^T x_i + b \leq -1 \;\; if \;\; y_i = -1$$

The objective is to separate the two classes by maximizing the margin, defined as the distance between the so called supporting hyperplanes:

$$w^T x + b = +1$$

$$w^T x + b = -1 \qquad (1.4)$$

A large margin favors the generalization necessary for the correct functioning of the model in classifying new examples. It is possible to show that the margin is computable as $\dfrac{2}{\|w\|}$; then the optimization problem P to be solved is:

$$\min \frac{1}{2} \|w\|^2$$

$$y_i(w^T x_i + b) \geq -1 \quad for \quad i = 1, ..., N \qquad (1.5)$$

where the expression $y_i(w^T x_i + b) \geq -1$ is just a compact way to write the two above constraints (1.3), and $\|w\|$ indicates Euclidean norm of vector w.

The solution of the problem P, obtained through w^* and b^*, is referred as statistical model, while the term training indicates the process of building the model. Assuming that feature vectors are two-dimensional, the problem and its solution can be visualized as in Figure 5.

Figure 5. SVM model for two-dimensional feature vectors

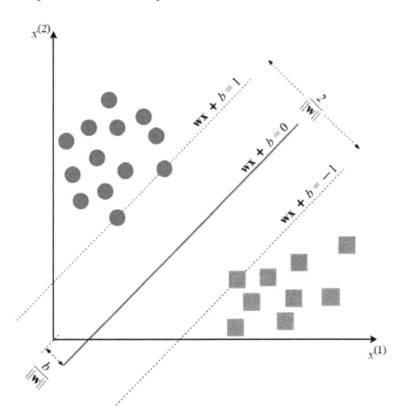

The blue and orange circles represent, respectively, positive and negative examples, and the line given by $w^T x + b = 0$ is the separating hyperplane.

Any classification learning algorithm that builds a model implicitly or explicitly creates a decision boundary. The decision boundary can be straight, or curved, or it can have a complex form, or it can be a superposition of some geometrical figures.

The form of the decision boundary determines the accuracy of the model, namely the ratio of examples whose labels are predicted correctly. The form of the decision boundary and the way it is computed differentiate a learning algorithm from any another type. An- other essential factor to be considered is the speed in building the model and in performing a prediction. In many practical cases, it is preferable to have a learning algorithm that builds a less accurate fast model.

Classification performances can be invalidated both by noise in data, because of the presence of outlier, or by the intrinsic nature of the data that cannot be linearly separated using a hyperplane. In fact, even though the maximum margin allows the SVM to select among multiple candidate hyperplanes, for many data sets, the SVM may not be able to find any separating hyperplane at all because the data contains misclassified instances.

Figure 6. Linearly non-separable cases: a) presence of noise, b) inherent nonlinearity

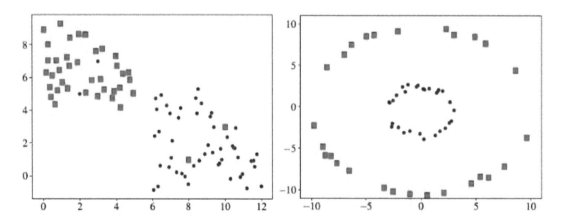

These situations can be effectively managed. In Figure 6 a), the data could be separated by a straight line except for the outliers with wrong labels. In the Figure 6 b), the decision boundary is a circle and not a straight line. The question of solving the optimization problem arises.

Dealing with Noise

To extend the SVM to cases in which the data is not linearly separable, the so called hinge loss function has been introduced:

$$max\{0, 1 - y_i(w^T x_i + b)\}$$

The hinge loss function is zero if the constraints of P are satisfied, that is xi lies on the correct side of the hyperplane. For data on the wrong side of the decision boundary, the function value is proportional to the distance from the decision boundary. The aim is to minimize the following cost function:

$$\frac{1}{2}\|w\|^2 + C\sum_{i=1}^{N} max\{0, 1 - y_i(w^T x_i + b)\} \tag{1.6}$$

where the parameter C determines the tradeoff between the maximization of the margin and the minimization of the hinge loss function. SVMs that optimize (1.6) are called *soft-margin SVMs*, while the original formulation P is referred to as a hard-margin SVM.

To effectively manage the non-smoothness in formulation (1.6) due to the presence of the maximum in the objective function, we introduce the auxiliary variables ξ by obtaining the following problem *P"*:

$$\min \frac{1}{2}\|w\|^2 + C\sum_{i=1}^{N} \xi_i$$

$$\xi_i \geq 0$$

$$\xi_i \geq 1 - y_i(w^T x_i + b) \tag{1.7}$$

The value of C is experimentally tuned: for small values of C, the second term in the cost function becomes negligible, so the SVM algorithm will try to find the highest margin by completely ignoring misclassification. On the other hand, increasing the value of C makes classification errors more costly, so the SVM algorithm will try to focus on minimizing the classification error, by sacrificing the margin.

In other words, since a larger margin is better for generalization, C tunes the tradeoff be- tween correctly classifying the training data (minimizing empirical risk) and correctly classifying future examples (generalization).

Dealing with Inherent Non-Linearity

The use of SVM is possible even when data sets are not separable in their original space via a hyperplane. The transformation of the original space into a higher dimensionality space could imply that the examples will become linearly separable in this transformed space. Using the kernel functions allows us to operate in a high-dimensional feature space, reducing the computational burden. In fact, it is sufficient to calculate the inner products between the images of all the pairs of data without calculating the coordinates of the data in the high- dimensional feature space. This approach is called kernel trick (Shawe-Taylor, J., & Cristianini, N., 2004), and is often cheaper than the computational burden associated with explicit computation of coordinates. The kernel functions have been adopted to deal with problems related to sequence data, graphics, text, images and vectors.

The effect of applying the kernel trick is illustrated in Figure 7, where a two-dimensional non-linearly-separable data are transformed into a linearly-separable three-dimensional data using a specific mapping $\Phi : x \mapsto \Phi(x)$, with $\Phi(x)$ being the vector x higher in dimensionality.

Figure 7. Data linearly separable after a transformation into a three- dimensional space

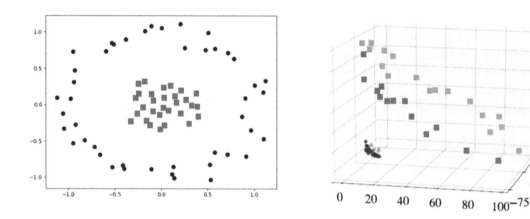

We don't know a priori which mapping Φ would work for a specific data-set. To under- stand how kernels work, it is necessary to understand how the optimization algorithm for SVM finds the optimal values for w and b. Problem (1.7), is generally solved by means of its Wolfe Dual, D defined as follows:

$$min_{\lambda_1,...\lambda_N} \frac{1}{2} \sum_{i=1}^{N} \sum_{k=1}^{N} \mathbf{y_i} \lambda_i (\mathbf{x_i}^T \mathbf{x_k}) \mathbf{y_k} \lambda_k - \sum_{i=1}^{N} \lambda_i$$

$$\sum_{i=1}^{N} \lambda_i \mathbf{y_i} = 0$$

$$0 \leq \lambda_i \leq C \quad i = 1,...N \tag{1.8}$$

where λ_i are the Lagrange multipliers. In this formulation, D is a convex quadratic optimization problem, efficiently solvable by quadratic programming algorithms. In the above formulation, the term $\mathbf{x_i}^T \mathbf{x_k}$ is the only place where the feature vectors are used. In order to transform a certain vector space into an higher dimensional space, it is necessary to transform x_i into $\Phi(\mathbf{x_i})$ and x_j into $\Phi(\mathbf{x_j})$ and then multiply $\Phi(\mathbf{x_i})$ and $\Phi(\mathbf{x_j})$.

Through kernel trick, the inner product $\mathbf{x_i}^T \mathbf{x_k}$ can be substituted by a kernel function such as the Radial Basic Function (RBF):

$$k(\mathbf{x}, \mathbf{x}') = \exp\left(\frac{\|\mathbf{x} - \mathbf{x}'\|^2}{2\sigma^2}\right)$$

where $\|\cdot\|^2$ is the squared Euclidean norm.

By varying the hyper-parameter σ, the data analyst can choose between getting a smooth or curvy decision boundary in the original space.

To summarize, kernels are a special class of functions that allow inner products to be calculated directly in the feature space, without performing the mapping described above (Burges, C. J., Smola, A. J., & Scholkopf, B., 1999). Once a hyperplane has been created, the kernel function is used to map new points into the feature space for classification. The selection of an appropriate kernel function is important, since the kernel function defines the transformed feature space in which the training set instances will be classified. In (Genton, M. G., 2001), the author described different classes of kernels, without however giving indications as to which class is most suitable for a given problem. It is a common practice to estimate a range of potential settings and use cross-validation over the training set to find the best one. For this reason, a limitation of SVMs is the low speed of the training.

The complexity of an SVM model is not affected by the number of features in training data. It follows that SVMs are suitable for dealing with learning tasks with large number of features compared to the number of instances used for model's training.

Neural *Networks*

In many real-world problems, the classification is non-linear and the number of features is very high. Artificial Neural Networks (ANNs), provide simpler and more efficient non-linear classifiers. The concept of "natural network" derives from electronic models in order to mimic the neural structure of human brain.

A neural network is a set of artificial neurons interconnected in order to obtain a complex global behavior, which is precisely determined by weighted connections and specific parameters of the neurons. In practical terms, ANNs are non-linear structures of statistical data organized as modeling tools. ANNs can be used to simulate complex relationships between inputs and outputs that other analytic functions fail to represent.

An artificial neuron is the basic unit of ANNs, and has a structure completely inspired by the biological neuron (see Figure 8), whose structure is emulated within a computer (Bengio, Y., 2009):

Due to its physiological and chemical properties, the biological neuron is able to integrate, receive and transmit nerve impulses, from/to other artificial neurons.

The dendrites in the biological neural network are analogous to the weighted inputs on their synaptic interconnection in the ANN. The cell body is comparable to the unity of artificial neurons, which also includes units of sum and threshold. Axon is analogous to the output unit of the artificial neural network. Thus, ANN is modeled using the functioning of basic biological neurons. Figure 9 reports more in detail the structure of the artificial neuron. We identify the following quantities:

- the inputs x_i: they represent the input signals of the neuron, which can come from other neurons or from the environment;

Figure 8. Mapping between the elements of the biological neuron and artificial neuron

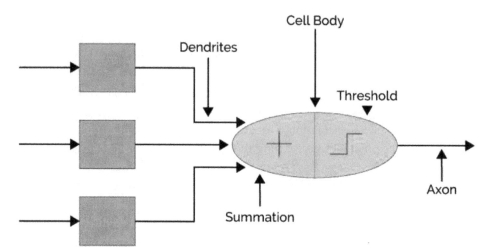

- the weights w_i: they are multipliers associated to the input values and used to weight them;
- the activation function φ: it is the mathematical function that determines the output value of the neuron on the basis of the inputs; there are several types of ϕ, each for specific cases;
- the transfer function sum: it generates the value to be submitted to the activation function ϕ and obtained by adding the input values previously multiplied by the corresponding weights w_i;
- the output: it represents the output signal of the neuron, which can be directed towards other neurons or in the environment.

Figure 9. Artificial neuron: inputs, activation function, weighted connections, calculation function

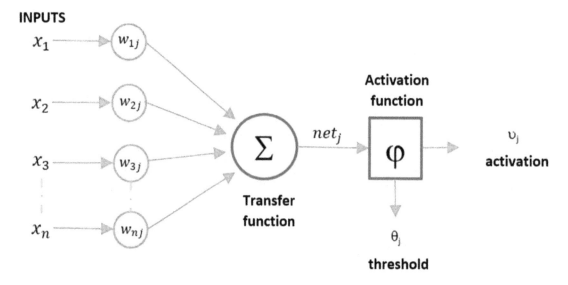

Thus, an artificial neuron receives input values x_i that are multiplied by a factor w_i, all the resulting values are added together; such sum constitutes the input for the activation function φ that determines the final output value of the neuron. The activation function is useful because it adds possibly non-linearity to the neural networks. In such sense, the ANNs are considered universal function approximators. There are different types of activation functions in the literature, each of which has its own advantages and application contexts (Specht, D. F., 1990). Some of them are plotted in Figure 10.

All the activation functions, are characterized by the fact that they can be treated, in practice, by minimizing the nonlinear error function of the back-propagation algorithm, useful for learning complex behaviors.

Figure 10. Types of activation function

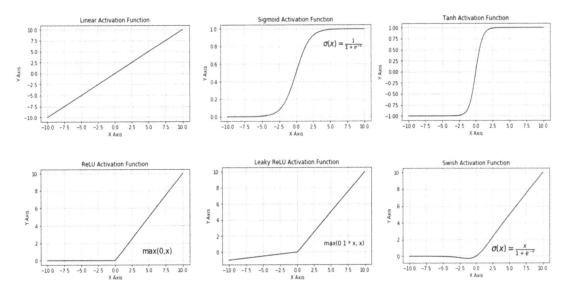

Summing up, in neural networks the basic unit is the neuron that work like simple processor. Each neuron receives the weighted sum of the input nodes and through the activation function generates the output of the next neuron. In neural networks, the neurons are grouped in the so called "layers".

In fact, more complex network topologies include a dedicated layer for input neurons and output neurons and one or more hidden layers (see Figure 11).

To design a neural network, the structure of the network (topology), the transfer function and the learning algorithm must be defined. The distinction of different topologies of neural networks depends on the directions of interconnection in the layer; among the most popular topologies, it is worth mentioning *Feed Forward Topology* (FFT) and *Recurrent Topology* (RNT).

In particular, in the FFT network, the nodes are "hierarchically arranged" in levels. The various levels follow one another starting from the input to the output, where the hidden levels provide most of the computational power of the network. *Multilayer Perception Network* (MPN) and *Radial Basic Function Network* (RBFN) (Haykin, S. S., 2009), represent typical applications in which the nodes of each level are connected to the nodes of the next level through unidirectional paths.

Figure 11. An example of Neural Networks

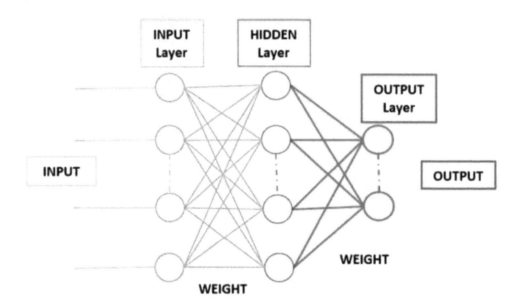

Nearest Neighbor

Among the simplest machine learning algorithms, Nearest Neighbor should be mentioned. Nearest Neighbor methods must be recalled for classification and regression problems, focusing on their performance for binary classification and on the efficiency of implementing these methods. The idea is to memorize the training set and then to predict the label of any new instance on the basis of the labels of its closest neighbors in the training set.

A sample will be assigned to the class of the "nearest neighbor", usually using metric such as Euclidean distance. It is clear that the algorithm will be more expensive depending on the size of training set and on the number of features to be considered: it is appropriate to find a fair compromise, because a larger training set tends to be more representative, and a high number of features allows to better discriminate between the possible classes. If, on the one hand we have these advantages, on the other hand we have an increase in the calculations. Some variations of the algorithm have therefore been elaborated, in order to reduce the number of distances to be calculated, for example partitioning the feature space and measuring the distance only with respect to some of the volumes thus obtained. k-Nearest Neighbor (kNN) is a variant that determines the k closest elements using a distance metric: each of these elements "votes" for the class to which it belongs, and a new unseen sample will be assigned to the most voted class. kNN is a non-parametric learning algorithm that, differently from other learning algorithms that allow discarding the training data after the model is built, keeps all training examples in memory.

Once a new, previously unseen example x comes in, the kNN algorithm finds k training examples closest to x and returns the majority label for classification problem or the average label for regression problem. A strategy often adopted, both for classification and regression problems, suggests the assignment of weights to the contributions of the neighbors: in this way the contribution provided by the nearest neighbors is greater than the average of the more distant ones. More precisely, a weighting scheme consists in giving each neighbor a weight of $1/d$, where d is the distance to the neighbor.

Apart the Euclidean distance, other popular distance metrics include Chebychev, Mahalanobis, and Hamming distance (Kumar, V., Chhabra, J. K., & Kumar, D., 2014). The choice of these hyper-parameters, i.e. the distance metric, and the value of k, is to be made before running the algorithm.

Clustering

Clustering is one of the most widely used techniques for exploratory data analysis. An approach adopted in various research areas involves a study of the reference data, trying to deduce the presence of some significant groups: this is an attempt to deduce intuitively possible cluster formations. Clustering is the task of grouping a set of objects such that similar objects end up in the same group and dissimilar objects are separated into different groups. There may be several very different conceivable clustering solutions for a given data set. As a result, there is a wide variety of clustering algorithms that, on some input data, will output very different clustering. Clustering algorithms can be categorized based on their cluster model.

There is no "correct" clustering algorithm in an absolute sense: "clustering is in the eye of the be-holder" (Estivill-Castro, V., 2002). The most appropriate clustering algorithm for a particular problem often has to be chosen in an experimental way, except for cases in which it is a mathematical model suggesting the adoption of a solution instead of others. In general, an algorithm designed for a particular context may not perform well when applied to a different data set. As reported in (Xu, R., & Wunsch, D., 2008) clustering methods can be classified as follows:

- Connectivity-based clustering
- Centroid-based clustering
- Distribution-based clustering
- Density-based clustering.

K-means algorithm

To effectively use the k-means algorithm, we need to define the distance between the clusters and to determine when the merging process between various clusters has to be stopped. The result of such an algorithm can be represented using the clustering dendrogram i.e. a tree structure of domain subsets (see Figure 12).

In clustering dendrogram, singleton sets are represented in its leaves and the entire do- main as its root. This view provides a visual summary of the data. More generally, the pursued approaches can be agglomerative or divisive, according to respectively bottom-up or top-down approach.

In the first case the algorithm starts by trying to aggregate single elements; at each step elements or sub-clusters that are more similar to each other in a cluster are merged into a cluster. In the second case, more complex and therefore less used, the algorithm starts with a single cluster and at each level the most different elements are subdivided into sub-clusters. In both cases the result can be represented through a tree.

Common stopping criteria include:

- Fixed the number of clusters k, and stop merging clusters as soon as the number of clusters is k
- Appropriately defined a limit distance $r \in R^+$ the process of generating clusters is interrupted as soon as all the distances between the clusters are greater than r. If $r = max\ d(x,y): x, y \in X$ for some $\alpha < 1$, the stopping criterion is referred as "scaled distance upper bound."

Figure 12. Hierarchical clustering

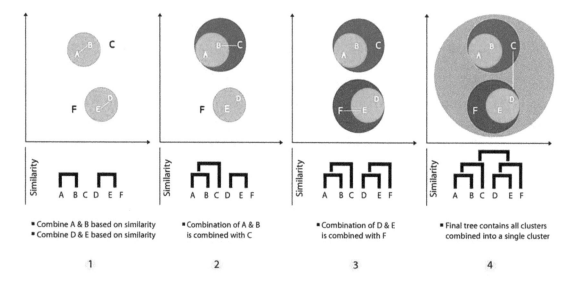

Another approach to clustering starts by defining a cost function over a parameterized set of possible clustering aiming to find a partitioning (clustering) of minimal cost. In this paradigm, the clustering task is turned into an optimization problem, and the solutions implies the use of some appropriate search algorithm. Many common objective functions require the number of clusters k as a parameter. Practically, it is often up to the user of the clustering algorithm to choose the parameter k that is most suitable for the given clustering problem.

The k-means objective function is quite popular in practical applications of clustering. However, it turns out that finding the optimal k-means solution is often computationally unfeasible (the problem is NP-hard, and even NP-hard approximated within some constant).

As an alternative, the following simple iterative algorithm is often used. Considering the Euclidean distance function $d(x,y) = x-y$, the algorithm can be represented by the following pseudo code reported in table 1:

This algorithm tends to converge rather quickly (it is rare that more than 10 steps are needed) and to give rather good results, starting from a reasonable initial solution (see Figure 13).

K-means has some disadvantages: first the number of K classes must be known a priori; furthermore, the optimization is iterative and local, therefore it is possible to have convergence on a local maximum of the solution. The fuzzy variant of k-means allows a pattern to belong with a certain degree of probability to different classes; this variant sometimes provides a more robust convergence towards the final solution, but suffers in essence from the same problems as the standard k-means.

Table 1. k-Means Algorithm

k-Means Algorithm
Step 1: Input $X \subseteq \mathbb{R}^n$; k = number of cluster; **Step 2: initialize:** Random choose of centroids $\mu_1, \ldots, \mu_k$; **Step 3: repeat until convergence:** **3.1:** $\forall i \in [k]$ set $C_i = \{x \in X \mid i = arg\min_j \quad x - \mu_j \quad \}$; **3.2:** break ties in some arbitrary manner; **3.3:** $\forall i \in [k]$ update $\mu_i = \dfrac{1}{\mid C_i \mid} \sum\limits_{x \in C_i} x$.

Several variants have been proposed to solve these problems: for example, to minimize the risk of convergence towards local minima, the algorithm can be performed many times starting from different initial solutions, random or perhaps produced by an evolutionary method (genetic algorithm).

Figure 13. K-means clustering approach

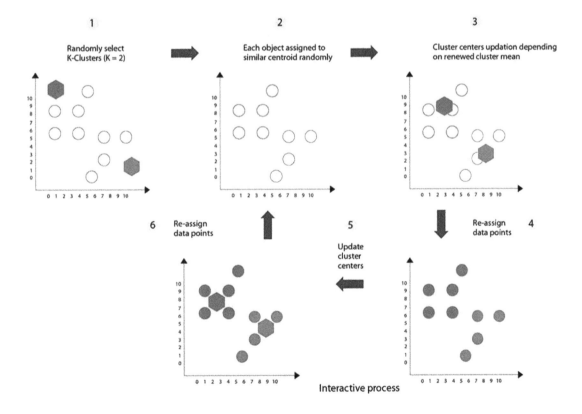

There are recent approaches that solve the problem faced by k-means. For example, in (Tao, P. D., 2009) the authors propose an approach based on the explicit expression of the clustering problem as a nonlinear, non-smooth, non-convex optimization problem. Such problem is treated by its reformulation as a DC (Difference of Convex) optimization problem, which in turn is numerically treated by a sequence of partial linearizations.

In (Khalaf, W., Astorino, A., d'Alessandro, P., & Gaudioso, M., 2017) a novel DCA algorithms for edge detection was proposed. This proposal adopted clustering on the pixels representing any given digital image into two sets i.e. the "edge pixels" and the "non-edge" ones. The process is based on associating to each pixel an appropriate vector representing the differences in brightness of surrounding pixels. Clustering is driven by the norms of such vectors, thus it takes place in R, which allows to use a (simple) DC (Difference of Convex) optimization algorithm to get the clusters.

Clustering validation techniques (the determination of the number of classes without this information being known), on the other hand, tend to evaluate *a posteriori* the goodness of the solutions produced for different K values, and to choose one on the basis of a validation criterion that takes account both of the goodness of the solution and of its complexity.

Decision Trees

"Decision tree" refers to a structure similar to a graph where each internal node represents a query on a specific attribute, each branch represents the result of the query and finally each leaf node represents a class label or the resulting decision. In fact, a classification tree is a classifier defined as a set of if-then. One of the main advantages of decision trees is the simplicity of the model. The classification rules are represented by the paths from the root to the leaves. Decision trees are used as a tool to calculate the expected values of several concurrent alternatives. A decision tree consists of three types of nodes that are differentiated in the graphic display (Kamiński, B., Jakubczyk, M., & Szufel, P., 2018):

1- Decision nodes - represented by squares
2- Probability nodes - represented by circles
3- End nodes - represented by triangles

To build the classifier, it is necessary to define the topology of its associated root tree, as well as the subdivision associated with each node. A decision tree can be understood as a predictor h: X → Y, which determines the label associated with a certain instance x ∈ X, moving through the decision tree from a root node to a leaf one. In the most immediate case of the binary classification, the label will assume dichotomous values, i.e. Y ={0, 1}; decision trees can also be applied to other forecasting problems. On each node of the root-leaf path, the successor child is chosen based on a subdivision of the input space. The tree is then constructed following a greedy procedure in which the new nodes are recursively created and connected to the previously defined ones until a stop criterion is defined.

A widespread rule of division in the internal nodes of the tree is realized considering the threshold of the value of a single function; starting from the root node, the algorithm chooses the right or the left child of the node based on $[x_i < \theta]$, where i is the index of the relevant feature and $\theta \in R$ is the threshold. The resulting decision tree corresponds to a cell division of the instance space, where each leaf of the tree corresponds to a specific cell. Considering decision trees of arbitrary dimensions, it is possible to obtain a class of hypotheses of infinite size; the risk inherent in this approach is the overfitting of the model on the considered data.

To remedy overfitting, the principle of minimum length of the description (MDL) can be used, aiming at learning a decision tree that adapts well to the data but is not too extensive (Rissanen, J., 1983). Unfortunately, solving this problem is computationally difficult. It follows that the decision-making tree learning algorithms are based on heuristics with a greedy approach, in which the tree is built gradually and locally optimal decisions are taken in the construction of each node. Although these algorithms do not guarantee the return of the optimal global decision tree, they work well in practice.

With reference to a generic tree, at the root of which a label is assigned based on the majority vote among all the labels on the training set. At each iteration, the effect of the division of a single leaf is evaluated by defining some gain measures able to quantify the improvement due to this division. Concerning all the possible divisions, the configuration that maximizes the gain is chosen, or one chooses not to divide the leaf at all. The features that best divide training data would be the root node of the tree.

There are numerous methods for determining the characteristic that best divide training data such as information acquisition and index data (Breiman, L., Friedman, J., Stone, C. J., & Olshen, R. A., 1984) but most studies have concluded that there is no single best method (Murthy, S. K., 1998). Considering a given data set, comparing individual methods can be important in deciding which metric to use. The process of generation of trees and sub-trees continues until all training data has been divided into subsets of the same classes. We report below the pseudo-code of a general decision tree algorithm as described in Kotsiantis, S. B., Zaharakis, I., & Pintelas, P., 2007) reported in table2:

Table 2. Decision Trees algorithm

Decision Trees algorithm
Step 1: Check for the above base cases; **Step 2:** For each attribute a, find the normalized information gain ratio from splitting on a;
Step 3: Let a^* be the attribute with the highest normalized information gain;
Step 4: Create a decision node that splits on a^*;
Step 5: Recur on the sub-lists obtained by splitting on a^* and add those nodes as children node.

A decision tree, or any learned hypothesis h, is said to overfit training data if another hypothesis h" exists that has a larger error than h when tested on the training data, but a smaller error than h when tested on the entire data set. There are two common approaches that can be used to avoid overfitting on training data:

- Interrupt the training algorithm before it reaches a point where it adapts perfectly to the training data;
- Prune the induced decision tree.

Many studies have been presented on techniques to manage overfitting: in general, with the same test and prediction accuracy, the tree with less leaves is preferred (Breslow, L. A., & Aha, D. W., 1997).

The easiest way to deal with overfitting is to pre-prune the decision tree by not allowing it to grow to its maximum size. Adopting termination criteria as a threshold test for the function quality metric is effective. Decision tree classifiers usually use post pruning techniques that evaluate the performance of decision trees, since they are pruned using a validation set. Any node can be removed and assigned to the most common class of training instances that are ordered to it (Bruha, I., 2000; Elomaa, T., & Rousu, J. 1999). To reduce the disadvantages and solve the problems of decision trees related to overfitting, many decision trees can be combined together.

The random forest is an ensemble of learning algorithm (Dietterich, T. G., 2000). An ensemble is a collection of different classifiers put together to create a more powerful model. In particular, the random forest is based on the bagging technique, which is a statistical method to create different training sets starting from just one. The random forest builds a decision tree on each training set, using only a subset of random features for each classifier. Since decision trees are very unstable, building them on different training sets with random characteristics would lead to very different classifiers. This reduces the correlation between the models, thus increasing overall performance. Indeed, to carry out the classification the random forest combines all decision trees with a voting system. Each tree "votes" a class for the record and therefore the random forest chooses the "most voted" as the final result (Breiman, L., 2001). The voting system averages the forecasts of the individual decision trees, which are affected by a high variance, therefore the results show greater accuracy, even with a large amount of data. This also means that the random forest is less prone to overfitting than a single decision tree, because it averages forecasts, leading to more robust results. Furthermore, it has only a few parameters to set, which is always desirable. The main disadvantage of this approach, however, is the calculation time, which increases proportionally to the number of trees.

Among the best known algorithms for decision trees construction, we should remember ID3 (Quinlan, J. R., 1979) and its extension C4.5 (Quinlan, J. R., 1993). Subsequently a more efficient version of the algorithm was implemented, called EC4.5, which is able to calculate the same decision trees as C4.5 with an increase in performance up to five times (Ruggieri, S., 2002).

One of the assumptions of C4.5 is that the training data adapt to the memory: this pro- vided the starting point for the creation of frameworks such as *Rainforest*, oriented to the development of fast and scalable algorithms to build decision trees that fit to the amount of main memory available (Gehrke, J., Ramakrishnan, R., & Ganti, V., 2000). The various proposals for the parallelization of the C.45 algorithm focused on proposing approaches based on features, nodes and data. Since a decision tree constitutes a hierarchy of tests, an unknown feature value during classification is usually treated by passing the example on all branches of the node where the unknown feature value was detected and each branch generates a distribution of class.

The output is a combination of several class distributions that add up to 1. In decision trees it is assumed that instances belonging to different classes have different values in at least one features. Decision trees work best when discrete and categorical features are used. Using decision trees allows to easily understand why an instance is classified as belonging to a specific class.

Multi-Classifiers

A multi-classifier is a system in which different classifiers are used (normally in parallel, but sometimes also in cascade or in a hierarchical manner) to perform pattern classification; the decisions of the individual classifiers are therefore merged to some level of the classification chain. Recently it has been shown that the use of combinations of classifiers (multi-classifier) can improve, sometimes very markedly, the performance of a single classifier. Therefore, it may be appropriate, instead of focusing on small improvement of the accuracy of a classifier, to add to it other classifiers based on different features and algorithms. The combination is in any case effective only if the individual classifiers are somehow independent of each other, that is, they do not all make the same type of errors. Independence (or diversity) is normally achieved by trying to:

- Use different features to identify patterns
- Use different algorithms for feature extraction
- Use different classification algorithms
- Train the same classification algorithm on different training sets (bagging)
- Insist on the training of some classifiers with the most frequently erroneously classified patterns (boosting).

The combination of classifiers is a solution that is gaining ground in the implementation of Computer Aided Diagnosis (CAD) systems that help doctors to take decisions swiftly. These solutions allow to classify particular images in their reference domain. Analysis of imaging in medical field is a very crucial task that allows to diagnose specific diseases at the earliest avoiding costly and invasive investigations (Li, Q., & Nishikawa, R. M., 2015). The combination of classifiers can be per- formed at the decision or at the confidence level.

Merger at decision level

Each individual classifier outputs his own decision, which consists of the class to which the pattern has be assigned and optionally of the reliability level of the classification performed (that is, of how much the classifier feels sure of the decision made). Decisions can be combined with each other in different ways like voting schemes and ranking-based schemes.

One of the most well-known and simple methods of fusion is the so-called majority vote rule: each classifier votes for a class, and the pattern is assigned to the most voted class; the reliability of the multi-classifier can be calculated by averaging the single confidences. On the other hand, another way is that each classifier produces a class ranking based on the probability that the model to be classified belongs to each of them. The rankings are converted into scores that are added together, and the class with the highest final score is the one chosen by the multi-classifier.

Confidence level fusion

Each individual classifier outputs the confidence in the classification of the pattern with respect to each of the classes, or a dimensionality vectors in which the $i - th$ element indicates the probability of the pattern belonging to the $i - th$ class. Different casting methods are possible, including sum, average, product, max, min.

The sum method is a well-known method used for its robustness: it expects to perform the vectorial sum of the different confidence vectors, and to classify the pattern on the basis of the major element. A very effective variant is using the weighted sum, where the sum of the confidence vectors is performed by weighting the different classifiers according to their degree of skill: the degrees of skill can be defined basing on the individual performances of the classifiers, for example inversely proportional to the classification error.

Take Away

The classifiers are widely used in various fields of computer vision, and many times they are used in conjunction with other geometric and probabilistic techniques of image analysis.

So far there are no standards or guidelines regarding the choice of the classifier type, nor for the configuration of a specific classifier.

It becomes important to know the classifiers that are widely used in various fields aiming at images classification. Recently, new approaches such as Active Learning, Multiple Instance Learning, and Transfer Learning are allowing extremely positive results especially in the classification of medical images.

In reference to the automatic recognition of melanoma, for example, Multiple Instance Learning it is establishing itself as an emerging approach among the various Machine Learning techniques (Vocaturo, E., Perna, D., & Zumpano, E., 2019). In this particular field, the union between the optimization of mathematical models and the proliferation of unlabeled images is favoring the spread of increasingly recognized approaches for pathology recognition (Astorino, A., Fuduli, A., Gaudioso, M., & Vocaturo, E., 2018, 2019; Gaudioso, M., Giallombardo, G., Miglionico, G., & Vocaturo, E., 2019).

The result highlights how the use of only color and texture features makes it possible to obtain classification performance of interest (Fuduli, A., Veltri, P., Vocaturo, E., & Zumpano, E., 2019; Astorino, A., Fuduli, A., Veltri, P., & Vocaturo, E., 2020).

The obtained results can be improved by considering appropriate pre-processing steps (Vocaturo, E., Zumpano, E., & Veltri, P., 2018,2019) and thus directing the research towards applications capable of supporting the diagnosis of new pathologies such as Dysplastic Nevi Syndrome (DNS) (Vocaturo, E., & Zumpano, E., 2019,2020).

Generally, the best approach is to evaluate the type of problem and try to use the most suitable classifier type, eventually even adjusting it and optimizing it with some trial and error steps. Many classifiers and related applications require deal of computations, and often good performance in terms of CPU times are not easy to achieve. On the other hand, good results seem to be obtainable with multi-classifiers and cascading classifiers like in real-time object detection.

REFERENCES

Astorino, A., Fuduli, A., Gaudioso, M., & Vocaturo, E. (2019, June). Multiple Instance Learning Algorithm for Medical Image Classification. SEBD.

Astorino, A., Fuduli, A., Veltri, P., & Vocaturo, E. (2020). Melanoma detection by means of Multiple Instance Learning. *Interdisciplinary Sciences, Computational Life Sciences*, *12*(1), 24–31. doi:10.100712539-019-00341-y PMID:31292853

Bengio, Y. (2009). *Learning deep architectures for AI*. Now Publishers Inc. doi:10.1561/9781601982957

Bishop, C. M. (2006). *Pattern recognition and machine learning*. Springer.

Breiman, L. (2001). Random forests. *Machine Learning*, *45*(1), 5–32. doi:10.1023/A:1010933404324

Breiman, L., Friedman, J., Stone, C. J., & Olshen, R. A. (1984). *Classification and regression trees.* CRC Press.

Breslow, L. A., & Aha, D. W. (1997). Simplifying decision trees: A survey. *The Knowledge Engineering Review*, *12*(1), 1–40. doi:10.1017/S0269888997000015

Bruha, I. (2000). From machine learning to knowledge discovery: Survey of preprocessing and postprocessing. *Intelligent Data Analysis*, *4*(3-4), 363–374. doi:10.3233/IDA-2000-43-413

Burges, C. J. (1998). A tutorial on support vector machines for pattern recognition. *Data Mining and Knowledge Discovery*, *2*(2), 121–167. doi:10.1023/A:1009715923555

Burges, C. J., Smola, A. J., & Scholkopf, B. (1999). *Advances in Kernel Methods-Support Vector Learning. MIT Press.*

Caroprese, L., Veltri, P., Vocaturo, E., & Zumpano, E. (2018, July). Deep learning techniques for electronic health record analysis. In *2018 9th International Conference on Information, Intelligence, Systems and Applications (IISA)* (pp. 1-4). IEEE. 10.1109/IISA.2018.8633647

Cristianini, N., & Shawe-Taylor, J. (2000). *An introduction to support vector machines and other kernel-based learning methods.* Cambridge University Press. doi:10.1017/CBO9780511801389

Dietterich, T. G. (2000, June). Ensemble methods in machine learning. In *International workshop on multiple classifier systems* (pp. 1-15). Springer.

Elomaa, T., & Rousu, J. (1999). General and efficient multisplitting of numerical attributes. *Machine Learning*, *36*(3), 201–244. doi:10.1023/A:1007674919412

Estivill-Castro, V. (2002). Why so many clustering algorithms: A position paper. *SIGKDD Explorations*, *4*(1), 65–75. doi:10.1145/568574.568575

Friedman, N., Geiger, D., & Goldszmidt, M. (1997). Bayesian network classifiers. *Machine Learning*, *29*(2-3), 131–163. doi:10.1023/A:1007465528199

Fuduli, A., Veltri, P., Vocaturo, E., & Zumpano, E. (2019). Melanoma detection using color and texture features in computer vision systems. Advances in Science. *Technology and Engineering Systems Journal*, *4*(5), 16–22. doi:10.25046/aj040502

Gaudioso, M., Giallombardo, G., Miglionico, G., & Vocaturo, E. (2019). Classification in the multiple instance learning framework via spherical separation. *Soft Computing*, 1–7.

Gehrke, J., Ramakrishnan, R., & Ganti, V. (2000). RainForest-a framework for fast decision tree construction of large datasets. *Data Mining and Knowledge Discovery*, *4*(2-3), 127–162. doi:10.1023/A:1009839829793

Genton, M. G. (2001). Classes of kernels for machine learning: A statistics perspective. *Journal of Machine Learning Research*, *2*(Dec), 299–312.

Harrington, P. (2012). *Machine learning in action.* Manning Publications Co.

Haykin, S. S. (2009). *Neural networks and learning machines.* Academic Press.

Kamiński, B., Jakubczyk, M., & Szufel, P. (2018). A framework for sensitivity analysis of decision trees. *Central European Journal of Operations Research*, *26*(1), 135–159. doi:10.100710100-017-0479-6 PMID:29375266

Khalaf, W., Astorino, A., d'Alessandro, P., & Gaudioso, M. (2017). A DC optimization-based clustering technique for edge detection. *Optimization Letters*, *11*(3), 627–640. doi:10.100711590-016-1031-7

Kotsiantis, S. B., Zaharakis, I., & Pintelas, P. (2007). Supervised machine learning: A review of classification techniques. *Emerging Artificial Intelligence Applications in Computer Engineering, 160*(1), 3-24.

Kumar, V., Chhabra, J. K., & Kumar, D. (2014). Performance evaluation of distance metrics in the clustering algorithms. *INFOCOMP Journal of Computer Science*, *13*(1), 38–52.

Lampinen, J., Laaksonen, J., & Oja, E. (1997). *Neural network systems, techniques and applications in pattern recognition*. Helsinki University of Technology.

Li, Q., & Nishikawa, R. M. (Eds.). (2015). *Computer-aided detection and diagnosis in medical imaging*. Taylor & Francis. doi:10.1201/b18191

Murthy, S. K. (1998). Automatic construction of decision trees from data: A multi-disciplinary survey. *Data Mining and Knowledge Discovery*, *2*(4), 345–389. doi:10.1023/A:1009744630224

Quinlan, J. R. (1979). Discovering rules by induction from large collections of examples. *Expert systems in the micro-electronics age*.

Quinlan, J. R. (1993). *Program for machine learning*. C4. 5.

Rissanen, J. (1983). A universal prior for integers and estimation by minimum description length. *Annals of Statistics*, *11*(2), 416–431. doi:10.1214/aos/1176346150

Ruggieri, S. (2002). Efficient C4. 5 [classification algorithm]. *IEEE Transactions on Knowledge and Data Engineering*, *14*(2), 438–444. doi:10.1109/69.991727

Russell, S. J., & Norvig, P. (2016). *Artificial intelligence: a modern approach*.

Shawe-Taylor, J., & Cristianini, N. (2004). *Kernel methods for pattern analysis*. Cambridge university press. doi:10.1017/CBO9780511809682

Specht, D. F. (1990). Probabilistic neural networks. *Neural Networks*, *3*(1), 109–118. doi:10.1016/0893-6080(90)90049-Q PMID:18282828

Tao, P. D. (2009, September). Minimum sum-of-squares clustering by DC programming and DCA. In *International Conference on Intelligent Computing* (pp. 327-340). Springer.

Vapnik, V. (2013). *The nature of statistical learning theory*. Springer Science & Business Media.

Vocaturo, E., Perna, D., & Zumpano, E. (2019, November). Machine Learning Techniques for Automated Melanoma Detection. In *2019 IEEE International Conference on Bioinformatics and Biomedicine (BIBM)* (pp. 2310-2317). IEEE. 10.1109/BIBM47256.2019.8983165

Vocaturo, E., & Veltri, P. (2017). On the use of Networks in Biomedicine. *FNC/MobiSPC, 2017*, 498-503.

Vocaturo, E., & Zumpano, E. (2019, November). Dangerousness of dysplastic nevi: a Multiple Instance Learning Solution for Early Diagnosis. In *2019 IEEE International Conference on Bioinformatics and Biomedicine (BIBM)* (pp. 2318-2323). IEEE. 10.1109/BIBM47256.2019.8983056

Vocaturo, E., Zumpano, E., & Veltri, P. (2018, December). Image pre-processing in computer vision systems for melanoma detection. In *2018 IEEE International Conference on Bioinformatics and Bio-medicine (BIBM)* (pp. 2117-2124). IEEE. 10.1109/BIBM.2018.8621507

Vocaturo, E., Zumpano, E., & Veltri, P. (2018, July). Features for melanoma lesions characterization in computer vision systems. In *2018 9th International Conference on Information, Intelligence, Systems and Applications (IISA)* (pp. 1-8). IEEE. 10.1109/IISA.2018.8633651

Xu, R., & Wunsch, D. (2008). *Clustering* (Vol. 10). John Wiley & Sons. doi:10.1002/9780470382776

Zhu, X. J. (2005). *Semi-supervised learning literature survey*. University of Wisconsin-Madison Department of Computer Sciences.

Zumpano, E., Iaquinta, P., Caroprese, L., Cascini, G., Dattola, F., Franco, P., ... Vocaturo, E. (2018, December). Simpatico 3d: A medical information system for diagnostic procedures. In *2018 IEEE International Conference on Bioinformatics and Biomedicine (BIBM)* (pp. 2125-2128). IEEE. 10.1109/BIBM.2018.8621090

Chapter 4
Prediction Models

Amit Kumar Tyagi

🆔 https://orcid.org/0000-0003-2657-8700

Vellore Institute of Technology, Chennai, India

ABSTRACT

Having/living convenient life through smart devices, people are more interested or more dependent on to predict something for future (i.e., with respect to their health, business, etc.). For that, many prediction models by several researchers are being used in many applications. Due to a vast (rapid) change in lifestyle, people are more prone to a number of life-threatening diseases when it comes to their well-being. Many of these diseases start developing their symptoms in their early stages. But, still many of these diseases like cancer, kidney damages remain unidentified in their developing stages. The earlier a disease is predicted, the easier it becomes to cure it and even prevent it. Predictive modeling provides a huge step forward in medical science in preventing the risk among patients. Prediction modeling is the process of analyzing current conditions to predict future results.

INTRODUCTION

The storage of data in digital form has provided an opportunity to efficient data usage and produce useful information. The data rich environment provides actionable information that can be processed using different models to predict the future outcomes. Predictive analytics (Galit & Otto, 2011) comprises of varied statistical trends and techniques ranging from machine learning and predictive modeling to data mining (Riccardo & Blaz, 2009) to efficiently analyze the historical data and information so as to process them to create predictions about the unknown future events. It deals in developing various models that can predict the future outcome of an event by describing a variety of statistical and analytical techniques (Borislava et al., 2011). Today predictive analysis is used in many industries to solve different problems. The choice of predictive model to be used depends on the type of field to which the model would be applied. The components related to prediction modeling or predictive analytics can be depicted in figure 1 and discussed as:

DOI: 10.4018/978-1-7998-2742-9.ch004

Data Mining: With the increasing sources of information, a huge amount of data is being fed into the databases daily. This data is in the form of raw facts. By analyzing the trends in the data, useful information can be articulated which could help in decision making. Data mining is the process of discovering patterns and anomalies form large sets of data through the application of statistics, machine learning and database systems. Data mining is used in extraction of potentially useful information that is still undiscovered in a large database. Data mining could be applied to identify multiple groups and clusters of data and forward them for further analysis through machine learning or predictive analytics.

Machine Learning: Machine leaning is the branch of artificial intelligence which provides computer the ability to learn. One of the important ways is to learn by examples. These days, it is being used in various statistical models and methods for prediction of risks and opportunities and is found applicable in various fields such as banking fraud detection, medical diagnosis, natural language processing and analysis over the stock market. Various learning techniques (Carbonneau et al., 2008; Ruchika, 2015) such as Neural Networks, Multilayer Perceptron, support vector machines, Naïve Bayes and other are being used according to the application areas.

Figure 1. Component of Predictive Analytics (Dean & Will, 2014)

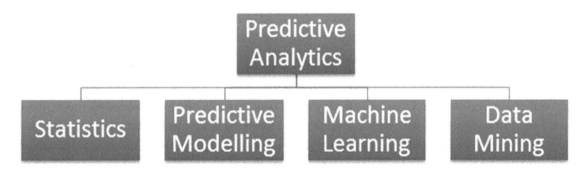

Here, figure 1 show that statistics, predictive modeling, machine learning and data mining are the part of predictive analytics. Predictive analytics and predictive modeling are two essential terms and used in many business applications like e-healthcare, retail/ customer relationship management (CRM), etc., for producing useful decisions. Prediction modeling is used in business applications like, fraud detection, spam mail detection, etc. Other applications include capacity planning, change management, Disaster Recovery (DR), engineering, physical and digital security management and city planning.

Analytics: Analytics is the scientific process of discovering and communicating the meaningful patterns which can be found in raw data or unstructured data (collected from many smart devices). There are four types of analytics (Wullianallur & Vijju, 2013) like data/ descriptive, predictive, prescriptive, diagnostic (refer figure 4 for explanation). Descriptive analytics put results in statistic form which can be easily understood by human-being.

Predictive Analytics: *Predictive analytics* is the use of data, statistical algorithms and machine learning techniques to identify the likelihood of future outcomes based on historical data. The evolution of predictive analytic can be found in figure 2.

Figure 2. Evolution of Predictive Analytics (Mariam, 2017)

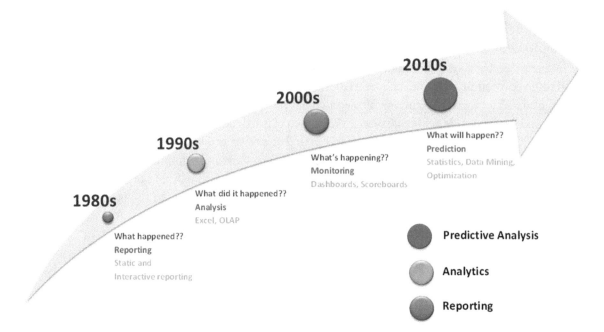

Need for Predictive Analytics: Human are always hungry to know about their future. They want to analyze their historical patterns and predict the best possible outcome/ decisions. In general, for making such analysis we require predictive analysis process. This process is being completed by predictive analytics. The goal of predictive analytics is to go beyond knowing what has happened to providing a best assessment of what will happen in the future. Figure 3 discuss complete process of predictive analytics. Serval component considered during predictive analytic which are included as:

a) Risk management (Stephanie, 2017): While developing a new system we need to consider the risks involved that may lead to system failure in future. Some factors may be hidden or ignored by us but may cause harm to the system in long term. The predictive models analyze the current and historical data and predict the forthcoming risks in an organization, so that they can be reduced and preventive measures could be taken on time.

b) Decision making (Foster & Tom, 2013): While making a decision huge amount of data is analyzed. This data may be from any source such as sensors, routers, servers and many other heterogeneous resources. Predictive modeling is used by a Decision Support System to predict the value of a variable. The predictive model realizes the current situation and makes the predictions to support the upcoming decisions and plans.

c) Resource management (Rahul & Vijay, 2012): predictive modeling analysis the daily usage of resources in an organization and provides with the appropriate quantity of resources that could be stocked so as to run the work smoothly. In case, the system observes any halt in work due to lack of resources, it informs the organization in advance.

d) Fraud detection (Gopinathan et al., 1998): with the increasing rate of networking, the cases of cybercrime are also increasing. The predictive model analyzes these networks continuously and warns the user in case of any threat or fraud.

Prediction Modeling: Prediction modeling is associated with meteorology and weather forecasting, but mostly used in business. Now days role of prediction modeling have moved towards e-healthcare to take care patients.

Figure 3. Process of Predictive Analytics (Credit: predictiveanalyticstoday.com)

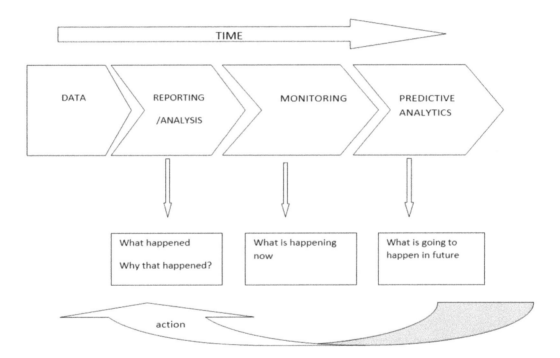

As discussed above, Predictive analytics uses historical data to predict future events. Typically, historical data is used to build a mathematical model that captures important trends. That *predictive* model is then used on current data to predict what will happen next, or to suggest actions to take for optimal outcomes. As this chapter is written toward predict best solution for a critical disease, we need historical data of patients and his/ her activity then we require to produce best possible outcome or solution or prediction for curing any diseases (which are yet to cure or take loner times). Note that predictive analytics and predictive modelling two are different terms, difference discussed in section 3.

Applications of Predictive Models (in general): There are different fields/ sectors/ applications where predictive modeling has made its mark. We are going to discuss a few of them.

a) Medical Science: The need for predictive modeling in medical science is growing day by day. The motive of such models is to predict the best diagnosis for a disease and to conclude the treatment outcomes. There are many areas, such as treatment of patients suffering from lung cancer, autism, diabetes, where prediction modeling is being practiced. Yet there are many other areas where it can be used.

b) Marketing analysis: due to increasing customer's demands for budget purchase, it has become very important to predict the discounted profit in future. Predictive modeling can also be used by investors to track the marketing index since the investor needs to buy all of the financial securities in the market and adjusts its weight to match with the market.

c) Business integrity: Fraud investigators can look into only a set number of cases each week. With predictive analytics, you can use your company's past experience with fraud cases to score transactions according to their level of risk. More precisely, narrowing the number of potential fraud cases more effectively uses investigators' time while leading to fewer false positives and more fraud cases detected.

d) Insurance Marketing: settling insurance claims involves many objections, human sentiments and unseen factors which are hard to be estimated. Predictive modeling can be used as a solution to predict the settlement amount of the claims. Also predictive modeling can be used to predict the average number of days for which a customer may be hospitalized per year. This can help health insurers to develop better plans and strategies.

e) Sales Distribution: In the Information Technology (IT) industry a study used predictive analytics to build a model that analyze the factors affecting the chances to loss or win the IT services deals for IT service providers. This study benefits could be to better take decisions for the preparation and allocation of needed resources, and the attributes of sales pursuit may give awareness to what to do to raise the chances to win sales pursuits in the future. The model provided early ranking list of deals with the chances of winning and then it was applied to obtain the ideal distribution of sales to following deals in order to increase the sales revenue.

f) Prediction of student's performance: Predicting the performance of students in advance can advantage both the institution and learner to take measurable steps in order to enhance the learning process.

Hence, now the remaining part of this chapter is organized as:

- Section 2 describes about literature work related to prediction models.
- Section 3 will explain difference between Predictive Modelling and Predictive Analytics.
- Section 4 will describe several models existed in machine learning and deep leaning domain/ area.
- Section 5 will explain difference between Predictive Modelling and Predictive Analytics.
- Section 6 will discuss the value of predictive modelling and analytics in current smart era.
- Further, section 7 will discuss predictive modelling for several use cases like retail, e-healthcare, Applications.
- Then, section 8 will discuss several issues and Challenges in Predictive Modelling/ Predictive Analytics.
- Section 9 will discuss about several research directions/ opportunities for future researchers.
- In last, this chapter will be summarized in brief in section 10.

LITERATURE WORK

So far we have concluding that predictive modeling basically means to design such models that can transform data into future insights. The concept of predictive analytics emerged in early 1940's with the origin of computational modeling. With the increase in data clouds it gained its popularity in many functional fields like insurance underwriting, fraud detection, risk management, direct marketing, customer retention, at-risk patient determination, and so much more.

It (such predictions) was also in 1940 when Alan Turing developed a machine to decode the German's Enigma communications during World War 2 (WW2). This machine was known as Bombe Machine (Donald, 1999) and acted as the precursor to the computer. During the period of World War 2 (WW2), the Manhattan Project team utilized Monte Carlo simulation (manually) to predict the behavior of atoms during a chain reaction. After observing the results they created the nuclear bombs. These bombs were made out of uranium and plutonium. In 1945, these bombs were dropped on Hiroshima and Nagasaki during the last stage of WW2.

1950's was the era when punch cards came into existence. These punch cards were now being used to store data generated by the computers. This was the year when the ENIAC (Electronic Numerical Integrator And Computer) ran a set of mathematical equations to predict the air flow in the upper levels of the atmosphere. These computations lead to the use of computers to help forecast the weather. In 1958, FICO applied predictive modeling to credit risk decisions.

In 1973 Robert C. Merton published a paper that elaborated the mathematical understanding of the options pricing model named as "Black–Scholes options pricing model". This model was used in financial marketing and to predict the optimal prices of stocks over time. During the period of 1980-1990, the race for online data management started. Amazon and eBay enhanced the online experience. This led to vast amount of data being collected online.

In 2000, the concept of Natural Language Processing gained its popularity. NLP was known for unlocking the analytical value of unstructured data. More and more data was being stored online daily which led to emergence of Big Data and Hadoop to manage the data.

Hence, this section discusses several attempted which have been tried in last century towards analytics or modeling process in medical care or other applications. Now, next section will discuss difference between predictive analytics and predictive modeling.

PREDICTIVE MODELLING VS PREDICTIVE ANALYTICS

As discussed in section 1, four types of data analytics exist for forecasting. The types of data analytics are: Descriptive Analytics (it describes the data), Diagnostic Analytics, Predictive Analytics and Prescriptive Analytics. Predictive analytics utilizes techniques such as machine learning and data mining to predict what might happen next (refer figure 4). It can never predict the future, but it can look at existing data and determine a likely outcome. Data analysts can build predictive models once they have enough data to make predicted outcomes. Predictive analytics (PA) differs from data mining (DM) because DM focuses on discovery of the hidden relationships between variables, while PA applies a model to determine likely outcomes. *Prescriptive analytics takes the final step and offers a recommendation based on a predicted outcome.* Once a predictive model is in place, it can recommend actions based on historical data, external data sources, and machine learning algorithms. Analytics can drive improvement in patient outcomes while providing in-depth information on clinical performance.

Predictive analytics encompasses a variety of statistical techniques from data mining, predictive modelling, and machine learning that analyze current and historical facts to make predictions about future or otherwise unknown events. Some examples of Predictive Analytics (PA) are: Retail, Health, Sports, Weather, Insurance/Risk Assessment, Financial modeling, Energy, and Social Media Analysis.

Note that there are two major ways in which Predictive Analytics differs from traditional statistics (and from evidence-based medicine):

- First, predictions are made for individuals and not for groups
- Second, PA does not rely upon a normal (bell-shaped) curve.

Predictive modeling is a process that uses data mining and probability to forecast outcomes. Each model is made up of a number of predictors, which are variables that are likely to influence future results. Once data has been collected for relevant predictors, a statistical model is formulated. Similarly, some uses of Predictive Modeling (PM) are: E-healthcare (Chuan, 2018), Retail, Fraud detection and many more. Predictive modeling is often performed using curve and surface fitting (Clenshaw & Hayes, 1965), time series regression (Clifford & Hurvich, 1989), or machine learning approaches. Regardless of the approach used, the process of creating a predictive model is the same across methods. The steps are:

- Clean the data by removing outliers and treating missing data
- Identify a parametric or nonparametric predictive modeling approach to use
- Preprocess the data into a form suitable for the chosen modeling algorithm
- Specify a subset of the data to be used for training the model
- Train, or estimate, model parameters from the training data set
- Conduct model performance or goodness-of-fit tests to check model adequacy
- Validate predictive modeling accuracy on data not used for calibrating the model
- Use the model for prediction if satisfied with its performance

Note that Predictive modeling is also often referred to as Predictive analytics, Predictive analysis and Machine learning. These synonyms are often used interchangeably. However, predictive analytics most often refers to commercial applications of predictive modeling, while predictive modeling is used more generally or academically. In practice, machine learning and predictive modeling are often used interchangeably. However, machine learning is a branch of artificial intelligence, which refers to intelligence displayed by machines. Hence, this section discusses essential difference between predictive analytics and predictive modeling. Now, next section will discuss several prediction models, existed in machine learning and deep learning techniques. In other words, we will share some prediction models in next section which work together with machine or deep learning techniques.

EXISTING PREDICTION MODELS IN MACHINE LEARNING AND DEEP LEARNING

As discussed in precious section, predictive and prediction modelling are different terms and connected towards purpose of prediction, fetches information from raw and historical data. Similarly, data analytics and predictive analytics are different terms and difference is included here as:

Data Analytics: Data analytics and predictive analytics both are dissimilar terms. *Data analytics* is primarily conducted in Business-to-Consumer (B2C) applications. It is the science of analyzing raw *data* in order to make conclusions about that information, the process for analyzing sets of data to guide business decisions and test scientific theories. In simple terms, Big *data analytics* (Amir& Murtaza, 2018) examines large amounts of data to uncover hidden patterns, correlations and other insights. Now, some important terms are discussed here as:

- Data analysis is a process of inspecting, cleansing, transforming and modeling data with the goal of discovering useful information, informing conclusions and supporting decision-making.
- Data science is a field comprises of everything that related to data cleansing, preparation, and analysis.
- Big data is somethings that can be used to analyze insights which can lead to better decision and strategic business moves.
- Data analytics involves automating insights into a certain dataset as well as supposes the usage of queries and data aggregation procedures.

In summary, data science refers to the process of extraction of useful insights from data. Machine Learning (ML), statistical methods are used to empower machines to learn without being programmed explicitly. Artificial Intelligence (AI) refers to the process of making machines enable to simulate the human brain function. ML and AI are a part and parcel of data science. Machine learning is used to make prediction, data science is used to produce insight and artificial intelligence is sued for making a decision.

Predictive analytics: It tells what will happen, like insight about in near future. For example, having large amount of data related to patients, we can be presented in a state to think what will happen in near future, if such things occurs with a such (constant/ rapid) rate. We can get shortage of bed in hospitals or if we did not find any optimal solution regarding to nay critical/ serious disease, then we may loss may live. Such kinds of possible results/ outcomes are being done using predictive analytics process/ mechanism. *Predictive analytics methodologies* rely on the following techniques:

- Logistic regression (Gary & Langche, 2001): a static analysis method used to predict a data value based on prior observation of a data-set.
- Time series analysis: an illustration of data points at successive time intervals.
- Decision trees (Safavian & Landgrebe, 1991): a graph that uses a branching method to illustrate every possible outcome of a decision.

Some other more complex predictive models include decision trees, k-means clustering (Amir & Lipikaand, 2007) Bayesian inference (John & Fredrik, 2001) to name just a few potential methods. Note that predictive analytics and predict modelling share some common techniques (like linear regression,

Figure 4. Data Analytics Vs Predictive Analytics (Daniel, 2016)

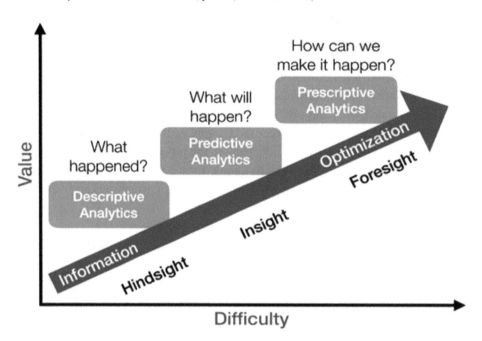

clustering) for making useful prediction for some critical applications like e-healthcare, fraud detection, customer relationship management, etc.

Predictive Modeling Methods/ Techniques

It is always difficult to select best predictive models for generating large amount of big data. Because, several measurements like accuracy of models, efficient statistical theorems matter a lot for selection in predictive model. But, at a point feeding more data into a predictive analytics model does not improve accuracy. Analyzing representative portions of the available information, i.e., sampling, it can help speed development time on models and enable them to be deployed more quickly. For that, first we collect sample data, and then select the right model. For example, Linear regressions (Astrid & Gerhard, 2010) are among the simplest types of predictive models (can be used to predict future occurrences of the dependent variable). Linear models essentially take two variables that are correlated, i.e., one independent and the other dependent and plot one on the x-axis and one on the y-axis. Moreover this, most complex area of predictive modeling is neural network. This type of machine learning model independently reviews large volumes of labeled data in search of correlations between variables in the data. It can detect even subtle correlations that only emerge after reviewing millions of data points. The algorithm can then make inferences about unlabeled data files that are similar in type to the data set it trained on. Today Neural networks used in many examples (of artificial intelligence (AI)) like image recognition, smart assistants and natural language generation (NLG) (Ehud & Robert, 1997). Note that Machine learning might or might not provide benefits and the data might not be robust enough to be useful to clinical teams. But, Prediction algorithms that combine the best clinical expertise with rigorous machine learning tools are the most promising for continued work. *This is a reason to be optimistic about the ability of machine learning to transform prediction in an array of medical fields.* Machine learning also used (have capabilities) in healthcare when the goal is to discover clusters in the data, such as imaging analysis for therapeutic selection. Here, the new features can be validated with expert evaluation from radiologists or neurologists, which differs from the prediction setting where observed labels exist in the data. Causal inference methods that incorporate machine learning are a burgeoning area, including techniques for treatment effect heterogeneity. Understanding heterogeneous treatment effects will likely be one path in the journey toward precision medicine (Euan, 2015). Hence, we can see machine learning and neural network has an essential role in prediction modeling, i.e., in solving complexing problems (related to healthcare applications). In this section, we have discussed some of the application areas where predictive modeling is being implemented. Medical science is the most popular area with growing need of predictive analytics. Next, we are going to discuss several predictive modeling requirements which may have essential role in many business applications.

RECOMMENDED PREDICTIVE MODELLING REQUIREMENTS FOR BUSINESS APPLICATIONS

Today's most of the devices are connected in form of IoT based Cloud (Fei Tao et al., 2015) or Cloud based IoT (Rodger & Michael, 2014). In simple terms, smart devices are being used and connected with internet to solve complex task in many applications like retail, e-healthcare, etc. Today these devices are generating a lot of data via communicating with each other (for solving any problem). For example, many social networking sites, or other popular websites like YouTube, etc., are generating a lot through uploading and sharing of audio and videos. Note that 90% of the data has been in last ten year/ decade by these smart devices. Most of the data 90% of the data is going to be useful for analytics/ analysis tools for making useful decision for healthcare field. Analytics is becoming very crucial (sensitive) in tracking different types of healthcare applications. Advanced analytics touches every aspect of healthcare software systems including clinical, operational and financial sectors. In continuation to this, we use several metrics **for e-healthcare, like** AUC, positive predictive values, sensitivity, and specificity. Hence now in this section, we will discuss some useful requirement like data, value of data, statistics, learning techniques, etc., for predictive modelling (i.e., required for business applications).

- Data: it is presented in two forms like internal and external. For this, predictive provides external data, which create a much more complete view of who the prospects are and whether they are in the market for solutions.
- Statistics: it is used to find patterns. Statistics and advanced algorithms allow marketers to identify patterns that identify buyers that would be otherwise invisible. Machine learning involves feedback loops embedded within statistical modelling processes to enable continuous models refinement.
- Prediction: it is used to discovered patterns. It is achieved by the combination of data and statistics. It is used by some companies/ vendors as additional services like enrichments to enable more effective marketing and sales tactics.
- Value of Data: Healthcare data management is the process of analyzing all the data collected from several sources. This helps the healthcare organizations treat their patients in a holistic manner, provide personalized treatments and enhance health outcomes (refer figure 5).

Figure 5. Value of Data in e-healthcare for Predictive Modeling in near future
(Credit: *hackernoon.com)*

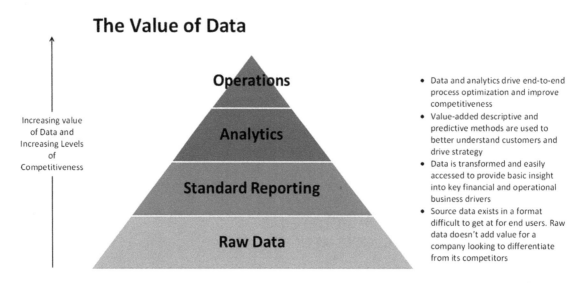

Today's healthcare application has become more competitive and complex, and it will be more complex in near future. We require efficient tools and methods to create value (useful decision/ prediction) from this data (collected from many devices in healthcare in unstructured form). By collecting the data, efficient technologies can help users in making informed decisions for improving quality in respective applications. Using analytics, we get bigger picture of the patient's condition, and eventually, we able to give more precision driven care and treatment, it leads to end-to-end process optimization and increased competitiveness. Hence, this section discusses several predictive modelling requirements for business applications. Now, next section will discuss about importance of predictive modeling or analytics in current smart era.

THE IMPORTANCE OF PREDICTIVE MODELLING/ ANALYTICS IN CURRENT SMART ERA

Today's healthcare industry (value-added business) or bio-medical imaging have a lot of work in finding best (optimal) solutions for critical diseases. This has in fact led to change in the cost structure, increased life expectancy and better control over chronic illnesses and infectious diseases. The benefits are not only for the patients, because it has touched several other entities as well facility providers, insurance providers, government entities, etc. For example, insurance companies are moving their models from a fee-for-service to value-based data-driven payments by making use of Electronic Medical Records (EMRs) (Robert & Ida, 2004). Electronic Medical Records can ensure high quality patient care, but also raises several security and privacy concern in it. Predictive modelling in healthcare is used to:

- Disease Intervention and Prevention: Prediction of disease and their prevention techniques often go hand in hand with analytics. This way, the organizations will be able to identify patients with high risk of developing serious diseases quite early in the condition and provide them with better outcomes so they don't have to face long-term health problems. This prevents long term care which could mean costly treatments and complications that might arise.

- Care Coordination: Analytics helps in delivering care coordination and this is really helpful in emergency care or intensive care. Especially, when there should be quick response time. This can save the patient's life. Apart from deploying care coordination strategies, analytics can even alert the caregiver of a readmission to the hospital in a 30-day window.

- Customer Service: Excellent customer service is extremely important in healthcare, and any discrepancies in that could prove to be fatal. Analytics can deeply impact customer service. And it helps you provide a personalized touch, understand the patient's needs accurately and even motivates them to improve their health. The personalized strategy delivered through analytics can really help the clinician provide better outcomes.

- Financial Risk Management: Artificial Intelligence is the key to financial risk management. According to a report by Hospitals and Health Networks, the biggest financial challenge in the fee-for-service to performance contract model is that it takes quite a lot of time in determining patient outcomes and to decide the payment. Other challenges include lower reimbursements, unpaid patient bills and underused billing and under-utilized record keeping technology. Predictive analytics can help the cash flow to the hospitals by determining the accounts that demand payment, and also predict which payments are likely to remain unpaid in the future.

- Fraud and Abuse: Leveraging data and analytics can help in detecting fraud and abuse. There can be several instances of fraudulent incidents in healthcare, and it could range from honest mistakes like erroneous billings, to wasteful diagnostic tests, false claims leading to improper payments and so on. Big Data helps in identifying the patterns that lead to potential patterns of fraud and abide in healthcare insurance as well. Sniffing out false claims is no longer the tedious process it once was.

- Operations: Healthcare has slowly begun to rely on technology to guide the decision making process. With improved technological infrastructure and proper analysis of data, it is possible for them to make key operational decisions. They have begun to shift away from a reactive approach to manage patient flow, making it easier to avoid operational bottlenecks and reduce clinical variations. Operational decision makers have started making informed decisions as they are able to garner powerful insights from the health system's data.

- Healthcare Reform: Through analytics, health organizations are able to drive healthcare reforms, and this will in turn drive impressive levels of reimbursement restructuring. This is powerful enough to bring about drastic changes in the present hospital-centric delivery model by making it deliver, not volume, but value, and not activity, but outcomes.

In summary, analytics on patient data can help us gain in-depth insights to each and every patient so caregivers can develop targeted patient engagement plans. Analytics can make patient's life easier and longer to live. Hence, this section discusses the importance of predictive modelling/ analytics in healthcare applications. Now, next section will discuss several predictive modelling or discussion of a prediction model with a use case, i.e., e-healthcare.

PREDICTIVE MODELLING FOR POPULAR APPLICATIONS: AN USE CASE

Predictive modelling is used to predict some valuable for curing or finding optimal solution for patients and reducing the workload of doctor and caregivers. The role of analytics in changing/ transforming working style in healthcare is too much. Healthcare organizations have begun to adopt technologies like PACS imaging systems and EMRs (Electronic Health Records) that attempts to make sense of the massive data that flows through the system (both structured and unstructured). We need to know, what are the tools can be useful in extracting information from the data to generate value and enjoy operational, financial and clinical insights. There are *genome analyzers and other analytics tools* in the market that help in understanding the facts, and eliminate unwanted/useless details to extract only what's needed. The end result of this is better clinical outcomes for the patient. There are several ways in which the healthcare organizations can make use of information collected through various sources.

Disease Surveillance and Preventative Management

Healthcare analysts work diligently on the data that's provided to them. Hence, they scour both structured and unstructured data, including the data that's readily available on non-traditional channels like social media messages, text messages and the like to discern any patterns. They convert all the information into actionable insights and work towards achieving better health outcomes. The proliferation of mobile devices has really helped in this regard too. It helps the analysts understand the path of infectious diseases (through the GPS coordinates obtained from the cell phone). This was how they were able to take preventive measure during the Ebola (Derek, 2014) outbreak in West Africa. Cell phone mobility data can help them understand not just present cases of outbreak and infectious diseases, but it will also shed light on diseases could spread in the future as well. The process of using and converting the data:

- Study the patterns presented in the data and check for any disease outbreaks. By correct analysis, the caregivers will be able to provide treatments and even respond to medical emergencies.
- Use the analyzed data to come up with preventive techniques, medicines and vaccines.
- Work towards preventing the spread of the crisis and reduce mortality rates caused by the disease by checking where prompt care should be provided.

It was difficult to control epidemics in the past because of lack of timely data, disparate datasets that you cannot collate, lack of experts with computational background who can help in epidemic planning, control and response. With big data analytics, the challenges and epidemics cans be monitored. For example, genome sequencing gives out huge quantities of big data, and you can use powerful analytics that would help you watch how microbes mutate during an outbreak in real time. Nexstrain (James, 2018) is a tool that enables the sharing and tracking of genome sequences as and when they happen to prevent and control outbreaks.

Develop Clinically Relevant and More Effective
Diagnostic and Therapeutic Techniques

Organizations depend on the expertise of the healthcare analytics to collaborate the data collected from various sources to monitor the efficacy of their processes. This would help them understand how the patients have responded to their program and what their condition is presently. Here are some areas where healthcare providers can enjoy the advantage of predictive analytics and healthcare informatics:

- Recognizing those patients that are likely to develop diseases or possess certain risks to their health.
- Develop specific wellness programs that can be catered to serve the interests of patients, so they can enjoy improved health.
- Identify inefficient programs and processes that do not generate desired results, so they can be removed completely. This ensures that only result-oriented programs are kept in the wellness program packages. The rest are all removed from it.
- In certain cases, the patient may have to be readmitted due to a relapse or adverse effect. The analytics will be able to identify what caused the relapse, and can make suggestions on how to prevent it.
- It is possible to optimize usage of resource, increase productivity, and throughput after analyzing.

While predicting the outcomes for the patients, the analytics will also consider the latest medical research through all the peer-reviewed journals and databases. The predictions can come up with analysis that the human brain can never perceive or suspect. This is why the predictions range from how the patient responds to medications to hospital readmissions. Artificial intelligence is also used to create a production profile (algorithms) collected from previous patients. A prediction model is created using this technique. This technique is then deployed to help new patients to get a new diagnosis.

Development of a Faster, Leaner, and More Productive R&D Pipeline

It is not easy to get a drug out to the patient. There is a thorough and overwhelming process of creating the drug, taking it through elaborate clinical trials and then finally, approval from the FDA. Every pharmaceutical company and healthcare provider must strictly go through this process before administering medicines to the patients. Companies use predictive modelling, statistical tools and algorithms, and healthcare analytics to shorten the time a drug stays in the R&D pipeline. The advantages are stated below:

- Advanced analytics play a major role in developing a low-attrition, leaner, faster and highly productive R&D pipeline.
- Looking for methods that would accelerate the process of drug development to improve patient health. Try procedures that would prevent failures in the clinical trials and improve patient recruitment processes.
- Analyze the patient records to see if there were any drug interactions in the past when new drugs were introduced in the market, and to identify the effects of such drugs.

In order to have a very fast productive pipeline, the healthcare organizations must have sophisticated tools and techniques that will help in analyzing all the information that's coming in.

Moreover this, *machine learning* for prediction in electronic health data has been deployed for many clinical questions during the last decade. Machine learning methods may excel at finding new features or nonlinear relationships in the data, as well as handling settings with more predictor variables than observations. *Electronic health data* often have quality issues (e.g., missingness, misclassification, measurement error), and machine learning may perform similarly to standard techniques for some research questions. Ensembles (running multiple algorithms and either selecting the single best algorithm or creating a weighted average) can help mitigate the latter concern. Using several machine learning tools, Wong et al. predicted delirium risk for newly hospitalized patients with high-dimensional electronic health record data at a large academic health institution. They compared these approaches with a questionnaire-based scoring system and found improved performance for machine learning with respect to several metrics calculated in a single holdout sample.

Figure 6. Role of Prediction Modeling in Healthcare Applications (hackernoon.com/)

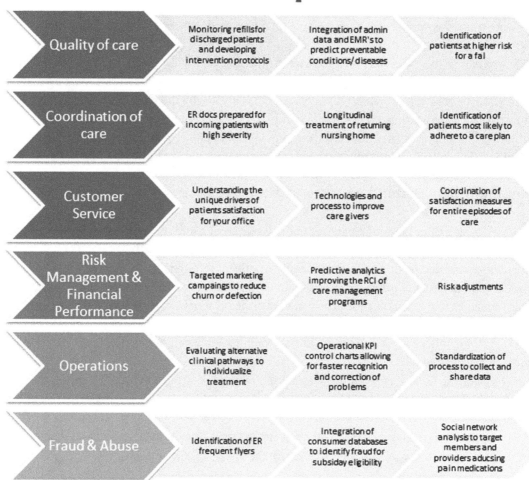

Predictive modeling (popular technique) uses mathematical and computational methods to predict an event or outcome. For that, a mathematical approach is used as an equation-based model to produce/ forecast an outcome for future. For example, time-series regression models for predicting airline traffic volume or predicting fuel efficiency based on a linear regression model of engine speed versus load.

Hence, this section discusses predictive modeling techniques for e-healthcare in detail (refer figure 6). Now, next section will discuss several issues and challenges in predictive modeling/ predictive analytics.

ISSUES AND CHALLENGES IN PREDICTIVE MODELLING/ PREDICTIVE ANALYTICS

Several key issues in machine learning for making prediction in electronic health data are: evaluation and generalizability. In continuation to this, with efficient prediction models, we always require efficient tools and algorithms which fail in analyzing current/ large amount of data (unstructured/ structured data). Also, we may optimize to achieve the best area under the receiver operating characteristic curve (AUC) (Alberto, 2011)but what a doctor might need is high sensitivity or positive predictive value. But, algorithms can have misleading performance when evaluated only along 1 or 2 dimensions or few sample data-sets. Selecting maximum data-set or re-sampling of data-sets will produce more valid and accurate results. For example, high AUC, accuracy, and positive predictive values can be accompanied by near-zero levels of sensitivity and specificity (Altman & Bland, 1994). Note that it is too essential to calculate metrics like the percentage of true cases for calculate higher risk in an application like e-healthcare (i.e., high-risk patients for interventions). Hence, accuracy is always a critical issue in prediction modeling and predictive analytics. Also, it (accuracy) matters a lot in critical applications like aerospace, defence, e-healthcare, etc.

Now coming to challenges in predictive modeling, selecting the right (useful) data to use with developing algorithms is a biggest challenge. In a study, we found that people/ researchers spend about 80% of their time on this step or in choosing right data from right source. Note that if we are unable to get valid, authentic and meaningful data for analytic purpose then we are moving forward towards to get inaccurate results which have no use. Another biggest challenges is building or required projects to solve real world' problems. Sometimes, data scientists discover correlations that seem interesting at the time and build algorithms to investigate the correlation further.

Hence, this section discusses several popular issues and challenges in predictive analytics or in current existing analysis mechanisms. Now, next section will discuss several research directions towards prediction modeling/ predictive analytics for future researchers.

RESEARCH DIRECTIONS/ SUGGESTIONS FOR FUTURE

Predictive analytics can support population health management, financial success, and better outcomes across the value-based care continuum. We can move forward to provide high value services to patients (or to customers, related to other applications) using Predictive Analytics/ Prediction Modeling in Healthcare (in near future). Some services we can provide:

- Risk scoring for chronic diseases, population health

- Avoiding 30-day hospital readmissions
- Getting ahead of patient deterioration
- Forestalling appointment no-shows
- Preventing suicide and patient self-harm
- Predicting patient utilization patterns
- Managing the supply chain
- Ensuring strong data security: Predictive analytics and artificial intelligence are also anticipated to play an important role in cybersecurity, especially as the complexity of attacks continues to increase. Using analytics tools to monitor patterns in data access, sharing, and utilization can give organizations an early warning when something changes, i.e., especially when those changes indicate an attacker/ intruder may have breached a network. In near future, we will calculate risk score in real-time and based on high risk, i.e., high risk score (using predictive analytics), and will block the access for respective events. On another hand, predictive can help with following services to healthcare sector in near future, where we can always try to provide some efficient services like:
- Predictive analytics increase the accuracy of diagnoses
- Predictive analytics will help preventive medicine and public health.
- Predictive analytics provides physicians with answers they are seeking for individual patients.
- Predictive analytics can provide employers and hospitals with predictions concerning insurance product costs.
- Predictive analytics allow researchers to develop prediction models that do not require thousands of cases and that can become more accurate over time.
- Pharmaceutical companies can use predictive analytics to best meet the needs of the public for medications.
- Patients have the potential benefit of better outcomes due to predictive analytics.

Hence, many big changes are coming in medicine area worldwide with predictive analytics. Moreover this with predictive analytics, prediction modeling with patient/ healthcare/ electronic healthcare data can be useful in:

- Developing precision medicine and new therapies
- Bolstering patient engagement and satisfaction

Today's Big data and predictive analytics are being used in making a decision/ management decisions which provide a good and stronger relationship between providers and patients. This plays a crucial role in generating long-term positive engagement, prevent readmission wherever possible and reduce risks of chronic diseases. Combining artificial intelligence (AI) with data analysis, machine learning, and IoT, it is easy to provide proactive care and robust (efficient) services to patients. Hence, it would be a good move to invest in analytical solutions that can control and mitigate clinical and financial risks, with new payment bundles and models to go with it.

Hence, terms predictive analytics, prediction modeling, data mining and machine learning (including deep learning) are very much useful in prediction or making useful decision for healthcare application. This section discusses several research directions or suggestions for future. Now, next section will summarize this chapter in brief.

SUMMARY

In this chapter, we get to know that Prediction analytics and prediction modeling used several techniques Logistic Regression, Random Forest, Ridge Regression, K-nearest Neighbor and XGBoost for forecasting/ prediction purpose. In this chapter, the term "predictive modeling" is used with predictive analytics, predictive analysis, and machine learning interchangeably. Also, in this chapter we discussed difference among popular terms like data analytics, predictive analytics, and prediction modeling. Predictive modeling is useful because it gives accurate insight towards any unstructured data (e.g., audio, video, etc.). For feeding predictive models, we collect data from internet of thing's devices/ smart devices implemented in many applications/ areas. We collect data (from various applications) like Transaction data, CRM data, Customer service data, Survey or polling data, Digital marketing and advertising data, Economic data, Demographic data, Machine-generated data (e.g., telemetric data or data from sensors), Geographical data and Web traffic data. Then, we discussed importance of prediction modeling in smart era and e-healthcare sector. Later, we discussed several critical and challenges towards prediction modelling. In that, selection of appropriate tolls, algorithms, and data (also at right time) is a biggest issue, also a biggest challenge. Also, early identification of patients at risk of developing complications during their hospital stay is currently one of the most challenging issues in healthcare. Note that by studying and analyzing structured and unstructured data it is possible for the organizations to predict illnesses, prevent epidemics and reduce mortality rates. So, we write this chapter, i.e., to provide entire information with respect to prediction modeling at a single place.

REFERENCES

Alberto, J. V. (2011). Insights into the area under the receiver operating characteristic curve (AUC) as a discrimination measure in species distribution modelling. *Journal of Microbiology (Seoul, Korea)*.

Altman, D. G., & Bland, J. M. (1994). Diagnostic tests. 1: Sensitivity and specificity. *BMJ*.

Amir, A., & Lipika, D. (2007). *A k-mean clustering algorithm for mixed numeric and categorical data*. Elsevier.

Amir, G., & Murtaza, H. (2015). *Beyond the hype: Big data concepts, methods, and analytics*. Elsevier.

Astrid, S., & Gerhard, H. (2010). Linear Regression Analysis. *Deutsches Ärzteblatt International*. PMID:21116397

Borislava, M., Andrew, B., Anthony, O., & Simon, G. T. (2011). Review of statistical methods for analysing healthcare resources and costs. *Health Economics*, *20*(8), 897–916. doi:10.1002/hec.1653 PMID:20799344

Camilla, L. W., Jayna, M. H., David, L. S., & Sharon, E. S. (2010). Does This Patient Have Delirium? Value of Bedside Instruments. *Journal of the American Medical Association*. PMID:20716741

Carbonneau, R., Kevin, L., & Rustam, V. (2008). *Application of machine learning techniques for supply chain demand forecasting*. Elsevier.

Chuan, Z. (2018). *PPDP: An efficient and privacy-preserving disease prediction scheme in cloud-based e-Healthcare system*. Elsevier.

Clenshaw, C. W., & Hayes, J. G. (1965). Curve and Surface Fitting. *IMA Journal of Applied Mathematics, 1*(2), 164–183. doi:10.1093/imamat/1.2.164

Clifford, M. H., & Chih-ling, T. (1989). Regression and time series model selection in small samples. *Biometrika*.

Daniel, B. K. (Ed.). (2016). *Big data and learning analytics in higher education: Current theory and practice*. Springer.

Dean, A., & Will, D. (2014). *Data mining and predictive analytics*. Abbottanalytics-blog.

Derek, G. (2014). The 2014 Ebola virus disease outbreak in West Africa. *Journal of General Virology*.

Donald, W. D. (1999). The bombe a remarkable logic machine. *J Cryptologia*.

Ehud, R., & Robert, D. (1997). Building applied natural language generation systems. *Natural Language Engineering, 3*(1), 57–87. doi:10.1017/S1351324997001502

Euan, A. A. (2015). The Precision Medicine Initiative-A New National Effort. *Journal of the American Medical Association*. PMID:25928209

Fei, T., Ying, C., LiDa, X., Lin, Z., & Li, B.H. (2015). CCIoT-CMfg: Cloud Computing and Internet of Things-Based Cloud Manufacturing Service System. IEEE.

Foster, P., & Tom, F. (2013). Data science and its relationship to big data and data-driven decision making. *Big Data*.

Galit, S., & Otto, R. K. (2011). Predictive Analytics in Information Systems Research. *MIS, 3*, 553–572.

Gary, K., & Langche, Z. (2001). Logistic Regression in Rare Events Data. *J Oxford*.

Gopinathan, K. M., Biafore, L. S., Ferguson, W. M., Lazarus, M. A., Pathria, A. K., & Jost, A. (1998). *Fraud detection using predictive modeling*. US Patent. 5,819,226. https://hackernoon.com/ http://predictiveanalyticstoday.com/

James, H., Colin, M., Sidney, M. B., John, H., Barney, P., Charlton, C., ... Richard, A. N. (2018). Nextstrain: Real-time tracking of pathogen evolution. *Bioinformatics (Oxford, England)*. PMID:29790939

John, P. H., & Fredrik, R. (2001). MRBAYES: Bayesian inference of phylogenetic tree. *Bioinformatics (Oxford, England)*.

Mariam,I. (2017). *UIC Health Informatics Health Data Sciences-blog*. Academic Press.

Rahul, G., & Vijay, K. N. (2012). *Predictive Analytics for Resource Over-commit in IaaS Cloud*. IEEE.

Riccardo, B., & Blaz, Z. (2009). *Predictive data mining in clinical medicine: Current issues and guidelines*. Elsevier.

Robert, H. M., & Ida, S. (2004). Physicians' Use of Electronic Medical Records: Barriers And Solutions. *Health Affairs*. PMID:15046136

Rodger, L., & Michael, B. (2014). *City Hub: A Cloud-Based IoT Platform for Smart Cities*. IEEE.

Ruchika, M. (2015). *A systematic review of machine learning techniques for software fault prediction*. Elsevier.

Safavian, S. R., & Landgrebe, D. (1991). *A survey of decision tree classifier methodology*. IEEE. doi:10.1109/21.97458

Stephanie, C., & Regan, F. (2017). *Risk assessment and decision making in child protective services: Predictive risk modeling in context*. Elsevier.

Wullianallur, R., & Viju, R. (2013). *An Overview of Health Analytics. J Health Med Informat*.

Chapter 5
Prediction Models for Healthcare Using Machine Learning:
A Review

Ayushe Gangal
https://orcid.org/0000-0002-7831-9682
G. B. Pant Government Engineering College, India

Sunita Kumari
https://orcid.org/0000-0002-9864-6584
G. B. Pant Government Engineering College, India

Peeyush Kumar
https://orcid.org/0000-0001-6771-740X
G. B. Pant Government Engineering College, India

Anu Saini
https://orcid.org/0000-0003-3683-2071
G. B. Pant Government Engineering College, India

ABSTRACT

Healthcare is always a sensitive issue for all of us, and it will always remain. Predicting various types of health issues in advance can lead us to a better life. Various types of health problems are there like cancer, heart diseases, diabetes, arthritis, pneumonia, lungs disease, liver disease, and brain disease, which all are at high risk. To reduce the risk of health issues, some suitable models are needed for prediction. Thus, it became as a motivational factor for the authors to survey the existing literature on this topic thoroughly and have consequently to identify suitable machine learning techniques so that improvement can be possible while selecting a prediction model. In this chapter, concept of survey is used to provide the prediction models for healthcare issues along with the challenges associated with each model. This chapter will broadly cover the following: machine learning algorithms used in health industry, study various prediction models for Cancer, Heart diseases, Diabetes and Brain diseases, comparative study of various machine learning algorithms used for prediction.

DOI: 10.4018/978-1-7998-2742-9.ch005

INTRODUCTION

We as human beings, stand the highest in the hierarchy of beings, acquire or broaden our existing knowledge by a difficult yet fruitful process called 'learning'. Mathematically, learning can be defined as acquiring wisdom or awareness by a process of studying, experiencing, analyzing or being taught all the above stated. But if given much thought, the process of learning cannot be defined by mere words, as the process is susceptible to change and is different for everyone.

Machine learning attends to computational learning by employing pattern recognition as it's base concept. It works by extracting knowledge or information from the data which is fed into it as input. Machine learning is a scopic field that acknowledges the concepts related to the study and formulation of algorithms that can learn from and make predictions on the given data or sets of data called as datasets. It is the crossroads between mathematics, which supplies with all the methods, concepts and theories required for the domain, statistics, a discipline which happens to specialize in the prediction making from the given data, and artificial intelligence, which is nowadays a shorthand for any task which a computer can perform just as well, if not better than humans. Machine learning has become an indivisible element of our lives, or to say it with even more clarity, our lives are strongly influenced by machine learning algorithms, be it a selection of a movie or a TV series to watch or chatbots instructing you on how to get your mixer running again, They've covered it all. Various fields which are being influenced are transportation, gaming, environmental protection, security, media, healthcare, and the list can go on. Some major breakthroughs have been witnessed in the field of medicine. A study by Consulting firm Frost & Sullivan claims that the use of Artificial Intelligence in the healthcare industry will most likely grow to $6.16 billion, at an annual rate of 68.55% between 2018 and 2022. 'Automatic diagnosis' using image recognition, disease spot identification using pattern recognition and the use of patient's data to generate personalized treatment plans for patients, are some of the highlights of the use of artificial intelligence in the healthcare sector. Here, the authors talk about the predictive models of machine learning in detail and look into their types, usage and limitations.

Dealing with diseases before their spread or even diagnosis is a better approach than combating these maladies, and for this purpose, artificial intelligence has proved to be provident. They have proved to be an exceptional resource for the healthcare industry by enabling it to achieve much higher accuracy and thus diagnosis results.

In this chapter, different types of machine learning algorithms are talked about and their implementation is studied on various diseases with the help of a survey conducted. The diseases selected to fulfil this purpose are distinctly general, so as to bolster the reader's understanding of the disease and thus, the predictive model explained later. The algorithms emphasized in this chapter are K-Nearest Neighbor, Classification and Regression Trees, Support Vector Machine (SVM), Naive Bayes, Gradient Boosted Regression Tree, Perceptron Back-Propagation, Random Forest in Supervised learning, Linear Regression and Logistic Regression in Semi Supervised learning, K-Means Clustering and Classification in Unsupervised Learning.

The chapter is divided into 5 sections. Section 2 talks about the various machine learning concepts, which are a prerequisite for the subsequent sections. Section 3 gives a brief introduction to the diseases taken for the study and survey. Section 4 illustrates the different machine learning algorithms by dividing them on the basis of the diseases they are used to predict. The results obtained from the survey are tabulated in a precise manner for enriching the reader's understanding. The final section presents the conclusions drawn and the possible future work in the field.

CONCEPTS USED

Supervised Machine Learning

Supervised machine learning is the most successful and mostly used type of machine learning. Supervised learning is used whenever someone wants to predict a certain outcome from a given input and examples of input/output pairs are present. These examples were used to train the algorithm, so as to make accurate predictions for new unknown data. In supervised learning human effort is required to build the dataset but afterward automates and often speeds up an otherwise laborious or infeasible task.

The machine learning algorithms which are considered to be the most successful kind of learning algorithms, are those that automates the process of decision making by generalizing from known examples. In supervised learning, the user provides the algorithm with pairs of inputs and desired outputs, and the algorithm finds a way to produce the desired output, given an input. Therefore, the algorithm is able to create an output for an input it has never seen before without any help from a human being.

A model which is able to generalize as accurately as possible should be built.

Classification

In classification, the goal is to predict the class label, using a predefined list of examples. Classification is different from Regression, as in Classification, the input data will completely belong to a particular class or will not belong at all, there is no partial belonging. Classification can be divided into two types:-

1. Binary Classification: In binary classification, there are only two types of classes. The input data can only be classified as one of these two classes. Binary classification is like predicting Yes/ NO. The classification of an email as a spam email or a non-spam email, is an example of Binary Classification. Classes are represented as 0 and 1.
2. Multi-class Classification: In multi-class classification, there are more than two classes. The task of representing a website's languages is an example of multi-class classification. Classes are represented as 0, 1, 2 and so on.

K-Nearest Neighbors

K-Nearest Neighbor is a very basic machine learning model. To make a prediction for a new data point, the algorithm finds the point that is closest to the new point in the training set. Then it assigns the label or output of this training point to the new data point. The k in k-nearest neighbors signifies that instead of using only the closest neighbor to the new data point, any fixed number k of neighbors in the training set can be considered (for example, the closest three or five neighbors). Then the prediction which is in majority is assigned to the new data point. Using only a single neighbor for classification may give very high accuracy on the training set but the model will be very complex and chances of overfitting is high. The number of neighbors for classification must be selected carefully, so that the kNN model is neither too complex nor too simple, and will be able to generalize. Building the kNN model is usually very fast, but for training set which is very large (either in number of features or in number of samples) prediction can be very slow.

Linear Regression

Linear regression is one of the major supervised machine learning algorithms. In regression, the goal is to predict a continuous number, or a floating-point number in programming terms. Predicting the weather, using weather reports and related data of previous years is an example of a regression task. In linear regression, a prediction formula with multiple parameters is used and parameters are selected in order to fit the learning model perfectly with respect to the dataset. The intuition behind the linear regression is that it is a linear model which determines the equation of a high dimensional plane by figuring out the values of parameters in the equation by using the training dataset. The model is tested by entering a new input, then the value of this input is put into the equation of the plane determined, and the value obtained after putting the values is the resulting prediction.

The general formula for linear regression model with multiple features or variables is given by:

$$H_\theta(X) = \theta_0 x_0 + \theta_1 x_1 + \theta_2 x_2 + \ldots + \theta_n x_n$$

Where $\theta_0, \theta_1, \theta_2 \ldots, \theta_n$ are parameters or weights for the model which are to be learned from our data set, so that our model fits perfectly with our data set.

Here $x_0 = 1$ and $x_1, x_2 \ldots, x_3$ are the features or the variables in our data set. $H_\theta(X)$ is also called a hypothesis.

Logistic Regression Model

The Logistic regression model is extensively used for classification. Despite its name, Logistic Regression is a classification algorithm and not a regression algorithm. In this model, the hypothesis has to lie between 0 and 1. The form of hypothesis used in this:

From linear regression, the general equation for hypothesis $H_\theta(X)$ is:

$$H_\theta(X) = \theta^T X$$

Where $\theta = \begin{bmatrix} \theta_0 & \theta_1 & \theta_2 \ldots \theta_n \end{bmatrix}$ and $X = \begin{bmatrix} x_0 & x_1 & x_2 \ldots x_n \end{bmatrix}$ here, $\theta_0, \theta_1, \theta_2 \ldots, \theta_n$ are parameters or weights for the model which are to be learned from the dataset, so that the model fits perfectly with the dataset and $x_0 = 1$ and $x_1, x_2 \ldots, x_3$ are the features or the variables in the data set.

But in Logistic Regression Model,

$$0 \leq H_\theta(X) \leq 1$$

so hypothesis $H_\theta(X)$ in it is: $H_\theta(X) = g(\theta^T X)$

Now here $g(\theta^T X)$ is a Sigmoid function or Logistic function. The equation for this sigmoid function is:

$$g\left(\theta^T X\right) = \frac{1}{1+e^{-\theta^T X}}$$

where g(x) is:

The value of this sigmoid function lies between 0 and 1. The logic behind using this sigmoid function is to restrict the hypothesis in an interval 0 to 1.

Neural Networks

In order to search for an algorithm that can mimic a human brain, the formation of neural networks model took place. The Neural networks were developed in order to use a non-linear hypothesis for machine learning classification problems. When dealing with a really large and complex dataset, the linear hypothesis fails to give gratifying results, so a non-linear hypothesis was needed and executing a non-linear hypothesis with the help of already existing linear model would cost more computation time and power. One of the main advantages of the neural networks is that they are able to capture the information contained in large amounts of data and build incredibly complex models. Neural Networks can often beat other machine learning algorithms if given enough time, data and careful tuning of the parameters.

Ensemble of Decision Trees

Ensemble is the method of creating a more powerful model by combining two or more models together. There are two ensemble models that have proven to be more effective on a wide range of datasets for classification and regression, both of which use decision trees as their building blocks: Random forests and Gradient boosted decision trees.

Random Forest

As the word 'forest' in name 'Random forest' suggests that the random forest model is a collection of multiple decision trees and each tree is somewhat slightly different from the other. The logic behind random forests model is that each tree might do a relatively good job of predicting, but will likely overfit on part of the data. If many trees are built, all of which work well and overfit in different ways, the amount of overfitting can be reduced by averaging their results. To implement the strategy behind the idea of random forests, many decision trees need to be built. Each tree should do an average or acceptable job of predicting the target, and should also be different from the other trees. Random forests get their name from injecting randomness into the tree building to ensure each tree is different. There are two ways in which the trees in a random forest are randomized: First, by selecting the features in each split test and second, by selecting the data points used to build a tree.

Gradient Boosted Decision Trees

The Gradient boosted decision tree is another ensemble model in which a powerful model is created by combining multiple decision trees together. These models can be used for classification and as well as for regression. In gradient boosting model, the trees are built in a serial manner and each tree tries to correct the errors done by the previous tree. The strong pre-pruning is used in gradient boosted, as by default there is no randomization in it. Gradient boosted trees often use very shallow or low depth trees, i.e., of depth ranging from one to five, which makes the model smaller in terms of memory and makes predictions faster. The main logic behind gradient boosting is to combine many simple models (in this context known as weak learners), like shallow trees. Each tree can only provide good predictions on part of the data, and so more and more trees are added to iteratively improve performance. Gradient boosted decision trees are widely used for supervised learning and also are among the most powerful models. Their main drawback is that they require careful tuning of the parameters and may take a long time to train. Just like random forest it also does not work well on high-dimensional sparse data.

Support Vector Machine (SVM)

The Support Vector Machines also called Kernelized Support Vector Machines (KSVMs) are considered as the most powerful 'Black Box' learning algorithm by many experts and is also one of the most widely used learning algorithms. Support vector Machine algorithm is used to determine a Non linear hypothesis. One can say that KSVMs are an extension that allows for more complex models that are not defined simply by hyperplanes in the input space. The Gaussian kernel corresponds to an infinite-dimensional feature space and is hard to explain. One simple way to explain is that it considers all possible polynomials of all degrees, but the importance of the features decreases for higher degrees. During all this computation, the SVM learns the importance of each data point in representing the decision boundary between the two classes. Actually, only a subset of the training points matter for defining the decision boundary: these are the points which lie at the border between the classes. These are called support vectors and give the support vector machine its name. In order to make a prediction for a new point, the distance to each of the support vectors is measured. A classification decision in KVSM is made based on the distances to the support vector and the importance of the support vectors that was learned during training. One thing to remember is that the scaling of data between 0 and 1 can increase the performance of KSVMs exponentially.

Naive Bayes Classifier

The Naive Bayes (in short NBC) classifiers are termed as a family of classifiers that are quite similar to the linear models. But Naive Bayes Classifier tend to be even faster in training. In order to achieve this efficiency the Naive Bayes models often provide generalization performance that is slightly worse than that of linear classifiers like Logistic regression. The reason behind this efficiency is that NBC learns parameters by looking at each feature individually and collecting simple per-class statistics from each feature.

Unsupervised Machine Learning

The Unsupervised learning subsumes all kinds of machine learning where no known output is provided to the algorithm. Input data is given to the learning algorithm and asked to extract knowledge from this given data. There are many successful applications for these methods but they are usually harder to understand and evaluate. There are two types of unsupervised learning, namely, transformations of dataset and clustering.

Unsupervised transformations of a dataset creates a new representation for the given data, so that humans or machine learning algorithms can easily understand them. Clustering algorithms partition the dataset into distinct groups of similar items. K-means clustering is one of the simplest and also most commonly used unsupervised algorithms for clustering. This algorithm finds clusters that contain data of similar type.

The algorithm loops between two steps, namely, Assigning each data point to the closest cluster center, and setting each cluster center as the mean of the data points that are assigned to it.

A major challenge in unsupervised learning is notifying whether the algorithm learned has learned something useful or not. In unsupervised learning there is no label or output provided for the given information, so it is not known what output should be right and thus it's hard to tell whether the unsupervised model did well or not. As a result of the problem, the unsupervised learning is used only for exploratory setting, for instance, to understand the data in a profound way. Another use for unsupervised algorithms is as a preprocessing step for supervised algorithms. Learning a new representation of the data can sometimes improve the accuracy of supervised algorithms.

DISEASES CONSIDERED

Cancer

Cancer may be defined as the rampant growth and division of aberrant cells on any part of the body. There are about 200 types of cancers known to man. Some types cause very quick cell growth, while others cause the cells to grow and divide at a slower rate. Tumor is the visible growth due to cancer, while in some kinds of cancers, visible growth may not present itself, in leukemia, for instance. The cells in the human body also follow some natural order and thus have a fixed lifespan. The cells are instructed to die when their work is done, so that the body can replace them with new cells. Cancerous cells have an absence of the components that instructs them to stop cell division and die.

Some of the major preventable risks involve smoking, heavy alcohol consumption, excess body weight, poor nutrition. The other risks are not preventable. Currently, the most dangerous and non-preventable risk factor is age. According to the American Cancer Society, "Doctors in the US diagnose 87% of the cancer cases in people above 50 years of age". Besides this, genetic agents can also be responsible for the occurrence of cancer in a person, as the genetic codes of a person decides or controls the cell's division and expiration. A person can also inherit an affinity for a particular type of cancer, which may also be referred to as having a 'hereditary cancer syndrome'. These inherited genetic disorders make up about 5-10% of the total cancer cases overall the world.

As the cancer type and therapy is personalized, the treatment varies for different cancer types. The treatment given depends upon the site of the tumor, distribution of cells and type of cells and the patient's overall condition and the presence of any other diseases.

Cancer can be segregated into various types, usually based on the target site and the type of cells, where it first develops. Following is a brief description about the various types of cancer. The data about the number of cases and estimated death tolls has been taken from the American Cancer SocietyCancer Facts and Figures, Estimated new cases and deaths by State, for the year 2019.

Table 1. Depicts the types of cancer, estimated cases per year and the number of deaths caused

Cancer type	No. Of cases	Estimated Deaths	Description of the disease
Prostate cancer	174,650	31,620	This type of cancer occurs in the prostate gland in men, responsible for the secretion of seminal fluid and transports sperm. Causes include mutations in cells' DNA. It doesn't show any signs or symptoms in its early stages, but trouble while urinating, blood in semen, bone pain, discomfort in the pelvic region are common in the later stages.
Lung cancer	228,150	142,670	This type of cancer develops in the lungs. It is the most common type of cancer and a major cause of deaths around the globe. The major causes include both active and passive smoking, exposure to radon gas, diesel exhaust and asbestos fibre or silicate fibre. Symptoms include persistent and worsening cough, chest pain, bronchitis, abrupt weight loss, fatigue, shortness of breath and blood in sputum.
Ovarian cancer	22,530	13,980	This type of cancer begins in the ovaries of the female. Ovarian cancer often goes undetected until it has spread to the pelvic region. At an early stage, symptoms are not visible, but advanced stage symptoms include abdominal bloating, weight loss, discomfort in pelvis area, bowel dysfunction and a continual need to urinate.
Cervical cancer	13,170	4,250	This type of cancer develops in the cells of the cervix, the lower part of the uterus that goes all the way to the vagina of the female reproductive system. Usually a sexually transmitted infection causes this. Signs and symptoms at an advanced stage include watery, bloody vaginal discharge having foul odor and pelvic pain. Human papillomavirus (HPV) is also believed to be one of the causes.
Oral cancer	53,000	10,860	This type of cancer develops inside any part, that constitutes the oral cavity of the body, for eg, gums, tongue, inner lining of cheeks, roof and floor of mouth etc. Symptoms may include a persistent mouth sore, loose teeth, a lump inside the oral cavity, painful swallowing, a white or reddish patch on the insides of the mouth. Tobacco of any kind and heavy alcohol consumption are the major risk factors.
Rectal cancer	145,600		This type of cancer develops in the rectum, which is the last several inches of the large intestine. As the rectum is present at a compact place, surgical removal is quite difficult. Symptoms include bowel dysfunction, diarrhea, dark or bloody stool, mucus in stool, painful bowel movements, fatigue, weight loss and anemia.

Heart Diseases

'Heart disease' is an elementary term, used to cover a wide range of problems associated with the heart. They can be related to the blood vessels or the circulatory system, heart rhythm problems, problems with the make of the heart itself, which can be by birth or due to an accident, and many more. The term 'cardiovascular diseases' hold the same meaning as the term 'heart diseases', and generally refers to a condition of narrowed or blocked arteries causing chest pains, heart attacks or strokes. The blood flow in the arteries is obstructed by a substance called plaque, which develops in the arterial walls. It is a wax-like substance, made up of fatty molecules, minerals and cholesterol. If the blood clots and blocks the arteries, it can cause a heart attack or a stroke. Some of the major risk factors are age, high blood pressure, which can damage the blood vessels, smoking or use of tobacco in any form, high cholesterol, diabetes, being overweight etc,. The various types of heart diseases are listed in the following table and their respective symptoms and description is also given. As different types of heart diseases have different symptoms.

Table 2. Types, description and symptoms of heart diseases

Types of heart diseases	Description	Symptoms
Atherosclerotic diseases	Narrowing of arteries due to plaque buildup in the arterial walls, causing obstruction in the flow of blood in the arteries.	Chest pain, Chest tightness, chest discomfort, shortness of breath, pain, numbness in legs, pain in jaw, neck, upper abdomen or back.
Arrhythmias	Abnormal rate or rhythm of the heartbeat. Heartbeat can be too slow, too quick or can be of an irregular pattern. If the heart beats too fast, it is called tachycardia. If the heart beats too slow, it is called bradycardia. Fibrillation, when the heart beats irregularly.	Fluttering in chest, racing heartbeat, slow heartbeat, chest pain or discomfort, shortness of breath, lightheadedness, dizziness, fainting.
Congenital heart defects	This is a general term coined for the deformities present in the heart in the heart since birth.	Pale gray or blue coloration of skin, swelling in the legs, abdomen or around eyes, shortness of breath.
Dilated cardiomyopathy	The chambers of the heart dilates due to weakness of heart muscles, thus cannot pump properly. This is usually caused by a lack of oxygen in the heart muscle due to coronary artery disease. Usually affects the left ventricle.	Shortness of breath, exertion, swelling of legs, ankles and feet, fatigue, irregular heartbeats-rapid pounding or fluttering, dizziness, lightheadedness and fainting.
Endocarditis	Infection of endocardium, generally due to bacteria, fungi or other germs that travel from other body parts like mouth to the bloodstream and attach to the damaged site in the heart.	Fever, shortness of breath, weakness or fatigue, swelling in legs or abdomen, changes in heart rhythm, dry cough, skin rashes.

Diabetes

A collection of diseases that affect how our body uses the blood sugar is called 'Diabetes Mellitus'. The causes of diabetes vary according to the types. Diabetes is of four major types, type 1, type 2, prediabetes and gestational. The presence of excessive sugar in the blood can lead to severe health issues. Table 3 enlists the types of diabetes and their respective risk factors. Gestational diabetes is caused during pregnancy. The placenta produces hormones to sustain pregnancy, which make the cells more resistant to insulin. The pancreas produces extra insulin to overcome this resistance, but sometimes the pancreas can't keep up. When this happens, the sugar gets dissolved in the blood, rather than going in the cells, which causes gestational diabetes. Some common symptoms of type 1 and type 2 diabetes are increased thirst, frequent need to urinate, extreme hunger, unexplained weight loss, fatigue, blurred vision, slow healing of wounds, frequent infections and presence of ketones in urine. As far as prevention of diabetes is concerned, type 1 diabetes can't be prevented. Some of the basic prevention steps include eating healthy and balanced diets, getting more physical exercise and losing extra weight.

Brain Diseases

Brain diseases or disorders can be defined as the damage, disruption or abnormality present in the brain, usually due to falls, accidents, concussion and other forms of trauma, lack of oxygen, alcohol, infectious diseases, degenerative diseases like Alzheimer's disease, Parkinson's disease, brain tumors, stokes, etc. brain diseases or disorders doesn't affect the intelligence of the person, but might cause problems with memory, concentration and attention. Brain diseases can be categorized as brain infections like men-

Table 3. Types, description and risk factors of diabetes

Type of diabetes	Description	Risk factors
Type 1 diabetes	It is also called insulin-dependent diabetes. Often starts to show up in childhood. It is an autoimmune condition in which the body attacks its own pancreas with antibodies. Thus, insulin is not produced by the pancreas and glucose doesn't get absorbed in cells.	Family History, Environmental factors like being exposed to a viral infection, presence of cells that damage the immune system
Type 2 diabetes	The most common type of diabetes. Called as adult-onset diabetes. It is the milder form of type 1 diabetes. In type 2, the pancreas produces some insulin, but it is rather insufficient or the cells become resistant to it. Can be controlled by weight management, nutrition and exercise	Weight, inactivity, family history, race, age, gestational diabetes, high blood pressure, abnormal cholesterol and triglyceride levels
Prediabetes	Condition where blood sugar levels are higher than normal but not alarmingly high enough to be called type 2 diabetes.	Weight, inactivity, family history, race, age, gestational diabetes
Gestational diabetes	Diabetes triggered during pregnancy, as pregnancy, to some extent it leads to insulin resistance.	Age, family history, weight, race

ingitis, trauma, stroke, seizures and degenerative brain diseases like Alzheimer's disease, Parkinson's disease, dementia, etc., different types of brain diseases and enlisted in the following table, along with their description and symptoms.

PREDICTIVE MODELS & APPROACHES USED SO FAR

An extensive survey is conducted on various predictive models, constructed using different machine learning algorithms for the anticipation of different diseases. A brief summary of the research papers and related materials surveyed, and the datasets considered by their respective authors is also discussed. This section is divided on the basis of diseases picked.

Cancer

(Aditya Singh 2017) proposed a novel Error guided Artificial Bee Colony (EABC), based on the operations of Artificial Bee Colony (ABC). ABC is an optimization algorithm that simulates the intelligent scouring behavior of honey bees. In this paper, an EABC trained neural network is used for the prediction of ovarian cancer. The dataset for this particular prediction model was taken from National Cancer Institute, USA, consisting of mass spectrometry reports of 216 patients.

(Saba Bashir, 2018) used machine learning algorithms like Support Vector Machine (SVM), Naive Bayes, Decision Tree, Neural Network, Auto Multi-Layer Perceptron (MLP), Gradient Boosted Tree, Random Forest and Majority Voting to predict the occurrence of lung cancer. The given set of algorithms were implemented using a dataset called 'Lung Cancer,' salvaged from the UCI (University of California, Irvine) online repository. The dataset consisted of 32 instances and 57 attributes.

(Rayavarapu, Krishana, 2018) used Voting Classifier and Deep Neural Network (DNN) for the prediction of cervical cancer. In this paper, classification was done by applying supervised algorithms to classify people with cervical cancer. Data for this particular research was taken from Cervical Cancer dataset from UCI (University of California, Irvine). The final results are passed into the Voting Classifier, supported by test data to generate class labels.

(Suman & Hooda, 2019) presented a case study on prediction of cervical cancer using machine learning algorithms. The algorithms considered were Random Forest, Neural Network, Support Vector Machine (SVM), AdaBoost, Naive Bayes and Bayesian Network. The dataset was taken from 'Hospital Universitario de Caracas', Caracas, Venezuela. The proposed method involved analyzing the biopsy results initially, and patient's traits, earlier pregnancies, smoking habits, usage of hormonal contraceptives etc, were also considered for this study.

(Andres M. Bur, 2019) presented a machine learning algorithm to predict the occurrence of oral cancer. This paper also compares the performance of DOI (depth of invasion) model to various machine learning algorithms. The algorithms taken into account were Kernel SVM (support vector machine), Gradient Boosting, Logistic Regression and Decision Forest. National Cancer database (NCDB) supplied with 1961 patients' data and University of Kansas Medical Center supplied with another 71 patients' data.

(Sunil Kumar Prabhakar, 2017) did a comparative study for prediction of oral cancer using Gaussian Mixture Measures and the classification accuracy of TNM (Tumor, Node, Metastasis) staging system using Multi Layer Perceptron. A total of 75 oral cancer patients were considered for this study. The dataset was taken from the Department of Oncology of G. Kuppuswamy Naidu Hospital (GKNM) Hospital, Coimbatore, India.. The results of the study were divided on the basis of the four stages of oral cancer T1, T2, T3 and T4.

Table 4. Types of brain diseases with their description and symptoms

Brain Disease	Description	Symptoms
Meningitis	It is an inflammation of the membranes surrounding the spinal cord and brain. It is usually caused by a viral infection, bacterial, fungal or parasitic infections. Keeping good hygiene can prevent this.	Sudden high fever, stiff neck, severe headache, nausea and vomiting, difficulty in concentrating, seizures, dizziness, sensitivity to light, loss of appetite and thirst, skin rashes, difficulty waking up
Concussion	A traumatic brain injury caused by a blow to the head or neck. It can cause the brain to slide back and forth forcefully against the inner walls of the skull.	Headaches or a feeling of pressure in the head, loss of consciousness, dizziness, nausea, vomiting, slurred speech, fatigue, ringing in the ears, delayed responses
Brain Tumor	Growth of abnormal cells or mass in the brain is a brain tumor. Usually occurs due to genetic causes or DNA mutations	Worsting and frequent headache, nausea, vomiting, loss of sensation, movement, speech difficulty, personality changes
Stroke	Stroke is a condition in which the blood supply to the brain is cut off or is reduced, bereaving the brain tissue of oxygen and nutrients. Causing the brain cells to die within a short period of time.	Sudden trouble in speaking (slurred speech), paralysis and numbness of the face, arm or leg, trouble in seeing with one or both the eyes, sudden and extreme headache, difficulty in walking
Brain Aneurysm	It is the bulging of a blood vessel in the brain, which can lead to a leak or rupture, causing bleeding in the brain. It has two types, namely, ruptured and unruptured aneurysm. A ruptured aneurysm is life threatening, if not cared	Ruptured aneurysm's symptoms include sudden and extreme headaches, nausea, stiff neck, blurred vision, seizures, sensitivity to light. Unruptured aneurysm's symptoms include change in vision, dilated pupils, numbness on face.
Alzheimer's Disease	It is a progressive disease that causes brain cells to degenerate and die. It is the most common cause of dementia. There is no cure for this, and it results in death.	Memory loss, difficulty in thinking, reasoning, making decisions and judgments, changes in personality like frequent mood swings, flashes of depression, social withdrawal.
Parkinson's disease	A nervous disorder that affects the movement. Symptoms start with barely noticeable tremors, face may not show any expressions.	Symptoms often begin on one side of the body and worsen with time, usually include, tremors, slowed movement, rigid muscles, stiffness all over, flawed posture and balance, changes in speech, writing.

(D. Padmini Pragna, 2017) proposed a health alert system to help identify oral cancer at an early stage. Computerized Tomography (CT) scanned images of the cancerous region were given as inputs, to detect malignancy. The CT images were preprocessed using several image processing techniques like Adaptive Median Filter, and features like texture, shape, water content etc, were extracted. Feature election was used to remove redundant features and Support Vector Machine algorithm was applied to classify the cancer as malignant or benign.

Heart Diseases

(D. R. Patil, 2014) presented a prediction system by making use of Multi Layer Perceptron Neural Network. 13 clinical features are given as input in the neural network and it is trained using back-propagation algorithm. Cleveland heart disease database taken from UCI repository database, was used for the evaluation of the performance of the prediction model. The database had 303 records with 13 clinical features each.

(Ismaeel, 2015) proposed a system using Extreme Learning Machine (ELM) to predict heart diseases. Cleveland Clinic Foundation database was used for this study. The output gave the exact presence value of the heart disease, instead of a typical yes/no response.

(Kamra, 2016) developed a framework using Associative Learning Technique for early prediction of heart based diseases. Cleveland heart diseases dataset from the University of California, Irvine (UCI) machine learning repository supplied with the required data for the predictive model.

(Karaylan, 2017) proposed a predictive system for the prediction of heart diseases using Artificial Neural Network back-propagation algorithm. Cleveland database was used for this purpose, which consisted of 303 records with 13 main clinical attributes.

(Indu Yekkala, 2017) proposed a predictive model for heart disease prediction using ensemble methods like Bagged Tree, Random Forest and AdaBoost, along with a Feature selection method, called the Particle Swarm Optimization (PSO). The heart disease dataset was taken from the UCI Repository, which consisted of 270 records and 14 features.

(Morteza Ghazanfari, 2017) proposed a prediction model using pattern recognition algorithms like Decision Tree, Neural Network, Rough Set, Naive Bayes and Support Vector Machine, for the detection of cardiovascular diseases in patients. The data was obtained from cardiovascular patients' data from the UCI Repository. It had 303 records and 14 features.

(Tahira Mahboob, 2017) used machine learning algorithms like Support Vector Machine (SVM), K-Nearest Neighbor (KNN) and Artificial Neural Network (ANN) for the prediction of coronary heart diseases. The proposed ensemble algorithm consisted of a combination of SVM, KNN and ANN using a voting technique. The data inputted consisted of risk factors collected from 50 people through case studies provided at the website of the American Heart Association.

(S. Sharmila, 2017) used Naive Bayes algorithm and proposed an improved version of Naive Bayes. The UCI Repository dataset is used as the input data, which consists of 303 records with 14 attributes each.

(Dinesh Kumar G., 2018) used pattern recognition algorithms like Support Vector Machine (SVM), Gradient Boosting, Random Forest, Naive Bayes and Logistic Regression for predicting cardiovascular diseases. Data used in this study was obtained from the Cleveland, Hungarian, Switzerland, Long Beach VA heart disease database from the UCI Machine Learning Repository.

Table 5. Analysis of machine learning algorithms based predictive models for cancer

Cancer Type	Author	Year of Publication	Machine Learning Algorithm	Source of Dataset	Accuracy
Cervical Cancer	K. Rayavarapu et al.	2018	• Voting Classifier • Deep Neural Network (DNN)	Cervical Cancer database from UCI	• 97% • 90%
	Sujay K. Suman et al.	2019	• Random Forest • Decision Tree • Neural Network • SVM • AdaBoost • Naive Bayes • Bayesian Network • Logistic regression • Decision Stump • J48	Hospital Universitario de Caracas, Venezuela	• 95.68% • 95.92% • 93.58% • 96.15% • 94.17% • 88.69% • 96.38% • 95.33% • 96.15% • 95.15%
Ovarian Cancer	Aditya Singh et al.	2017	Error guided Artificial Bee Colony (EABC)	National Cancer Institute, USA	91.2%
Lung cancer	Saba Bashir et al.	2018	• SVM • Naive Bayes • Decision Tree • Neural Network • Auto MLP • Gradient Boosted Tree • Random Forest • Majority Voting (MLP+GBT+SVM)	UCI online repository, called 'Lung Cancer'	• 79.17% • 85.00% • 78.33% • 71.67% • 78.33% • 90.00% • 79.17% • 88.57%
Oral Cancer	• Rajaguru, Prabhakar • D. Padmini Pragna et al. • Andres M. Bur et al	2017 2017 2019	• Gaussian Mixture Measures (GMM) • Multi Layer Perceptron (MLP) • SVM • KNN • Depth of Invasion (DOI) • Kernel SVM • Gradient Boosting • Logistic Regression • Decision Forest	Department of Oncology of G.Kuppuswamy Naidu Hospital, Coimbatore, India A set of 29 CT scanned images verified by an Oncologist • National Cancer Database (NCDB) • University of Kansas Medical Center	Stage T1 • 100% • 92% Stage T2 • 100% • 89% Stage T3 • 85.56% • 87% Stage T4 • 91.17% • 90% • 96.55% • 85.71% • 55.80% • 64.25% • 62.70% • 63.25% • 62.25% • 60.40% • 69.60% • 73.80% • 77.20% • 74.65%

(Rajiwall, 2018) employed predictive algorithms like Neural Network, Support Vector Machine, Naive Bayes, Bagging, K-Nearest Neighbor, Ensemble and Logistic Regression for the prediction of cardiovascular diseases on fuzzy data. The data used for the study was obtained from two databases, namely, Framingham Heart Study (FHS) and National Health and Nutrition Examination dataset (NHANES).

(M. Raihan, 2019) proposed the use of Artificial Neural Network (ANN) for the prediction of Ischemic Heart Diseases. The patient's history and diagnostic data were collected from. Data of 917 instances with ECG and ETT results were acquired. About 506 instances from AFC Fortis Escorts Heart Institute, Khulna, Bangladesh, data of 281 instances from the general population and the data of 130 instances from Rural Health Progress Trust, India were collected and recorded for the study.

Diabetes

(Rachita Mishra, 2014) described and compared the performance of back-propagation neural network and extreme learning machine (ELM) algorithms for the prediction of diabetes mellitus. The data used was obtained from the Pima Indians diabetes dataset from UCI learning repository. The dataset consisted of 768 instances, 8 attributes and one class attribute.

(Lin Li, 2014) combined three classifiers, namely, Support Vector Machine (SVM), Artificial Neural Network (ANN) and Naive Bayes to diagnose diabetes. The Pima Indians diabetes dataset was used for this study. The authors proposed a new method of voting for combining the decisions of the individual classifiers. The prediction of subjects as diabetic, was considered as positive votes and prediction of subjects as non-diabetic was considered to be negative votes. The idea of the method was in favor of positive votes rather than the negative votes.

(Suharjito, 2014) implemented Extreme Learning Machine (ELM) for predicting diabetes mellitus. The data used in this study was taken from the UCI Repository, by Vincent Sigillito from The Johns Hopkins University. The data consisted of 769 women population which lives in Phoenix, Arizona, and was taken according to the criteria of WHO.

(Ayush Anand, 2015) aimed to establish a relation between the occurrence of diabetes to be developed from a person's daily habits and activities. Data for this study was collected manually using questionnaires, made specifically with the help of two diabetologists. Two types of questionnaires were made, one for diabetic and the other for non-diabetic people. The Chi-Squared Independence Test was performed on the data acquired, followed by the application of Classification and Regression Trees (CART) machine learning algorithm.

(Anjali C, 2015) proposed the use of Decision Stump with AdaBoost to predict the occurrence of diabetes mellitus. Support Vector Machine (SVM), Naive Bayes and Decision Tree were also implemented. The UCI learning repository dataset, consisting of 768 instances and 9 attributes was used for this study. A local dataset consisting of 200 records was collected and used for the purpose of validation.

(Zhilbert Tafa, 2015) proposed a joint implementation of Support Vector Machine and Naive Bayes for the prediction of diabetes mellitus. The dataset consisting of 402 records was taken. It was created using information from three different places in Kosovo.

(Aparimita Swain, 2016) proposed the use of Artificial Neural Network (ANN) and hybrid Adaptive Neuro-Fuzzy Inference System (ANFIS) for the prediction and classification of Diabetes Mellitus. The network was trained by using the data of 100 individuals collected from the local inhabitants of Bhubaneswar, Odisha, India.

(S. Pranavi, 2017) compared different machine learning algorithms like Random Forest (RF), Support Vector Machine (SVM), K-Nearest Neighbor (KNN), Classification and Regression Trees (CART) and Latent Dirichlet Allocation (LDA). The dataset considered for this work had 650 records of diabetic patients of different age groups which were collected from Diagnosis Lab located in Warangal, TS, India.

(Maham Jahangir, 2017) used Automatic Multi-Layer Perceptron (AutoMLP) combined with an outlier detection method Enhanced Class Outlier Detection using distance based algorithm to predict the occurrence of diabetes mellitus. The Pima Indians Diabetes Dataset (PIDD) from UCI machine learning repository was used for this study. It consisted of 768 instances and 8 attributes.

Table 6. Analysis of machine learning algorithms based predictive models for heart

Year of Publication	Author	Machine Learning Algorithms	Source of Dataset	Accuracy
2014	D. R. Patil et al.	Multi Layer Perceptron Neural Network with n neurons, where • n = 5 • n = 10 • n = 15 • n = 20	Cleveland Heart disease dataset from UCI Repository database	• 92.92% • 95.75% • 96.69% • 98.58%
2015	Salam Ismaeel et al.	Extreme Learning Machine	Cleveland Clinic Foundation database	86.5%
2016	Amit Kamra et al.	Associative Learning Technique ★ Using Apriori • Naive Bayes • K-Nearest Neighbor • J48	Cleveland Heart Disease dataset from the UCI Repository database	• 97.55% • 99.19% • 97.85%
		★ Using FP-Growth • Naive Bayes • K-Nearest Neighbor • J48	Cleveland Heart disease dataset from UCI Repository database	• 97.55% • 94.84% • 96.56%
2017	• Tülay Karaylan et al.	Artificial Neural Network back-propagation using n neurons, for • n = 3 • n = 4 • n = 5 • n = 6 • n = 7 • n = 8 • n = 9 • n = 10 • n = 11 • n = 12	Cleveland Heart disease dataset from UCI Repository database	• 91.11% • 88.88% • 88.88% • 89.66% • 93.33% • 95.55% • 91.11% • 91.11% • 95.55% • 91.11%
	• Indu Yekkala et al.	• Bagged Tree + Particle Swarm Optimization • Random Forest + PSO • AdaBoost + PSO	Cleveland Heart disease dataset from UCI Repository database	• 100% • 90.37% • 88.89%
	• Morteza Ghazanfari et al.	• Decision Tree • Neural Network • Rough Set • Naive Bayes • Support Vector Machine	Cardiovascular patients' data present in the UCI Repository	• 74.80% • 86.90% • 88.10% • 86.90% • 75.40%
	• Tahira Mahboob et al.	• Support Vector Machine • K-Nearest Neighbor • Artificial Neural Network	50 case studies' data from American Heart Association	• 88.24% • 88.24% • 87.50%
	• S. Sharmila et al.	• Naive Bayes • Proposed method (Improved Naive Bayes)	UCI Repository database	• 89% • 97%

continues on following page

Table 6. Continued

Year of Publication	Author	Machine Learning Algorithms	Source of Dataset	Accuracy
2018	• Dinesh Kumar G. et al.	• Support Vector Machine • Gradient Boosting • Random Forest • Naive Bayes • Logistic Regression	Cleveland, Hungarian, Switzerland and LongBeach VA databases from UCI Repository National Health and Nutrition Examination dataset (NHANES)	• 88.26% • 90.70% • 89.53% • 90.50% • 91.61%
	• Rachel DaveyRajiwall et al. et al.	• Neural Network • Support Vector Machine • Naive Bayes • Bagging • K-Nearest Neighbor • Decision Tree • Logistic Regression • Random Forest • Neural Network • Support Vector Machine • Naive Bayes • Ensemble • K-Nearest Neighbor • Decision Tree • Logistic Regression • Random Forest	Framingham Heart Study (FHS)	• 98.80% • 95.40% • 95.70% • 96.50% • 80.80% • 97.60% • 96.40% • 98.50% • 89.00% • 90.20% • 89.90% • 89.30% • 90.10% • 90.00% • 90.00% • 90.10%
2019	M. Raihan et al.	Artificial Neural Network	AFC Fortis Escorts Heart Institute, Khulna, Bangladesh and Rural Health Progress Trust, India.	84.47%

(Ayman Mir, 2018) used Support Vector Machine (SVM), Naive Bayes, Random Forest and Classification and Regression Trees (CART) machine learning algorithms for the prediction of diabetes. The dataset chosen for this purpose was Pima Indians Diabetes Database.,

(Shobitha, 2018) used photoplethysmogram (PPG) signals to predict blood glucose level (BGL) using Relevance Vector Machine (RVM), which is a supervised learning algorithm. To carry out a comparative study, Random Forest was implemented to predict the BGL. The data used in this study was obtained from Biomedical research lab, Universiti Kebangsaan Malaysia. The blood glucose levels obtained were validated using Cohen Kappa Statistics.

(Asaduzzaman, 2019) employed popular machine learning algorithms like Support Vector Machine (SVM), Naive Bayes, K-Nearest Neighbor (KNN) and C4.5 (Decision Tree) for the prediction of diabetes mellitus. The data was obtained from the diagnostics of Medical Centre Chittagong (MCC), Bangladesh. It consisted of 200 records and 16 risk factors as attributes.

Brain Diseases

(Adrien Payan, 2015) used deep learning methods and 3D convolutional neural networks to predict the presence of Alzheimer's disease in patients, using the MRI (magnetic resonance imaging) scans. The dataset used for this particular study was obtained from the ADNI data set consisting of 2,265 historical scans. A clear cut comparison was made between the performance of the 2D neural networks and 3D neural networks on the basis of accuracy.

(Pan Zhou, 2016) used Deep Learning for the diagnosis of Alzheimer's disease, using magnetic resonance imaging (MRI) scans as input. The data used for the study was obtained from the Alzheimer's disease neuroimaging association (ADNI). The predictive models were trained using time series data and correlation coefficient data individually.

Table 7. Analysis of machine learning algorithms based predictive models for diabetes

Year of Publication	Author	Machine Learning Algorithms	Source of Dataset	Accuracy
2014	• Rachita Mishra et al. • Lin Li et al. • Suharjito et al.	• Back-propagation neural network • Extreme Learning Machine • Support Vector Machine (SVM) • Artificial Neural Network (ANN) • Naive Bayes (NB) • SVM + ANN + NB • Extreme Learning Machine • Back-propagation	Pima Indians Diabetes Dataset from the UCI repository Pima Indians Diabetes Dataset from the UCI repository UCI repository	• 68.00% • 75.72% • 75.20% • 77.30% • 74.00% • 74.40% • 60.70% • 28.36%
2015	• Ayush Anand et al. • Anjali C et al. • Zhilbert et al.	Classification and Regression Trees (CART) • Support Vector Machine • Naive Bayes • Decision Tree • Decision Stump • SVM + AdaBoost • Naive Byes + AdaBoost • Decision Tree + AdaBoost • Decision Stump + AdaBoost • Support Vector Machine • Naive Bayes • SVM + Naive Bayes	Manually collected data using two types of questionnaires created. UCI learning repository Dataset manually from three different locations in Kosovo	75% • 79.68% • 78.10% • 76.00% • 74.47% • 79.68% • 79.68% • 77.60% • 80.72% • 95.52% • 94.53% • 97.60%
2016	Aparimita Swain et al.	• Artificial Neural Network (ANN) • Adaptive Neuro-Fuzzy Inference System (ANFIS)	Collected from local inhabitants of Bhubaneswar, Odisha, India	• 71.10% • 90.32%
2017	• S. Pranavi et al. • Maham Jahangir et al.	• Random Forest • Latent Dirichlet Allocation (LDA) • Support Vector Machine • CART • K-Nearest Neighbor Automatic Multi Layer Perceptron (AutoMLP)	Data collected from Diagnosis Lab located in Warangal, TS, India. Pima Indians Diabetes Dataset from the UCI repository	• 100% • 94.57% • 96.90% • 93.02% • 59.69% 88.70%
2018	• Ayman Mir et al. • Shobitha et al., 2018	• Support Vector Machine • Naive Bayes • Random Forest • CART Relevance Vector Machine (RVM)	Pima Indians Diabetes Dataset from the UCI repository Data collected from Biomedical research lab, Universiti Kebangsaan Malaysia	• 78.75% • 76.85% • 76.50% • 76.23% 95.50%
2019	Asaduzzaman et al.	• Support Vector Machine • Naive Bayes • K-Nearest Neighbor • C4.5 (Decision Tree)	Data collected from the diagnostics Medical Centre Chittagong (MCC), Bangladesh	• 96.40% • 67.80% • 70.20% • 73.50%

Table 8. Analysis of machine learning algorithms based predictive models for brain diseases

Year of Publication	Author	Disease Targeted	Machine Learning Algorithms	Source of Dataset	Accuracy
2015	Adrien Payan et al.	Alzheimer's disease	• 2D neural network • 3D neural network	ADNI dataset	• 85.52% • 89.47%
2016	Pan Zhou et al.	Alzheimer's disease	• SVM • Logistic Regression • Auto encoder	ADNI dataset	• 62.90% • 59.70% • 67.50%
2017	• Xiao Zheng et al. • Ammarah Farooq et al.	Alzheimer's disease Alzheimer's disease	• SVM • SVM + LUPI • RBM + LUPI • (SVM+LUPI) +(RBM+LUPI) Deep Convolutional neural network (CNN)	ADNI dataset ADNI dataset	• 85.27% • 87.16% • 87.17% • 88.52% 98.01%
2018	• Srishti Grover et al. • Kim Younga et al. • Hajra F. Syed et al. • Charles Laidi et al.	Parkinson's disease Parkinson's disease Parkinson's disease Schizophrenia	Deep Neural Network (DNN) • SVM • Random Forest • C4.5 (Decision Tree) • Regression Tree • Boosted C5.0 • NNge default • NNge optimized • Default NNge with AdaBoost • Optimized NNge with AdaBoost • SVM • ElasticNet • GraphNet • TV-Enet	Parkinson's Tele-Monitoring Voice dataset from the UCI repository Max Little University Oxford and National Centre for Voice and Speech, Denver, Colorado Parkinson's dataset from the UCI repository COBRE, NMorphCH, NUSDAST and VIP cohort	62.73% • 97.57% • 95.25% • 79.85% • 82.82% • 83.10% • 85.13% • 89.23% • 90.95% • 96.30% • 69.00% • 71.00% • 70.00% • 68.00%
2019	P. J. Moore et al.	Alzheimer's disease	Random Forest	TADPOLE grand challenge	73%

(Xiao Zheng, 2017) developed a new predictive model to predict Alzheimer's disease using MRI scans. The authors used a Learning Using Privileged Information (LUPI) algorithm with Support Vector Machine (SVM) and Restricted Boltzmann Machines (RBM). An ensemble LUPI algorithm, integrating SVM with LUPI and RBM with LUPI was also developed by multiple kernel boosting strategy. The MR and PET scanned images, used as dataset for this study, were taken from the Alzheimer's Disease Neuroimaging Initiative (ADNI) database.

(Ammarah Farooq, 2017) used a Deep Convolutional Neural Network (DeepCNN) based pipeline for the prediction of Alzheimer's disease using MRI scans. The dataset used for the study was taken from the Alzheimer's Disease Neuroimaging Initiative (ADNI).

(Srishti Grover, 2018) used Deep Learning (DNN) for the prediction of the severity of Parkinson's disease. The dataset used for this study was the Parkinson's Tele-monitoring Voice Data Set, acquired from the UCI Machine Learning Repository. The dataset contains 5,875 voice recordings of these patients. The data obtained was normalized using min-max normalization. The neural network constructed had 16 units in the input layer, and 10,20 and 30 neurons in each of the three hidden layers respectively.

(Kim Younga, 2018) proposed a machine learning model for the prediction of Parkinson's disease using Random Forest, Support Vector Machine (SVM), C4.5 (Decision Tree), Bagging Classification, Regression Tree (Bagging CART) and Boosted C5.0. The dataset used for the study was acquired from the dataset created by Max little University Oxford, in collaboration with the National Centre for Voice and Speech, Denver, Colorado.

(Hajra F. Syed, 2018) used NNge (Non-Nested Generalized Exemplars) for the prediction of Parkinson's disease using voice signals. The data used for this study was acquired from the Parkinson's Dataset from UCI machine learning repository, and it comprised of the biomedical voice measurements of 31 individuals, out of which 23 were diseased.

(Charles Laidi, 2018) used standard Support Vector Machine (SVM) with structured sparsity on a large dataset of schizophrenic subjects. 3D maps of the grey matter density of the brain were used to obtain inter-site prediction performance. The dataset was assembled from four different independent studies (COBRE, NMorphCH, NUSDAST from the schizophrenia public repository and VIP cohort). The complete dataset consisted of 276 schizophrenic patients and 330 healthy controls.

(P. J. Moore, 2019) used Random Forest algorithm for the prediction of Alzheimer's disease using pairwise selection from time series data. The dataset used for this proposed method was taken from the TADPOLE grand challenge, an initiative which aims to predict the progression of subjects at risk of Alzheimer's disease using demographic, physical and cognitive input data.

REFERENCES

Aich, S., Kim, H. C., Hui, K. L., Al-Absi, A. A., & Sain, M. (2019, February). A Supervised Machine Learning Approach using Different Feature Selection Techniques on Voice Datasets for Prediction of Parkinson's Disease. In *2019 21st International Conference on Advanced Communication Technology (ICACT)* (pp. 1116-1121). IEEE. 10.23919/ICACT.2019.8701961

Alqahtani, E. J., Alshamrani, F. H., Syed, H. F., & Olatunji, S. O. (2018, April). Classification of Parkinson's Disease Using NNge Classification Algorithm. In *2018 21st Saudi Computer Society National Computer Conference (NCC)* (pp. 1-7). IEEE. 10.1109/NCG.2018.8592989

Anand, A., & Shakti, D. (2015, September). Prediction of diabetes based on personal lifestyle indicators. In *2015 1st International Conference on Next Generation Computing Technologies (NGCT)* (pp. 673-676). IEEE. 10.1109/NGCT.2015.7375206

Bur, A., Holcomb, A., Goodwin, S., Woodroof, J., Karadaghy, O., Shnayder, Y., Kakarala, K., Brant, J., & Shew, M., (2019, March). Machine learning to predict occult nodal metastasis in early oral squamous T cell carcinoma. In *2019 Elsevier* (pp. 20-25). Elsevier.

De Pierrefeu, A., Löfstedt, T., Laidi, C., Hadj-Selem, F., Leboyer, M., Ciuciu, P., ... Duchesnay, E. (2018, June). Interpretable and stable prediction of schizophrenia on a large multisite dataset using machine learning with structured sparsity. In *2018 International Workshop on Pattern Recognition in Neuroimaging (PRNI)* (pp. 1-4). IEEE. 10.1109/PRNI.2018.8423946

Dinesh, K. G., Arumugaraj, K., Santhosh, K. D., & Mareeswari, V. (2018, March). Prediction of Cardiovascular Disease Using Machine Learning Algorithms. In *2018 International Conference on Current Trends towards Converging Technologies (ICCTCT)* (pp. 1-7). IEEE. 10.1109/ICCTCT.2018.8550857

Esfahani, H. A., & Ghazanfari, M. (2017, December). Cardiovascular disease detection using a new ensemble classifier. In *2017 IEEE 4th International Conference on Knowledge-Based Engineering and Innovation (KBEI)* (pp. 1011-1014). IEEE. 10.1109/KBEI.2017.8324946

Faisal, M. I., Bashir, S., Khan, Z. S., & Khan, F. H. (2018, December). An Evaluation of Machine Learning Classifiers and Ensembles for Early Stage Prediction of Lung Cancer. In *2018 3rd International Conference on Emerging Trends in Engineering, Sciences and Technology (ICEEST)* (pp. 1-4). IEEE. 10.1109/ICEEST.2018.8643311

Farooq, A., Anwar, S., Awais, M., & Rehman, S. (2017, October). A deep CNN based multi-class classification of Alzheimer's disease using MRI. In *2017 IEEE International Conference on Imaging systems and techniques (IST)* (pp. 1-6). IEEE. 10.1109/IST.2017.8261460

Faruque, M. F., & Sarker, I. H. (2019, February). Performance Analysis of Machine Learning Techniques to Predict Diabetes Mellitus. In *2019 International Conference on Electrical, Computer and Communication Engineering (ECCE)* (pp. 1-4). IEEE. 10.1109/ECACE.2019.8679365

Grover, S., Bhartia, S., Yadav, A., & Seeja, K. R. (2018). Predicting Severity of Parkinson's Disease Using Deep Learning. *Procedia Computer Science*, *132*, 1788–1794. doi:10.1016/j.procs.2018.05.154

Hu, C., Ju, R., Shen, Y., Zhou, P., & Li, Q. (2016, May). Clinical decision support for Alzheimer's disease based on deep learning and brain network. In *2016 IEEE International Conference on Communications (ICC)* (pp. 1-6). IEEE. 10.1109/ICC.2016.7510831

Ismaeel, S., Miri, A., & Chourishi, D. (2015, May). Using the extreme learning machine (ELM) technique for heart disease diagnosis. In *2015 IEEE Canada International Humanitarian Technology Conference (IHTC2015)* (pp. 1-3). IEEE. 10.1109/IHTC.2015.7238043

Jahangir, M., Afzal, H., Ahmed, M., Khurshid, K., & Nawaz, R. (2017, September). An expert system for diabetes prediction using auto tuned multi-layer perceptron. In *2017 Intelligent Systems Conference (IntelliSys)* (pp. 722-728). IEEE. 10.1109/IntelliSys.2017.8324209

Junifer, J., & Suharjito, P. (2014). Diagnosis of Diabetes Mellitus Using Extreme Learning Machine. In *International Conference on Information Technology Systems and Innovation (ICITS)* (pp. 1-6). Academic Press.

Karaylan, T., & Kılıç, Ö. (2017, October). Prediction of heart disease using neural network. In *2017 International Conference on Computer Science and Engineering (UBMK)* (pp. 719-723). IEEE. 10.1109/UBMK.2017.8093512

Kumar, P. S., & Pranavi, S. (2017, December). Performance analysis of machine learning algorithms on diabetes dataset using big data analytics. In *2017 International Conference on Infocom Technologies and Unmanned Systems (Trends and Future Directions) (ICTUS)* (pp. 508-513). IEEE. 10.1109/ICTUS.2017.8286062

Li, L. (2014, November). Diagnosis of diabetes using a weight-adjusted voting approach. In *2014 IEEE International Conference on Bioinformatics and Bioengineering* (pp. 320-324). IEEE. 10.1109/BIBE.2014.27

Mahboob, T., Irfan, R., & Ghaffar, B. (2017, September). Evaluating ensemble prediction of coronary heart disease using receiver operating characteristics. In *2017 Internet Technologies and Applications (ITA)* (pp. 110-115). IEEE.

Mir, A., & Dhage, S. N. (2018, August). Diabetes Disease Prediction Using Machine Learning on Big Data of Healthcare. In *2018 Fourth International Conference on Computing Communication Control and Automation (ICCUBEA)* (pp. 1-6). IEEE. 10.1109/ICCUBEA.2018.8697439

Moore, P. J., Lyons, T. J., & Gallacher, J. (2019). Random forest prediction of Alzheimer's disease using pairwise selection from time series data. *PLoS One, 14*(2), e0211558. doi:10.1371/journal.pone.0211558 PMID:30763336

Payan, A., & Montana, G. (2015). *Predicting Alzheimer's disease: a neuroimaging study with 3D convolutional neural networks.* arXiv preprint arXiv:1502.02506

Pragna, D. P., Dandu, S., Meenakzshi, M., Jyotsna, C., & Amudha, J. (2017, March). Health alert system to detect oral cancer. In *2017 International Conference on Inventive Communication and Computational Technologies (ICICCT)* (pp. 258-262). IEEE. 10.1109/ICICCT.2017.7975198

Priyadarshini, R., Dash, N., & Mishra, R. (2014, February). A Novel approach to predict diabetes mellitus using modified Extreme learning machine. In *2014 International Conference on Electronics and Communication Systems (ICECS)* (pp. 1-5). IEEE. 10.1109/ECS.2014.6892740

Raihan, M., Mandal, P. K., Islam, M. M., Hossain, T., Ghosh, P., Shaj, S. A., ... More, A. (2019, February). Risk Prediction of Ischemic Heart Disease Using Artificial Neural Network. In *2019 International Conference on Electrical, Computer and Communication Engineering (ECCE)* (pp. 1-5). IEEE. 10.1109/ECACE.2019.8679362

Rajaguru, H., & Prabhakar, S. K. (2017). Performance comparison of oral cancer classification with Gaussian mixture measures and multi layer Perceptron. In *The 16th International Conference on Biomedical Engineering* (pp. 123-129). Springer. 10.1007/978-981-10-4220-1_23

Rajliwall, N. S., Davey, R., & Chetty, G. (2018, December). Machine learning based models for Cardiovascular risk prediction. In *2018 International Conference on Machine Learning and Data Engineering (iCMLDE)* (pp. 142-148). IEEE. 10.1109/iCMLDE.2018.00034

Rayavarapu, K., & Krishna, K. K. (2018, March). Prediction of Cervical Cancer using Voting and DNN Classifiers. In *2018 International Conference on Current Trends towards Converging Technologies (ICCTCT)* (pp. 1-5). IEEE. 10.1109/ICCTCT.2018.8551176

Sharmila, S. (2017). *Analysis of Heart Disease Prediction Using Data mining Techniques. International Journal of Advanced Networking & Applications.*

Shobitha, S., Amita, P. M., Niranjana, K. B., & Ali, M. A. M. (2018, April). Noninvasive Blood Glucose Prediction from Photoplethysmogram Using Relevance Vector Machine. In *2018 3rd International Conference for Convergence in Technology (I2CT)* (pp. 1-4). IEEE. 10.1109/I2CT.2018.8529481

Singh, A., & Kumar, D. (2017, May). Novel ABC based training algorithm for ovarian cancer detection using neural network. In *2017 International Conference on Trends in Electronics and Informatics (ICEI)* (pp. 594-597). IEEE. 10.1109/ICOEI.2017.8300771

Singh, J., Kamra, A., & Singh, H. (2016, October). Prediction of heart diseases using associative classification. In *2016 5th International Conference on Wireless Networks and Embedded Systems (WECON)* (pp. 1-7). IEEE. 10.1109/WECON.2016.7993480

Sonawane, J. S., & Patil, D. R. (2014, February). Prediction of heart disease using multilayer perceptron neural network. In *International Conference on Information Communication and Embedded Systems (ICICES2014)* (pp. 1-6). IEEE. 10.1109/ICICES.2014.7033860

Suman, S. K., & Hooda, N. (2019). Predicting risk of Cervical Cancer: A case study of machine learning. *Journal of Statistics and Management Systems*, 22(4), 689–696. doi:10.1080/09720510.2019.1611227

Swain, A., Mohanty, S. N., & Das, A. C. (2016, March). Comparative risk analysis on prediction of Diabetes Mellitus using machine learning approach. In *2016 International Conference on Electrical, Electronics, and Optimization Techniques (ICEEOT)* (pp. 3312-3317). IEEE. 10.1109/ICEEOT.2016.7755319

Tafa, Z., Pervetica, N., & Karahoda, B. (2015, June). An intelligent system for diabetes prediction. In *2015 4th Mediterranean Conference on Embedded Computing (MECO)* (pp. 378-382). IEEE. 10.1109/MECO.2015.7181948

Vijayan, V. V., & Anjali, C. (2015, December). Prediction and diagnosis of diabetes mellitus—A machine learning approach. In *2015 IEEE Recent Advances in Intelligent Computational Systems (RAICS)* (pp. 122-127). IEEE.

Yekkala, I., Dixit, S., & Jabbar, M. A. (2017, August). Prediction of heart disease using ensemble learning and Particle Swarm Optimization. In *2017 International Conference On Smart Technologies For Smart Nation (SmartTechCon)* (pp. 691-698). IEEE. 10.1109/SmartTechCon.2017.8358460

Zheng, X., Shi, J., Zhang, Q., Ying, S., & Li, Y. (2017, April). Improving MRI-based diagnosis of Alzheimer's disease via an ensemble privileged information learning algorithm. In *2017 IEEE 14th International Symposium on Biomedical Imaging (ISBI 2017)* (pp. 456-459). IEEE. https://www.mayoclinic.org/diseases-conditions/alzheimers-disease/symptoms-causes/syc-20350447

Chapter 6
Chronic Kidney Disease Prediction Using Data Mining Algorithms

Devesh Kumar Srivastava
Manipal University Jaipur, India

Pradeep Kumar Tiwari
ⓘ https://orcid.org/0000-0003-0387-9236
Manipal University Jaipur, India

ABSTRACT

In today's contemporary world, it is important to know about the odds of having a disease because of changing living standards of the population overall in the continent. The disease on which the authors are working is chronic kidney disease. Once the person gets chronic kidney disease (CKD), his working capability decreases along with other adverse effects. It is possible to get rid of diseases like CKD with new methodologies that will help us to predict the stage of kidney disease at an early stage. Under big data analytics, data may be structured, unstructured, quasi- or semi-structured. The CKD detected and predicted by applying classification models: support vector machine (SVM), K-nearest neighbor (KNN), and logistic regression algorithm. It helps in predicting the likelihood of occurrence of disease on various different features. The two algorithms KNN and SVM are compared to find the algorithm that gives better accuracy. Further regression technique has been used to detect the disease based on, which the stages are classified by using GFR (glomerular filtration rate) formula.

INTRODUCTION

India is vast country with the population of more than 133 crores out of which there are more than 10 million cases are found approximately of chronic diseases per year as per survey result. Diagnosis of such chronic diseases like cardiac failure, kidney disease, HIV, diabetes mellitus etc. is important at an early stage as it may be controlled to a certain stage but cannot be cured. Some of the most common

DOI: 10.4018/978-1-7998-2742-9.ch006

diseases are: - Alzheimer's, Arthritis, Asthma, Cancer, Diabetes, Heart diseases, Chronic Kidney (Suprarenal Gland) disease. There is an increase in death rate in developing countries. As digitalization is growing widely from cities to remote villages, it has become important to use these new technologies for prediction, detection and prevention of such diseases (Ameta & Jain 2017). People putting up in small villages may not get access to proper medical facilities. 60% of all deaths worldwide are caused due to chronic kidney disease. Data mining is the process to extract meaningful information from the large amount of data sets in order to attain knowledge. In this work data mining algorithms are used for analyzing the different stages of chronic suprarenal gland disease. Before applying the algorithms, it is checked the feasibility by two-step process: Learning Step (Training Phase) and Construction of Classification Model. Various Algorithms are utilized to assemble a classifier by making the Model to get the hang of utilizing the preparation set accessible. Model is used to foresee class names and testing the developed model on test information and thus gauge the exactness of the arrangement rules. It has been developed to foresee class marks (Example: Label – "ckd" or "Not ckd" for the endorsement of some occasion). Utilizing mining based strategies are savvy and effective. They help foreseeing illness, Helps Banks and Financial Institutions to recognize defaulters with the goal that they may endorse Cards, Loan, and so forth (Dubey 2015)..

Chronic Kidney Disease (ckd) is referred to Chronic Suprarenal Gland Failure. When this disease occurs in human's body what happens is that kidneys get damaged and in turn toxics cannot be filtered out easily from our body. To classify this disease's likelihood, KNN and SVM data mining algorithms are implemented on the dataset. Important features are extracted which is required for the classification and to execute the work (Devi, 2014; Dubey 2015).

Text mining is the route toward investigating and dissecting a lot of unstructured information supported by programming that can distinguish ideas, designs, points, watchwords and different properties in the information. It is the way toward extricating the concealed learning from the content report. Content mining is characterized as learning serious procedure in which a client cooperates with the report gathering utilizing a suite of examination apparatus. It manages changing over unstructured information into organized information. Content mining fuses and incorporates the apparatuses of data recovery, information mining, AI, measurements, and computational etymology, and thus, it is out and out a multidisciplinary field. Content mining manages characteristic language messages either put away in semi-organized or unstructured organizations.5 fundamental steps involved in the text mining are:

1. Gathering unstructured data from numerous information sources like plain content, pages, pdf documents, messages, and online journals, to give some examples.
2. Detect and expel inconsistencies from information by directing pre-preparing and purifying activities. Information purifying enables you to separate and hold the significant data covered up inside the information and to help recognize the foundations of explicit words.
3. Convert all the important data separated from unstructured information into organized arrangements.
4. Analyze the examples inside the information through Management Information System (MIS).
5. Store all the significant data into a safe database to drive pattern investigation and upgrade the basic leadership procedure of the association (Arasu, & Thirumalaiselvi 2017; Bala, & Kumar (2014).

Content or Text mining is a subfield of NLP (Natural Language Processing) dedicated to empowering computational investigation of content bolted information. The content mining work process by and large includes distinguishing proof of explicit elements in surface content, for example, illnesses, quali-

Figure 1. Pictorial representation of process of text mining

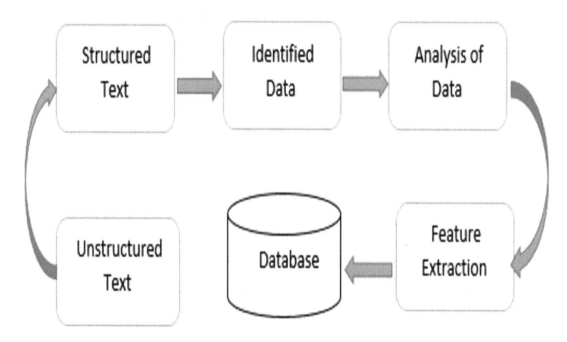

ties, or social terms and the profound standardization of these substances to institutionalized ontologies. Information accordingly handled become the information esteems for an assortment of calculations. There are two center elements of content mining: (1) data extraction and; (2) speculation age through relationship extraction. A viable strategy to separate the information from the huge measure of reports is proposed utilizing content mining. Disease Prediction system has data sets collected from different health related sites. With the help of Disease Predictor, the user will be able to know the probability of the disease with the given symptoms. Using text-mining techniques, the required data are extracted in the structured format.

Motivation

In health care sector, information mining strategies is ending up progressively mainstream in sickness finding. It has been selected because these days' way of life has turned out to be unfavorably influencing the well-being from numerous points of view where in one of them prompting constant maladies. Indeed, even youngsters in the present situation has been experiencing such illnesses and are analyzed late. To foresee the illness at a beginning time, information-mining strategies are utilized

Objective

Due to several seasonable time changes, more and more vulnerable diseases affect people. This can be predicted in advance using prediction model. The occurrence of the diseases in a particular area and at a particular time can be predicted. There are various techniques used for the prediction of diseases. Among the different strategies, content mining assumes a significant job in the restorative field. Step by step, huge number of patients visit the emergency clinics with the end goal of different medicines. In medical field, text-mining algorithms are used to mine the hidden knowledge in the dataset of the medical domain. Various prediction algorithms are available like text mining, image mining, web mining and processing but text mining is selected to predict the disease to measure high precision vales and accuracy to analyze and reduce the effect of various diseases. It plays significant in the field of medical science and health care. Prediction of chronic kidney disease (CKD) with the help of collective information gathered with the help data mining techniques.

Literature Review

Ramya and Radha (2016) discussed, Diagnosis of Chronic Kidney Disease using Machine Learning Algorithms, the classification algorithms considered for foreseeing constant kidney sickness are Back spread Neural Network, Random Forest and Radial Basis Function. The models are assessed with four distinct estimates like Kappa, Accuracy, Sensitivity and Specificity. The Radial Basis Function is the better exactness for anticipating ceaseless kidney ailment and it achieves the precision of 85.3%.

Vijayarani, Dhayanand and Phil (2015) discussed in this research work Correlation of Support Vector Machine and Naïve Bayes grouping calculations depend on the presentation factors order exactness and execution time. From the outcomes, it very well may be reasoned that the SVM accomplishes expanded arrangement execution, generate results that are exact, consequently it is considered as best classifier when contrasted and Naïve Bayes classifier calculation.

Arasu and Thirumalaiselvi (2017) discussed, Review of Chronic Kidney Disease based on Data Mining Techniques, this paper aims to analyze the various data mining techniques in medical domain and some of the algorithms used to predict kidney diseases eventually. From the above survey, it is proven that results may vary for different stages of kidney disease diagnosis based on the tools and techniques used.

Kunwar et al. (2016) discussed Chronic Kidney Disease using Data Mining Techniques, cluster similar kind of affected patient's records and to further classify the affected patient's records as per the variations and severity of the disease being affected. For analysis and prediction of Chronic Kidney Disease (CKD) Data mining techniques have been used. Expectation Maximization [EM] is the clustering algorithm, which is used to cluster similar type of person into one group. Artificial Neural Network [ANN] and C4.5 are classification algorithm which is used for prediction of the disease.

Gharibdousti et al. (2017) discussed, Prediction of Chronic Kidney Disease Using Data Mining Techniques, Different classification algorithm like decision tree, logistic regression, neural network and are compared to each other and are applied to normalized data.

Patil (2016) explored, review on prediction of chronic kidney disease using data mining techniques. According to the perception of various trials there are a few classifiers which gave most noteworthy precision are Random Forest, Multilayer Perceptron, Support Vector Machine Naïve Bayes, Radial Basis Function and K-nearest neighbor.

Kaur and Sharma (2017) discussed, Prediction of chronic kidney disease using data mining algorithms in Hadoop, they got trial results are appeared as two information mining calculations which are K-Nearest Neighbor and Support Vector Machine. Highlight assessment or extraction and order is done based on the dataset that is being utilized. Every one of the results are examined in the graphical grouping based on exactness, mistake, accuracy and slipped by time.

Bala and Kumar (2014) discussed, Information Mining Techniques to Predict Chronic Kidney Disease and its Stages, From the assessment, it is understood that Naïve Bayes game plan estimation gives

100% accuracy when appeared differently in relation to ANN. Consequently, Naïve Bayes is utilized to foresee the nearness of CKD and dependent on Glomerular Filtration Rate, CKD stages are anticipated.

Ameta and Jain (2017) discussed, it gives the solutions to diagnose the disease by analysing the data through different classification techniques. This helps to give quick and proper treatment to the patients. The major challenge is to find the best classification technique algorithm on the basis of type accuracy and execution time overall performance elements. The algorithm with better accuracy and minimal execution time is selected as the great algorithm. In this classification, different rate of accuracy charge is proven by means of every classifier. ANN has the maximum classification accuracy and ANN algorithm is considered as a better set of rules for classification technique

Devi (2014) discussed the creator depicts that C4.5 grouping calculation manages numerical properties and additionally all out characteristics. Information mining is the broad zone wherein the dataset beneath tests are examined and designs are removed. Dataset is the social event of characteristics and its cost for various cases. Properties speak to the qualities of the insights and occasions are the estimations of the measurements. Each dataset has an ascribe that should be recognized. This trait is named on the grounds that the class name. Result can be a decision tree display, arrangements mining, realities class and so on. Different comprehensively utilized methods in information mining are Association rules mining, Classification, Clustering, Temporal mining, spatial mining and so on. Among the strategies, Classification assumes a basic part in information mining. Neural people group based class, Decision tree, Likelihood assessment, Naïve Bayes order are few class methods employed. In this paper, choice tree based absolutely arrangement is mulled over. A whole dataset is required in ID3 while C4.5 would paintings be able to with the dataset with lacking realities esteems. For decision tree generation, the C4.5 classifier erases the occurrences whose characteristic esteems are deficient. C4. Five classifier can handle each numeric and express quality. In the event that particular quality has unmistakable esteems, at that point the split on the characteristic will brings about n brilliant hubs. On the off chance, that n is enormous; the choice tree will have high many-sided quality. This paper reasons that the paired decision tree classification construct absolutely with respect to C4.5 classifiers is far innovative access to the general determination tree built. [10]

Kumar, and Abhishek (2012) have used two neural network techniques, Radial Basis Function and Back Propagation Algorithm (BPA), and one non-direct classifier Support Vector Machine (SVM) and contrasted in agreement and their productivity and precision. They utilized WEKA 3.6.5 instrument for execution to locate the best procedure among the over three calculations for Kidney Stone Diagnosis. The primary reason for their proposition work was to propose the best device for therapeutic conclusion, similar to kidney stone distinguishing proof, to diminish the analysis time and improve the productivity and exactness. From the test results they closed, the back spread (BPA) essentially improved the traditional order strategy for use in therapeutic field.

Kusiak, Dixon and Shah (2005) discussed Back Propagation Algorithm, Radial Basis Function and one non-direct classifier Support Vector Machine and contrasted in agreement and their productivity and precision. They utilized WEKA 3.6.5 instrument for execution to locate the best procedure among the over three calculations for Kidney Stone Diagnosis. The primary reason for their proposition work was to propose the best device for therapeutic conclusion, similar to kidney stone distinguishing proof, to diminish the analysis time and improve the productivity and exactness. From the test results they closed, the back spread (BPA) essentially improved the traditional order strategy for use in therapeutic field.

Kharya (2012) depicted different audit, specialized articles on bosom disease analysis, and forecast. The flow research is being completed utilizing the information mining systems to improve the bosom malignancy analysis and guess. Among the different information mining classifiers and delicate registering approaches, Decision tree is observed to be better indicator with 93.62% precision on benchmark dataset (UCI AI dataset) and furthermore on SEER dataset.

Dubey (2015) discussed about the robotized recognition of sicknesses utilizing Machine Learning Techniques. The K-Means Algorithm with a solitary mean vector of centroids, to order and make groups of changing likelihood of likeliness of suspect being inclined to CKD. The outcomes are acquired from a Real Data-Set from UCI Machine Learning Repository Lambodar Jena and Kamila (2015) have broken down interminable kidney malady dataset by different grouping methods like Naïve Bayes, Multilayer Perceptron, Support Vector Machine, J48, Conjunctive Rule, Decision table. They have utilized a weka programming. They have utilized 25 unique characteristics for arrangement. Their examination demonstrates that for perpetual kidney ailment forecast similarly Multilayer Perceptron give higher exactness than different procedures for example 99.75% of precision.

Sinha and Sinha (2015) built up a choice emotionally supportive network to foresee endless kidney malady. They have looked at consequences of two methods Support Vector machine and KNN (K Nearest Neighbor). Their test result demonstrates that KNN has higher exactness than Support Vector Machine

Methodology

The following steps will depict our methodology:

- Learning data mining techniques and machine learning algorithms.
- Review the research papers.
- Studying the existing methods available properly.
- Designing methods and algorithm to predict chronic kidney diseases.
- Then the model is tested using a small data set and eliminate errors.
- After eliminating errors, we will test our project using larger data set.

Techniques Used

Classification: Enormous databases are turning into the standard in this day as a huge information. Envision a database with numerous terabytes of information — a terabyte is one trillion bytes of information. The essential test of huge information is the means by which to understand it. What's more, sheer volume is not the main issue: huge information additionally will in general be assorted, unstructured and quick evolving. Think about sound and video information, online networking posts, 3D information or geospatial information. This kind of information is not arranged or composed effectively. To address this difficulty, a scope of programmed techniques for extricating helpful data has been created, among them. KNN Classification and Support Vector Machine_Classification algorithms are used to predict the kidney disease.

K Nearest Neighbor (KNN) is an exceptionally basic, straightforward, flexible and one of the highest AI calculations. KNN utilized in the assortment of uses, for example, money, human services, political theory, penmanship discovery, picture acknowledgment and video acknowledgment. In Credit appraisals, budgetary organizations will foresee the FICO score of clients. In credit payment, banking organizations will anticipate whether the advance is sheltered or hazardous. In political theory, characterizing potential voters in two classes will cast a ballot or will not cast a ballot. KNN calculation utilized for both order

Figure 2. KNN Representation for cluster K=2 and k=6

	A	B	C	D	E	F	G
1	id	bp	sg	al	su	sc	classification
2	0	80	1.02	1	0	1.2	ckd
3	1	50	1.02	4	0	0.8	ckd
4	2	80	1.01	2	3	1.8	ckd
5	3	70	1.005	4	0	3.8	ckd
6	4	80	1.01	2	0	1.4	ckd
7	5	90	1.015	3	0	1.1	ckd
8	6	70	1.01	0	0	24	ckd
9	7		1.015	2	4	1.1	ckd
10	8	100	1.015	3	0	1.9	ckd
11	9	90	1.02	2	0	7.2	ckd
12	10	60	1.01	2	4	4	ckd
13	11	70	1.01	3	0	2.7	ckd
14	12	70	1.015	3	1	2.1	ckd
15	13	70				4.6	ckd
16	14	80	1.01	3	2	4.1	ckd
17	15	80	1.015	3	0	9.6	ckd
18	16	70	1.015	2	0	2.2	ckd
19	17	80				5.2	ckd
20	18	100	1.025	0	3	1.3	ckd
21	19	60	1.015	1	0	1.6	ckd
22	20	80	1.015	2	0	3.9	ckd
23	21	90				76	ckd
24	22	80	1.025	4	0	7.7	ckd

Sheet1 ⊕

Legends

bp = blood pressure

sg = specific gravity

al =albumin

su = sugar

sc = serum creatinine

and relapse issues. KNN calculation dependent on highlight likeness approach. The representation of KNN is shown in Figure 2.

SVM (Support Vector Machine)

A Support Vector Machine (SVM) is a discriminative classifier authoritatively described by a disengaging hyperactive plane. In two-dimensional spaces this hyper-plane is a line isolating a plane in two areas where in each class lay in either side. In this calculation, we plot every datum thing as a point in n-dimensional space (where n is number of highlights you have) with the estimation of each part being the estimation of a specific sort out. By at that point, we perform assembling by finding the hyper-plane that distinctive the two classes extraordinary. Our goal is to locate a plane that has the extreme edge, i.e. the greatest separation between information purposes of the two classes. Amplifying the edge separation gives some support so future information focuses can be grouped with more certainty. Hyper- planes are choice limits that help order the information focuses. Information focuses falling on either side of the hyper-plane can be credited to various classes. Additionally, the component of the hyper-plane relies on the quantity of highlights. In the event that the quantity of information highlights is 2, at that point the hyper-plane is only a line. On the off chance that the quantity of info highlights is 3, at that point the hyper-plane turns into a two-dimensional plane. We have following steps for SVM.

1. Import library
2. Create a svm object
3. Train the model using the training sets

Figure 3. SVM Representation

```
In [10]: from sklearn.metrics import confusion_matrix
    ...: cm = confusion_matrix(labels_test, labels_pred)
    ...: print("Confusion matrix by knn:\n",cm)
    ...: classifier.score(features_test, labels_test)
    ...: print("Accuracy by knn:",classifier.score(features_test, labels_test))
Confusion matrix by knn:
 [[59  3]
 [ 0 38]]
Accuracy by knn: 0.97
```

4. Predict the response for test dataset
5. Find accuracy for the applied algorithm

Decision Tree: Decision tree comes under supervised machine learning algorithm. This algorithm can be used for regression as well as classification problems. The aim of decision tree is to predict the value of target variable by the decision rules, which are trained to the model by creating some training data. This algorithm is easy to understand as compared to other classification algorithms. It uses tree representation to solve the problem, wherein, each internal node corresponds to the attribute and each leaf node corresponds to a class label. The primary cause of concern in decision tree is to select an attribute for root node from the dataset. Handling this concern is known as attribute selection, which, can be done by two methods, one is by information gain method and second is Gini impurity method. In this project, we use decision tree to predict whether or not a continent is having a particular disease. It uses various economic factors of each country in the continent to predict the occurrence of the disease over the continent. It predicts diseases like Hepatitis B, diphtheria, HIV/AIDS, polio and measles on the factors like adult mortality, infant deaths, percentage expenditure, total expenditure, GDP, population, schooling and average BMI of people and alcohol consumption in the countries of that continent. Decision tree is easy to explain and it follows the same concept as humans follow while making the decisions themselves. Along with pros come the cons which are that there is high probability of over fitting in this algorithm. Calculations become complex with multi class labels.

Naïve Bayes: A Naive Bayes classifier is a probabilistic AI model that is utilized for arrangement task. The essence of the classifier depends on the Bayes hypothesis. Utilizing Bayes hypothesis, we can discover the likelihood of an occasion. An incident, given that event B has happened. Here, B is the evidence and A is the hypothesis. The presumption made here is that the indicators/highlights are free. That is nearness of one specific element does not influence the other. Subsequently, it is called Naive. Innocent Bayes is an order calculation for parallel (two-class) and multi-class characterization issues.

Figure 4. Decision Tree Representation

```
    ...: from sklearn.metrics import classification_report, confusion_matrix
    ...: print("Confusion matrix by SVM:\n",confusion_matrix(labels_test,labels_pred))
    ...: print(classification_report(labels_test,labels_pred))
    ...: from sklearn import metrics
    ...: print("Accuracy by SVM:",metrics.accuracy_score(labels_test, labels_pred))
Confusion matrix by SVM:
[[60  2]
 [ 0 38]]
            precision    recall  f1-score   support

         0       1.00      0.97      0.98        62
         1       0.95      1.00      0.97        38

avg / total       0.98      0.98      0.98       100

Accuracy by SVM: 0.98
```

The procedure is least demanding to comprehend when portrayed utilizing double or clear cut information esteems.

Regression: Relapse is an information mining method used to foresee a scope of numeric qualities (additionally called persistent qualities), given a specific dataset. For instance, relapse may be utilized to anticipate the expense of an item or administration, given different factors. Relapse is utilized over different ventures for business and promoting arranging, budgetary estimating, ecological demonstrating and examination of patterns.

Logistic Regression: Calculated relapse is a measurable strategy for breaking down a dataset in which there are at least one free factors that decide a result. The result is estimated with a dichotomous variable (wherein there are just two potential results). It is utilized to foresee a double result (1/0, Yes/ No, True/False) given many autonomous factors. To speak to paired / clear cut result, we utilize sham factors. You can likewise consider strategic relapse as a unique instance of straight relapse when the result variable is clear-cut, where we are utilizing log of chances as reliant variable. In basic words, it predicts the likelihood of event of an occasion by fitting information to a rationale work. The steps are to implement the logistic regression is

1. Import library
2. Create a svm object
3. Train the model using the training sets
4. Predict the response for test dataset
5. Find accuracy for the applied algorithm

DATA IMPUTATION:

The data collection from various patients get a lot of missing data due to human error. Thus, we need to fill in the structured data and make it appropriate according to our requirements. We first collect appropriate data and modify or delete them to improve the data quality. Thereafter, we use data integration for data preprocessing. Afterwards, we perform one hot encoding, scale the data properly for the use, and finally check that there is no error in the data and we are ready to implement different algorithms on the data set. As shown in figure first data is pre-processed and by implementing statistical expression a model is experienced. When model or method is created, testing must be done by test data set.

Figure 5. Formula of Naïve Bayes classifier

```
In [18]: labels_pred = classifierLR.predict(features_test)

In [19]: from sklearn.metrics import confusion_matrix

In [20]: cm1 = confusion_matrix(labels_test, labels_pred)
    ...: print("Confusion matrix by logistic regression:\n",cm1)
    ...:
    ...: from sklearn import metrics
    ...: print("Accuracy by Logistic Regression:",metrics.accuracy_score(labels_test,
labels_pred))
Confusion matrix by logistic regression:
 [[60  2]
 [ 0 38]]
Accuracy by Logistic Regression: 0.98
```

Once the data is imputed and fit for the use then we perform KNN and SVM on chronic kidney disease and perform Naïve Bayes, KNN and Decision Tree on heart disease. These various classification algorithms are used in order to classify whether or not, disease is likely to occur. The decision is taken by using KNN classifier with higher significance in the first layer of classification model. The dataset is divided into training and testing dataset. First, we train the model on our training dataset and then test the accuracy of the model on the testing data set. We implemented both the algorithms on the training dataset and then test it on testing dataset. After this we analyzed the results of both of them and find the best fit algorithms which produce the most accurate results. The ckd dataset is first obtained from the repository. The data is then preprocessed i.e noise, missing values and redundant values are removed. The new dataset or normalized dataset is obtained after preprocessing. Data mining techniques are applied on it for knowledge; find a new pattern or useful information.

Figure 6. Naïve Bayes Representation

```
GFR:  32.468190979864815
STAGE 3B:Moderately reduced kidney function
 Ways to slow kidney damage in Stage 3B kidney disease:
1. Control your blood sugar if you have diabetes.
2. Keep a healthy blood pressure.
3. Eat a healthy diet.
4. Do not smoke or use tobacco.
5. Exercise 30 minutes a day, 5 days a week.
6. Keep a healthy weight.
7. Ask your doctor if there are medicines you can take to protect your kidneys.
8. Make an appointment to see a nephrologist, even if you already have a general doctor.
9. Visit a nephrologist to make a treatment plan that is right for you. Your nephrologist
will tell you how often you will need to have your kidneys checked.
10. Meet with a dietitian, who will help you follow a diet that will keep you healthy.
11. If you have diabetes or high blood pressure, ask your doctor about special kinds of
blood pressure medicines called ACE inhibitors and ARBs. Sometimes these medicines can
help keep kidney from getting worse.
```

Initially, the sentences that contained any term from the lexical profile were marked with Y, and, in the subsequent steps, the evidence was tested and conceivably turned into negative (N), questionable (Q), or unmentioned (U) dependent on the setting in which they were utilized. The sentence-based forecasts were then joined at the record level. The four preparing ventures in this module are portrayed quickly underneath (further subtleties are given in the online enhancement).

Step T1: Text coordinating. To provide food for phrased variety, terms that describe a sickness were coordinated against the content roughly, considering morphological variations, and if fundamental overlooking word request and enduring the separation between the words inside a term (e.g., both "stent arrangement" and "situation of coronary stent" alluded to a similar treatment for CAD).

Step T2: Sentences separating. Sentences that did not make reference to an ailment related term were sifted through. We additionally disposed of sentences from the segments considered less significant for the literary undertaking (to be specific "Social/Family History" and "Other"), sentences that possibly alluded to relatives, and sentences containing uncertain disease terms.

Step T3: Text labeling. After filtering, the remaining sentences were initially considered to support the judgment of disease presence yes (Y). We then applied a set of lexico-semantic patterns potentially re-label them with N, Q, or U judgments, using a pattern matching algorithm. The patterns generalized the structure of manually collected examples that indicated negative (N), questionable (Q) or unmentioned (U) status of diseases. If any of these patterns was matched successfully, the disease status was changed using the label associated with the pattern

Step T4: Result Integration. At the point when a report contained various sentences with clashing names related, we utilized a weighted casting a ballot conspire. The score for every infection status mark was gotten by gathering all sentences with the given name, and including the loads related with the compartment segments. The most astounding scored name was proposed as the last explanation, with potential tie cases named as Q.

Step T5: Textual Prediction: Depending on these qualities, we anticipate the outcome utilizing different calculations. We partition the information in preparing and testing informational collection. Execution of every one of the three calculations is assessed and we think about the three calculations dependent on the precision they produce on the testing dataset. We select that calculation which furnishes us with the higher precision on examination with others.

Figure 7. Pre-processing steps to learn the Model

```
    ...: elif GFR<15 and GFR>1:
    ...:     print("STAGE 5:Very severe, or end-stage kidney failure")
    ...:     print("Once your kidneys have failed, you will need to start dialysis or have
a kidney transplant to live.")
['notckd']
NO FURTHER EVALUATION
```

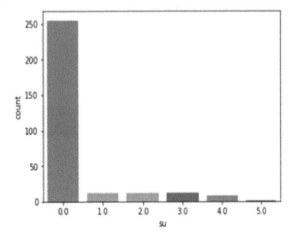

GFR Formula Used for the Prediction of Stages

GFR = 186 * (Creatinine)$^{-1.154}$ * (Age)$^{-.203}$*(0.742 if female) * (1.210 if black) [18]

GFR (Glomerular Filtration Rate) is equal to the total of the filtration rates of the functioning nephrons in the kidney. There is different estimated levels of GFR for African Americans, males and females, and people of different ages.

- For African American patients: The CKD Study conditions incorporate a term for the African-American that African Americans have a higher GFR than Caucasians at a similar degree of serum creatinine. This is because of higher normal bulk and creatinine age rate in African Americans. Clinical research centers may not gather information on race and accordingly may report GFR evaluations utilizing the condition for Caucasians. For African Americans, increase the GFR gauge by 1.21 for the CKD Study condition.
- For Male and female patients: The CKD Study conditions incorporate a term for female sex to represent the way that men have a higher GFR than ladies at a similar degree of serum creatinine. This is because of higher normal bulk and creatinine age rate in men. 0.7 For females and 0.9 for guys are increased in the equation for exact outcomes.
- Age: The CKD Study conditions incorporate a term for age to represent the way that more youthful individuals have a higher GFR than more seasoned individuals at a similar degree of serum creatinine. This is because of higher normal bulk and creatinine age rate in more youthful individuals.

Figure 8. Steps to prediction the disease

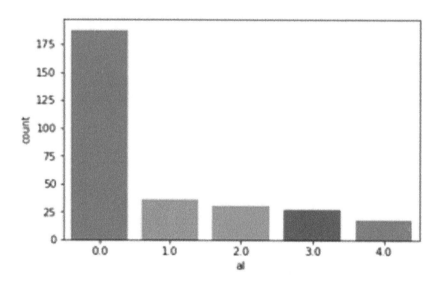

Classification into Various Stages

Stage 1: If GFR > 90ml/min - for normal and high value
Stage 2: If GFR = 60-89ml/min - Mild CKD value
Stage 3: If GFR = 45-59ml/min - Moderate CKD value
Stage 4: If GFR = 30-44ml/min Mild CKD value
Stage 5: If GFR = 15-29ml/min - Severe CKD value
Stage 5: If GFR < 15ml/min End Stage CKD (GFR < 15ml/min)

RESULTS AND DISCUSSION

Data preprocessing is done on the dataset by filling the missing values. We have used various data mining techniques like classification and regression such as SVM, KNN and logistic regression for the detection of chronic disease and for the prediction of stages based upon GFR (Glomerular Filtration Rate). It helps the patients to know their health condition at an early stage. Dataset used has 400 observations and 25 variables.

Figure 9. Dataset used

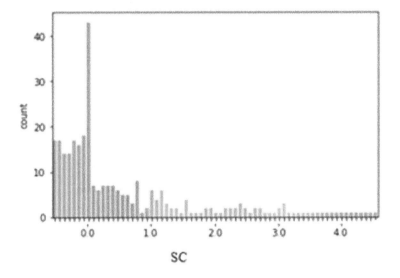

Figure 10. Features and labels used in the project

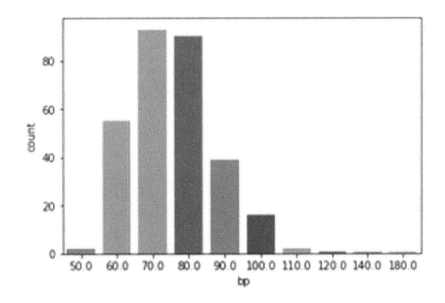

It is observed that SVM data mining classifier gives 98% accuracy, which is more as compared to KNN, which gives 97% accuracy. Comparison is made for the classification techniques: it indicates that the degree of accuracy of SVM is more than KNN algorithm hence SVM is more accurate for prediction of chronic kidney disease whether the patient is affected from the disease or not. The code is developed in python programming by implementation of algorithm.

Figure 11. Accuracy by KNN (97%)

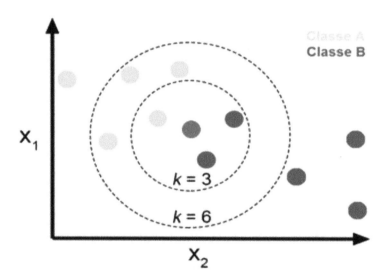

Figure 12. Accuracy by SVM (98%)

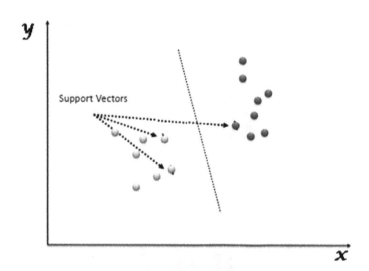

Figure 13. Accuracy by Logistic Regression (98%)

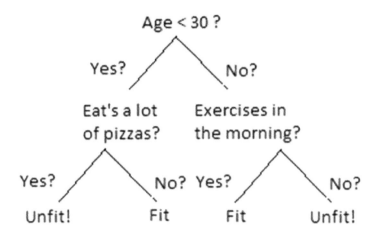

If the person is suffering from chronic kidney disease, the user inputs patients age, gender, race, serum creatinine for the prediction by the GFR formula.

Case Study 1: Let us input these values
Blood pressure=75; Specific gravity =1.015; Albumin =3; Sugar =4; Serum creatinine=2

Figure 14. The output for GFR is 32.46 ml/min

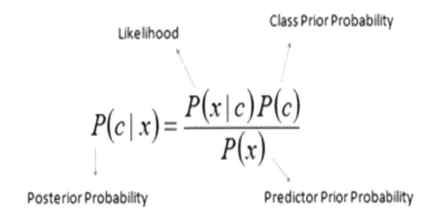

$$P(c \mid X) = P(x_1 \mid c) \times P(x_2 \mid c) \times \cdots \times P(x_n \mid c) \times P(c)$$

This predict the stage is 3 B i.e. moderately reduced kidney functions

Case Study 2: Let us assume that
Blood pressure=80, Specific gravity =1.025, Albumin =0, Sugar =0, Serum creatinine=0.6

Figure 15. Frequency of Sugar representation through graph

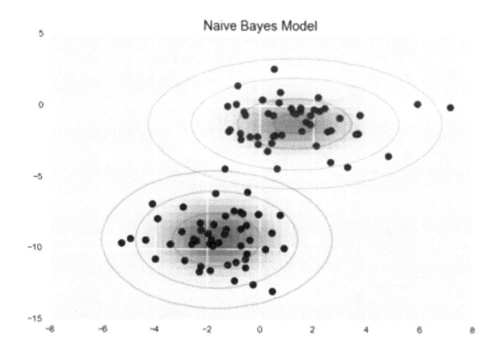

The x-axis of the graph indicates the range (i.e. 0-5) between which the value of sugar lies and the y-axis denotes the count of people having a particular value of sugar (Figure 16).

The x-axis of the graph indicates the range (i.e. 0-4) between which the value of Albumin lies and the y-axis denotes the count of people having a particular value of albumin (Figure 17).

The x-axis of the graph indicates the range (i.e. 0-50 mgs/dl) between which the value of Serum Creatine lies and the y-axis denotes the count of people having a particular value of Serum Creatine (Figure 18).

The x-axis of the graph indicates the range (i.e. 50-180 mm/Hg) between which the value of Blood Pressure lies and the y-axis denotes the count of people having a particular value of blood pressure.

Figure 16. Count for Albumin representation through graph

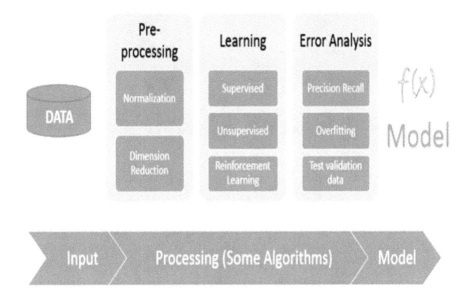

Figure 17. Count of Serum Creatinine

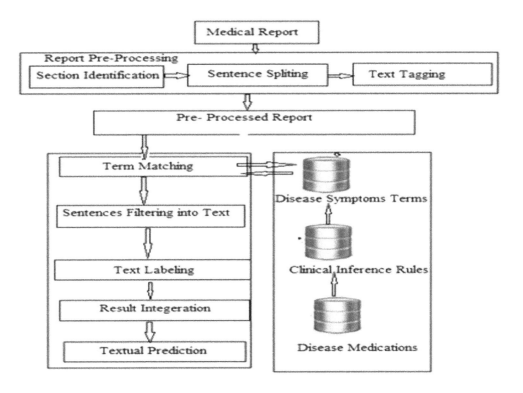

Figure 18. Count for Blood Pressure

id	age	bp	sg	al	su	rbc	pc	pcc	ba	bgr	bu	sc	sod	pot	hemo	pcv	wc	rc	htn	dm
0	48	80	1.02	1	0		normal	notpreser	notpreser	121	36	1.2			15.4	44	7800	5.2	yes	yes
1	7	50	1.02	4	0		normal	notpreser	notpresent		18	0.8			11.3	38	6000		no	no
2	62	80	1.01	2	3	normal	normal	notpreser	notpreser	423	53	1.8			9.6	31	7500		no	yes
3	48	70	1.005	4	0	normal	abnormal	present	notpreser	117	56	3.8	111	2.5	11.2	32	6700	3.9	yes	no
4	51	80	1.01	2	0	normal	normal	notpreser	notpreser	106	26	1.4			11.6	35	7300	4.6	no	no
5	60	90	1.015	3	0			notpreser	notpreser	74	25	1.1	142	3.2	12.2	39	7800	4.4	yes	yes
6	68	70	1.01	0	0	normal		notpreser	notpreser	100	54	24	104	4	12.4	36			no	no
7	24		1.015	2	4	normal	abnormal	notpreser	notpreser	410	31	1.1			12.4	44	6900		5	no	yes
8	52	100	1.015	3	0	normal	abnormal	present	notpreser	138	60	1.9			10.8	33	9600		4	yes	yes
9	53	90	1.02	2	0	abnormal	abnormal	present	notpreser	70	107	7.2	114	3.7	9.5	29	12100	3.7	yes	yes
10	50	60	1.01	2	4		abnormal	present	notpreser	490	55	4			9.4	28			yes	yes
11	63	70	1.01	3	0	abnormal	abnormal	present	notpreser	380	60	2.7	131	4.2	10.8	32	4500	3.8	yes	yes
12	68	70	1.015	3	1		normal	present	notpreser	208	72	2.1	138	5.8	9.7	28	12200	3.4	yes	yes
13	68	70						notpreser	notpreser	98	86	4.6	135	3.4	9.8				yes	yes
14	68	80	1.01	3	2	normal	abnormal	present	present	157	90	4.1	130	6.4	5.6	16	11000	2.6	yes	yes
15	40	80	1.015	3	0		normal	notpreser	notpreser	76	162	9.6	141	4.9	7.6	24	3800	2.8	yes	no

CONCLUSION

In the end, we can sum up by saying that text mining plays a vital role in the field of medical care and health care. We need to develop effective models, which can save lives of people by taking proper actions as soon as possible. We use different techniques available to us and perform the classification process. These diseases have seen an exponential rise within past few years. Most people have been suffering from these diseases and need proper cure of it. By the time we need to go to the doctor to get it cured, using the various content-mining techniques we can develop a model which can indicate people on an early stage about the disease and that can be taken care of at an initial stage. We picked up different datasets for this disease from www.kaggale.com and performed different algorithms to measure the accuracy of each applied algorithm. We selected the one, which gave us the highest accuracy and better prediction results. We firstly studied the chronic kidney disease dataset and performed the three classification models, which are KNN and SVM and Linear Regression. After implementation, we found out that SVM produces better results and better accuracy for the particular disease.

REFERENCES

Ameta, M. A., & Jain, M. K. (2017, Feb.). Data Mining Techniques for the Prediction of Kidney Diseases and Treatment: A Review. *International Journal of Engineering and Computer Science.*

Arasu, S. D., & Thirumalaiselvi, R. (2017, February). A novel imputation method for effective prediction of coronary Kidney disease. In *2017 2nd International Conference on Computing and Communications Technologies (ICCCT)* (pp. 127-136). IEEE. 10.1109/ICCCT2.2017.7972256

Bala, S., & Kumar, K. (2014). A literature review on kidney disease prediction using data mining classification technique. *International Journal of Computer Science and Mobile Computing, 3*(7), 960–967.

Devi, J. C. (2014). Binary Decision Tree Classification based on C4. 5 and KNN Algorithm for Banking Application. *International Journal of Computational Intelligence and Informatics, 4*(2), 125–131.

Dubey, A. (2015). A classification of ckd cases using multivariate k-means clustering. *International Journal of Scientific and Research Publications, 5*(8), 1–5.

Gharibdousti, M. S., Azimi, K., Hathikal, S., & Won, D. H. (2017). Prediction of chronic kidney disease using data mining techniques. In *IIE Annual Conference. Proceedings* (pp. 2135-2140). Institute of Industrial and Systems Engineers (IISE).

Jena, L., & Kamila, N. K. (2015). Distributed data mining classification algorithms for prediction of chronic-kidney-disease. *Int. J. Emerg. Res. Manag. &Technology, 9359*(11), 110–118.

Kaur, G., & Sharma, A. (2017, November). Predict chronic kidney disease using data mining algorithms in hadoop. In *2017 International Conference on Inventive Computing and Informatics (ICICI)* (pp. 973-979). IEEE. 10.1109/ICICI.2017.8365283

Kharya, S. (2012). *Using data mining techniques for diagnosis and prognosis of cancer disease.* arXiv preprint arXiv:1205.1923

Kumar, K., & Abhishek, B. (2012). *Artificial neural networks for diagnosis of kidney stones disease.* GRIN Verlag. doi:10.5815/ijitcs.2012.07.03

Kunwar, V., Chandel, K., Sabitha, A. S., & Bansal, A. (2016, January). Chronic Kidney Disease analysis using data mining classification techniques. In 2016 6th International Conference-Cloud System and Big Data Engineering (Confluence) (pp. 300-305). IEEE. doi:10.1109/CONFLUENCE.2016.7508132

Kusiak, A., Dixon, B., & Shah, S. (2005). Predicting survival time for kidney dialysis patients: A data mining approach. *Computers in Biology and Medicine, 35*(4), 311–327. doi:10.1016/j.compbiomed.2004.02.004 PMID:15749092

Patil, P. M. (2016). Review on Prediction of Chronic Kidney Disease using Data Mining Techniques. *International Journal of Computer Science and Mobile Computing, 5*(5), 135.

Ramya, S., & Radha, N. (2016). Diagnosis of chronic kidney disease using machine learning algorithms. *International Journal of Innovative Research in Computer and Communication Engineering, 4*(1), 812–820.

Vijayarani, S., Dhayanand, S., & Phil, M. (2015). Kidney disease prediction using SVM and ANN algorithms. *International Journal of Computing and Business Research, 6*(2).

Chapter 7
A Machine Learning Approach to Prevent Cancer

Ahan Chatterjee
https://orcid.org/0000-0001-5217-4457
The Neotia University, India

Swagatam Roy
https://orcid.org/0000-0002-8012-5529
The Neotia University, India

Rupali Shrivastava
The Neotia University, India

ABSTRACT

One of the most talked about diseases of the 21st century is none other than cancer. In this chapter, the authors take a closer look to prevent cancer through machine learning approach. At first, they ran their classifier models (e.g., decision tree, K-mean, SVM, etc.) to check which algorithm gives the best result in terms of choosing right features for further treatment. The classified results are compared, and then various feature reduction algorithm is being used to identify exactly which features affects the most. Various data mining algorithms are being used, namely rough-based theory, graph-based clustering, to extract the most important features which influence the results. In the next section they take a look in the cancer analytics part. A simulation model has been designed that can easily manage the patient flow in OPDs and a bed rotation model also have been designed to give patients an insight that how much time they will spend in the queue. Further they analyzed a risk analysis model for chemotherapy treatment, and finally, an econometric discussion has been drawn in how it affects the treatment.

INTRODUCTION

"We have two options, medically and emotionally: give up or fight like hell." – Lance Armstrong
7 Times Tour De France Winner and a Cancer Survivor

DOI: 10.4018/978-1-7998-2742-9.ch007

In the last year 2018, 9.6 million deaths have been recorded due to cancer. It has been estimated that every 1 out of 6 people die due to cancer. This disease is considered as heterogeneous disease as there are many subtypes of it. Early detection of this disease is much needed as it can be cured partially if detected early. Classification of cancer has moved various research organizations around the globe, and nowadays classifying the disease using Machine Learning approach is in the business. The paper is majorly divided into two sections in the first section we look into the machine learning tools to extract insights from the data by which it can be prevented and in the next section we take a closer look in the cancer analytics domain.

Machine Learning allows us to detect and extract key features or hidden patterns which are there in the complex datasets of cancer patients. Thus use of machine learning gives us an upper hand in this field detecting the disease. Classification and data mining are an effective way to classify the data. Especially in bio-medical field where based upon the classification results analyses are done and decisions are being taken. In this paper we aim to find a performance comparison between various algorithms namely, Support Vector Machine (SVM), Decision Tree, Naïve Bayes (NB) and K-Nearest Neighbor (KNN). All the algorithms are being applied on Wisconsin Breast Cancer (Original) Dataset. Then the breast cancer underwent a feature selection process to extract the key features which influences the most. All the features don't affect the result equally thus in this step we will cancel out the irrelative features to get better results. Rough Based Theory and Graph Based Clustering have been used to extract the features. PCA algorithm is also being used to reduce the dimension. The aim of this paper is to evaluate the correctness in classifying data for each algorithm with parameters namely, efficiency and effectiveness in terms of accuracy and precision. From the experiments and results we can say that use of machine learning models can improve our vision and understanding in progression of cancer cells, but we need a proper validation of this works to practice this in everyday clinical practice. In the next section we mainly focus on the analytics part of the healthcare. In easy words, we can say that how much care needed for the patients for better and stable health required it is analyzed in this step. We can say minimizing the queue time for a patient will return a better health status than being harassed by going here and there for different things. Other various factors has also been considered as the economic background to carry on the treatment, as the cancer treatment is still a costly one being one of the most dreadful disease in the modern times. The investment from the government in the treatment for cancer is also an important factor by which it influences the treatment rate or cost. In this limelight we will also analyze the waiting time and success rate for a patient undergo surgery or chemotherapy and how can we increase the success rate by risk analysis by Bayesian Modeling. A set of questions arise when we talk about the healthcare part, that is there timely detection, proper diagnosis, does the patients getting proper care from the industry specialties, in this section we will put a limelight in these sections to get an data insight which can be analyzed better performance in near future. Further we would design a patient flow model which can easily manage the flow timeliness manner, and the impact of rapid diagnosis is being measured. A patient when diagnosed with cancer it is not only the physical pain that they go through, various other factors is also closely related with those which directly or indirectly creates an impact over the health of the patient, *viz.* physical, psychological, financial, and spiritual as well plays a role. A patient can go under huge debt due to their treatment for which they go in depression which surely affects their health condition. We will go into a closer look how they affect the health and would try to frame a solution for these solutions. (Wait et al., 2017; Zhou et al., 2004)

BACKGROUND HISTORY OF CANCER

As we know cancer is a broad and generic term and one of the most dreadful diseases in the world which claims majority of lives, which is basically defined as the uncontrolled growth of abnormal cells in the body resulting in diseases that occurs when malignant forms of abnormal cell growth develop in one or more body organs. The most effective way to reduce cancer deaths is to detect it an early stage .Certain forms of cancer result in visible growths called tumors.

Figure 1. Represents difference between normal cell and cells having a tumor
Source: Dash, Kumar (2018)

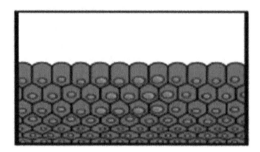 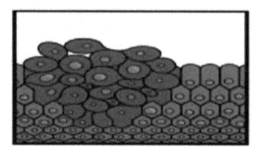

Normal cells   Cells forming a tumour

Cancer is being characterized as a heterogeneous disease consisting of many different subtypes. Predicting the outcome of a disease is one of the most interesting and challenging tasks where machine learning has to be applied. As cancer progresses, treatments techniques includes radiation, chemotherapy, hormone ablation therapy and appropriate targeted therapies .The combined genetic and non genetic changes induced by environmental factors causes cancer which triggers the inappropriate activation or inactivation of specific genes and thus leading to neoplastic transformations, or abnormal cell growth .The most unique feature of cancer is that it can occur at any age and in any organ. They follow two ways, one is aggressive course where the cancer grows rapidly and the other type is where it grows slowly or remains dormant for several years .It is being estimated that 80% of cancers are caused due to environment or lifestyle and so we can potentially prevent them. The stage of cancer at the time of diagnosis, the rate of its progression, and the treatment options vary significantly with the type of cancer it is. (Racz et al., 2016)

Classification of Cancer

There are many types of cancer. Different parts of India are affected by different types of cancer. Table 1 represents that.

Figure 2. Represents the world wide cancer distribution
Source: Created by Author, based on data

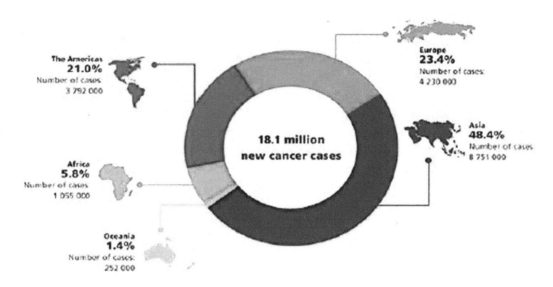

Table 1. Different region of India affected different cancer

Regions	Type of Cancer	Risk
Punjab	Kidney, urinary bladder, breast cancer	Pollution, pesticide, toxin in food
Gujarat & Rajasthan	Head & throat	Tobacco & paan masala
Madhya Pradesh(MP)	Oral	Tobacco & paan masala
Goa	Colon	Red meat, alcohol, tobacco
South and Coastal	Stomach	Diet rich in spices and salt
West Bengal	Lung, urinary bladder	Pollution
North-East	Oral and stomach	Tobacco, household burning of firewood
Gangetic plain(UP, Bihar)	Gall bladder, head, neck cancer	Water pollution, diet rich in animal protein

Source: Created by author, based on dataset

BRIEF DISCUSSION ON DIFFERENT TYPES OF CANCER

Breast Cancer

History: Breast cancer has been known to mankind since very ancient times. The visible symptoms especially at later stages, the lumps that form tumors have been recorded by physicians from early times. This is because, unlike other internal cancers, breast lumps tend to manifest themselves as visible tumors. By mid of nineteenth century, surgery was the only remedy for breast cancer. The reason behind the reduction of the tumor after removal of the ovaries was the fact that estrogen from ovaries helped in growth of the tumor and their removal helped reduce the size of the tumor.

Causes: Breast cancer occurs when some breast cells starts to form lumps. These cells divide rapidly than healthy cells do and accumulate at one place, forming a lump or mass. Breast cancer most often begins with cells in the milk-producing ducts called invasive ductal carcinoma. Breast cancer can start forming in the glandular tissue called lobules (invasive lobular carcinoma) or in other cells within the breast. Researchers have identified hormonal, lifestyle and environmental factors which are responsible for increasing the risk of breast cancer.

It's likely that breast cancer is caused by a complex interaction of the genetic makeup and environment. It is estimated that about 5 to 10 percent of breast cancers are linked to gene mutations passed through generations of a family. The most well-known are breast cancer gene 1 (BRCA1) and breast cancer gene 2 (BRCA2), both of which significantly increase the risk of both breast and ovarian cancer. (Alharthi, 2018)

Figure 3. Graph represents the mortality and incidence rate of breast cancer
Source: Dash, Kumar (2018)

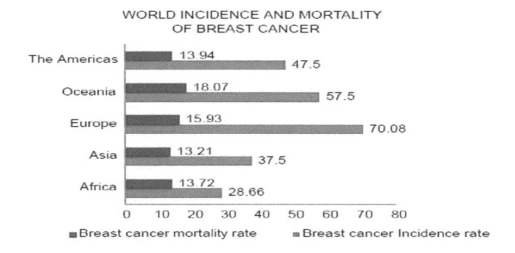

Symptoms

(i)   A breast lump or thickening that feels different from the surrounding tissue
(ii) Change in the size, shape or appearance of a breast
(iii) Changes to the skin over the breast, such as dimpling
(iv) A newly inverted nipple
(v)   Peeling, scaling, crusting or flaking of the pigmented area of skin surrounding the nipple (areola) or breast skin
(vi) Redness or pitting of the skin over your breast, like the skin of an orange

Blood Cancer

Although the specific cause of cancer in blood is also unknown, various factors are associated with its onset. Some causes are aging, family history, weak immune system, certain infections

Types

- Leukemia – It is caused by the abnormal blood cells in the bone marrow. These blood cells affect the bone marrow's ability to produce red blood cells and platelets.
- Lymphoma - This type of blood cancer affect the lymphatic system, which is responsible for the removal of excess fluids from your body and producing immune cells. Lymphocytes are a type of white blood cell that fights infection. Abnormal lymphocytes become lymphoma cells, which grow uncontrollably in your lymph nodes and other tissues.
- Myeloma - This type of blood cancer affects the plasma cells, which are white blood cells responsible for the production of disease-fighting antibodies in the body.

Symptoms

Blood cancer affects blood, bone marrow, or lymphatic system. Some of the common symptoms include:

- Shortness of breath
- Minimal body strain results in bone fractures
- Excessive or easy bruising

Figure 4. Difference between normal blood cell vs. cell affected by Leukemia
Source: Dash, Kumar (2018)

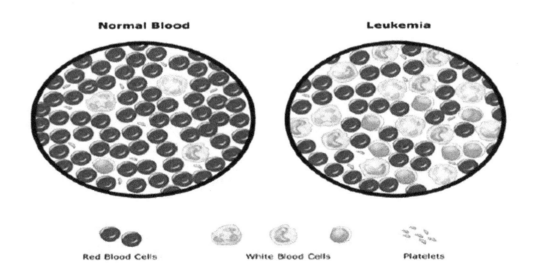

Colon Cancer

Colon cancer is visible in large intestine, thus named colon cancer. As screening practices have increased, colon cancer is now often detected before it starts to cause symptoms. In advanced cases, symptoms include iron-deficiency anemia, abdominal pain, rectal bleeding, change in bowel habits, and intestinal obstruction or perforation. The lesions on right side are likely to bleed and cause diarrhea, while tumors on the left side present as bowel obstruction. (Wang et al., 2011)

Figure 5. Represents the graph between the number of patients and age
Source: Dash, Kumar (2018)

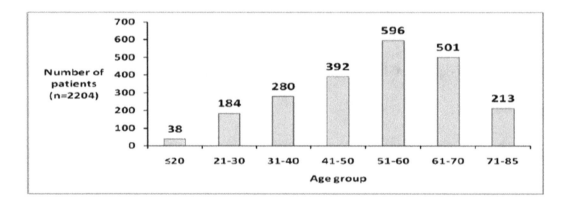

Causes: Generally, colon cancer begins when the healthy cells in the colon develop causes mutations in their DNA. Healthy cells grow and divide in an orderly way to keep your body functioning normally. But when a cell's DNA is damaged and becomes cancerous, cells continue to divide despite of the fact that new cells aren't needed. The accumulation of cells leads to development of tumor and like this way as time passes, the cancer cells can grow to invade and destroy normal tissue present nearby.

Symptoms

- A persistent change in the bowel habits, including diarrhea or constipation or in the consistency of the stool
- Unexplained weight loss
- Persistent abdominal discomfort, such as cramps, gas or pain
- Rectal bleeding or blood in stool

Skin Cancer

Causes: Ultraviolet (UV) radiation from the sun is the major cause of skin cancer. Exposure to sunlight during the winter months puts at the same risk as exposure during the summer time. Cumulative sun exposure mainly causes basal cell and squamous cell skin cancer, while severe blistering sunburns, mostly before age 18, can cause melanoma later in life. Other less common causes are repeated X-ray exposure, scars from burns, and occupational exposure to certain chemicals.

Figure 6. Layers of skin
Source: Dash, Kumar (2018)

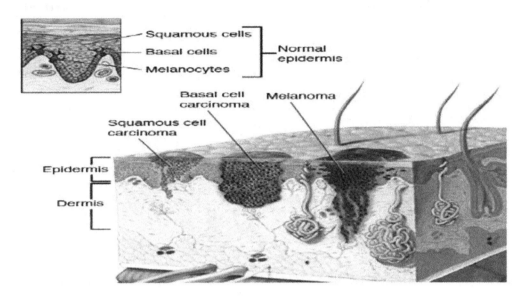

Symptoms

- Skin is smooth and pearly or waxy.
- Develop a crust or scab
- Appear as a firm, red lump or may look sunken in the middle.
- Appear as a pearly brown or black lump if you have darker skin.
- Feel itchy and bleed sometimes.
- Begin to heal but never completely heal.

DATA UNDERSTANDING AND DATA PREPARATION

The dataset is being collected from UCI repository, and this breast cancer dataset contains 699 instances of data with 11 features, they are being tabulated in table 2. The dataset is being split into 65% of cancerous cell and rest 35% into non cancerous cells.

INTRODUCTION TO MACHINE LEARNING IN CANCER TREATMENT

Nowadays, artificial intelligence is one of the emerging fields. Machine learning is one of the building blocks of it. It has many applications in medical fields and with the help of ML model and different algorithm biomedical research has been done.

Table 2. Description of Dataset

Attribute Number	Attribute Name	Value (Range)	Mean	Standard Deviation
1	Clump Thickness	1-10	4.44	2.83
2	Uniformity of Cell Size	1-10	3.15	3.07
3	Uniformity of Cell Shape	1-10	3.22	2.99
4	Marginal adhesion	1-10	2.83	2.86
5	Single epithelial cell size	1-10	2.23	2.22
6	Bare nuclei	1-10	3.54	3.64
7	Bland chromatin	1-10	3.45	2.45
8	Normal nucleoli	1-10	2.87	3.05
9	Mitoses	1-10	1.60	1.73

Source: Created by the Author, based on the dataset

Figure 7. Increase of ML models in various scientific domain
Source: Building Energy Information: Demand and Consumption Prediction with Machine Learning Models for Sustainable and Smart Cities by Amir Mosavi

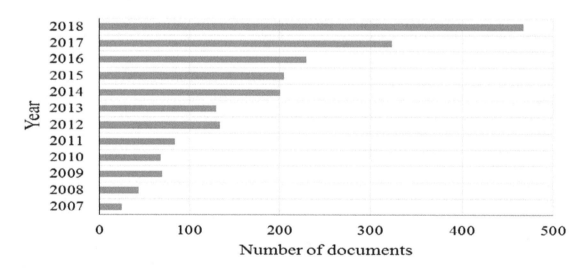

The main target of Machine learning is to find out the dependency or relation between the variable, it is defined as learning of algorithm and development of particular program having goal of learning work i.e. 'task' T with experience E and performance task or measure accuracy P with the improvement in the learning and experience E. 6[-8]

There are mainly 6 different stages of creating a model.

- Problem Definition
- Hypothesis generation & testing
- Data Extraction

- Data exploration
- Modelling
- Model Implementation

With the advent of new technologies in the field of medicine, large amounts of cancer data have been collected and are available to the medical research community. However, the accurate prediction of a disease outcome is one of the most interesting and challenging tasks for physicians. As a result, ML methods have become a popular tool for medical researchers. These techniques can discover and identify patterns and relationships between them, from complex datasets, while they are able to effectively predict future outcomes of a cancer type.

ML, a branch of Artificial Intelligence, relates the problem of learning from data samples to the general concept of inference. Every learning process consists of two phases: (i) estimation of unknown dependencies in a system from a given dataset and (ii) use of estimated dependencies to predict new outputs of the system. ML has also been proven an interesting area in biomedical research with many applications, where an acceptable generalization is obtained by searching through an n-dimensional space for a given set of biological samples, using different techniques and algorithms. There are two main common types of ML methods known as (i) supervised learning and (ii) unsupervised learning. In supervised learning a labeled set of training data is used to estimate or map the input data to the desired output.

An extensive search was conducted relevant to the use of ML techniques in cancer susceptibility, recurrence and survivability prediction. Majority of the studies use different types of input data: genomic, clinical, histological, imaging, demographic, epidemiological data or combination of these. Papers that focus on the prediction of cancer development by means of conventional statistical methods (e.g. chisquare, Cox regression) were excluded as were papers that use techniques for tumor classification or identification of predictive factors. (England, 2019)

Use of Machine Learning Algorithms

Here we want to classify cancer into its different types and with the help of artificial intelligence and machine learning. In case of supervised learning, different algorithms like logistic regression, classification, decision tree, etc. classify with accuracy into set of classes and so they can be easily distinguishable. For unsupervised learning, if we consider clustering algorithms, it will categorize by clustering in a distinguishable way.

Here the target or dependent variable is discrete in nature. So it will have only certain values i.e. not a range of values. So by those values we can get a certain class or a particular type. So data of many people and corresponding type of cancer is noted and dataset is made. The dataset has many independent variables but there is only one dependent variable. So for using machine learning algorithms we have to split the dataset into train and test in a particular ratio.

MACHINE LEARNING ALGORITHMS USED TO COMPUTE CANCER CELLS

In this experiment target variable is discrete in nature i.e. it will have a particular value and not a range of value. Therefore algorithms like *Linear Regression* cannot be used. The discrete values may be an integer value or string or character which during the experiment or running the code is transformed by

Figure 8. Represents use if different algorithm in this field
Source:

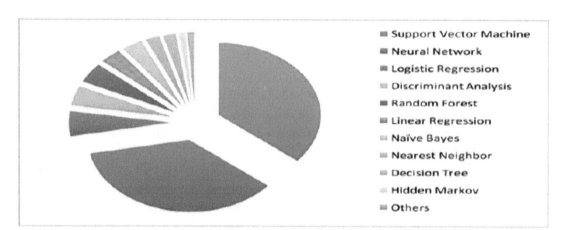

one hot encoding and then the experiments are performed. The brief introductions about the algorithms used to do the experiment and used in prediction are stated below:

Naïve Bayes Algorithm

It is a classification technique based on Bayes' theorem with an assumption of independence between predictors. The classifier assumes that the predictors/ features are independent of one another, i.e. the presence of one feature doesn't affect the presence of other features. That is why it is termed as naïve. Naïve Bayesian model is easy and particularly useful for very large datasets and outperforms even many other highly sophisticated classification models.

Mathematical Background

Naïve bayes algorithm gives us probability of a point x which can belong to a specified class C. The probability is calculated based on conditional probability model $P(x_i|C_K)$. The classification involves assigning the value to a class thus the proportion can be found using equation 1.

$$p(C_a)\prod_{i=1}^{n}p(x_i|C_a) > p(C_b)\prod_{i=1}^{n}p(x_i|C_b) => p(x_1, x_2 ..., x_n|C_a) > p(x_1, x_2 ..., x_n | C_b).$$ (1)

Thus the class can be found by mathematical notation given in equation 2.

$$C = \arg\max p(C_k)\prod_{i=1}^{n}p(x_i | C_K), \ k \in \{1, 2, ..., k\}.$$ (2)

Application of Naïve Bayes: Naïve Bayes segments the whole dataset into various classes and the new element is being inserted on the basis of higher probability wrt. to each classes, and the prediction on whether the cell is malignant or benign is being selected on the base of conditional probability.

Decision Tree Algorithm

It is a type of supervised learning used for classification problem. It works for both continuous and categorical dependent variables. In this model, we split the population in two or more homogenous sets (or, sub-populations) which is done on the basis of most significant attributes/ independent variables to make as many distinct group(s) as possible. (Dash et al., 2019)

Mathematical Background:

The Decision tree model works on the count of impurity and the split occurs in the direction where the impurity is least. The count of impurity is measured by 2 factors namely gini index and entropy. Entropy is described as the amount of information needed to correctly describe a sample. Homogenous sample will give o entropy while heterogeneous will yield 1. It's calculated as represented in equation 3. Similarly Gini index is measured using inequality in sample. Gini index value 0 denotes that the sample is perfectly homogenous and 1 shows it has maximal inequality. It's calculated as represented by equation 4.

$$Entropy = -\sum_{i=1}^{n} p_i \times \log(p_i) \tag{3}$$

$$Gini\ Index = 1 - \sum_{i=1}^{n} p_i^2. \tag{4}$$

KNN Clustering Algorithm

It is a type of unsupervised algorithm which solves the clustering problem. The objective of the algorithm is to group similar data points together and find the underlying patterns. The algorithm searches for a fixed number (k) of collections of data points aggregated together due to similarities among them, known as clusters, in a dataset. The 'means' refers to the averaging of the data, i.e. finding the centroids. (Ramachandran et al., 2013)

Mathematical Background:

The cluster is being formed using the Euclidian Distance, it is calculated for each value and then clusters are being formed. Centroid of clusters changes with each iteration and continues until they reach the same, the formula to calculate Euclidian distance is given in equation 5.

If $p=(p_1,p_2)$ and $q=(q_1,q_2)$ then Euclidian distance is

$$d(p,q) = \sqrt{(q_1 - p_1)^2 + (q_2 - p_2)^2} \tag{5}$$

$$Centroid = \arg\min dist(c_i, x)^2, \; c_i \in C. \tag{6}$$

Support Vector Machine (SVM) Algorithm

Support Vector Machine (SVM) is a supervised machine learning algorithm which is applicable for both regression rather logistic regression and classification. It makes a non probabilistic binary discriminative linear classifier. It basically creates hyper planes in infinite dimension and output or prediction is done on the basis of optimal hyper plane. So basically when the target variable is given along with labeled features then it creates set of hyper planes and each planes denotes each hyper planes and on basis of that it separates into different classes.

Mathematical Background

Kernel function $k(x,y)$ is defined.

In higher dimension hyper plane considered as bunch of observable points whose scalar product is constant. So for higher dimension $k(x,y)$ modifies to $k(x_i, y)$ and so for the hyperplane we can say that

$$\sum_{i=0}^{n} \beta.k(x_i, y) = C. \tag{7}$$

Higher value of k is preferable. Also the functional margin has to be maintained. If there are n points then $w.x - b = 0$ is the equation of hyper plane where w is the normal vector and $\dfrac{b}{w}$ is the offset of hyper plane.

NECESSITY OF FEATURE SELECTION AND FEATURE SELECTION ALGORITHMS

The dataset contains several features but for making correct prediction with high accuracy we take care of the quality of data. But to ensure high quality of data we face some problems. The dataset contains noise, outliers, missing value etc. So pre-processing of data is required for removal of noise and to sort out other factors. Some techniques used to resolve these matters are

- Dimension Reduction
- Feature selection
- Feature extractor

Dimension reduction helps in reduction of noise to improve the quality of data. It is a subset of feature selection

Feature selection is defined as the process of identifying and selecting relevant features from a collection of data or a dataset. This improves the accuracy of the model by reducing irrelevant features.

Figure 9. General flow of machine learning

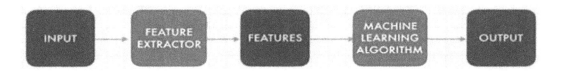

By feature selection we get an idea about the relation between target and independent variable and how they are correlated. More the correlation, more it will affect the target variable and thus small change in independent will also reflect. (Liu et al., 2010; Rajpal et al., 2018)

Figure 10. Steps of feature selection

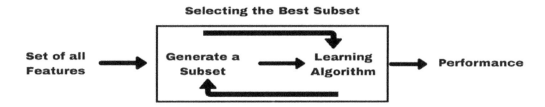

Rough Set Theory

It is basically approximation of conventional set. It helps to handle blurriness. It basically uses mathematical approaches for feature selection. It identifies boundary regions of set and by that it sets the upper approximation and lower approximation. Rough set theory removes redundant and irrelevant information from the dataset.

Algorithm of Rough Set Theory

Here, reduct R is minimal set of features when $\gamma R_{(}D)=\gamma F(_{D})$. It means R will be reduct if and only if the dependency of decision class D on feature subset R is exactly equal to that of D on whole feature set F. Firstly, the method takes the highest ranked feature as the initial reduct R. Then, in every iteration, the next most important feature will be added until the condition $\gamma R(D_{)}=\gamma F(D)$ is satisfied. Thus, final reduct R is generated. (Islam et al., 2018; Kritchanchai & Hoeur, 2018; Maher et al., 2018; Stafinski & Menon, 2017)

The detailed algorithm is mentioned below:

```
Algorithm: Reduct-Generation (U, F, D)
Input: U = the set of samples, F = set of features arranged based on their
rank and D= Decision class
Output: R = Reduct, reduced feature subset
Begin
```
F = { $f_{i_1} f_{i_2} ... f_{i_n}$. be the n features arranged in descending order of their rank;

R = { f_{i_1} . // core, [Assued as initial reduct];

For all f . (F − R)

If $^3{}_{R \cup \{f\}}(D) > {}^3{}_R(D)$. R = RU { f .};

If $^3{}_R(D) = {}^3{}_F(D)$. Return R;

```
End-if
End-for
Return R;
End
```

Principal Component Analysis (PCA) Algorithm

PCA is a dimension reduction technique because by PCA some most significant features are only selected which is useful for training the model. Moreover, more the number of features more are the computation time and complexity and EDA is convoluted. So PCA is needed. PCA identifies patterns and highly correlated features by applying correlation methods and then apply reduction techniques to remove inconsistency and produce a redutant data without loss of information.

Mathematical Background

If the dataset be $m \times q$ where m is observation serial and q is predictor. Then scatter plot required to find relation is $\dfrac{\{q \times (q-1)\}}{2}$. The dataset with reduced dimension should be formed by taking the mean and it should have the highest variance. It mainly finds a linear combination of features and by this method it finds the maximum variance. Variance is calculated as shown in equation 8.

$$V(x) = \sum x^2 . p - \mu . \tag{8}$$

Then we compute the correlation or covariance matrix which is defined as in equation 9.

$$C(X) = \frac{1}{n-1} \sum_{i=1}^{n} (x_i - \mu_1).(y_i - \mu_2).$$

Σx and Σy forms square matrix and square symmetric matrix is preferable. After this Eigen vectors is computed as

$$\det(x) = \left(M(A) - \lambda I\right).$$

Then accordingly $d \times k$ i.e. Eigen vector matrix W is formed. Then it is transformed into new subspaces $y = W' - x$ .and thus points are transformed into new space.

Now the new-subspace helps to predict/reconstruct the original dimensions and projection error is minimized. (Kourou et al., 2015; Liang et al., 2015; McCarthy et al., 2008)

Graph Based Clustering Algorithm

All the features are not important thus we perform this feature reduction for more precise results.

Let U the whole dataset and each object a in U is characterized by a set $F = \{F_1, F_2,..., Fn\}$ of n extracted features. Then we normalize the data into (Wait et al., 2017). Then all the values are being are formulated by $(x, x + 0.1]$. In this step all the values are being discrete.

Then all the similar points are being partitioned. $P_{Fi} = \{ P_{i_1}, P_{i_2},..., P_{i_{10}} \}$ .where, all the images in a group have same value for feature F_i and two images of two different groups have distinct feature values.

Let the two partitions obtained using features F_i and F_j are $P_{Fi} = \{P_{i_1}, P_{i_2},..., P_{i_{10}}\}$ .and $P_{Fj} = \{P_{j_1}, P_{j_2},..., P_{j_{10}}\}$ respectively. Similarity of F_i to F_j is computed using eq. (10).

$$S_{ij} = \frac{1}{10} \sum_{k=1}^{10} \max_{1 \leq l \leq 10} \left\{ \frac{\left| P_{i_k} \cap P_{j_l} \right|}{\left| P_{i_k} \cup P_{j_l} \right|} \right\}. \tag{10}$$

Then graphs are being drawn with $G=(F,E,W)$ where F is the features, E is the nodes of the graph and W is being the set of edges. Weights in the graph is assigned as $w_{ij} = (S_{ij} + S_{ji})/2$

RESULTS AND ANALYSIS ON THE BACKDROP OF THE RESULTS

We have implemented 4 types of classifier model in our Wisconsin breast cancer dataset to retrieve the results and gain insights from the raw data for better treatment procedure. Table 3 denotes result obtained by running our classifier model on the whole dataset and on the reduced dataset using rough set theory.

From this result we can see that the reduced dataset gives us more accuracy in this model. The highest accuracy in the reduced part came for the features namely, Uniformity of Cell Shape, Uniformity of Cell Size, Bland Chromatin, Clump Thickness, Normal Nucleoli, Marginal Adhesion.

The decision tree model has been visualized in figure 11.

The decision tree model finds the output by splitting into nodes and going to the lowest impurity state.

In table 4, we compute the result which was obtained by using Graph Based Clustering Algorithm.

Figure 12, describes the clusters which were formed using spectral based clustering model, and how the elements are being split in the clusters.

Table 3. Comparison of accuracy before and after reduction using rough set theory

Classifier Name	Accuracy *(Whole Dataset)* [In percentages]	Accuracy *(Reduced Dataset)* [In percentages]
KNN	95.57	97.14
Decision Tree	95.91	96.62
Naïve Bayes	97.14	98.26
SVM	95.42	97.14

Figure 11. Visualization of Decision Tree Model
Source: Created by the Author

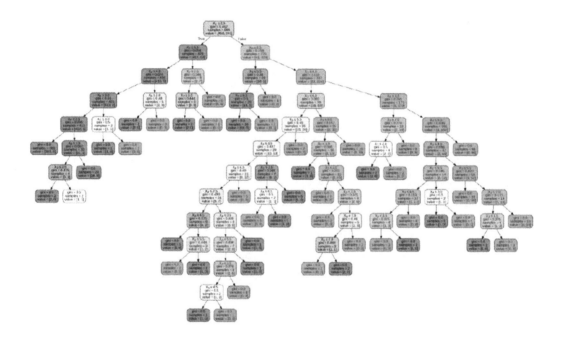

In table 4, we have computed the accuracy for PCA Model.

Figure 13, denotes the classes separated through PCA Algorithm.

CANCER HEALTHCARE ANALYTICS

A patient when diagnosed with cancer it is not only the physical pain that they go through, various other factors is also closely related with those which directly or indirectly creates an impact over the health of the patient, *viz.* physical, psychological, financial, and spiritual as well plays a role. A patient can go under huge debt due to their treatment for which they go in depression which surely affects their health condition. We will go into a closer look how they affect the health and would try to frame a solution for these solutions. (Mihaylov et al., 2019)

Table 4. Accuracy for Graph Based Clustering

Model Name	Accuracy [In percentage]
Graph Based Clustering Algorithm	97.56

Figure 12. Visualization of Spectral Based Clustering
Source: Created by the Author

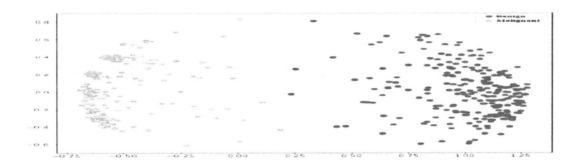

Table 5. Accuracy for PCA

Model Name	Accuracy [In percentage]
Principal Component Analysis (PCA)	98.18

Framework for Effective Patient Flow and Bed Occupancy Model

One of the most challenging jobs for cancer treatment in OPD section is to maintain the flow of patient in an effective mode, and the same for nursing section is to manage to bed occupancy model. There should be a good communication in between the administrative section and the specialist so that the time could be minimized as possible.

In general the patients have their appointment with the doctors, but when they visit the chamber or the OPD's of the hospital they go through an unacceptable long queue time. In recent times many hospitals have framed a 2 day model where patient in day 1 go through doctor visit and blood test and on next day they go through the chemotherapy checkup.

The growth has been phenomenal in terms of patients visiting oncologists. A statistics report from Tata Memorial Institute, Mumbai shows that around 14,000 patients visit this institute in a month in the year of 2018. And the number of patients receiving chemotherapy on the same month is stated as 1261 and 10,7600 patients go through laboratory test on the same month.

From table 1, we can say that there is a good crowd present for the treatment purpose thus we need a good model to satisfy all the patients and maintain a good flow in the setup.

Figure 13. Visualization of PCA
Source: Created by the Author

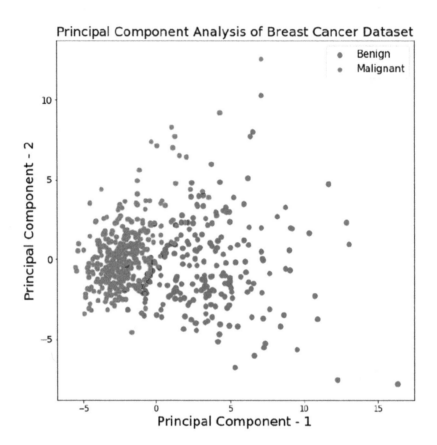

The efficiency of an OPD centre or a hospital can be easily measured by its efficiency to outflow the crowd of the patient. In this context we have created an event-simulation model to check and improve the flow of patients. (Zoullouti et al., 2019)

In cancer treatment, the time factor plays a huge role. Thus we aim to divide the primary treatment zone in one part and the other sections in the other part in which it will have the registration and cashier section which simply doesn't affect the treatment of the patient. We aim to reduce the processing time by implementing this model.

Proposed Pseudo Algorithm

```
Begin
P regs T
P gs rp Ct
Case 1: Ct Dr
If (Dr = = C)
P gs C₂
If (C₂ = = 0)
```

```
C Dr && P lvs
Case 2: Ct Blood
Rpt Dr
If (Chemo = = 1)
P gs C₃
Else P lvs
Case 3: Ct Chemo
Tr p
P lvs
End
```

The algorithm is proposed, and it aims to serve better patient flow the variable names have been explained below.

Table 6. Showing trends of Patients Visiting Oncologists

Total Patients Visiting TMC, Mumbai	Patients go through Chemotherapy (*In Percentages*)	Patients go laboratory test Chemotherapy (*In Percentages*)
13,991	9.01	76.94

Source: Created by the Author, Based on the dataset

The flowchart of the proposed algorithm is shown in figure 14. It implements that every registered patient will go directly to the specified counter which is needed, and thus the crowd will be easily split up. Then the patients will go to their respective needed departments, and the patients who will consult the doctors can move to blood test and chemo therapy section if and only if they are being suggested by the medicos. In this way the crowd can be easily moved out and a better flow of patients can be designed in the OPDs which supports cancer treatment. (Stojadinovic et al., 2011)

Table 7. Meaning of the variables used in our proposed algorithm

Variable Name	Meaning
P	Patient
regs	Registration
T	Token
gs	Goes
rp	Respective
Lvs	Leave
Rpt	report

Source: Created by the Author

Figure 14. Flowchart of Model
Source: Created by the Author

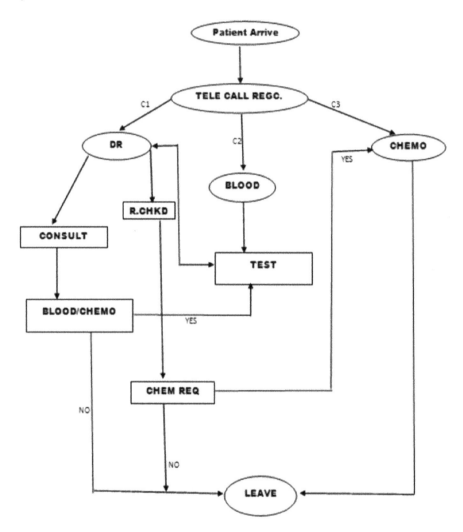

Event Simulation Results and Analysis on the Backdrop of the Results

The simulation model has been built on 5000 iteration count. As we all know that treating cancer patients can be tricky as all have different levels of priority. Thus we have simulated our model keeping in mind that the high priority patients will be given first chance and the scene goes as follows. In this case the patient with most critical condition will first get the call from the hospital authority to visit the doctor. (Wongthanavasu, 2011)

Implementing the aforesaid algorithm with this condition not only fastens our patient flow but also the factor of humanity is also kept in our mind. The patients are broadly classified into 3 levels of priority, priority 1, 2, 3.

In the figure 1 and 2 we will visualize our results based on the simulation model.

In figure 15(a) we can see the queuing time for different priority of patients, from the results we can say that our model has been implemented for good. We can clearly see that the queuing time for the patients belonging to the priority 1 section has the least waiting time to visit the medico, while the patients belonging to the priority 3 class have comparatively maximum waiting time in the queue.

Figure 15. (a) Graph showing time required for each priority of patient (time in minutes), (b) Graph showing waiting time of patients (c) Graph showing availability of doctors
Source: Created by the Author

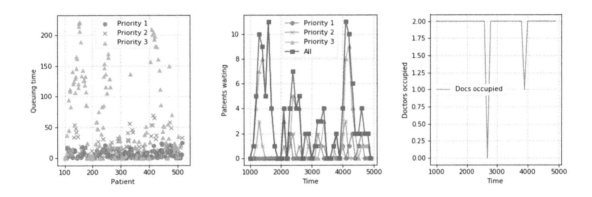

In figure 15(b) also supports our model's claim and figure 2(c) shows the rate of doctors being occupied for a particular treatment of a patient through all priorities taken.

The patient flow model have been effective in the cases of patients coming to consult doctors and having their blood test done and leaving the zone, but in the case of patients coming for chemotherapy they will be counted in the admit section of the hospital. In this case our patient flow model will not work, for this a bed occupancy model has been designed to provide beds to patients in effective manner. In a hospital there is a restricted count of beds, here we aim to simulate the model to visualize the waiting time for patients to get the beds. Patients having chemotherapy all belongs to critical stage of health thus here no priority model have been designed the model is based on first come first serve order. (Asri et al., 2016; Suss et al., 2017)

This model simulates the random arrival of patients at a hospital. Patients stay for a random time (given an average length of stay). Both inter-arrival time and length of stay are sampled from an inverse exponential distribution. At intervals the numbers of beds occupied are counted in an audit, and a chart of bed occupancy is plotted.

Figure 16(a) and 16(b) shows how our simulation model yields result for the bed occupancy model and queue time for a bed for the patients. Using these kinds of results the patients can be mentally prepared for their time requirement while going to the hospitals, because as a cancer patient the mental health also plays a key role in reshaping the health.

Figure 16. (a) Graph showing occupied beds with respect to days (b) Graph showing queue time for beds
Source: Created by the Author

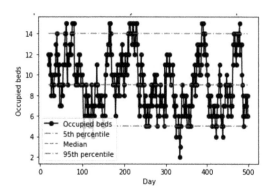
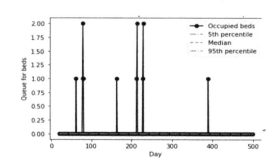

Risk Analysis for Chemotherapy Treatment

The patients who undergo the chemo treatment have their disease in very critical zone, in this section we will try to compute the risk model and risk analysis for the patients of survival rates in the chemo treatment. Significant advances have been made in the early detection phase of breast cancer. Despite these advances Ductal Carcinoma in situ is still in count of patients affecting in

The patients who undergo the chemo treatment have their disease in very critical zone, in this section we will try to compute the risk model and risk analysis for the patients of survival rates in the chemo treatment. Significant advances have been made in the early detection phase of breast cancer. Despite these advances Ductal Carcinoma in situ is still in count of patients affecting in breast cancer and it's one of the rarest part of breast cancer. The survival rate of cancer treatment varies across many factors and types of cancer it's visualized in the figure 4.

In the early detection of cancer the most important tool which is being used is the mammography. This tool can't state the cell is malignant or benign surely but it's used for preliminary test. The proper treatment can only be carried out if the doctors can analyze the risk factors associated with the mammography can carry out their treatments.

In recent time, the use of Bayesian Hierarchical Model (BHM) gained a lot of grounds in statistical modeling and analysis. Using this we can predict the uncertainty in the terms of both input and output. We have used this model to analyze and to get insights regarding the risks related to the treatment. Through BHM analysis of risk associated with a parameter can be better understood, over traditional subjective predictions. BHM represents and can solve hierarchical, complex and multilevel data structures. Through this model we can easily predict the death chances and can analyze and reduce the numbers of deaths.

Let, p be the probability of deaths occurred, i.e. an unsuccessful event occurs.

In order to determine the value of p we will implement models like event trees and fault trees.

p, is being computed using some parameterized function f, with parameters q. This is stated as $p=f(q)$.

Here, q is a vector which includes the probabilities for human failure or human mistake and infrastructural error or failure. This model is represented by the true parameters between p and q. Now, we will be analyzing death stats using Bayesian Model. Figure 18 suggests the parameters which are the main cause of the cancer causing.

Figure 17. Variation in survival rates for different stages of Cancer
Source: Mahe, Petchey, Greenfield, Levit, Freser (2018)

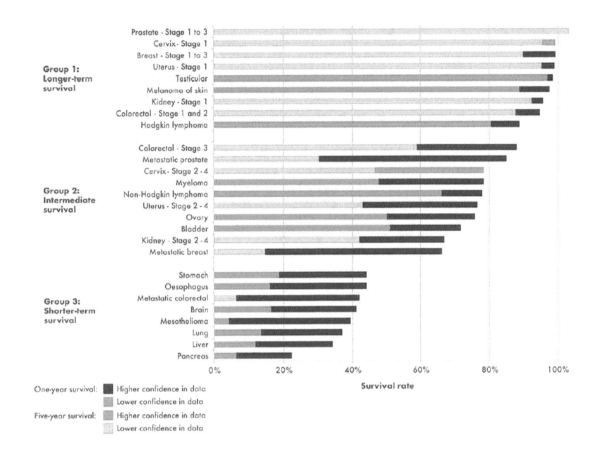

In this limelight we have trained the Bayesian classifier model, for the preliminary assessment of the patient and the risk associated with the treatment it will take from the medical experts. The classifier model gives us the probabilistic result regarding the variables affecting the disease and the chances of survival of the patient. Table 2 summarized the accuracy result of the classifier based on the parameters given through the dataset.

From the table 2, we can clearly visualize that we will conclude our model wrt. To 95% CI High section as the accuracy of the classifier model is significantly high in this section.

From the results we can say that with a loss of less than 10% of weight with mild or low problems assure you a high survival rate but with loss of more than 10% of weight with high pain or problems arising is a danger sign and the survival rates falls significantly in this case.

Econometric View on Cancer Treatment Aspect

The major public health concern of people across not only in India but across the world is cancer. Cancer is one of the fastest growing diseases across the world. The associated treatment is pretty hefty and for a middle class man the cost is growing rapidly and there is no hope for capping in the expenses in near future.

Figure 18. Mammography Parameters of Breast Cancer Risk Analysis
Source: Mahe, Petchey, Greenfield, Levit, Freser (2018)

Category	Node (variables)	States
Diagnosis	Age (years)	<20, 20-30, 31-40, 41-50, 51-60, >60
Patient History	Breast Cancer	present, absent
	Age at Menarche (years)	<12, 12-13, >13
	Age at First Live Birth (years)	<20, 20-24, 25-29, >29
	Number of First-Degree Relatives with Breast Cancer	0, 1, 2
	Age at First Live Birth (years)	<20, 20-24, 25-29, >29
	Age at Menopause (years)	<40, 40-44, 45-40, >49
	Number of Pregnancy	<2, 2-3, >3
Physical Findings	Pain	present, absent
	Nipple Discharge	present, absent
	Axilla	present, absent
	Inflame	present, absent
Indirect Mammographic Findings	Breast Composition	present, absent
Direct Mammographic Findings	Mass	malignant, benign, none
	Mass Present	yes, no
	Mass Lympnode	present, absent
	Mass Size (cm.)	1,2,3,4
	Calcification	malignant, benign, none
	Calcification Present	yes, no

The standardized result in this field shows that every 97 persons out of 10,0000 has a high chance of affecting by cancer leaving in the urban areas. Reports from Rural Health Statistics and DLHS IV report shows cancer affects mostly the aged persons and the females in the reproductive group. The average expense of treatment of cancer in private healthcare section is around 3 times higher than the public healthcare sections. In this backdrop we can analyze the current infrastructural condition and treatment facility in the public sectors is below standard condition thus the patients generally don't opt for treatment in the public healthcare domain.

Reports further shows that around 60% costs goes in treatment comes from selling assets and borrowing money. This leads to burden, and we can say that cancer is now becoming and burden for Indian middle class people. In this limelight we call for various healthcare policies to support this kind of burdens.

Reports from WHO suggests that the total count of deaths registered in India due to cancer will touch the figure of 900,000 by the end of this decade. This kind of figures is definitely is an eye opening for various sectors, reports further suggests that most of the deaths will occur due to breast and uterine cancer. The treatment of the cancer is being highly feared in India due to primarily two reasons. One, low survival rates and two, huge financial burden on the family as the current expense model is huge for the treatment.

Reports indicate that at an average of around Rs. 36,800 is being spent by any Indian household in non medical treatment for cancer. The catastrophic expenditure in the treatment is due to poor facility in the public healthcare sector, and poor designing of the healthcare policies. Figure 5 shows the average hospitalization expenditure for different sections.

Table 8. Accuracy of Bayesian Model

Test Set	Predicted Value (Accuracy of Model)	
	Dead	Alive
95% CI Low	55.45%	65.12%
95% CI High	86.63%	82.81%

Source: Created by the Author, Based on the dataset

Figure 19. Average Healthcare Expenses
Source: Rajpal, Kumar, Joe (2018)

Background characteristics	Average Hospitalization Expenditure			
	Public sector		Private sector	
	Medical	Total	Medical	Total
Age				
0–5 years	19805	30041	55136	61096
6–14 years	32391	36577	56102	67044
15–24 years	18083	20947	97068	100445
25–59 years	31084	36665	85441	91156
60+ years	16758	19912	65060	71936
Sex				
Male	22782	27427	101194	108062
Female	26448	30835	64562	70235
Education				
Illiterate	17641	23176	51754	57130
Primary	20495	24760	88644	93358
Secondary	20057	23413	37718	41202
Higher	37331	42232	121714	133020
MPCE quintile				
Lowest	-	-	-	-
Second	22064	27308	44500	48083
Third	21667	24226	44948	48857
Fourth	23117	27138	83933	92169
Highest	28645	34638	89809	95422
Social group				
Scheduled tribe	8596	10941	103079	108338
Scheduled caste	24306	27977	48389	53502
Other backward classes	23710	29528	74766	80430
Others	29994	34015	94923	103361
Place of residence				
Rural	26897	32202	72654	77903
Urban	20686	24044	86941	94443
All India	24523	29066	78045	84320

Figure 20. Average Healthcare Expenses
Source: Rajpal, Kumar, Joe (2018)

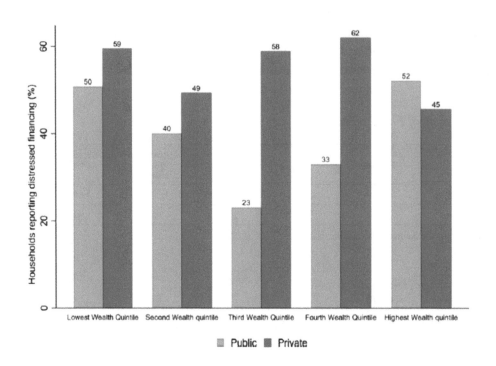

The result shows that the average healthcare expenditure in the public sector domain is around Rs. 29,000 and the same for private sector domain is Rs. 84,320. The high inclination in the private healthcare sector can be explained by the unavailability of proper facility in the public sector thus many people opting for higher expense but more assurance in the survival rates.

The financial hardship is also observed in the families with low household incomes. Around 50% families from low quintile income sector has a huge proportion of distressed income. The figures which shows high support of distressed financing is not a good indicator for a family as well as the country. Figures showing that around 40% families go through distressed income and around 50% household finds hardship to ensure medical support in private healthcare sector.

Increase in the count of cancer and the related medical expenses are now a major public health concern. The higher burden of expense is on the elderly people and the current scenario demands strong requirement of public healthcare facilities. The private healthcare sections attract major number of patients due to better facilities and economically higher families go for that sector while the households with relatively low family household income rely on the public healthcare treatment, our statements is also being supported by the research of Chatterjee, Roy, and Sinha, 2018. Various studies suggest that maximum cancer cases can be successfully cured if they are detected in right stages and go through proper treatment. The treatment have to ensure that the patient's survivorship will depend on the early detection i.e. in stage I and II, but on the contrary the early detection rate in India is mere 20% - 30% in early stages.

CONCLUSION

In this paper we took a deeper look into various aspects of cancer and how it can be treated in the preliminary stages and how can machine learning and advancements of artificial intelligence can help us to prevent cancer and how can the medicos treatment take the right path. Initially in section 1, we have introduced with the background history of cancer and subsequently various types of cancer has been defined in the following sections. In section 2, we have took a closer look in to the machine learning part in cancer treatment and following that various machine learning algorithms have been discussed with its mathematical background. Then the need of feature selection algorithm is been discussed and algorithms are also being taken care. In the next section cancer healthcare analytics have been draws. A patient flow model has been created along with bed model simulation which will certainly help the patients to be mentally prepared for their queue time in the hospital or OPDs. Next, a risk analysis has been carried out on the chemotherapy treatment model, where the risk associated with the treatment is shown and analyzed. Finally, an econometric view of expenses in cancer treatment is shown and what are the changes can be made to make better condition is also being suggested.

ACKNOWLEDGMENT

We would like to thank Mr. Aniruddha Mandal, of The Neotia University, Department of Computer Science and Engineering, 1st Year for his invaluable contribution in this paper. He processed all the images and graphs included in this paper. I, Ahan Chatterjee thank him on the behalf of the entire team.

REFERENCES

4.   Alharthi, H. (2018). Healthcare predictive analytics: An overview with a focus on Saudi Arabia. *Journal of Infection and Public Health*, *11*(6), 749–756. doi:10.1016/j.jiph.2018.02.005 PMID:29526444

27. Asri, H., Mousannif, H., Al Moatassime, H., & Noel, T. (2016). Using machine learning algorithms for breast cancer risk prediction and diagnosis. *Procedia Computer Science*, *83*, 1064–1069. doi:10.1016/j.procs.2016.04.224

6.   Botje, D., Ten Asbroek, G., Plochg, T., Anema, H., Kringos, D. S., Fischer, C., Wagner, C., & Klazinga, N. S. (2016). Are performance indicators used for hospital quality management: A qualitative interview study amongst health professionals and quality managers in The Netherlands. *BMC Health Services Research*, *16*(1), 1–9. doi:10.118612913-016-1826-3 PMID:27733194

10. Dash, S., Shakyawar, S. K., Sharma, M., & Kaushik, S. (2019). Big data in healthcare: Management, analysis and future prospects. *Journal of Big Data*, *6*(1), 54. doi:10.118640537-019-0217-0

9.   England, N. H. S. (2019). *Clinically-led Review of NHS Access Standards: Interim Report from the NHS National Medical Director*. NHS England.

16. Islam, M. S., Hasan, M. M., Wang, X., & Germack, H. D. (2018, June). A systematic review on healthcare analytics: Application and theoretical perspective of data mining. *Health Care*, 6(2), 54. PMID:29882866

19. Kourou, K., Exarchos, T. P., Exarchos, K. P., Karamouzis, M. V., & Fotiadis, D. I. (2015). Machine learning applications in cancer prognosis and prediction. *Computational and Structural Biotechnology Journal*, 13, 8–17. doi:10.1016/j.csbj.2014.11.005 PMID:25750696

17. Kritchanchai, D., & Hoeur, S. (2018). Simulation modeling for facility allocation of outpatient department. *International Journal of Healthcare Management*, 11(3), 193–201. doi:10.1080/20479700.2 017.1359920

7. Kumari, M., & Singh, V. (2018). Breast cancer prediction system. *Procedia Computer Science*, 132, 371–376. doi:10.1016/j.procs.2018.05.197

18. Liang, B., Turkcan, A., Ceyhan, M. E., & Stuart, K. (2015). Improvement of chemotherapy patient flow and scheduling in an outpatient oncology clinic. *International Journal of Production Research*, 53(24), 7177–7190. doi:10.1080/00207543.2014.988891

13. Liu, H., Liu, L., & Zhang, H. (2010). Ensemble gene selection by grouping for microarray data classification. *Journal of Biomedical Informatics*, 43(1), 81–87. doi:10.1016/j.jbi.2009.08.010 PMID:19699316

15. Maher, J., Petchey, L., Greenfield, D., Levitt, G., & Fraser, M. (2018). Implementation of nationwide cancer survivorship plans: Experience from the UK. *Journal of Cancer Policy*, 15, 76–81. doi:10.1016/j. jcpo.2018.01.002

20. McCarthy, M., Gonzalez-Izquierdo, A., Sherlaw-Johnson, C., Khachatryan, A., Coleman, M. P., & Rachet, B. (2008). Comparative indicators for cancer network management in England: Availability, characteristics and presentation. *BMC Health Services Research*, 8(1), 45. doi:10.1186/1472-6963-8-45 PMID:18304315

21. Mihaylov, I., Nisheva, M., & Vassilev, D. (2019). Application of machine learning models for survival prognosis in breast cancer studies. *Information*, 10(3), 93. doi:10.3390/info10030093

3. Racz, J. M., Holloway, C. M. B., Huang, W., & Hong, N. L. (2016). Improving patient flow and timeliness in the diagnosis and management of breast abnormalities: The impact of a rapid diagnostic unit. *Current Oncology (Toronto, Ont.)*, 23(3), e260. doi:10.3747/co.23.3017 PMID:27330363

12. Rajpal, S., Kumar, A., & Joe, W. (2018). Economic burden of cancer in India: Evidence from cross-sectional nationally representative household survey, 2014. *PLoS One*, 13(2), e0193320. doi:10.1371/ journal.pone.0193320 PMID:29481563

11. Ramachandran, P., Girija, N., Bhuvaneswari, T., Enathur, K., & Ponneri, C. (2013). Cancer spread pattern-an analysis using classification and prediction techniques. *Cancer*, 2(6).

8. Seow, H., Snyder, C. F., Mularski, R. A., Shugarman, L. R., Kutner, J. S., Lorenz, K. A., Wu, A. W., & Dy, S. M. (2009). A framework for assessing quality indicators for cancer care at the end of life. *Journal of Pain and Symptom Management*, 38(6), 903–912. doi:10.1016/j.jpainsymman.2009.04.024 PMID:19775860

14. Stafinski, T., & Menon, D. (2017). Explicating social values for resource allocation decisions on new cancer technologies: We, the jury, find···. *Journal of Cancer Policy*, *14*, 5–10. doi:10.1016/j.jcpo.2017.09.002

23. Stojadinovic, A., Nissan, A., Eberhardt, J., Chua, T. C., Pelz, J. O., & Esquivel, J. (2011). Development of a Bayesian Belief Network Model for personalized prognostic risk assessment in colon carcinomatosis. *The American Surgeon*, *77*(2), 221–230. doi:10.1177/000313481107700225 PMID:21337884

26. Suss, S., Bhuiyan, N., Demirli, K., & Batist, G. (2017). Toward implementing patient flow in a cancer treatment center to reduce patient waiting time and improve efficiency. *Journal of Oncology Practice / American Society of Clinical Oncology*, *13*(6), e530–e537. doi:10.1200/JOP.2016.020008 PMID:28471694

1. Wait, S., Han, D., Muthu, V., Oliver, K., Chrostowski, S., Florindi, F., ... Wierinck, L. (2017). Towards sustainable cancer care: Reducing inefficiencies, improving outcomes—A policy report from the All. Can initiative. *Journal of Cancer Policy*, *13*, 47–64. doi:10.1016/j.jcpo.2017.05.004

5. Wang, J. C., Huan, S. K., Kuo, J. R., Lu, C. L., Lin, H., & Shen, K. H. (2011). A multivariable logistic regression equation to evaluate prostate cancer. *Journal of the Formosan Medical Association*, *110*(11), 695–700. doi:10.1016/j.jfma.2011.09.005 PMID:22118313

24. Wongthanavasu, S. (2011). A Bayesian Belief Network Model for Breast Cancer Diagnosis. In *Operations Research Proceedings 2010* (pp. 3–8). Springer. doi:10.1007/978-3-642-20009-0_1

2. Zhou, X., Liu, K. Y., & Wong, S. T. (2004). Cancer classification and prediction using logistic regression with Bayesian gene selection. *Journal of Biomedical Informatics*, *37*(4), 249–259. doi:10.1016/j.jbi.2004.07.009 PMID:15465478

22. Zoullouti, B., Amghar, M., & Nawal, S. (2019). Using Bayesian Networks for Risk Assessment in Healthcare System. In *Bayesian Networks-Advances and Novel Applications*. IntechOpen. doi:10.5772/intechopen.80464

Chapter 8
Machine Learning Perspective in Cancer Research

Aman Sharma

IT Department, Jaypee University of Information Technology, Solan, India

Rinkle Rani

ⓘ https://orcid.org/0000-0002-5970-1026

Computer Science and Engineering Department, Thapar Institute of Engineering and Technology, Patiala, India

ABSTRACT

Advancement in genome sequencing technology has empowered researchers to think beyond their imagination. Researchers are trying their hard to fight against various genetic diseases like cancer. Artificial intelligence has empowered research in the healthcare sector. Moreover, the availability of opensource healthcare datasets has motivated the researchers to develop applications which can help in early diagnosis and prognosis of diseases. Further, next-generation sequencing (NGS) has helped to look into detailed intricacies of biological systems. It has provided an efficient and cost-effective approach with higher accuracy. The advent of microRNAs also known as small noncoding genes has begun the paradigm shift in oncological research. We are now able to profile expression profiles of RNAs using RNA-seq data. microRNA profiling has helped in uncovering their relationship in various genetic and biological processes. Here in this chapter, the authors present a review of the machine learning perspective in cancer research.

INTRODUCTION

Bioinformatics is playing a vital role in fighting against various stringent diseases such as cancer, diabetics, Alzheimer's, etc.. Cancer is one of the genetic diseases caused due to mutation and variation in genes of the patient's cells. Complexity in tumor microenvironment makes cancer difficult disease from the treatment perspective. Patients with homogeneous cancer type show heterogeneous responses toward the same type of targeted therapies. Clinical trials and the traditional drug discovery process is

DOI: 10.4018/978-1-7998-2742-9.ch008

a time demanding and tedious task. Hence, researchers are trying their hard to design optimal treatment options for such stringent diseases. Availability of huge amount of oncological and pharmacogenomics online data sources have boosted the research in this field. Unlike traditional statistical and computational approaches, bioinformaticians are using artificial intelligence and machine learning to improve the treatment options in genetic diseases.

Cells are the basic building block of all living organisms. There are different types of cells available in the human body such as blood cells, muscle cells, fat cells, etc. Genes are responsible for variation in these cells. Gene helps to carry heredity information and are responsible for various physical and functional processes in the body. Genes are responsible for heterogeneity in genotype and phenotype traits among species. All the information regarding the inheritance of phenotypic traits is carried by genes. Overall if one wants to fight against genetic disease then their root cause i.e. genes need to be studied. Advancement in computational biology and high throughput sequencing is helping to find biomarkers (genes) which are responsible for various diseases.

Further, chip technology in healthcare is considered as the future of the healthcare industry which also provided lab-on-a-chip devices. These chips help in proper diagnosis and prognosis of patients based on their genetic profiles. Various researchers are working in the field of genetics to identify genes which are responsible for the inheritance of diseases. Microarray technology helps to measure the gene expression levels of particular micro-environment. Along with gene expression data, we can collect (genome, transcriptome, and proteome) data such as copy number variations, gene mutation, etc.. Gene expression, drug response data is extensively used in identifying anti-cancer drugs, drug targets, and biomarkers. Some researchers are working to explore various biological pathways corresponding to genetic diseases.

The ratio of the expression level of an individual gene under two variable conditions, obtained by DNA microarray hybridization is called gene expression value. The quantity of mRNA released by gene determines the gene expression value of the individual gene. This quantity may vary based on external stimuli. mRNA helps to carry the information from the genes about protein synthesis. Gene expression data is an asset to various biological research outcomes. It maps the genotype traits to phenotype traits and hence helps to differentiate between various phenotype articulations. It is used to distinguish between different disease phenotypes and identify potential disease biomarkers. Machine learning models take this data as input from genomic assays like m-RNA, DNase-seq, MNase-seq. Active research on various chronic diseases like cancer has exploited its potential and waved various new research outcomes.

Cancer is a complex genetic disease involving various subtypes. There is a need to develop computational approaches which could aid in early diagnosis and prognosis of tumor subtypes. Over the past decade, oncological research has gained serious attention and researchers are trying to personalize treatment therapies for cancer patients (Błaszczyński & Stefanowski, 2015). Apart from biomarker identification researchers are also working for developing computational (in-silico) models/algorithms that can predict disease-specific drug responses, drug synergy, and drug-target interactions.

Many researchers are using supervised and unsupervised machine learning algorithms to solve biological research problems. There are specifically three stages for any supervised machine learning method. First stage deal with the development of a machine learning algorithm that can lead to successful learning. The second stage provides the algorithm with a large amount of data to build a machine learning model. The Model is the generalized summary of rules that came out from the input data set. Third, if any new data point is given to the algorithm, it should predict the label corresponding to it (e.g. classification problems). Whereas, in unsupervised learning, data points are given but no labels are provided. The problem is to partition the data point in such a way that there should be maximum relevance and minimum redundancy.

APPLICATION OF GENOMIC DATA USING MACHINE LEARNING

Microarray data analysis deals with gene classification, clustering using statistical approaches. Apart from statistical approaches, machine learning algorithms such as Support Vector Machine (SVM), Neural Networks, Decision Tree, and Random Forest are also used for microarray data analysis. Moreover, various computational approaches using machine learning are proposed in the literature for drug synergy prediction, drug response prediction, and drug-target interaction prediction and biomarker identification. All these computational approaches help in identifying potential drug molecules for various diseases. Cancer is one of the most researched diseases which have gained huge attention from academia and pharmacy industries.

Cancer Classification

Gene expression profiles have been used from decades for interpreting biological significance and correlation of genes with diseases. These profiles are obtained under different biological environments and from a variety of patients. To obtain better insight into the disease state, these expression profiles are compared between normal and diseased environment. Quantity of mRNA produced by a gene in a particular condition describes the gene expression or state (active or inactive) of a gene. Advancement in biological computational techniques has sparked analysis of microarray data and further research on cancer classification. Classification of tumor samples and their subtypes serves great importance in diagnosis and prognosis of different types of cancer. It helps in the precise prediction of cancer types and further identifying sub-type specific drug treatments.

Various authors have proposed different classification techniques using gene expression data (Lu & Han, 2003). These methods vary from statistical approaches to machine learning algorithms for cancer classification. High dimensional nature of gene expression data makes classification an arduous task; hence genes selection is a preliminary step in most of the classifiers (Okun, 2013). It helps in improving time complexity and classification accuracy by filtering irrelevant features. However, existing "feature selection algorithms" suffers from constraints of scalability and generalization; also classifier build using one feature selection method on a given data may not be able to give accurate results on new datasets. In such a scenario Deep Neural Networks (DNN) can help in automatic feature extraction and build generalized and scalable classifiers.

Technological advancement in DNA-microarray has widely pushed the research in bioinformatics. Further, with the introduction of NGS (Next Generation Sequencing) we can sequence the whole genome structure of any individual. Scientists are performing parallel screening of gnomonic data to fetch the hidden patterns which could help in drug discovery. Such a parallel screening helps to identify gene-gene relationships, potential biomarkers for different genetic diseases and genetic mutations/alterations. This parallel screening helps to early detect various stringent diseases such as cancer. Over the last two decades, various bioinformaticians have collaborated to contribute to open-source tumor data sets (Alon et al., 1999; Golub et al., 1999; Van't Veer et al., 2002) to boost cancer research. These datasets are generally microarray data of thousands of genes for different tissues (Patients). These are used as benchmark datasets to carry out data analysis/prediction for personalized medication and cancer classification. Machine learning is also used to exploit the potential of these datasets. Various researchers have proposed cancer classification techniques using machine learning (Chu et al., 2005; Furlanello et al., 2003; Guyon et al., 2002; Shevade & Sathiya Keerthi, 2003). Machine learning majorly focuses on identifying hidden patterns in data that could help to generalize the biological process/system. The key idea in cancer classification is to improve the prediction accuracy of the classification model and to find a minimum set of potential gene biomarkers.

Although all this seems to very interesting and easy the reality is that there are many key issues involved while designing the biological predictive modeling. Genes identification for tumor sub-type analysis is a tedious task as it depends on feature selection algorithms. These feature selection algorithms are dependent on optimization algorithms or statistical approaches which need to be defined very carefully for proper results. Broadly feature selection algorithms are categorized as a filter, wrapper, and hybrid methods. Filter method depends on the statistical background on data to identify the key genes which could serve as biomarkers (Saeys et al., 2007). Wrapper methods depend on suitable learning approach to filter out the most relevant genes (Saeys et al., 2007). Wrapper methods have the benefit of delivering higher accuracy (Inza et al., 2004).

Microarray data suffers from the issue of high-dimensionality and this makes cancer classification non-deterministic polynomial-time (NP-hard) problem. To solve such problems meta-heuristic algorithms are treated as an optimal choice (Saeys et al., 2007). Multi-objective functions are the real beauty of these algorithms as they help to find the global best solution. Conflicts between different objective functions have been resolved to fetch the optimal results. Many of these algorithms are bio-inspired optimization algorithms (Boussaï, 2013; Chakraborty & Kar, 2017; Li et al., 2008; Shen et al., 2008). Broadly they are classified as posterior-based (Marler & Arora, 2004) and prior-based (Branke et al., 2004) approaches. The concept of weighted multi-objective functions is used in prior approaches. Posterior approaches focus on the performance of problem for finding an optimal solution.

Drug Synergy Prediction

Targeted drug therapy is the most commonly used treatment given to cancer patients. These drugs are specially designed based on their targets which help to suppress cancer. These targets are known as anti-oncogene which is responsible for tumor suppression by suppressing mitosis (cell-division) (Weinberg, 1991). Any alteration, changes in these genes lead to uncontrollable cell growth. Unlike these genes, there are oncogenes which promote tumor growth. Most of the targeted drug therapies are designed considering oncogenes as anti-oncogenes are hard to target. Various studies revealed the resistance of targeted drug therapies and hence results in nonresponsive drug behavior (Knoechel et al., 2014; Rini & Atkins, 2009). This resistance may have occurred because of many reasons such as cell death inhibition, change in drug targets, etc.. Heterogeneous tumor microenvironment can also result in drug resistance (Housman et al., 2014). Combination drug therapy is considered a better alternative to avoid drug resistance. It helps in overcoming the drug resistance by delaying the tumor growth. It includes the usage of two or more drugs in fixed-dose proportion and as a single-dose formulation. Combination therapy is showing excellent results in tumor suppression by reducing the chances of multiple mutations (Fitzgerald et al., 2006) and single mutation (Cokol et al., 2011) that can escape all the drugs. Additionally, combination therapy helps in lowering drug dosage, side-effects (Fitzgerald et al., 2006). Combination of two or more drugs is considered effective if the tumor suppression rate of combination is higher than individual drugs. Such a combination of drugs is known as synergistic drugs otherwise antagonistic. The proposition of dose also matters in drug synergy, we cannot mix them in any random proportions. Quantify drug synergy is a very complex task but still few researchers have given metrics to measure it. Some of the quantitative methods for drug synergy are the Bliss independence model (Foucquier & Guedj, 2015), Dose equivalence, Isobolographic analysis (Tallarida, 2011) and Chou-Talalay (Ashton, 2015).

Drug Response Prediction

Cancer is a genetic disease caused due to mutation and variation in genes of the tumor cells. Genes are responsible for various cellular activities; hence mutation in genes directly affects cellular functioning. Most of the mutations occur because of exposure to an unfavourable environment which promotes tumor growth. Complexity in tumor microenvironment makes cancer difficult disease from the treatment perspective. Patients with the same type of cancer show heterogeneous treatment responses toward the same type of targeted therapies. Such differences in responses are because of genetic variations among individuals. We cannot provide optimal cancer treatment options just based on their anatomical origin. Precision medicine aims to consider the individual's genomic profile to provide tailor treatment options that could control cancer progression (Xiao et al., 2014). Identification of optimal treatment for various types of cancers is a challenging task; still, researchers are trying their hard to make the ends meet.

Various large-scale throughput drug screenings have been performed to reveal the relationship between genomic profiles and drug responses. These screens provide pharmacogenomics datasets, including a large number of human cancer cell lines and their corresponding drug responses. Genomics of Drug Sensitivity in Cancer (GDSC) (Garnett et al., 2012)and Cancer Cell Line Encyclopedia (CCLE) (Barretina et al., 2012) are two such large-scale databases aim to promote oncological research. These datasets help in predicting drug (responses/combinations/repositioning) and play a very critical role in modern-day drug discovery. There is a need to develop computational methods which could utilize these large-scale screening datasets and build effective predictive models. One of the important tasks is to predict potential drugs for a given cell-line by exploiting the relationship between existing cancerous genomic profiles and their drug responses.

Recently several machine learning approaches have been proposed to predict anti-cancer drug responses and their potential genomic biomarkers in cancerous profiles. These approaches are based on the common assumption that similar drugs (similarity in chemical structure) will have similar drug-targets. Most of the methods defined in literature exploit the drugs structure similarity and similarity in cell-lines (genomic characterization). Random forest and elastic net regularization are most frequently used machine learning algorithms to predict drug sensitivity (response) in cancerous cell lines. Apart from these machines learning algorithms matrix factorization technique has been used recently to predict toxicological drug responses (Yamada et al., 2017). This method is mostly used in recommender systems where there are a group of users (P) and items (Q). Ratings are given to each item by an individual user. There might be some missing ratings in the final response matrix. The task of recommender based systems is to predict the missing entries or new ones. Matrix factorization solves this problem by finding some latent features (k) that determines the relationship between users and items. This method has numerous application areas, such as computer vision, Image processing, recommender systems, and computational biology. In general practice matrix factorization is to find low-rank matrices P&Q, such that $P \times QT \gg R$, where R is our target response matrix. P and Q are calculated in such a way that k should be kept minimum $(k<m,n)$. Stochastic gradient descent is the most commonly used method for finding matrices P and Q. Regular-

ization is also one of the most important parts of matrix factorization as it helps in avoiding over-fitting. Matrix factorization has shown significant performance in recommendation based applications and other research domains. Jamali et al. have proposed trust prorogation based models for the recommendation within social networks (Jamali & Ester, 2010). Makoto et al. have proposed convex factorization method for predicting toxic drug responses (Yamada et al., 2017). Moreover, various complex predictions related to brain activities, bioinformatics are also performed using regularized factorization methods (Wang et al., 2017). Similarity-based matrix factorization technique has gained much attention among researchers working in the domain of image processing, computational biology. The idea is to consider similarity among users(pi-pj similarity) and item(qi-qj similarity) as the important parameters for predicting the final target response. Based on this notion we can exploit this technique to predict optimal drug responses by considering similarity among drugs (chemical structure) and cell-lines (genomic characterization).

Drug-Target Interaction Prediction

Drug discovery involves finding new drugs and their potential targets. Identifying such drug-target interaction out of pool of drug and targets is a tedious task. Current research on drugs aims to repurpose an already existing drug for new diseases and targets. Repurposing a drug for new disease and target helps in saving time and money as the repurposed drugs are already approved. Drug-target interactions involve two sets of agents: Chemical compounds from the drug set and Protein (amino acid) form a target set. This research problem has a vital role in discovering new drugs and to recognize new potential targets of it. They play an important role to understand the mechanism of drugs and their side effects. However, there exist some key issues related to drug discovery such as drug resistance, time-consuming clinical trials, and toxicity towards patients. Heterogeneous drug effects on different people (Evans & McLeod, 2003; Wei et al., 2008) and to map drug effect with the drug interaction pathway (Kotelnikova et al., 2010) is one of the issues discussed in literature.

We can predict Drug-target interactions using either of the two methods: clinical/experimental (in vivo) or with the help of computational (in silico) methods. These methods are further classified into four broad categories: Docking methods (Rarey et al., 1996; Xie et al., 2011), ligand-based methods (Jacob & Vert, 2008), literature text mining (Zhu et al., 2005) and pharmacogenomics methods (Wang et al., 2011; Yamanishi et al., 2008). Clinical methods are time-consuming, tiresome and even difficult to reproduce (Fakhraei et al., 2014). However, clinical docking methods are well-accepted methods and more reliable than others but it as some major drawbacks because of the unavailability of the 3-D structure of proteins and time-consuming simulations. These methods take information about protein 3-D structure into consideration and then approximate the possibility of using simulations that if it will interact with the given drug or not. There exist some more methods known as ligand-based that use the similarity between targets (ligands). But due to the lack of proper information about target ligands of these methods they are not so popular. One another method Literature text mining explore literature to find out the relationship between the given drug and target. However, they also suffer from limited available information that exists for predicting new interactions. The next category i.e. pharmacogenomics utilizes features of drugs' and targets' simultaneously to find out potential drug-target interactions. These approaches investigate computational methods such as machine learning technique and kernel-based similarity approaches to decrease the problem related to the complexity involved in DTI. In recent research, for the prediction of DTI, various computational methods have been proposed (van Laarhoven et al., 2011; Zheng et al., 2013). Various online databases are available that provide access to the data related to compounds and target proteins. PubChem (Bolton et al., 2008) consists of 35 million compounds but, approximately 7000 compounds possess information regarding target protein. There are several other databases such as DrugBank (Knox et al., 2010), ChEMBL (Gaulton et al., 2011), KEGG DRUG (Kanehisa et al., 2011). These databases help to boost the research related to DTI. Various researches have used these databases in their studies to identify novel drug-target interactions (Yamanishi et al., 2008).

CHALLENGES IN HEALTHCARE PREDICTIVE ANALYSIS

1. High dimensionality and imbalance class problem: Cancer data classiðcation suffers from several issues like high dimensionality, imbalanced class problem. High dimensionality in data refers to the presence of an exceptionally large number of features as compared to samples. To deal with high dimensionality feature selection algorithms are designed. There are various methods and techniques (Bolón-Canedo et al., 2016; Hira & Gillies, 2015) proposed in the literature for feature selection. However, still, no generic approach is developed which could handle all types of datasets and domains.

In class imbalance problem there is miss-match between the numbers of samples available for each class. It results in the biasedness of predictive models towards majority class samples. Various researchers have contributed solutions to this problem (Haixiang et al., 2017; Krawczyk et al., 2016). But most of the existing work on cancer data classification is done using binary imbalanced classes; there is a need to address the imbalance problem in multi-class paradigm.

2. Heterogeneity: Heterogeneity of drug responses to cancer patients with the same cancer type has raised a major challenge of precision medication (Dagogo-Jack & Shaw, 2018). There is a need to develop a drug prediction model which could help in strengthening the present status of precision medication. There is no effective method to predict the drug responses of individual patients precisely and reliably. Genetic instability and variations among individuals are responsible for varied drug responses.

3. Further, there is a need to propose a computationally efficient feature selection technique that could eliminate the need for the data cleaning procedures while generating high cancer prediction accuracy with an optimal set of protein properties for drug design.

4. Scalability: Gene classiðcation suffers from the issue of feature selection. There is a need to develop scalable feature selection methodology which could consider maximum genetic aberrations simultaneously and efficiently (Tadist et al., 2019). There is a need to predict sensitive drugs for individual patients. As cancer is a complex disease and its complexity varies from patient to patient and one cannot rely on generalized medication and hence a scalable drug sensitivity criterion need to be taken into consideration.

5. Drug Synergy Prediction: Machine learning capabilities for optimal drug synergy prediction are unexplored hence relevant machine learning models need to be developed for the proper diagnosis and treatment of stringent diseases like cancer. Drug synergism helps in designing novel drug combinations which could complement each other to suppress the progression of the disease. There is a need to extract potential drug combination features to understand drug-disease interaction in a holistic manner.

6. Next Generation Sequencing (NGS): Analyzing NGS dataset using machine learning is also one of the biggest challenges that researchers are facing. Advancement in genome sequencing technology has empowered researchers to think beyond their imagination. Next-generation sequencing has helped to look into detailed intricacies of biological systems. It has provided an efficient and cost-effective approach with higher accuracy. Advent of microRNAs also known as small non-coding genes has begun the paradigm shift in oncological research. We are now able to profile expression profiles of RNAs using RNA-seq data. microRNA profiling is helping in uncovering their relationship in various genetic and biological processes.

FUTURE OF HEALTHCARE PREDICTIVE ANALYSIS

In this section, we will discuss the future of anti-cancer drug prediction approaches in context to big data and Next Generation Sequencing (NGS). We will discuss the use of deep learning in anti-cancer drug prediction and how it will help to foster the research in this domain.

MicroRNAS

microRNAs are small non-coding RNAs that bind to 3 UTR regions of their target mRNA. They are newly discovered types of RNAs, shorter in length as compared to other RNAs. Generally, mature microRNAs are single-stranded and 18-24 nucleotide long. They play an important role in controlling the post transcription regulation of coding genes, either by degrading them or inhibiting their translation. Translation is post transcription cellular mechanism for protein synthesis with the help of ribosomes. Ribosomes decode the mRNA produced by DNA transcription. On the other hand, degradation is the process of ceasing mRNA translation. Their initial research gained momentum because of the keen interest of some researchers but later they were identified as a predominant component in cellular mechanism. Each microRNA has been identified as a controller of a wide range of target genes (Bartel, 2009). These microRNAs regulate mRNAs but there is also a regulatory body known as polymerase-2 which regulates microRNAs (Lee et al., 2004; Xie et al., 2005). It is an enzyme used in the catalysis of DNA transcription during the synthesis of microRNA and other RNAs. Biological synthesis of microRNA is a seamlessly regulated process where multiple sub-processes are involved.

High Throughput Sequencing(HTS)

High throughput sequencing(HTS) is the use of modern technologies in the field of sequencing. It is also popularly known by another name, that is Next-generation sequencing(NGS). Advancement in computational capabilities has brought a radical change in the field of genome sequencing. These HTS technologies can generate a large amount of biological data at a much faster rate and in a cost-effective manner. We can perform deep sequencing and quantification of complete genome sequence transcriptomes. HTS has led to evolutionary insight into various biological processes and macromolecules identification. These sequencing technologies are used to profile various genomic profiles to reveal the underlying biological aspects and interactions. It has provided the ability to look into interactions between proteomes, transcriptomes and genomes. HTS technology has fostered research in characterizing small RNA transcriptomes. There are various platforms and technologies such as Illumina (Solexa), SOLID sequencing for HTS. RNA-seq is the most widely used RNA sequencing method using HTS, it allows wide-scale transcriptome analysis with higher resolution and lesser errors. Mostly RNA-seq experiments are based on common protocol. The basic principle for NGS is identical to Electrophoresis sequencing, the only difference lies in the incorporation of parallelization in the sequencing of DNA fragments by NGS. Illumina sequencing is the most preferred chemistry in academics and industry because of its accuracy. In RNA-seq experiments firstly complete RNA is extracted from sample under consideration

Figure 1. Biogenesis of microRNA. Image from Olga Barca-Mayo et al. (Lu & Barca, 2012)

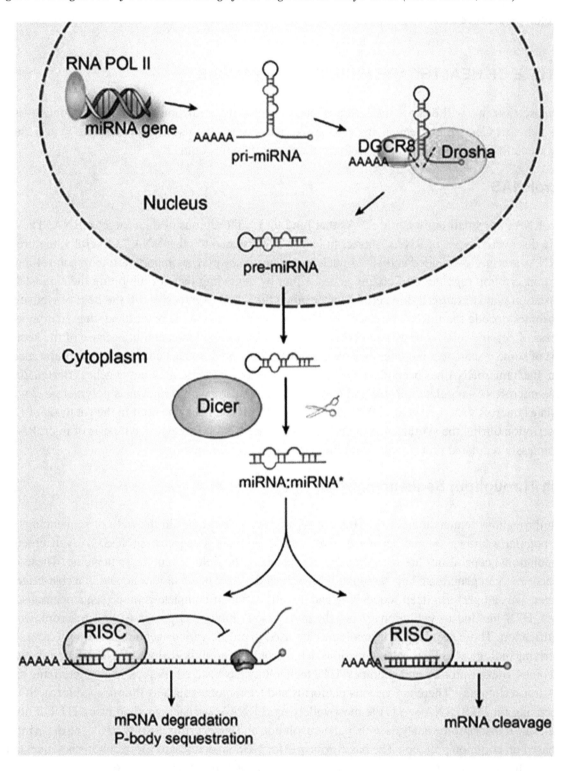

and further, it can be profiled to fetch individual microRNAs and mRNAs before library preparation. There are various steps involved in library preparation such as RNA fragmentation, reverse transcription, amplification, quantification, and quality control. Further, we can perform downstream analysis of fetched sequences to find differential expressions, novel transcripts (Mortazavi & Brian, 2008).

Importance of HTS Over Microarray

Microarray technology is serving the biological community from the last two decades, researchers have found their expertise in this technology hence most of the traditional sequencing was based on hybridization profiling. But with the advancement in Next-generation sequencing (NGS) technology and reduction in its cost has pushed researchers interest in it. NGS has the advantage of delivering more accurate profiling results as compared to microarray technology. Microarray has limitation in identifying novel microRNAs and moreover biasing in results can be introduced. Various comparative studies have identified NGS a better microRNA profiling approach as compared to microarray. Results showed that many microRNAs would have remained undetected if they used microarray technology (Murakami et al., 2014). Profiling of microRNA expressions using NGS serves potential in uncovering their relationship in many disease and predicting their role in precision medication.

MicroRNA as Cancer Biomarkers

As cancer is a stringent disease with complex and inexpedient diagnosis procedure, so an inefficient diagnosis can lead to serious health impact to patient. A cancer biomarker can be any variation in biological process, tissue, or molecules which can predict cancer or its subtype significantly (Daniel, 1996). So there is an urgent need for good cancer markers which could strengthen the present state of diagnosis. Various studies revealed microRNAs as potential biomarkers for diagnosis and prognosis of cancer (Garzon et al., 2010). microRNAs modulates their target genes (Ambros, 2003) by suppressing their normal expression state (Doench & Sharp, 2004; Zhang et al., 2002). microRNAs can serve as biomarkers for different kinds of cancer. The presence of circulating microRNA (plasma and serum) in blood tissues of cancer patients has embossed it as an optimal diagnostic marker (Kosaka et al., 2010). Other than these microRNA biomarkers, urinary microRNA are also considered potentially viable for prostatic cancer (Ploussard & de la Taille, 2010). Recent advancement in high throughput technologies have raised the possibility of easy identification of microRNA and their targets. Assays/Sequences generated through these technologies are platform-independent and provides better analytical and statistical inference. Table 1. describes the various microRNAs as potential cancer diagnostic biomarkers in blood.

Recent Research Related to MicroRNA in Cancer

As we have already discussed the significant role of microRNA in various diseases and drug therapies, still identification of novel microRNAs and their targets is a challenging issue. Although various tools and pipelines have been developed but inconsistency between their results and no standardized approach has raised a serious issue among researchers in this field. Still, researchers are trying their hard to relate these newly identified disease predictors with targeted drug therapies. Recently microRNA 374b is identified as a resistive agent in pancreatic cancer drug therapy (Schreiber et al., 2016). The major goal of new generation drug prediction is to predict novel drugs that could be useful in a wide range of diseases. The

Table 1. microRNAs as potential Cancer Diagnostic Biomarkers in Blood

S.No	Cancer Type	microRNAs	Author (s)
1	Pancreas	miR - 2001, 200b, 210, 155, 18 a	Li A., et al. (Li et al., 2010); Ho AS, et al. (Allen, 2010); Wang J, et al. (Wang et al., 2009); Morimura R, et al. (Morimura et al., 2011)
2	Prostate	miR - 141	Mitchell PS, et al. (Mitchell et al., 2008)
3	Breast	miR - 21,155,195 and let-71	Zhu W, et al. (Zhu et al., 2009); Heneghan HM, et al. (Heneghan et al., 2010); Asaga S (Asaga et al., 2011); Zhao H (Zhao et al., 2010)
4	Lung	miR - 21, 25, 126, 223, 155, 197 and 182	Chen X, et al. (Chen et al., 2008); Shen J, et al. (Shen et al., 2011); Zheng D, et al. (Zheng et al., 2011)
5	Ovarian	miR - 21, 141, 200c, 203, 205, 214, 200a, 200b, 92, 93, 126, 155, 127, 99b	Taylor DD, et al. (Taylor & Gercel-Taylor, 2008); Resnick KE, et al. (Resnick et al., 2009)
6	Gastric	miR - 17-5p, 106a, 106b, 32, 182, 143 and 21	Tsujiura M, et al. (Tsujiura et al., 2010); Li X, et al. (Li et al., 2011)
7	Liver	miR - 199, 195, 16, 500	Yamamoto Y, et al. (Yamamoto et al., 2009); Qu KZ, et al. (Qu et al., 2011)
8	Esophageal	miR - 223, 133a, 127-3p, 22, 10a, 100 and 148b	Zhang C, et al.(Zhang et al., 2010)
9	Squamous cell-Tongue	miR-184	Wong TS, et al. (Wong et al., 2008)
10	Colorectal	miR-92, 29, 17-3p	Ng EK, et al. (Ng et al., 2009); Huang Z, et al. (Huang et al., 2010)

Scripps Research Institute (TSRI) researchers have designed a drug that has shown tumor suppressor capabilities in breast cancer animal models (Velagapudi et al., 2016). Breast cancer is one of the most researched cancer type because of its intricacy and commonality among women, therefore deeper knowledge about its subtypes and drug therapies can help to fight against it. Circulating microRNAs have been identified as potential biomarkers for early detection of breast cancer (Hamam & Arwa, 2016). Recently a study revealed the deregulation of microRNAs in tumor environment and their role in cancer cell line (Rupaimoole et al., 2016). Laura Cantini, et al. have proposed a pipeline for subtype identification and analysis of colorectal cancer using an interaction network of mRNA-microRNA (Cantini et al., 2015).

MicoRNA Gene Prediction

microRNAs are essence and indeed need to present biomedical research. We have already discussed the importance and role of microRNAs in various biological systems. Many microRNAs have been identified but still many more to be discovered. Due to the limitation of biological experimental approaches microRNA identification suffers from serious bottleneck and hence efficient computational approaches are needed for identification and prediction of novel microRNAs. Most of the real-world problems are complex in nature, which makes them difficult to model.

ML approaches can help in modeling such complex problems and to incorporate data-driven decision-making capabilities in resultant models. We can apply ML approaches on microRNA data for their identification, their target genes and then further analysis of microRNA expression data. NGS has given a powerful platform for discovering new microRNAs and their targets. NGS platforms like Illumina/

Figure 2. Generalized Workflow for machine learning microRNA gene prediction

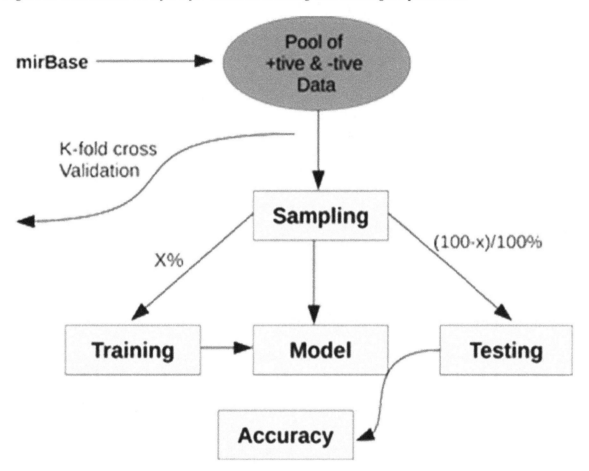

Solexa GA are popularly used platforms which give more accurate expression values as compared to hybridization-based technologies. As a result, significant improvement has been seen in microRNA identification and their targets. ML approaches can classify candidate target genes corresponding to identified microRNA. Classifiers such as Random Forest, SVM, and Decision Trees are used popularly. Figure 2 describes the generalized workflow for microRNA gene prediction using ML. The basic idea here is that ML will generalize the prediction rules based on the positive and negative data sets. A positive data set contains microRNA sequences which have been already identified and a negative dataset contains microRNA look-alike sequences, that are not microRNAs. Most of the available methods for microRNA gene prediction rely on structure similarity of the hairpin structure of pre-microRNA. They are based on the principle of homologous structure identification, if we could find microRNA in one genome, then there is a possibility of identifying it in another genome too. Homology modeling and ab-initio are presently available methods for microRNA prediction in bioinformatics. Homology technique is a simple method which predicts microRNAs based on existing information from already identified microRNAs. It is the sequence alignment technique, nothing new can be predicted regarding microRNAs.

There are various tools available based on homology technique and ML such as ProMir (Nam et al., 2005) and MirFinder (Huang et al., 2007). In contrast to homology-based methods, ab-initio methods are not similarity-based, they do not require any additional reference sequence for predicting microRNAs. Proper parameter selection can lead to the prediction of new microRNAs but if not selected properly can result in high false-positive predictions. Ab-initio methods also use ML capabilities and there are software such as MiPred (Kwang & Santosh, 2007), MiRenSVM (Ding et al., 2010), Triplet-SVM (Xue et al., 2005) based on it. The availability of a huge amount of biological data has raised the need for new data handling, prediction and classification algorithms. Traditional methods are no more reliable enough to handle such an enormous growth of data. In such a scenario ML approaches are considered an optimal choice for better results. ML approaches are used in various fields of bioinformatics such as genomics, proteomics, transcriptomics, and system biology. ML algorithms for prediction of microRNAs starts with training step to build an expert model. A model is designed based on the learning it gathers from sequence data, microRNA structure and intensity data of microRNAs. Based on learning from these features it can classify unknown sequence as microRNA or not. But these ML algorithms suffer from serious class imbalance problem and most of the algorithms consider fixed loop size stems, reducing the overall prediction accuracy. Learning in ML models for microRNA predictions is based on positive and negative data. Majority of the time these datasets are derived from mirBase (Kozomara & Griffiths-Jones, 2014), although a little of pre-processing is needed before actually using it.

Role of Deep Learning in MicroRNA Analysis in NGS

"Big Data" has been a buzz topic in the recent years, it has gained huge interest from academics as well as industry. Rate at which data is being produced has increased to many folds and so is the research in this field. Data related to bioinformatics has also evolved over many years. Increase in computational capabilities and the emergence of HTS technology has lead to sudden outburst of biomedical data. This data serves a great potential in identifying disease biomarkers, discovering new drugs, but unfortunately, it is not effectively utilized. NGS technologies have created a serious need for new technologies and algorithms. In such a scenario deep learning using neural networks are considered an effective choice. Although ML approaches have been used for many years but they have limitation of processing raw data. Deep learning is a new version of ML algorithms, that incorporate artificial intelligence using multilayer neural networks. In contrast to traditional ML approaches, deep learning can extract features from data itself. In efforts to apply deep learning algorithms to microRNA prediction, researchers have proposed various deep learning algorithms. Seunghyun Park, et al. have proposed deepMiRGene (Park et al., 2016) an algorithm to predict microRNA precursor. They used RNN, there is no need to input features manually, the algorithm automatically identifies features from input data. This approach leads to the discovery of various new features too which can be used in future research. Similarly Cheng S., et al. developed MiRTDL (Cheng et al., 2015) an algorithm for microRNA target prediction using CNN. It automatically extracts desired information from the data itself rather than relying on information fed manually. These algorithms have shown efficient results and have improved prediction results. The use of deep learning techniques in microRNA and their target prediction can help in novel microRNA predictions and one can investigate better knowledge about the underlying mechanism.

CONCLUSION AND FUTURE DIRECTIONS

Although various researchers are working in the field of anti-cancer drug prediction but still there are various possible future directions which are discussed in this section. Heterogeneous omic data can be considered to further improve the performance of cancer classification. In the case of drug synergy prediction, there is a need to extract potential drug combination features to understand drug-disease interaction in a holistic manner. The existing approaches can be validated in heterogeneous contexts involving a variety of cancer patients with distinctive genomic profiles. Genomic features of cell lines such as copy number variation, somatic mutation and pathways can be further considered in predicting drug responses. Multiple types of similarity measures can be used to improve the performance of existing approaches. In the future, predicting drug synergism can be extended for handling large datasets for scalability. Genomic data integration can be performed to further improve prediction results.

Further, apart from microarray data, we can use microRNAs which are small non-coding RNAs that bind to 3 UTR regions of their target mRNA. They play an important role in controlling the posttranslational regulation of coding genes, either by degrading them or inhibiting their translation. Various microRNA have been identified and many more to be discovered from a pool of genomic data. Various computational and statistical approaches are proposed to leverage the best results out of sequencing data. NGS technology is popularly used these days due to cost reduction, higher accuracy, as a result, we need efficient algorithms and pipelines which could cater to the present need. Machine learning and deep learning algorithms can prove useful in handling NGS data and develop biomedical applications. Using these technologies we can predict promising microRNA biomarkers which could later be used as drug targets for a variety of diseases. Hence microRNAs have paved the path for precision medication in fighting against cancer. Identifying novel and tissue-specific microRNA can help to differentiate significantly between healthy and diseased cell state. This paper attempts to highlight the possible application areas of anti-cancer drug prediction using machine learning, NGS data using machine learning and how microRNAs can help in better diagnosis and prognosis of cancer.

REFERENCES

72. Allen, S. (2010). Circulating mir-210 as a novel hypoxia marker in pancreatic cancer. *Translational Oncology*, *3*(2), 109–113. doi:10.1593/tlo.09256 PMID:20360935

5. Alon, U., Barkai, N., Notterman, D. A., Gish, K., Ybarra, S., Mack, D., & Levine, A. J. (1999). Broad patterns of gene expression revealed by clustering analysis of tumor and normal colon tissues probed by oligonucleotide arrays. *Proceedings of the National Academy of Sciences of the United States of America*, *96*(12), 6745–6750. doi:10.1073/pnas.96.12.6745 PMID:10359783

66. Ambros, V. (2003). Microrna pathways in ies and worms: Growth, death, fat, stress, and timing. *Cell*, *113*(6), 673–676. doi:10.1016/S0092-8674(03)00428-8 PMID:12809598

78. Asaga, S., Kuo, C., Nguyen, T., Terpenning, M., & Armando, E. (2011). Direct serum assay for microrna-21 concentrations in early and advanced breast cancer. *Clinical Chemistry*, *57*(1), 84–91. doi:10.1373/clinchem.2010.151845 PMID:21036945

28. Ashton, J. C. (2015). Drug combination studies and their synergy quantification using the Chou–Talalay method. *Cancer Research*, *75*(11), 2400–2400. doi:10.1158/0008-5472.CAN-14-3763 PMID:25977339

33. Barretina, J., Caponigro, G., Stransky, N., Venkatesan, K., Margolin, A. A., Kim, S., Wilson, C. J., Lehár, J., Kryukov, G. V., Sonkin, D., Reddy, A., Liu, M., Murray, L., Berger, M. F., Monahan, J. E., Morais, P., Meltzer, J., Korejwa, A., Jané-Valbuena, J., ... Garraway, L. A. (2012). The Cancer Cell Line Encyclopedia enables predictive modelling of anticancer drug sensitivity. *Nature*, *483*(7391), 603–607. doi:10.1038/nature11003 PMID:22460905

60. Bartel. (2009). Micrornas: target recognition and regulatory functions. Cell, 136, 215-233.

1. Błaszczyński, J., & Stefanowski, J. (2015). Neighbourhood sampling in bagging for imbalanced data. *Neurocomputing*, *150*, 529–542. doi:10.1016/j.neucom.2014.07.064

55. Bolón-Canedo, V., Sánchez-Maroño, N., & Alonso-Betanzos, A. (2016). Feature selection for high-dimensional data. *Progress in Artificial Intelligence*, *5*(2), 65–75. doi:10.100713748-015-0080-y

49. Bolton, E. E., Wang, Y., Thiessen, P. A., & Bryant, S. H. (2008). PubChem: integrated platform of small molecules and biological activities. In *Annual reports in computational chemistry* (Vol. 4, pp. 217–241). Elsevier.

19. Boussaï, D. (2013). A survey on optimization metaheuristics. *Information Sciences*, *237*, 82–117. doi:10.1016/j.ins.2013.02.041

17. Branke, J., Deb, K., Dierolf, H., & Osswald, M. (2004). Finding knees in multi-objective optimization. In *International conference on parallel problem solving from nature*, (pp. 722-731). Springer.

97. Cantini, L., Isella, C., Petti, C., Picco, G., Chiola, S., Ficarra, E., Caselle, M., & Medico, E. (2015). Microrna-mrna interactions underlying colorectal cancer molecular subtypes. *Nature Communications*, *6*(1), 6. doi:10.1038/ncomms9878 PMID:27305450

20. Chakraborty, A., & Kar, A. K. (2017). Swarm intelligence: A review of algorithms. In *Nature-Inspired Computing and Optimization* (pp. 475–494). Springer. doi:10.1007/978-3-319-50920-4_19

80. Chen, X., Ba, Y., Ma, L., Cai, X., Yin, Y., Wang, K., Guo, J., Zhang, Y., Chen, J., Guo, X., Li, Q., Li, X., Wang, W., Zhang, Y., Wang, J., Jiang, X., Xiang, Y., Xu, C., Zheng, P., ... Zhang, C.-Y. (2008). Characterization of micrornas in serum: A novel class of biomarkers for diagnosis of cancer and other diseases. *Cell Research*, *18*(10), 997–1006. doi:10.1038/cr.2008.282 PMID:18766170

107. Cheng, S., Guo, M., Wang, C., Liu, X., Liu, Y., & Wu, X. (2015). MiRTDL: A deep learning approach for miRNA target prediction. *IEEE/ACM Transactions on Computational Biology and Bioinformatics*, *13*(6), 1161–1169. doi:10.1109/TCBB.2015.2510002 PMID:28055894

10. Chu, W., Ghahramani, Z., Falciani, F., & Wild, D. L. (2005). Biomarker discovery in microarray gene expression data with Gaussian processes. *Bioinformatics (Oxford, England)*, *21*(16), 3385–3393. doi:10.1093/bioinformatics/bti526 PMID:15937031

26. Cokol, M., Chua, H. N., Tasan, M., Mutlu, B., Weinstein, Z. B., Suzuki, Y., & Nergiz, M. E. (2011). Systematic exploration of synergistic drug pairs. Molecular Systems Biology, 7(1), 544-553. doi:10.1038/msb.2011.71

58. Dagogo-Jack, I., & Shaw, A. T. (2018). Tumour heterogeneity and resistance to cancer therapies. *Nature Reviews. Clinical Oncology*, *15*(2), 81–94. doi:10.1038/nrclinonc.2017.166 PMID:29115304

64. Daniel, F. (1996). Tumor marker utility grading system: A framework to evaluate clinical utility of tumor markers. *Journal of the National Cancer Institute*, *88*(20), 1456–1466. doi:10.1093/jnci/88.20.1456 PMID:8841020

14. Dhiman, G., & Kumar, V. (2017). Spotted hyena optimizer: A novel bio-inspired based metaheuristic technique for engineering applications. *Advances in Engineering Software*, *114*, 48–70. doi:10.1016/j.advengsoft.2017.05.014

103. Ding, J., Zhou, S., & Guan, J. (2010). Mirensvm: Towards better prediction of microrna precursors using an ensemble svm classifier with multi-loop features. *BMC Bioinformatics*, *11*(11), 1. doi:10.1186/1471-2105-11-S11-S11 PMID:21172046

67. Doench, J. G., & Sharp, P. A. (2004). Specificity of microrna target selection in translational repression. *Genes & Development*, *18*(5), 504–511. doi:10.1101/gad.1184404 PMID:15014042

37. Evans, W. E., & McLeod, H. L. (2003). Pharmacogenomics—Drug disposition, drug targets, and side effects. *The New England Journal of Medicine*, *348*(6), 538–549. doi:10.1056/NEJMra020526 PMID:12571262

46. Fakhraei, S., Huang, B., Raschid, L., & Getoor, L. (2014). Network-based drug-target interaction prediction with probabilistic soft logic. IEEE/ACM Transactions on Computational Biology and Bioinformatics, 11(5), 775-787. doi:10.1109/TCBB.2014.2325031

25. Fitzgerald, J. B., Schoeberl, B., Nielsen, U. B., & Sorger, P. K. (2006). Systems biology and combination therapy in the quest for clinical efficacy. Nature Chemical Biology, 2(9), 458-466. doi:10.1038/nchembio817

29. Foucquier, J., & Guedj, M. (2015). Analysis of drug combinations: Current methodological landscape. *Pharmacology Research & Perspectives*, *3*(3), e00149. doi:10.1002/prp2.149 PMID:26171228

9. Furlanello, C., Serafini, M., Merler, S., & Jurman, G. (2003). Gene selection and classification by entropy-based recursive feature elimination. In *Proceedings of the International Joint Conference on Neural Networks* (vol. 4, pp. 3077-3082). IEEE. 10.1109/IJCNN.2003.1224063

32. Garnett, M. J., Edelman, E. J., Heidorn, S. J., Greenman, C. D., Dastur, A., Lau, K. W., Greninger, P., Thompson, I. R., Luo, X., Soares, J., Liu, Q., Iorio, F., Surdez, D., Chen, L., Milano, R. J., Bignell, G. R., Tam, A. T., Davies, H., Stevenson, J. A., ... Benes, C. H. (2012). Systematic identification of genomic markers of drug sensitivity in cancer cells. *Nature*, *483*(7391), 570–575. doi:10.1038/nature11005 PMID:22460902

65. Garzon, R., Marcucci, G., & Carlo, M. (2010). Targeting micrornas in cancer: Rationale, strategies and challenges. *Nature Reviews. Drug Discovery*, *9*(10), 775–789. doi:10.1038/nrd3179 PMID:20885409

51. Gaulton, A., Bellis, L. J., Bento, A. P., Chambers, J., Davies, M., Hersey, A., & Light, Y. (2011). ChEMBL: a large-scale bioactivity database for drug discovery. Nucleic Acids Research, 40(D1), D1100-D1107.

4. Golub, T. R., Slonim, D. K., Tamayo, P., Huard, C., Gaasenbeek, M., Mesirov, J. P., & Coller, H. (1999). Molecular classification of cancer: class discovery and class prediction by gene expression monitoring. Science, 286(5439), 531-537.

7. Guyon, I., Weston, J., Barnhill, S., & Vapnik, V. (2002). Gene selection for cancer classification using support vector machines. *Machine Learning*, *46*(1-3), 389–422. doi:10.1023/A:1012487302797

56. Haixiang, G., Li, Y., Shang, J., Gu, M., Huang, Y., & Bing, G. (2017). Learning from class-imbalanced data: Review of methods and applications. *Expert Systems with Applications*, *73*, 220–239. doi:10.1016/j.eswa.2016.12.035

95. Hamam, R., & Arwa, M. (2016). Microrna expression profiling on individual breast cancer patients identifies novel panel of circulating microrna for early detection. *Scientific Reports*, 6.

77. Heneghan, Miller, Kelly, Newell, & Kerin. (2010). Systemic mirna-195 differentiates breast cancer from other malignancies and is a potential biomarker for detecting noninvasive and early stage disease. *The Oncologist*, *15*(7), 673–682. doi:10.1634/theoncologist.2010-0103 PMID:20576643

54. Hira, Z. M., & Gillies, D. F. (2015). A review of feature selection and feature extraction methods applied on microarray data. Advances in Bioinformatics, 2015(198363), 1-13. doi:10.1155/2015/198363

24. Housman, G., Byler, S., Heerboth, S., Lapinska, K., Longacre, M., Snyder, N., & Sarkar, S. (2014). Drug resistance in cancer: An overview. *Cancers (Basel)*, *6*(3), 1769–1792. doi:10.3390/cancers6031769 PMID:25198391

101. Huang, T.-H., Fan, B., Max F Rothschild, Z.-L. H., Li, K., & Zhao, S.-H. (2007). Mirfinder: An improved approach and software implementation for genome-wide fast microrna precursor scans. *BMC Bioinformatics*, *8*(1), 1. doi:10.1186/1471-2105-8-341 PMID:17868480

92. Huang, Z., Huang, D., Ni, S., Peng, Z., Sheng, W., & Du, X. (2010). Plasma micrornas are promising novel biomarkers for early detection of colorectal cancer. *International Journal of Cancer*, *127*(1), 118–126. doi:10.1002/ijc.25007 PMID:19876917

12. Inza, I., Larrañaga, P., Blanco, R., & Cerrolaza, A. J. (2004). Filter versus wrapper gene selection approaches in DNA microarray domains. *Artificial Intelligence in Medicine*, *31*(2), 91–103. doi:10.1016/j.artmed.2004.01.007 PMID:15219288

42. Jacob, L., & Vert, J.-P. (2008). Protein-ligand interaction prediction: An improved chemogenomics approach. *Bioinformatics (Oxford, England)*, *24*(19), 2149–2156. doi:10.1093/bioinformatics/btn409 PMID:18676415

35. Jamali, M., & Ester, M. (2010). A matrix factorization technique with trust propagation for recommendation in social networks. In *Proceedings of the fourth ACM conference on Recommender systems*, (pp. 135-142). ACM. 10.1145/1864708.1864736

52. Kanehisa, M., Goto, S., Sato, Y., Furumichi, M., & Tanabe, M. (2011). KEGG for integration and interpretation of large-scale molecular data sets. Nucleic Acids Research, 40(D1), D109-D114.

22. Knoechel, B., Roderick, J. E., Williamson, K. E., Zhu, J., Lohr, J. G., Cotton, M. J., Gillespie, S. M., Fernandez, D., Ku, M., Wang, H., Piccioni, F., Silver, S. J., Jain, M., Pearson, D., Kluk, M. J., Ott, C. J., Shultz, L. D., Brehm, M. A., Greiner, D. L., ... Bernstein, B. E. (2014). An epigenetic mechanism of resistance to targeted therapy in T cell acute lymphoblastic leukemia. *Nature Genetics*, *46*(4), 364–370. doi:10.1038/ng.2913 PMID:24584072

50. Knox, Law, Jewison, Liu, Ly, Frolkis, & Pon. (2010). DrugBank 3.0: a comprehensive resource for 'omics' research on drugs. *Nucleic Acids Research, 39*(S1), D1035-D1041.

69. Kosaka, N., Iguchi, H., & Ochiya, T. (2010). Circulating microrna in body uid: A new potential biomarker for cancer diagnosis and prognosis. *Cancer Science*, *101*(10), 2087–2092. doi:10.1111/j.1349-7006.2010.01650.x PMID:20624164

30. Kotelnikova, E., Yuryev, A., Mazo, I., & Daraselia, N. (2010). Computational approaches for drug repositioning and combination therapy design. Journal of Bioinformatics and Computational Biology, 8(3), 593-606. doi:10.1142/S0219720010004732

105. Kozomara, A., & Griffiths-Jones, S. (2014). mirbase: Annotating high confidence micrornas using deep sequencing data. *Nucleic Acids Research*, *42*(D1), D68–D73. doi:10.1093/nar/gkt1181 PMID:24275495

57. Krawczyk, B., Galar, M., Jeleń, Ł., & Herrera, F. (2016). Evolutionary undersampling boosting for imbalanced classification of breast cancer malignancy. *Applied Soft Computing*, *38*, 714–726. doi:10.1016/j.asoc.2015.08.060

102. Kwang, L. S. N., & Santosh, K. (2007). De novo svm classification of precursor micrornas from genomic pseudo hairpins using global and intrinsic folding measures. *Bioinformatics (Oxford, England)*, *23*(11), 1321–1330. doi:10.1093/bioinformatics/btm026 PMID:17267435

61. Lee, Y., Kim, M., Han, J., Yeom, K.-H., Lee, S., Baek, S. H., & Narry Kim, V. (2004). Microrna genes are transcribed by rna polymerase ii. *The EMBO Journal*, *23*(20), 4051–4060. doi:10.1038j.emboj.7600385 PMID:15372072

71. Li, A., Omura, N., Hong, S.-M., Vincent, A., Walter, K., Griffith, M., Borges, M., & Goggins, M. (2010). Pancreatic cancers epigenetically silence sip1 and hypomethylate and overexpress mir-200a/200b in association with elevated circulating mir-200a and mir-200b levels. *Cancer Research*, *70*(13), 5226–5237. doi:10.1158/0008-5472.CAN-09-4227 PMID:20551052

16. Li, S., Wu, X., & Tan, M. (2008). Gene selection using hybrid particle swarm optimization and genetic algorithm. *Soft Computing*, *12*(11), 1039–1048. doi:10.100700500-007-0272-x

86. Li, X., Luo, F., Li, Q., Xu, M., Feng, D., Zhang, G., & Wu, W. (2011). Identification of new aberrantly expressed mirnas in intestinal-type gastric cancer and its clinical significance. *Oncology Reports*, *26*(6), 1431–1439. PMID:21874264

63. Lu, R., & Barca, O. (2012). Fine-tuning oligodendrocyte development by micrornas. *Frontiers in Neuroscience, 6,* 13. PMID:22347159

2.   Lu, Y., & Han, J. (2003). Cancer classification using gene expression data. *Information Systems*, *28*(4), 243–268. doi:10.1016/S0306-4379(02)00072-8

18. Marler, R. T., & Arora, J. S. (2004). Survey of multi-objective optimization methods for engineering. Structural and Multidisciplinary Optimization, 26(6), 369-395. doi:10.100700158-003-0368-6

75. Mitchell, Parkin, Kroh, Fritz, Wyman, Pogosova-Agadjanyan, Peterson, Noteboom, O'Briant, & Allen. (2008). Circulating micrornas as stable blood-based markers for cancer detection. *Proceedings of the National Academy of Sciences*, *105*(30), 10513-10518.

39. Mizutani, S., Pauwels, E., Stoven, V., Goto, S., & Yamanishi, Y. (2012). Relating drug–protein interaction network with drug side effects. *Bioinformatics (Oxford, England)*, *28*(18), i522–i528. doi:10.1093/bioinformatics/bts383 PMID:22962476

74. Morimura, R., Komatsu, S., Ichikawa, D., Takeshita, H., Tsujiura, M., Nagata, H., Konishi, H., Shiozaki, A., Ikoma, H., Okamoto, K., Ochiai, T., Taniguchi, H., & Otsuji, E. (2011). Novel diagnostic value of circulating mir-18a in plasma of patients with pancreatic cancer. *British Journal of Cancer*, *105*(11), 1733–1740. doi:10.1038/bjc.2011.453 PMID:22045190

98. Mortazavi, A., & Brian, A. (2008). Mapping and quantifying mammalian transcriptomes by rna-seq. *Nature Methods*, *5*(7), 621–628. doi:10.1038/nmeth.1226 PMID:18516045

99. Murakami, Y., Tanahashi, T., Okada, R., Toyoda, H., Kumada, T., Enomoto, M., Tamori, A., Kawada, N., Taguchi, Y. H., & Azuma, T. (2014). Comparison of hepatocellular carcinoma miRNA expression profiling as evaluated by next generation sequencing and microarray. *PLoS One*, *9*(9), e106314. doi:10.1371/journal.pone.0106314 PMID:25215888

100.   Nam, J.-W., Shin, K.-R., Han, J., & Lee, Y. (2005). Human microrna prediction through a probabilistic co-learning model of sequence and structure. *Nucleic Acids Research*, *33*(11), 3570–3581. doi:10.1093/nar/gki668 PMID:15987789

91. Ng, Chong, Lam, Shin, Yu, Poon, Ng, & Sung. (2009). Differential expression of micrornas in plasma of colorectal cancer patients: A potential marker for colorectal cancer screening. *Gut*.

3.   Okun, O. (2013). *Survey of Novel Feature Selection Methods for Cancer Classification. In Biological Knowledge Discovery Handbook: Preprocessing*. Mining, and Postprocessing of Biological Data.

106.   Park, S., Min, S., Choi, H., & Yoon, S. (2016). *deepmirgene: Deep neural network based precursor microrna prediction.* arXiv preprint arXiv:1605.00017

70. Ploussard, G., & de la Taille, A. (2010). Urine biomarkers in prostate cancer. *Nature Reviews. Urology*, *7*(2), 101–109. doi:10.1038/nrurol.2009.261 PMID:20065953

88. Qu, Zhang, Li, Afdhal, & Albitar. (2011). Circulating micrornas as biomarkers for hepatocellular carcinoma. *Journal of Clinical Gastroenterology*, *45*(4), 355–360. doi:10.1097/MCG.0b013e3181f18ac2 PMID:21278583

40. Rarey, M., Kramer, B., Lengauer, T., & Klebe, G. (1996). A fast flexible docking method using an incremental construction algorithm. Journal of Molecular Biology, 261(3), 470-489. doi:10.1006/jmbi.1996.0477

84. Resnick, Alder, Hagan, Richardson, Croce, & Cohn. (2009). The detection of di_erentially expressed micrornas from the serum of ovarian cancer patients using a novel real-time pcr platform. *Gynecologic Oncology*, *112*(1), 55–59. doi:10.1016/j.ygyno.2008.08.036 PMID:18954897

23. Rini, B. I., & Atkins, M. B. (2009). Resistance to targeted therapy in renal-cell carcinoma. The Lancet Oncology, 10(10), 992-1000. doi:10.1016/S1470-2045(09)70240-2

96. Rupaimoole, R., George A Calin, G. L.-B., & Anil, K. (2016). Mirna deregulation in cancer cells and the tumor microenvironment. *Cancer Discovery*, *6*(3), 235–246. doi:10.1158/2159-8290.CD-15-0893 PMID:26865249

13. Saeys, Y., Inza, I., & Larrañaga, P. (2007). A review of feature selection techniques in bioinformatics. Bioinformatics, 23(19), 2507-2517. doi:10.1093/bioinformatics/btm344

93. Schreiber, R., Mezencev, R., Matyunina, L. V., & McDonald, J. F. (2016). Evidence for the role of microrna 374b in acquired cisplatin resistance in pancreatic cancer cells. *Cancer Gene Therapy*, *23*(8), 241–245. doi:10.1038/cgt.2016.23 PMID:27229158

81. Shen, J., Liu, Z., & Nevins, W. (2011). Diagnosis of lung cancer in individuals with solitary pulmonary nodules by plasma microrna biomarkers. *BMC Cancer*, *11*(1), 1. doi:10.1186/1471-2407-11-374 PMID:21864403

15. Shen, Q., Shi, W.-M., & Kong, W. (2008). Hybrid particle swarm optimization and tabu search approach for selecting genes for tumor classification using gene expression data. *Computational Biology and Chemistry*, *32*(1), 53–60. doi:10.1016/j.compbiolchem.2007.10.001 PMID:18093877

8. Shevade, S. K., & Sathiya Keerthi, S. (2003). A simple and efficient algorithm for gene selection using sparse logistic regression. *Bioinformatics (Oxford, England)*, *19*(17), 2246–2253. doi:10.1093/bioinformatics/btg308 PMID:14630653

59. Tadist, K., Najah, S., Nikolov, N. S., Mrabti, F., & Zahi, A. (2019). Feature selection methods and genomic big data: A systematic review. *Journal of Big Data*, *6*(79), 1–24. doi:10.118640537-019-0241-0

27. Tallarida, R. J. (2011). Quantitative methods for assessing drug synergism. *Genes & Cancer*, *2*(11), 1003–1008. doi:10.1177/1947601912440575 PMID:22737266

83. Taylor, D. D., & Gercel-Taylor, C. (2008). Microrna signatures of tumor-derived exosomes as diagnostic biomarkers of ovarian cancer. *Gynecologic Oncology*, *110*(1), 13–21. doi:10.1016/j.ygyno.2008.04.033 PMID:18589210

85. Tsujiura, M., Ichikawa, D., Komatsu, S., Shiozaki, A., Takeshita, H., Kosuga, T., Konishi, H., Morimura, R., Deguchi, K., Fujiwara, H., Okamoto, K., & Otsuji, E. (2010). Circulating micrornas in plasma of patients with gastric cancers. *British Journal of Cancer*, *102*(7), 1174–1179. doi:10.1038j. bjc.6605608 PMID:20234369

47. van Laarhoven, T., Nabuurs, S. B., & Marchiori, E. (2011). Gaussian interaction profile kernels for predicting drug–target interaction. *Bioinformatics (Oxford, England)*, *27*(21), 3036–3043. doi:10.1093/bioinformatics/btr500 PMID:21893517

6.   Van't Veer, L. J., Dai, H., Van De Vijver, M. J., & He, Y. D. (2002). Gene expression profiling predicts clinical outcome of breast cancer. Nature, 415(6871), 530-536.

94. Velagapudi, Cameron, Haga, Rosenberg, Lafitte, Duckett, Phinney, & Disney. (2016). Design of a small molecule against an oncogenic noncoding rna. *Proceedings of the National Academy of Sciences*.

73. Wang, J., Chen, J., Chang, P., LeBlanc, A., Li, D., & James, L. (2009). Micrornas in plasma of pancreatic ductal adenocarcinoma patients as novel blood-based biomarkers of disease. *Cancer Prevention Research (Philadelphia, Pa.)*, 2(9), 807–813. doi:10.1158/1940-6207.CAPR-09-0094 PMID:19723895

36. Wang, L., Li, X., Zhang, L., & Gao, Q. (2017). Improved anticancer drug response prediction in cell lines using matrix factorization with similarity regularization. *BMC Cancer*, 17(1), 513–524. doi:10.118612885-017-3500-5 PMID:28768489

45. Wang, Y.-C., Zhang, C.-H., Deng, N.-Y., & Wang, Y. (2011). Kernel-based data fusion improves the drug–protein interaction prediction. Computational Biology and Chemistry, 35(6), 353-362. doi:10.1016/j.compbiolchem.2011.10.003

38. Wei, D.-Q., Wang, J.-F., Chen, C., Li, Y., & Chou, K.-C. (2008). Molecular modeling of two CYP2C19 SNPs and its implications for personalized drug design. *Protein and Peptide Letters*, 15(1), 27–32. doi:10.2174/092986608783330305 PMID:18221009

21. Weinberg, R. A. (1991). Tumor suppressor genes. *Science*, 254(5035), 1138–1146. doi:10.1126cience.1659741 PMID:1659741

90. Wong, T.-S., Liu, X.-B., Wong, B. Y.-H., Ng, R. W.-M., Yuen, A. P.-W., & Wei, W. I. (2008). Mature mir-184 as potential oncogenic microrna of squamous cell carcinoma of tongue. *Clinical Cancer Research*, 14(9), 2588–2592. doi:10.1158/1078-0432.CCR-07-0666 PMID:18451220

31. Xiao, G., Ma, S., Minna, J., & Xie, Y. (2014). Adaptive Prediction Model in Prospective Molecular Signature–Based Clinical Studies. *Clinical Cancer Research*, 20(3), 531–539. doi:10.1158/1078-0432.CCR-13-2127 PMID:24323903

41. Xie, Evangelidis, Xie, & Bourne. (2011). Drug discovery using chemical systems biology: weak inhibition of multiple kinases may contribute to the anti-cancer effect of nelfinavir. *PLoS Computational Biology, 7*(4).

62. Xie, Z., Allen, E., Fahlgren, N., Calamar, A., & Scott, A. (2005). Expression of arabidopsis mirna genes. *Plant Physiology*, 138(4), 2145–2154. doi:10.1104/pp.105.062943 PMID:16040653

104.   Xue, C., Li, F., He, T., Liu, G.-P., Li, Y., & Zhang, X. (2005). Classification of real and pseudo microrna precursors using local structure-sequence features and support vector machine. *BMC Bioinformatics*, 6(1), 310. doi:10.1186/1471-2105-6-310 PMID:16381612

34. Yamada, M., Lian, W., Goyal, A., Chen, J., Wimalawarne, K., Khan, S. A., Kaski, S., Mamitsuka, H., & Chang, Y. (2017). Convex factorization machine for toxicogenomics prediction. In *Proceedings of the 23rd ACM SIGKDD International Conference on Knowledge Discovery and Data Mining*, (pp. 1215-1224). ACM.

87. Yamamoto, Y., Kosaka, N., Tanaka, M., Koizumi, F., Kanai, Y., Mizutani, T., Murakami, Y., Kuroda, M., Miyajima, A., Kato, T., & Ochiya, T. (2009). Microrna-500 as a potential diagnostic marker for hepatocellular carcinoma. *Biomarkers*, *14*(7), 529–538. doi:10.3109/13547500903150771 PMID:19863192

44. Yamanishi, Y., Araki, M., Gutteridge, A., Honda, W., & Kanehisa, M. (2008). Prediction of drug–target interaction networks from the integration of chemical and genomic spaces. *Bioinformatics (Oxford, England)*, *24*(13), i232–i240. doi:10.1093/bioinformatics/btn162 PMID:18586719

89. Zhang, C., Wang, C., Chen, X., Yang, C., Li, K., Wang, J., Dai, J., Hu, Z., Zhou, X., Chen, L., Zhang, Y., Li, Y., Qiu, H., Xing, J., Liang, Z., Ren, B., Yang, C., Zen, K., & Zhang, C.-Y. (2010). Expression profile of micrornas in serum: A fingerprint for esophageal squamous cell carcinoma. *Clinical Chemistry*, *56*(12), 1871–1879. doi:10.1373/clinchem.2010.147553 PMID:20943850

68. Zhang, H., Fabrice A Kolb, V. B., Billy, E., & Filipowicz, W. (2002). Human dicer preferentially cleaves dsrnas at their termini without a requirement for atp. *The EMBO Journal*, *21*(21), 5875–5885. doi:10.1093/emboj/cdf582 PMID:12411505

79. Zhao, H., Shen, J., Medico, L., Wang, D., & Christine, B. (2010). A pilot study of circulating mirnas as potential biomarkers of early stage breast cancer. *PLoS One*, *5*(10), e13735. doi:10.1371/journal.pone.0013735 PMID:21060830

82. Zheng, D., Haddadin, S., Wang, Y., Gu, L.-Q., & Michael, C. (2011). Plasma micrornas as novel biomarkers for early detection of lung cancer. *International Journal of Clinical and Experimental Pathology*, *4*(6), 575–586. PMID:21904633

48. Zheng, X., Ding, H., Mamitsuka, H., & Zhu, S. (2013). Collaborative matrix factorization with multiple similarities for predicting drug-target interactions. In *Proceedings of the 19th ACM SIGKDD international conference on Knowledge discovery and data mining*, (pp. 1025-1033). ACM. 10.1145/2487575.2487670

43. Zhu, Okuno, Tsujimoto, & Mamitsuka. (2005). A probabilistic model for mining implicit 'chemical compound–gene' relations from literature. *Bioinformatics*, *21*(2), ii245-ii251.

76. Zhu, W., Qin, W., Atasoy, U., & Edward, R. (2009). Circulating micrornas in breast cancer and healthy subjects. *BMC Research Notes*, *2*(1), 89. doi:10.1186/1756-0500-2-89 PMID:19454029

Chapter 9
A Pathway to Differential Modelling of Nipah Virus

Dheva Rajan S.

https://orcid.org/0000-0002-4377-4423

Almusanna College of Technology, Oman

ABSTRACT

This chapter is devoted to the study of mathematical modelling part of infectious diseases, especially the nipah virus. In the past few decades, one cannot deny that enormous new unanticipated diseases have been the cause of serious concern among the human community and that so many viruses have begun emerging and re-emerging though people are trying all means to get rid of diseases. It can even be said that diseases of all sorts are ruling the world. Early prediction of diseases that spread in humans plays a vital role to protect living beings. Most of such diseases are highly infectious, get transmitted from human to human or through some other vectors. Several research and developments take place in the pharma industry notably after the Second World War. Hence, the predictions are not just for theoretical purposes as quite a number of pharma industries use mathematical models for their findings in new medicines and even to decide the quantity of medicine production. This chapter gives an overview of the different researches conducted in mathematical modelling of nipah virus.

INTRODUCTION

A virus is called zoonotic if it spreads to humans from animals. Nipah is one of the virulentzoonotic viruses that is reasoned to be the cause of deadly Nipahfever. This virus can also be spread directly through people themselves or consumption of filthy food. This virus attacks not only humans but also animals. It is notated popularly by NiVand this notation will be used throughout this chapter to denote Nipah Virus. NiV can cause severe diseases in animals like pigs. The study of infections is called infectionology and the study deals withinfectionology concept towards mathematical modelling. At the time of first outbreak of NiV, infection not only in pigs but other household creatures, for example, horses, goats, sheeps, etc were also reported. NiV profoundly infectious in pigs as they are irresistible during the

DOI: 10.4018/978-1-7998-2742-9.ch009

incubation period, which keeps going from 4 to 14 days. A contaminated pig can display no indications, yet some create intense fever, issues in breathing, and neurological side effects like trembling, jerking and muscle fits. But the mortality is low with the exception of youthful piglets. NiV ought to be suspected if pigs additionally have an abnormal woofing hack or if human instances of encephalitis are available. The virus develops in the bladder, saliva, and face of fruit bats and is harbored naturally in fruit bats and microbats of numerous species. The fruit bat is also called as flying fox. It also infects bats when they eat the bites of the other bats and their urine and saliva. When humans come in close contact with infected domestic animals, they too become infected. Apart from pigs, the virus is also found in domestic cats, dogs, and horses. Also, bats can often live in high altitudes. Accordingly, in the pots tied to tall palm trees if the saliva and urine of the bats get mixed, it would spread quickly when humans drink it. This will result in significant economic loss for farmers. Post-mortem inspection showed critical NiV to be a systemic infection (Wong et al 2002)Canines were observed to be frequentlydiseasedas well (Field H et al. 2001). Anotherhazard factor was found with caninesdying on farms frequently (Parashar UD et al. 2000). It also can be transmitted from human to human (H-H). It was Rahman SA et al. (2010) who discovered that Pteropus bats were exposed to be the reservoir of such a poisonous infection in Malaysia which diseased the magnifying hosts and vectors too by ingestion of bat-nibbled fruit and there is no proof of H-Htransmission from these epidemics but later Stephen P. et al (2009) proposed the evidence of H-H transmission of disease. Here, especially in epidemiology modelling, one should know the few terminologies like host, vector, etc., (Source: Centers for Disease Control and Prevention. "Division of Vector-Borne Diseases")

Host (Intermediate stage): A living being tainted by a parasite whereas the parasite is in aninitial formative structure, not explicitly developed.

Host (Primary stage): An essential host is a life form that gives sustenance and haven to a parasite while enabling it to turn out to be explicitly full grown, while an auxiliary host is one involved by a parasite during the larval or agamic phases of its life cycle.

Reservoir: The creature or living being in which the infection or parasite regularly exist in.

Vector: Any mediator, living or something else, acting as a carrier and spreads parasites and infections. Likewise, a living being or chemical used to transporta gene into anotherhost.

de Wit, E., & Munster, V. J. (2015) have given animal models of disease that shed light on NiV pathogenesis and transmission. A beginner to such modelling can read this, to get more insight about the channels for the spread of the diseases, the factors causing it and how to develop a non-mathematical model initially. Hammoud, D. A et al (2018) proposed the model to determine the Aerosol exposure to intermediate size NiV particles that induces nervous illness in African green monkeys, though this work has deviated from the current objective.One might be interested in creating models and forecasting, hence, the author wishes to suggest this article for such aspirants whereas earlier Johnston, S (2015) has given a wonderfully detailed analysis of the African Green Monkey Model of NiV Disease.Middleton et al., (2007) detailed in their work based on an Investigational taint of Pteropus that bats with NiVhave not affected or given the disease in the fruit bats. Examinations of rodents and other faunae have not perceived further natural life repositories for NiV (Hsu VP 2004 & Yob JM 2001). Nowak (1994) stated in the work that around 50 kinds of Pteropus bats live in the South East Side of Asia.

Outbreaks

Despite the fact that NiV has caused just a couple of known flare-ups in Asia, it taints a wide scope of creatures and causes extreme illness and demise in individuals, making it a general wellbeing concern. At the Malaysian peninsula, the pig farmers suffered due to encephalitis(brain inflammation). That is the first known human outbreak in the world in 1998-1999 where around 257 people suffered among which 157 died (Goh KJ et al 2000). NiV is a type of RNA the genus being Henipavirus order Mononega-virales. (Source: WHO NiV Infection 2018). The other genus and viruses of this genus are as follows respectively: Cedar henipavirus,Cedar virus (CedV), Ghanaian bat henipavirus, Kumasivirus (KV), Hendrahenipavirus, Hendra virus (HeV), Mojiang virus (MojV). In 1947, the probable origin of this virus was found. The 95% confidence interval for this virus statistically is between 1888 to 1988. The virus evolved two times; one in 1985 and another in 2002. The mutation rate was estimated to be 6.5×10^{-4} substitution/site/year with 95% confidence interval 2.3×10^{-4} -1.18×10^{-3}. (Lo Presti A et al 2015).The fatal death rate was estimated at50% to 75%. (Broder, C2013) NiV is named after the village Sungai Nipah, a river village in the Negeri Sembilan state in Malaysia. (Nipah Virus CDC 2017). To save people (infact the other animals too from infection) from the spread of the disease, more than 10 lakh pigs were euthanized (set to death without pain). Infact, that caused a great business loss to Malaysia. The reason for business trade loss is, the Pork consumption per capita in Malaysia from 2009 to 2018 (in kilograms) varies from 5.85 to 6.83, forecasted for 2020 and 2025 almost to 6 (Source: Statistica.com). Apart from this pork consumption, the adjoined business too encountered a great loss. After the euthanasia, there was no other outbreak reported neither from Malaysia nor from Singapore. The NiV but with different strains than identified in 1999 and found in 2001, again emerged in Bangladesh to give another outbreak. In 2014, an epidemic of NiV arose in Philippines. 17 cases were confirmed with the fatality rate of 82% in humans. It was observed that out of 17, 10 had adjacent connection with horses or consumption of horse meat. It was reported the deaths of 10 horses were found dead at 2014 epidemic of NiV in Philippines. Five health care nurses were infected at the same time while treating infected patients. (Ching PKG et al 2015)

Figure 1. Nipah Epidemics in Bangladesh

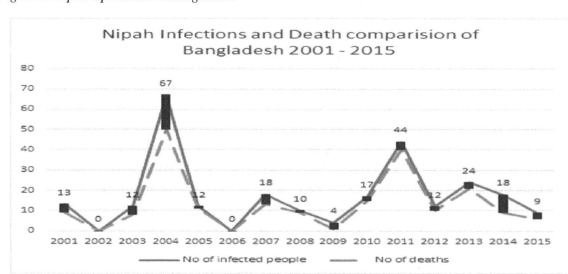

Symptoms and Remedy

The incubation period (interval from infection to the onset of symptoms) of NiVvaries from 5 to 14 days. The infection later becomesan exposed state that varies from 3 to 14 days though reports say it can be till 45 days. The symptoms ofNiV begins with mild fever. The virus affects the Blood vessels and parenchymal cells in most of the foremost organs.The symptomsof level exposing may include, drowsiness, mental confusion, fever, headache, disorientation etc. This exposure leads to infection and severe infection can lead to coma stage within 1 to 2 days. Few have shown pulmonary (related to lungs) signs and more than 50% have shown neurological symptoms. Other few have shown respiratory illness before reaching the exposed state of infections. It can lead to sequela (death as a result of nipa after the disease run out), and a sudden contraction in muscles and personality changes. It is to be noted that even after years of exposed state of the disease, latent infections with ensuring renaissance of NiV and morbid were also reported. ("Signs and Symptoms NiV", CDC, 2018). There were many people who recovered from coma. But those who went to the extent of coma to attack the virus must eventually die. No specific drugs have been found yet and there are currently only pharmaceuticals to partially control them. Doctors say the best medicine is to give full support to those infected with virus. The victims should be away from food and others should not eat the leftovers of their food. Friends and relatives should personally take care of cough and colds if the victim has any. . It is also good that others do not use the affected victim's clothes.. So far, 75 percent of those infected with the virus have died, as per reports. .

InSiliguri, India, the NiVwas reported in2001, in the meantime, it was reported in Bangaladesh too. The outbreak emerged again in the years 2003,04,and 05 in districts, Naogaon, Rajbari, Manikganj, Tangail, and Faridpur. (Chadha et al 2006& Hsu 2004). In Kerala, India, at MalappuramKozhikode district an outbreak was reported in May 2018 in which 17 people died. The crucial thing is, out of 17 who were reported dead, one included a anurse (healthcare worker) who treated the infected people. (source: https://www.ndtv.com/kerala-news/nurse-lini-who-treated-kerala- Nipah-victim- left-heartbreaking - note-for-husband- 1855625). Though in June 2018, the govt announced officially that the outbreak was over, it emerged again in May 2019. This shows the severity and re-emerging speed of the disease. A student admitted at Ernakulam, Kerala was infected and his treatment was confirmed with 2 months at the hospital. The infection of NiV was inveterate from RT-PCR tests. The communication rotations of NiV in Malaysia and Bangladesh are somewhat different. In Bangladesh, Nipah infection is believed to be communicated through the utilization of crude date palm sap. While date palm sap is gathered, bats enter the sap stream or accumulation pots and pollute the sap with NiV through their spit or pee. People become tainted with NiV after the utilization of this dingy date palm juice. Later these contaminated individuals can transmit NiV to others by means of close contact. In Malaysia, Nipah infection was transmitted from bats perching in organic product trees or on pig homesteads.. Pigs mainly inflicted NiV to people in close contact with them. (de Wit, Emmie, and Vincent J Munster, 2015). Figure 2 explains the way how NiVspreads among fruit bats, pigs, and humans.

Ayush Kumar (2019) found many standards in the classical texts of Ayurveda, that can be compared with the concepts of epidemiology. Also, he stated that "Ayurveda labelsidea of the prevalence of disease and that can be compared with Janapadodhwans. Ayurveda summarizes the entire relevant concept in a single word as JanapadopdhwansaRogas". Though, being anorthodoxtherapeutic doctrine, it has its allure that can't be compared with the modern concepts of study of disease transmission.

Figure 2. Schematic diagram of NiV infection

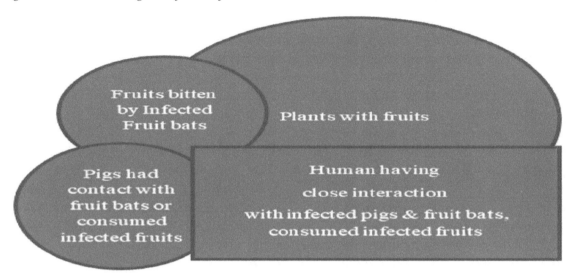

Currently, neither vaccines nor medicines have been proven to be effective in treating NiV infection. However, health care providers may offer supportive therapy to manage symptoms. At this time duration of fever and the severity of diseases can be reduced and also may alleviate the symptoms of nausea, vomiting, and convulsions by ribavirin.

Mathematical Modeling

An abstract model is said to be a Mathematical model if that utilizes the mathematical language to explain the behavior of a proposed system and it is likewise a helpful device for the estimation of the impact of various methodologies for controlling the spread of communicable diseases within a populace.There is no limitation discipline wise for the usage of Mathematical models. It is widely used in all disciplines, viz., computer science, engineering, management, all science and humanities, even political science too. Eykhoff(1974) defined a mathematical model as 'a representation of the essential aspects of an existing system (or a system to be constructed) which presents knowledge of that system in usable form'. Mathematical modeling has turned into a significant tool for analyzing the spread and for the control of communicable diseases. It is a helpful tool for the estimation of the impact of various methodologies for controlling the spread of irresistible infections within a population.One of the major epidemics in the U.S.A. was the Yellow Fever prevalent in Philadelphia in 1793. About 5000 individuals expired out of about 50,000, despite the fact that approximations propose that about 20,000 escaped the city; see the intriguing artifact by Foster et al. (1998) and the book by Powell (1993). The milestone book by McNeill (1989) is an enthralling story of the connection between diseases and individuals. The modeling literature is now extensively growing rapidly.Several kinds of modeling include claims about causality. This is typically (but not always) factual models concerning differential equations. The purpose of modeling is to upsurge the understanding of real-world problems. The validity of the models always sail on fitting it to the empirical data. It should have the ability to extrapolate to different circumstances. Mathematical modeling can be classified into two types based on the quantity of prior available information of the system which requires examination.

- Black box model - With no prior data
- White box model or glass box or clear box - all essential data

In the real scenario, all the examinations are in the intermediate stage between black and clear box model. So, the classification of the model concept acts as an intuitive guide to approaching a problem, not for the entire solution of the problem proposed. To propose an accurate model with high predictive power, it is advisable to use the available prior information as much as possible. One can use that information for better prediction and for checking the reliability of the modal. For example, if a researcher proposes a forecasting model for rainfall, the usage of the prior data can be used to check the reliability and error in the model. Based on that data, it is possible to check the current scenario and predict future values. On such predictions, the error obtained from the past data is useful to propose the limitations. A regularly utilized methodology for modeling is neural systems which for the most part don't accept nearly anything about the prior information. The issue with utilizing a huge arrangement of capacities to portray a framework is that evaluating the parameters turns out to be progressively troublesome when the number of parameters (and various kinds of capacities) increases. In recent years, the epidemiological modeling of such communicable disease transmission has had an upsurge impact on the various theories, spread and control management of the disease. Dheva Rajan et al (2013a) proposed a two compartmental model for the spread of Dengue fever. The model consists of set of 7 ordinary differential equations 4 for human and 3 for mosquito. The model is based on SEIR type model, which can be abbreviated as Susceptible, Exposed, Infectious and Recovered. There is no recovery of mosquito from infections, hence for mosquitoes it was only 3 states except recovery. The model was then developed to arbitrary n regions (Dheva Rajan et al 2013b). Again, with the help of work done by DhevaRajan et al (2013c,d)the stability analysis of the said model was discussed. The Bifurcation and sensitivity analysis has been performed by the same author in which the mosquito biting has the highest sensitive parameter value. (Dheva Rajan et al 2014 a,b,c,d). Though the model was proposed particularly for Dengue fever spread, it can also be used for other communicable diseases, by varying the respective parameters. As a future development, Dheva Rajan et.al (2014) proposed the inclusion of rainfall, climatic factors, temperature, humidity, impact of awareness programs, seasonality, self-prevention, etc., The said model is based on population dynamics model and is a reflection of the use in serving to comprehend the dynamic processes and in making predictions. It was developed from the basic concept birth-death, which people called as birth and death model. Consider any species. Let $TP(t)$ be the population at time t, then the rate of change $\dfrac{d(TP)}{dt}$ is the equation for the population. Hence,

$$\frac{d(TP)}{dt} = births \; - \; deaths \; + \; migration \ldots \tag{1}$$

The Right-hand side of the equation (1) demands to demonstrate the situation with which the proposers are concerned. The simplest model that has birth (b) and death (μ) terms are proportional to the total population (TP) with the absence of migration.

That is,

$$\frac{d(TP)}{dt} = b(TP) - \mu(TP) \ldots \tag{2}$$

On integrating the equation 2, one can get,

$$TP(t) = (TP)_0 e^{(b-\mu)t} \ldots \tag{3}$$

The RHS of Equation 3 is the abstract mathematical solution of LHS of 2 with $TP(0) = (TP)_0$ the initial value of the population, b, $\mu > 0$ & constants. Hence, for 3 one can get the following interpretation.

$$\begin{cases} b > \mu & \text{grows exponentially} \\ b < \mu & \text{out} \end{cases}$$

This approach proposed by Malthus (1790), is honestly impractical. A very good starter of reading the diverse problems and models for the spread and control of communicable diseases is the volume by Bailey (1975).

Mathematical modeling of communicable disease commenced in 1911 with Ross's (Ross 1911). The most important biological incorporations are described in a book (MacDonald 1957). Let $S(t)$, $I(t)$ and $R(t)$ denote the number of individuals in the susceptible, infectious and recovered classes at time t respectively. Hence, these susceptible, infectious and recovered classesare represented as a function of t, however, for the sake of simplicity, hereafter in this chapter it follows the notations by omitting the independent variable t, viz, Susceptible (S), Infection (I), and Recovery (R)and it is applicable for other state variables, if any defined for either host or vector. The total population at time t is represented by $TP(t) = S + I + R$. In this book it is assumed that the total population is $TP(t) = N$ and inconvenience is regretted for the usage of two parameters to denote the population. It is used only for the sake of convenience. This becomes asystem of non-linear differential equations. The advancement of the human population is schematically characterized by SIR. This SIR is one of the furthermost uncomplicated fundamental infectious disease model from 1927. Equation 2 gives a better idea to the ancient type of mathematical model SIR.

The basic SIR model can be expressed as follows with the parameters:

$$\frac{dS}{dt} = -\beta * S * I \ldots \tag{4}$$

$$\frac{dI}{dt} = \beta SI - \gamma * I \ldots \tag{5}$$

$$\frac{dR}{dt} = \gamma * I \ldots \tag{6}$$

Equations 4,5 and 6 constitute a type of standard SIR model. Remember that, when giving the initial conditions on these type of models, values S & I should be at least one, and R is non-negative. The epidemic like fever is usually faster than that of birth and death, hence, birth and death in the above set of equations is omittedwith $S + I + R = N$, as assumed earlier. It is the choice of the experimenter to use the value of S,I and R directly or as the fraction value after dividing by the total number of population N. This is based on the basic logic that, in order to spread the disease, there should be at least one infective population and if found susceptible, it is evident that the recovery can be zero and cannot be in negative. This SIR type of model is a standard disease model that consists of a set of equations and can be used to explain the dynamics of NiV infections in society.

Figure 3. SIR model with assumed values β =400, γ =365/13, S=0.999,I=0.001,R=0.000

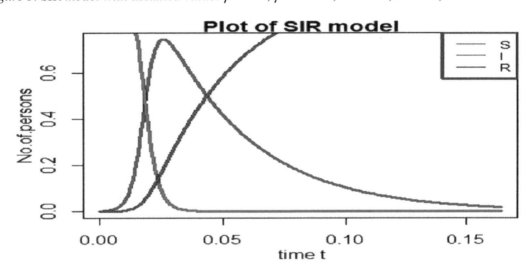

The set of equations 4,5 and 6 together represents the SIR model. This model was proposed first by O. Kermack and Anderson Gray McKendrick. Hethcote H (2000) mentioned this as a specific case of the Kermack-McKendrick theory. (Kermack, W&McKendrick, A (1991a,b,c). Figure 1 describes the graph of the SIR model with different parameter values. To generate the graph like figure 3, one can use any mathematical programming language such as Matlab, Julia, Mathematica, etc., Usage of Mathematica is advisable but researchers have to think of the cost of the software also. Matlab is a widely used one to solve ODEs, especially using ODE 45 solver. Here, R programming language is used to generate as it is an open-source software. By seeing figure3, one can immediately find that the system is non-linear, hence it cannot have a standard plausible solution. However, the outcomes can be obtained using the replication methods specifically like Monte Carlo Simulation techniques and/or by using the process like Gillespie Algorithm (Gillespie D.T, 1976, 1977). Aron & May (1982) andNedelman (1985)have proposedafew analyses on the Mathematical modeling of communicable diseases. Initially, the models are of two compartments, one for human and another one for vector-borne diseases. A significant accumulation of variables & parameters to the said replicas was the insertion of acquired immunity proposed by Dietz et.al (1990).Anderson & May (1991) and Koella (2003) have proposednotable contributions to the incorporation of biological factors and analyseson the SIR modeling of communicable diseases.

For the communicable diseases like yellow fever or malaria one can use the parameters for birth and death for better prediction. The model is given below with birth and death.

$$\frac{dS}{dt} = \text{birth} - \beta * S * I - \text{death} * S \dots \tag{7}$$

$$\frac{dI}{dt} = \beta * S * I - \gamma * I - \text{death} * I \dots \tag{8}$$

$$\frac{dR}{dt} = \gamma * I - \text{death} * R \dots \tag{9}$$

The equations 7, 8 and 9 constitute a set representing the SIR model system with incorporation of birth and death parameters. Figure 2 shows the solution of the SIR model with the incorporation of birth and death parameters.

Figure 4. SIR model with birth and death & assumed values S = 0.9, I = 0.1, R = 0.005, beta = 0.1, death = 0.001, birth = 0.001

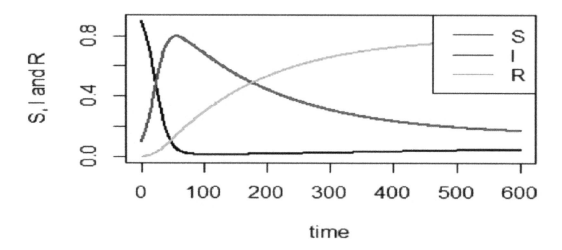

Also, the assumption of values of birth and death may be equal or unequal. In equations 7,8 and 9 it is assumed to have different parameters for birth and death values. However, few researchers use the same parameters too. Though it is preferable to use the birth and death values separately, due to circumstances, the value becomesthe same or at the start of the disease, the parameter value may not be available. Hence, few researchers use same value for birth and death parameters. The equations and the solution graph generated is given below. Usually a simple SIR Mathematical model forever forecasts hindered fluctuations for an equilibrium position. This is usually at odds among periodic epidemics which people can observe in various real circumstances with pathogens. Persistent fluctuations necessitate a few extra catalystparameters for the proposed mathematical model. For instance, the infection of measles among children's contact rate follow seasonality as the children accumulate or gather at schools and there is a high chance during such gathering. Such circumstances can be explored by incorporating the seasonality parameters. It is the usual practice of assuming the sinusoidal curve forcing on β and can be defined as $\beta(t) = \beta_0\left(1 + \beta_0 Cos 2\pi t\right)$.

The SIR model along with the seasonality is given.

$$\frac{dS}{dt} = \text{birth}*(1\text{-S}) - \beta * S * I \dots \tag{10}$$

$$\frac{dI}{dt} = \beta * S * I - \gamma * I - \text{birth} * I \dots \tag{11}$$

$$\frac{dR}{dt} = \gamma * I - \text{birth*R} \dots \tag{12}$$

Figure 5. SIR model with values S=0.999,I=0.001,R=0.000, μ =1/50, β =400, γ =365/12 without seasonal parameter

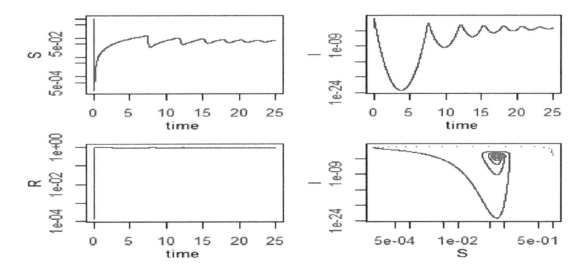

If one wants to incorporate the rainfall as a parameter, the rainfall, $\log[R_A(t)] = \dfrac{a * R_A(t)}{b + R_A(t)}$, where $R_A(t)$ is the rainfall data with respect to time t, a and b are the respective parameters.If one replaces the value of β in equations 10,11 and 12 with the rainfall parameter $R_A(t)$, the one can change the model. Here it is to be noted that, by using programming, one can interpolate, especially extrapolate or predict the rainfall values using forecasting models. One such visualization is found in figure 7. The

Figure 6. SIR model with initial conditions $\mu = 1/50$, $\beta_0 = 400$, $\beta_1 = 0.15$, $\gamma = 365/12, S = 0.07, I = 0.00039,$
R=0.92961, $\beta(t) = \beta_0 \left(1 + \beta_1 Cos 2\pi t\right)$

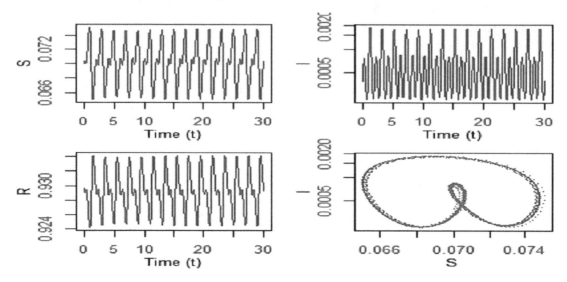

solution of the SIR model with respect to time for *S, I,* and *R* with incorporated rainfall data with forecasting is shown in figure 8.

As the seasonality becomes a specific case of SIR model formulation, it is continued without the sinusoidal assumption hereafter. There are various strategies for ascertaining the ideal control for a particular Mathematical model. As an example, Pontryagin's (1962) extreme principle permits the computation of the ideal control for a system of ordinary differential conditions with given restrictions. The ideal control approach is used to minimize the infected people and to amplify the number of recovered people. The book by Diekmann and Heesterbeek (2000) discusses the usage of biological assumptions in building replicas and current applications. The interesting thing is, the book covers both deterministic and stochastic modeling. The vaccinated population (v_a) has more immunity power and should be removed from the susceptible population and can be included in the recovered population. Since still no vaccination has been found for the deadly disease NiV, this variable v_a can be considered as the awareness level and /or self-prevention along with the immunity coefficient.

$$\frac{dS}{dt} = \text{birth} - \beta * S * I - \text{death} * S - v_a * S \ldots \tag{13}$$

$$\frac{dI}{dt} = \beta * S * I - \gamma * I - \text{death} * I \ldots \tag{14}$$

$$\frac{dR}{dt} = \gamma * I + v_a * S - \text{death} * R \ldots \tag{15}$$

Figure 7. Sample forecasting for rainfall with respect to time

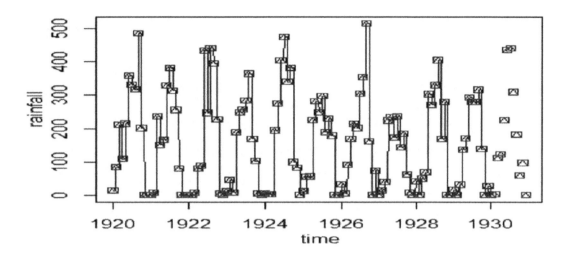

Figure 8. SIR solution with forecasted rainfall with respect to time with different initial conditions

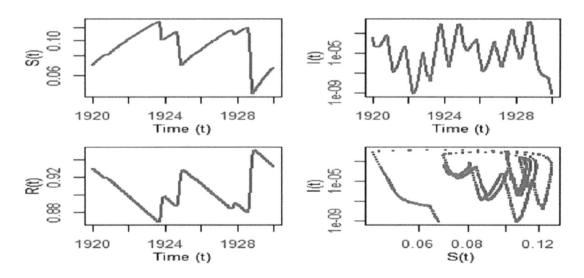

Here, it is assumed that the value of $v_a = 0.1$, as people don't have much awareness initially with the disease. Only after the spread of the disease, the Government and other organizations can start the awareness to people and provide vaccination if any. Hence, assumption of $v_a = 0.1$ is reasonable. As days roll on, the value of v_a can be increased which impact the decrease in S and increase in R. One can include the vaccination strategies in different aspects, and it can be expressed as the accumulation of awareness, vaccinations if any, cleanliness, self-awareness, etc., One can observe that figure 9 has quick and greater recovery than that of recovery curve in figure 4. The environmental effects for the spread and resistance to drug, evolution of immunity was proposed by Yang (2000) and Chen & Wilson (2006) for communicable diseases.

Figure 9. SIR model with birth, death, vaccination & assumed values S=0.9, I=0.1, R=0, beta = 0.1, recovery = 0.005, death = 0.001, birth = 0.001, vaccination = 0.1

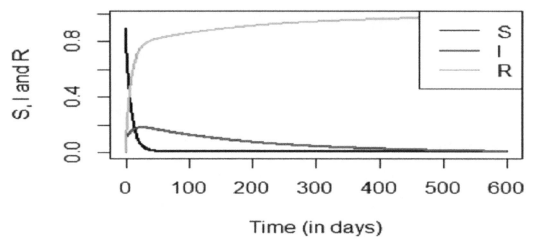

Sultana, J et al (2016) propose a model for NiVthat incorporates the awareness among people as conveyed by Dheva Rajan et al (2014d) too. A new design was proposed by Ngwa and Shu (2000) and Ngwa (2004) which consists of ordinary differential equation (ODE) compartmental model, a susceptible-exposed-infectious-recovered-susceptible (SEIRS) model for humans and a susceptible-exposed-infectious (SEI) pattern for vector. It is the choice of the researcher to propose the appropriate pattern for host and vector. The presumptions made about the transmission of the disease and incubation period are pivotal in any model; these are reflected in the terms of equations and parameters. One may get attracted to the modelling parameters of Heesterbeek, H (2015) due to his wonderful explanations in the article. In his article, he discussed several factors for notable achievements in control management of communicable diseases. The most significant factors like human connectivity, dynamic behavior of humans, etc., has been discussed in his work wonderfully.

Reproductive Number

The reproductive number R_0 is the most important parameter in studies related to the prevalence of disease and the respective mathematical models. By assuming all the individuals being susceptible to the disease infection, this number R_0 can be defined as the number of infected personalities (either host or vector) with one infected host results during its infectious period. The concept of R_0 was formerly established (1886) for the independent study for malaria 1911 and 1927 and & is nowcommonly applied and aimed at almost all communicable illness (1975) (Heesterbeek & Dietz, 1996).If the value R_0 is greater than 1, each infected person produces more than one new illness and, on average. Hence the disease can conquer the entire susceptible people. If the value R_0 is less than 1, the disease may go out of the population in the short run and that shows the effectiveness of the optimal control measures and the strategies followed. The effective reproduction rate is the average infection triggered by an infected person when only a cluster of a populace is susceptible. As discussed earlier,if $R_e > 1$, then the disease remains spreading or otherwise vanishes. The resisting power of people says immunity can be taken into account, whereas this becomes a challenging one while modeling initially at the time of emerging disease. The state of a population where the portion saved is enough to avert epidemics say $R_e < 1$. Perilous removal edge p_c is a part of the vulnerable people's desires to be hoarded with effective measures or actions. For instance, one can obtain the perilous removal edge through vaccination. If the hosts are assumed to be mixed randomly, then p_c can be defined as $1 - \dfrac{1}{R_0}$. Nikolay B (2019) at PubMed published an article about 14 years examination for the Spread of NiV in Bangladesh. It is one of the most interesting articles that involves case studies and provides the following results. These results will be highly useful for future mathematical model developers while choosing the parameters and the values of different parameters. 82 caused by P-P transmission. This PP transmission yields $0.33 R_0$. Nikolay B (2019) predicted the R_0 value as 1.1 for the infected people of age 45 and above along with struggle in breathing, which has a confidence interval of 0.4 to 3.2 at 95%. 0.05 times of association has been observed amongst the patients who did not have trouble breathing. Around 14% of the infected people are close spouses of the infected, 1.3% are close relatives and around 1% were others. It was observed that there was high positive correlation between infection and the body fluid.

Modelling with Controls

Using the ideal philosophy of rheostat, Jakia& Chandra (2016) proposed a Mathematical model and did the analysis for NiV. Here, the classical SIR model is designed with incorporated parameters; different natural birth rate (b) and death rates (μ), disease-induced death rate (α), effective contact rate or transmission coefficient (β), and the recovery rate (γ). Hence, the equations 16, 17 and 18 can be enhanced with the incorporation of control strategies. Only two parameters namely awareness $u_1(t)$, and treatment $u_2(t)$ are included here as there is no vaccination found still now, hence one cannot include the effect of vaccination. The parameter $u_1(t)$ gives the decrease in β and the measure of $u_2(t)$ is required and determined by analyzing the health care facilities for the infected people, hence such measurements yield reduction in the infected stage I. Based on the above argument, the model has been proposed along with the initial conditions $S(0) = S_0 \geq 0, I(0) = I_0 \geq 0, R(0) = R_0 \geq 0, N(0) = N_0 \geq 0$.

$$\frac{dS}{dt} = b*N - \beta*S*I - \mu*S - u_1*S \ldots \tag{16}$$

$$\frac{dI}{dt} = \beta*S*I - \gamma*I - \mu*I - \alpha*I - u_2*I \ldots \tag{17}$$

$$\frac{dR}{dt} = \gamma*I - \mu*R + u_1*S + u_2*I \ldots \tag{18}$$

With

$$\frac{dN}{dt} = b*N - \alpha*I - \mu*N \ldots \tag{19}$$

This definition of the total population N gives a different idea to new researchers as infection and death are totally eliminated from the population. Bakare, E.A (2014) proposed the integration technique for minimization of the infected people, hence one can adopt the technique for the minimization of I. It is used in weight parameters say W_1 and W_2 which is required for the cost of treatment. After computation, the cost of awareness and cost of treatment is calculated as $W_1 * \frac{u_1^2}{2}$ and $W_2 * \frac{u_2^2}{2}$ respectively.

For the set of ODE, it is mandatory to prove the existence of the solution and uniqueness, and it is the choice of the reader to adopt the different techniques to prove the same. Bakare, E.A (2014) used the assumed initial values of 0.90, 0.05, 0.05, 0.03, 0.002, 0.005, 0.01, and 6 for S, I, R, b, μ α, γ and number of years respectively. Bakare, E.A (2014) calculated the effective contact rate or the transmission coefficient β as 0.75, weight parameters W_1 and W_2 as 1 and 2 respectively. The model is proposed with simulated solutions, and one can develop by comparing it with actual data. Also, several assumed values are used in the model. As days roll by, one can get the epidemics and the much essential information with which the parameters can be updated with the current scenario. It was observed that the epidemic incidence is high during monsoon time and so the incorporation of seasonal parameters like rainfall, humidity, and temperature can be considered. One can think of next-generation reproductive number for NiVepidemics for better prediction. Though there is no significant predictions and publications on gender-wise differences in NiV epidemics, it is evident that women and children were affected more than males and a greater number of female infections is observed due to human interaction concerning social and family responsibilities. Hence, one can consider modelling with the inclusion of gender and age-wise infection levels.

Biswas (2014) has performed an investigation on "Optimal Control of NiV Infections: A Bangladesh Scenario". In his work, he used the scholastic campaigns and public dissociating as control measurement tools to prevent individuals from being affected by the epidemics of NiV. Nita et al (2018) proposed a two-compartment SEIR model with control strategies as a developmental work of Biswas (2014). In this work, Nita et al (2018) considered separate SEIR models for host and vector, that is, humans and bats. It is proposed to divide the human population to susscepible, exposed, infected, hospitalized and death and bat population as susscepible, exposed, infected, and removed. Figure 10 describes the transmission cycle, pathway and the stages of spread of NiV comprising of human and bat population. Nita et al (2018) proposed a model where the death stage is included in infectious stage. This assumption seems to be unrealistic, as the entire human death population cannot be included in the human exposed population, whereas the coefficient or parameter or additional transmission coefficient comprising of the spread of infections to human from the human death can be considered to incorporate. Hence, the future researcher may incorporate or modify the death stage to improve the predictive power of the proposed model. In the model, natural death rate is removed from every stage of human SEIHD while it is common to the total human and bat population. Hence one can get the accuracy error if the total death rate is removed from every stage and for future modelling one can think of removing different death rates at every stage.

The control strategies are divided into four parts in this model, spraying insecticides, buried bats, self-prevention and hospitalization denoted by u_1, u_2, u_3 and u_4 respectively. Such a division is an appreciable move, so that, one can evaluate each strategy separately to analyze its impact on the spread of the disease and to improve the model. The transmission coefficient α of bats is divided into five parts as susceptible to exposed, exposed to infected, infected to removed, infected to susceptible and infected to removed denoted by $\alpha_1, \alpha_2, \alpha_3$ α_4 and α_5 respectively. The transmission coefficient β of humans

Figure 10. Two-compartment model for Human and Bat

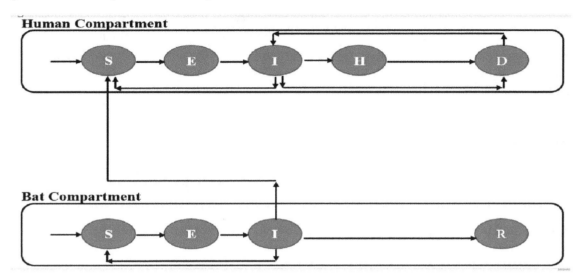

is divided into seven parts as susceptible to exposed, exposed to infected, infected to death (removed), infected to susceptible, infected to hospitalized, hospitalized to death, and death to exposed denoted by $\beta_1, \beta_2, \beta_3, \beta_4, \beta_5, \beta_6$ and, β_7 respectively. Modelling the transmission coefficients separately like this definitely will increase the predictive power, as the coefficients and the impacts are calculated separately. The local & global stability is discussed and it has been proved that the model is locally and globally asymptotically stable. The optimality is also discussed with strong mathematical calculations, shreds of evidence and numerical simulations with the effect of control strategies. The entire solution of the said model is not discussed here,as the reader can refer the work of Nita et al (2018) whenever necessary, however it is discussed the loop wholes and future development for the upcoming researchers.

Challenges

Lloyd-Smith, J. O (2015) enlightened 9 most significant points in detail in modelling the novel pathogens. The challenges includes, finding the illness dynamics in non-human proximal types of species, intensifying the model for cross-species, detection of adaption and human-animal interface to map the transmission, incorporation of analyzation methods like stochasticity after pathogen introduction leads to observation errors, the data collection from the sporadic types, develop specific theories and case studies for intermediate hosts, incorporation of immunity of host in the models, developing a model that measure the fatality measurements of the diseases, designing the empirical studies of emerging pathogens for the most accurate scheming of risk.

This detailing by Grant, C (2016) traces the advantages of utilizing various ways to deal to improve a model and encourage multidisciplinary investigation into communicable illnesses, just as appearing and proposing down to earth instances of powerful incorporation. It takes a look at the advantages of utilizing participatory research related to conventional demonstrating techniques to possibly improve illness research, control, and the board. Incorporated methodologies can prompt increasingly reasonable numerical models which thusly can help with settling on strategy choices that lessen malady and advantage nearby individuals.Huyvaert, K. P (2018) analyzed the gaps of Lloyd-Smith, J. O (2015) and provided the most significant points in developing mathematical models. He discussed the challenges and opportunities too while modelling the pathogens of both wild and domestic animals. Also, Huyvaert, K. P (2018) suggested incorporating the separate mortality and birth rates of wild and domestic animals separately with the force of infection. Also, he suggested separating the population by gender-wise since there were changes in the immunity levels.

REFERENCES

Anderson, R. M., & May, R. M. (1991). *Infectious Diseases of Humans: Dynamics and Control*. Oxford University Press.

Aron, J. L., & May, R. M. (1982). *The Population Dynamics of Infectious Disease: Theory and Applications*. Chapman and Hall.

Bailey, N. T. J. (1975). *The Mathematical Theory of Infectious Diseases*. Griffin.

Bakare, E. A., Nwagwo, A., & Danso-Addo, E. (2014). Optimal Control Analysis of an SIR Epidemic Model with Constant Recruitment. *International Journal of Applied Mathematical Research*, *3*(3), 273–285. doi:10.14419/ijamr.v3i3.2872

Biswas, M. H. A. (2014). Optimal Control of Nipah Virus (NiV) Infections: A Bangladesh Scenario. *Journal of Pure and Applied Mathematics: Advances and Applications*, *12*(1), 77–104.

Broder, C. C., Xu, K., Nikolov, D. B., Zhu, Z., Dimitrov, D. S., Middleton, D., & Wang, L. F. (2013). A treatment for and vaccine against the deadly Hendra and NipahViruses. *Antiviral Research*, *100*(1), 8–13. doi:10.1016/j.antiviral.2013.06.012 PMID:23838047

Chadha, M. S., Comer, J. A., Lowe, L., Rota, P. A., Rollin, P. E., Bellini, W. J., & Mishra, A. (2006). Nipah virus-associated encephalitis outbreak, Siliguri, India. *Emerging Infectious Diseases*, *12*(2), 235–240. doi:10.3201/eid1202.051247 PMID:16494748

Chen, L. H., & Wilson, M. E. (2006). Dengue and chikungunya infections in travelers. *Current Opinion in Infectious Diseases*, *5*, 438–444. PMID:20581669

Ching, P. K. G., de los Reyes, V. C., Sucaldito, M. N., Tayag, E., Columna-Vingno, A. B., Malbas, F. F. Jr, Bolo, G. C. Jr, Sejvar, J. J., Eagles, D., Playford, G., Dueger, E., Kaku, Y., Morikawa, S., Kuroda, M., Marsh, G. A., McCullough, S., & Foxwell, A. R. (2015). Outbreak of henipavirus infection, Philippines, 2014. *Emerging Infectious Diseases*, *21*(2), 328–331. doi:10.3201/eid2102.141433 PMID:25626011

de Wit, E., & Munster, V. J. (2015). Animal models of disease shed light on Nipah virus pathogenesis and transmission. *The Journal of pathology*, 235(2), 196–205. doi:10.1002/path.4444de

Dheva Rajan, S., IyemPerumal, A., Kalpana, D., & Rajagopalan, S.P. (2013a). SPR_SODE Model for dengue fever.*International Journal of Applied Mathematical and Statistical Sciences*, 2(3), 41-46.

Dheva Rajan, S., IyemPerumal, A., Kalpana, D., & Rajagopalan, S.P. (2013b). Improved SPR_SODE Model for dengue fever. *International Journal of Advanced Scientific and Technical Research*, *5*(3), 418–425.

Dheva Rajan, S., IyemPerumal, A., Kalpana, D., & Rajagopalan, S.P. (2013c). Asymptotic Stability Of SPR_SODE Model for Dengue. *International Journal of Research in Applied.Natural and Social Sciences*, *1*(6), 59–64.

Dheva Rajan, S., Iyemperumal, A., Kalpana, D., & Rajagopalan, S.P. (2013d). A support investigation for SPR_SODE Model for dengue. *American Journal of Sustainable City and Society*, *1*(2), 204-212.

Dheva Rajan, S., IyemPerumal, A., Kalpana, D., & Rajagopalan, S.P. (2014a). Existence of the solution and disease-free equilibrium of SPR_SODE Model. *International Journal of Pure and Applied Mathematical Sciences, 7*(1), 1-7.

Dheva Rajan, S., Iyemperumal, A., Kalpana, D., & Rajagopalan, S.P. (2014b). A Critical analysis on bifurcation of SPR_SODE Model for the spread of dengue. *International Journal of Advanced Natural Sciences*, *3*(1), 33-40.

Dheva Rajan, S., IyemPerumal, A., Kalpana, D., & Rajagopalan, S.P. (2014c). Bifurcation Analysis of SPR_SODE Model for the spread of dengue. *International Journal Applied Engineering Research*, *9*(6), 643–651.

Dheva Rajan, S., IyemPerumal, A., Kalpana, D., & Rajagopalan, S.P. (2014d). Sensitivity Analysis of SPR_SODE Model for the spread of dengue. *International Journal Applied Environmental Sciences*, *9*(4), 1237–1250.

Diekman, O., Heesterbeek, J. A. P., & Metz, J. A. J. (1990). On the definition and the computation of the basic reproduction ratio R_0 in models for infectious diseases in heterogeneous populations. *Journal of Mathematical Biology*, *28*, 365–382. PMID:2117040

Diekmann, O., & Heesterbeek, J. A. P. (2000). *Mathematical Epidemiology of Infectious Diseases: Model Building, Analysis and Interpretation*. John Wiley.

Dietz, K., Molineaux, L., & Thomas, A. (1990). A dengue model tested in the African Savannah. *Bulletin of the World Health Organization*, *50*, 347–357. PMID:4613512

Eykhoff, P. (1974). *System Identification: Parameter and State Estimation*. Wiley & Sons.

Field, H., Young, P., Yob, J. M., Mills, J., Hall, L., & Mackenzie, J. (2001). The natural history of Hendra and Nipah viruses. *Microbes and Infection*, *3*(4), 307–314. doi:10.1016/S1286-4579(01)01384-3 PMID:11334748

Foster, K. R., Jenkins, M. E., & Toogood, A. C. (1998). The Philadelphia Yellow Fever Epidemic of 1793. *Scientific American*, *279*(2), 88–93. doi:10.1038cientificamerican0898-88 PMID:9674172

Garg, A. K., Chouhan, P., & Sharma, B. (2019). Fundamental Tenets of Nipah Virus Infection in Ayurveda and its Management:A Multidisciplinary Investigation. *International Journal of Ayurveda and Pharmaceutical Chemistry*, *10*(2), 48–64.

Gillespie, D.T. (1976). A general method for numerically simulating the stochastic time evolution of coupled chemical reactions. *Journal of Computational Physics, 22*, 403–434. doi:10.1016/0021-9991(76)90041-3

Gillespie, D. T. (1977). Exact stochastic simulation of coupled chemical reactions. *Journal of Physical Chemistry, 81*(25), 2340–2361. doi:10.1021/j100540a008

Goh, K. J., Tan, C. T., Chew, N. K., Tan, P. S. K., Kamarulzaman, A., Sarji, S. A., Wong, K. T., Abdullah, B. J. J., Chua, K. B., & Lam, S. K. (2000). Clinical features of Nipah virus encephalitis among pig farmers in Malaysia. *The New England Journal of Medicine, 342*(17), 1229–1235. doi:10.1056/NEJM200004273421701 PMID:10781618

Grant, C., Lo Iacono, G., Dzingirai, V., Bett, B., Winnebah, T. R., & Atkinson, P. M. (2016). Moving interdisciplinary science forward: Integrating participatory modelling with mathematical modelling of zoonotic disease in Africa. *Infectious Diseases of Poverty, 5*(1), 17. doi:10.118640249-016-0110-4 PMID:26916067

Hammoud, D. A., Lentz, M. R., Lara, A., Bohannon, J. K., Feuerstein, I., Huzella, L., Jahrling, P. B., Lackemeyer, M., Laux, J., Rojas, O., Sayre, P., Solomon, J., Cong, Y., Munster, V., & Holbrook, M. R. (2018). Aerosol exposure to intermediate size Nipah virus particles induces neurological disease in African green monkeys. *PLoS Neglected Tropical Diseases, 12*(11), e0006978. doi:10.1371/journal.pntd.0006978 PMID:30462637

Heesterbeek, H., Anderson, R. M., Andreasen, V., Bansal, S., De Angelis, D., Dye, C., Eames, K. T. D., Edmunds, W. J., Frost, S. D. W., Funk, S., Hollingsworth, T. D., House, T., Isham, V., Klepac, P., Lessler, J., Lloyd-Smith, J. O., Metcalf, C. J. E., Mollison, D., Pellis, L., ... Viboud, C. (2015). Isaac Newton Institute IDD Collaboration (2015). *Modeling infectious disease dynamics in the complex landscape of global health. Science, 347*(6227), aaa4339. Advance online publication. doi:10.1126cience.aaa4339 PMID:25766240

Hethcote, H. (2000). The Mathematics of Infectious Diseases. *SIAM Review, 42*(4), 599–653. doi:10.1137/S0036144500371907

Host and Vector. (2019). *Infectious Diseases: In Context*. Retrieved August 27, 2019 from Encyclopedia.com: https://www.encyclopedia.com/media/educational-magazines/host-and-vector

Hsu, V. P., Hossain, M. J., Parashar, U. D., Ali, M. M., Ksiazek, T. G., Kuzmin, I., Breiman, R. F., & ... . (2004). Nipah virus encephalitis reemergence, Bangladesh. *Emerging Infectious Diseases, 10*(12), 2082–2087. doi:10.3201/eid1012.040701 PMID:15663842

Huyvaert, K. P., Russell, R. E., Patyk, K. A., Craft, M. E., Cross, P. C., Garner, M. G., & Walsh, D. P. (2018). Challenges and Opportunities Developing Mathematical Models of Shared Pathogens of Domestic and Wild Animals. *Veterinary Sciences, 5*(4), 92. doi:10.3390/vetsci5040092 PMID:30380736

Johnston, S. C., Briese, T., Bell, T. M., Pratt, W. D., Shamblin, J. D., Esham, H. L., & Honko, A. N. (2015). Detailed analysis of the African green monkey model of Nipah virus disease. *PLoS One, 10*(2), e0117817. doi:10.1371/journal.pone.0117817 PMID:25706617

Kermack, W., & McKendrick, A. (1991a). Contributions to the mathematical theory of epidemics—I. *Bulletin of Mathematical Biology, 53*(1–2), 33–55. doi:10.1007/BF02464423 PMID:2059741

Kermack, W., & McKendrick, A. (1991b). Contributions to the mathematical theory of epidemics—II. The problem of endemicity. *Bulletin of Mathematical Biology, 53*(1–2), 57–87. doi:10.1007/BF02464424 PMID:2059742

Kermack, W., & McKendrick, A. (1991c). Contributions to the mathematical theory of epidemics—III. Further studies of the problem of endemicity. *Bulletin of Mathematical Biology, 53*(1–2), 89–118. doi:10.1007/BF02464425 PMID:2059743

Koella, J. C., & Boete, C. (2003). A model for the co-evolution of immunity and immune evasion in vector-borne disease with implications for the epidemiology of malaria. *American Naturalist, 161*(5), 698–707. doi:10.1086/374202 PMID:12858279

Lo Presti, A., Cella, E., Giovanetti, M., Lai, A., Angeletti, S., Zehender, G., & Ciccozzi, M. (2015). Origin and evolution of Nipah virus. *Journal of Medical Virology, 88*(3), 380–388. doi:10.1002/jmv.24345 PMID:26252523

Luby, S. P., Gurley, E. S., & Hossain, M. J. (2009). Transmission of Human Infection with Nipah Virus. *Clinical Infectious Diseases, 49*(11), 1743–1748. doi:10.1086/647951 PMID:19886791

MacDonald, G. (1957). *The Epidemiology and Control of Malaria.* Oxford University Press.

Malthus, T. R. (1970). *An essay on the Principal of Population.* Penguin Books. (Original work published 1798)

McNeill, M. (1989). *' Plagues and People.* Anchor Books.

Middleton, D. J., Morrissy, C. J., van der Heide, B. M., Russell, G. M., Braun, M. A., Westbury, H. A., Halpin, K., & Daniels, P. W. (2007). Experimental Nipah virus infection in pteropid bats (*Pteropus-poliocephalus*). *Journal of Comparative Pathology, 136*(4), 266–272. doi:10.1016/j.jcpa.2007.03.002 PMID:17498518

Nikolay, B., Salje, H., Hossain, M.J., Khan, A.K.M.D., & Sazzad, H.M.S. (2019). *Transmission of Nipah Virus - 14 Years of Investigations in Bangladesh.* Doi:10.1056/NEJMoa1805376

Nipah Virus (NiV) CDC. (n.d.). www.cdc.gov

Nowak, R. (1994). *Walker's bats of the world.* Johns Hopkins University Press.

Parashar, U. D., Sunn, L. M., Ong, F., Mounts, A. W., Arif, M. T., Ksiazek, T. G., Kamaluddin, M. A., Mustafa, A. N., Kaur, H., Ding, L. M., Othman, G., Radzi, H. M., Kitsutani, P. T., Stockton, P. C., Arokiasamy, J., Gary, H. E. Jr, & Anderson, L. J. (2000). Case-control study of risk factors for human infection with a new zoonotic Paramyxovirus, Nipah virus, during a 1998–1999 outbreak of severe encephalitis in Malaysia. *The Journal of Infectious Diseases, 181*(5), 1755–1759. doi:10.1086/315457 PMID:10823779

Pontryagin, L. S., Boltyanskii, V. G., Gamkrelize, R. V., & Mishchenko, E. F. (1962). *The Mathematical Theory of Optimal Processes.* Wiley.

Powell, J.H. (1993). *Bring Out Your Dead: The Great Plague of Yellow Fever in Philadelphia in 1793.* University of Pennsylvania Press.

Rahman, S. A., Hassan, S. S., Olival, K. J., Mohamed, M., Chang, L.-Y., Hassan, L., Saad, N. M., Shohaimi, S. A., Mamat, Z. C., Naim, M. S., Epstein, J. H., Suri, A. S., Field, H. E., & Daszak, P. (2010). Characterization of Nipah virus from naturally infected Pteropusvampyrus bats, Malaysia. *Emerging Infectious Diseases*, *16*(12), 1990–1993. doi:10.3201/eid1612.091790 PMID:21122240

Ross, R. (1911). *The Prevention of Malaria*. John Murray.

Shah, N. H., Trivedi, N. D., Thakkar, F. A., & Satia, M. H. (2018). Control Strategies for Nipah Virus. *International Journal of Applied Engineering Research*, *13*(21), 15149–15163.

Signs and Symptoms Nipah Virus (NiV). (n.d.). www.cdc.gov

Sultana, J., & Podder, C. N. (2016). Mathematical Analysis of Nipah Virus Infections Using Optimal Control Theory. *Zeitschrift für Angewandte Mathematik und Physik*, *4*, 1099–1111. doi:10.4236/jamp.2016.46114

Sultana, J., & Podder, C. N. (2016). Mathematical Analysis of Nipah Virus Infections Using Optimal Control Theory. *Zeitschrift für Angewandte Mathematik und Physik*, *4*, 1099–1111. doi:10.4236/jamp.2016.46114

WHO Nipah Virus (NiV) Infection. (n.d.). www.who.int

Wong, K. T., Shieh, W. J., Kumar, S., Norain, K., Abdullah, W., Guarner, J., Goldsmith, C. S., Chua, K. B., Lam, S. K., Tan, C. T., Goh, K. J., Chong, H. T., Jusoh, R., Rollin, P. E., Ksiazek, T. G., & Zaki, S. R. (2002). Nipah virus infection: Pathology and pathogenesis of an emerging paramyxoviral zoonosis. *American Journal of Pathology*, *161*(6), 2153–2167. doi:10.1016/S0002-9440(10)64493-8 PMID:12466131

Yang, H. M. (2000). Malaria transmission model for different levels of acquired immunity and temperature-dependent parameters (vector). *Revista de Saude Publica*, *34*(3), 223–231. doi:10.1590/S0034-89102000000300003 PMID:10920443

Yang, H. M., & Ferreira, M. U. (2000). Assessing the effects of global warming and local social and economic conditions on the malaria transmission. *Revista de Saude Publica*, *34*(3), 214–222. doi:10.1590/S0034-89102000000300002 PMID:10920442

Yob, J. M., Field, H., Rashdi, A. M., Morrissy, C., van der Heide, B., Rota, P., bin Adzhar, A., White, J., Daniels, P., Jamaluddin, A., & Ksiazek, T. (2001). Nipah virus infection in bats (order Chiroptera) in peninsular Malaysia. *Emerging Infectious Diseases*, *7*(3), 439–441. doi:10.3201/eid0703.017312 PMID:11384522

Chapter 10
Application of AI for Computer–Aided Diagnosis System to Detect Brain Tumors

Poulomi Das

OmDayal Group of Institutions, India & Maulana Abul Kalam Azad University of Technology, India

Rahul Rajak

iD https://orcid.org/0000-0001-6978-6839

University of Calcutta, India

Arpita Das

iD https://orcid.org/0000-0002-5939-2382

University of Calcutta, India

ABSTRACT

Early detection and proper treatment of brain tumors are imperative to prevent permanent damage to the brain even patient death. The present study proposed an AI-based computer-aided diagnosis (CAD) system that refers to the process of automated contrast enhancement followed by identifying the region of interest (ROI) and then classify ROI into benign/malignant classes using significant morphological feature selection. This tool automates the detection procedure and also reduces the manual efforts required in widespread screening of brain MRI. Simple power law transformation technique based on different performance metrics is used to automate the contrast enhancement procedure. Finally, benignancy/ malignancy of brain tumor is examined by neural network classifier and its performance is assessed by well-known receiver operating characteristic method. The result of the proposed method is enterprising with very low computational time and accuracy of 87.8%. Hence, the proposed method of CAD procedure may encourage the medical practitioners to get alternative opinion.

DOI: 10.4018/978-1-7998-2742-9.ch010

INTRODUCTION

The main objective of a new AI based CAD system is to analyze the brain MRI to detect the lesion characteristics in early stage. In most of the cases, existence of different brain tumors including gliomas, meningiomas, medulloblastomas, pituitary tumors in a patient is diagnosed after long suffering from the symptoms of unexplained nausea, headaches, vision problems, speech difficulties, personality changes, Seizures etc (Ricard et al., 2012). However, in most of the cases these symptoms are very common to other diseases and hence neglected to encounter the early detection procedure. During last few decades, death rates due to brain tumor are increasing rapidly as compared to any other diseases among the men, women and children. The 5-year survival rate is also very poor for people with a cancerous brain or CNS tumor. It is approximately 34% for men and 36% for women. However, survival rates vary widely and depend on several factors, including the type of brain or spinal cord tumor.

The primary tumors start in the brain and are inclined to stay in the brain, the metastatic or malignant tumors may also be developed and spread out in the brain from other parts of the body (Davies & Clarke, 2004). Brain tumors are classified from grade I to IV. Generally, grade I and grade II are benign (non-cancerous) brain tumors which are also called as low-grade. Grade III and grade IV are malignant (cancerous) brain tumors which are called as high-grade.

Patients having stage II (cancerous) tumors in brain need continuous monitoring and observations by magnetic resonance imaging (MRI) or computed tomography (CT) scan by every 6 months (Herholz et al., 2012). However, from the previous studies we have found that the composition of gray matter/ white matter density of brain substantially varies from relative smooth to complex patterns of brightness (Rogowska, 2000)-(Simmons et al., 1994). Regarding this, appearance of tumors may also be obscured by the surrounding soft tissues, presence of cerebral cortex, ventricles etc. As we know that the composition of MRI depends on the differing relaxation times of water contents within various tissues, noises during MRI mainly caused due to field strength variations with time, presence of RF pulses, and receiver bandwidth variation pattern (McVeigh et al., 1986). All these factors may provide serious inaccuracies regarding the location and exact boundaries of tumors. Sometimes recent technology undergoes MRI with contrast for obtaining better contrast which in turn occasionally introduces many side effects including allergic reactions. Few researchers also found that this toxic contrast agent is deposited and retained in the brain (Rogosnitzky & Branch, 2016). Hence there is a biggest concern in radiology about the safety of these agents. Nevertheless, cost of so-called safe contrast agents in MRI is also expensive.

All these factors arise because of visual inspection and interpretation of MRI is performed to find out the presence of abnormalities. Decision made by this examination is going to be much difficult for radiologists to provide accurate and uniform interpretation due to the enormous number of images generated in a widespread screening. Yearly routine check-up of MRI also demands automated computer assisted interpretation system to find out the risk factors. So, the radiologists turn to automated and accurate detection approach prescribed by the specialized computer algorithms which in turn safe, non-invasive and fast. Obscured nature of normal brain MRI also alternatively bypasses the requirement of invasive contrast agent technique. Therefore, enhancement of brain MRI followed by proper segmentation approach is very important and emerging demand for visual interpretation and therapeutic planning of tumors by the radiologists.

In a successful CAD based detection procedure, inhomogeneous nature of brain MRI requires an appropriate contrast enhancement technique followed by a segmentation approach and then significant features to be extracted to distinguish the benignancy/malignancy of the tumors. This proposal will provide a general framework of an intelligent CAD system to detect brain tumor in the early stage which may help the radiologists for alternative review option. More specifically, in this work feature characterization and 2D/3D scatter distribution of extracted features also helps to visualize the benignancy/malignancy of the tumors. Moreover, performances of the CAD system will be analyzed in this work in terms of different classification indices such as sensitivity, specificity, accuracy, receiver operating characteristics and so on.

The rest of the article is arranged as follows. Background of the work is discussed briefly in section 2. Proposed methodology of the present work is described in section 3. We show the efficiency of the proposed method through experimental results on brain tumor images in section 4. We have drawn some conclusions in section 5.

BACKGROUND

AI introduces different algorithmic approaches to estimate and analyze the medical information similar to human reasoning. Nowadays acceptance of AI in biomedical image/signal analysis is rising and it may resolve a variety of problems of patients, medical practitioners and the healthcare industry. However, initial and important challenging step of AI in biomedical image/signal processing is to design a computer aided diagnosis (CAD) system for therapeutic planning of patients. Now a days, therapeutic procedure is fully operated by the expert's inspection and hence enormous human resources are exploited for this purpose. A CAD based biomedical image analysis and monitoring system may provide a second opinion to the medical practitioners in a short time and also improve the therapeutic planning in a greater sense. In this study, AI is applied to develop a flow algorithm of a CAD system for brain lesion detection, classification and performance analysis.

A large number of survey work have been conducted by the researcher to explore better detection of the lesion characteristics in early stage. Poor visibility of MRI may misguide the radiologists to predict prognosis of the disease. So, the radiologists turn to various computer assisted analysis systems as an alternative reviewing process. Various filtering technique (Gonzalez & Woods, 2003) can be adopted to improve the image resolution and image de-noising. Apart from various filtering technique, many local and global intensity-based contrast enhancement (Kim et al., 2014),(Kamil & Ahmet, 2016) methods, wavelet-based techniques (Tang et al., 2009), fuzzy logic approaches have also been used for contrast enhancement of medical images (Cheng & Xu, 2002). After contrast enhancement of medical images, the goal of AI based CAD system is to choose those significant features of segmented lesion that allow the classifier to categorize the masses into benign/malignant stages.

Segmentation is the process of partitioning an image into a set of homogeneous regions. Several segmentation methods are available in the literature to segment suspicious region depending on grey level, color, or texture (Gonzalez & Woods, 2003). Apart from this, many automated segmentation methods have been proposed which incorporates intensity-based method, region-growing methods and deformable contour models. Region growing algorithm is a bottom-up iterative approach proposed by Adam et al. (Adams & Bischof, 1994), in which neighboring image pixels of the initial seed region are compared based on a similarity criterion and if adjacent regions are found, then those regions are added by a region-merging process in which weak edges are dissolved and strong edges are left intact (Meenalosini et al., 2012). K-means clustering algorithm (Qiao et al., 2019), Fuzzy C-means algorithm (Alruwaili et al., 2019),(Adhikari et al., 2015), and folded Kernal based Fuzzy C-Means algorithm,

(Das & Das, 2019) Genetic algorithms (Chandra & Dr. Rao, 2016) are used in automated segmentation process. Rangayyan et al (Rangayyan et al., 1997) proposed changes of shape patterns from benign to malignant lesion expresses the prognosis of cancer stages. Bruce (Bruce & Adhami, 1999) proposed discrete wavelet transform modulus-maxima (mod-max) method based multiresolution analysis, which exploits shape features of suspicious region. Local and discrete texture features are also useful to determine the prognosis of malignancy (Wanga et al., 2019). Based on feature selection, classifiers are to be modeled to classify the benignancy/malignancy of lesions. The choice of classifier will depend on the nature of available feature space. However, faulty characteristics of selected features may mislead the classification process. Design of classifier may adopt statistical Bayesian approach to hybrid soft computing approaches in order to obtain satisfactory results (Bruce & Adhami, 1999),(Dadabada & Vadlamani, 2018),(Bhaumik et al., 2016). However, accuracy and efficiency of classifiers mostly depends on the choice of significant features.

Present study enhances the MRI of brain images by applying γ based power law transformation to improve the visual quality. However, determination of appropriate γ value is based on the quantitative measuring parameter, which automates the enhancement procedure without any prior knowledge. Then we segment the suspicious region and emphasize on feature extraction methodology. In this study, we attempt to select the significant shape describing features which are able to convey the precise information about benignancy/malignancy. Following this feature selection approaches, classification result with conventional multilayer neural network is able to produce satisfactory detection accuracy. Small but significant feature dimension also relieves the necessity of high computational facility and time. Therefore, it is also convenient to use in the clinical purposes.

METHODOLOGY

Poor visibility of MRI may misguide the radiologists to predict prognosis of the disease. So, the radiologists turn to various computer assisted analysis systems as an alternative reviewing process. The main objective of a new AI based CAD system is to analyze the brain MRI to detect the lesion characteristics in early stage. For improving that poor visibility, brain MRI requires the automated and efficient enhancement technique. Proposed approach exploits very simple power-law transformation technique based on some quantitative parameter measurement in an iterative manner to achieve the best enhancement results. Followed by this automated enhancement procedure, suspicious regions (ROI) are extracted segmentation using K-means algorithm. Since malignancy implies the abnormal and uncontrolled growth of brain cells, significant shape representing features are appropriate for describing the prognosis of malignancy. Using significant morphological feature artificial neural Network classifier is designed to classify benignancy/malignancy of lesions.

A typical overview of the proposed methodology is given in Fig. 1. New concepts of automated contrast enhancement procedure and shift invariant feature selection methodology are focused in the figure.

Each of the processing blocks of Fig.1 is discussed in the following section —

Preprocessing

The preprocessing step improves the standard of the brain tumor MR images and makes these images suited for future processing. Preprocessing includes the removal of irrelevant noise and contrast en-

Figure 1. Schematic diagram of the proposed methodology to determine benignancy/ malignancy

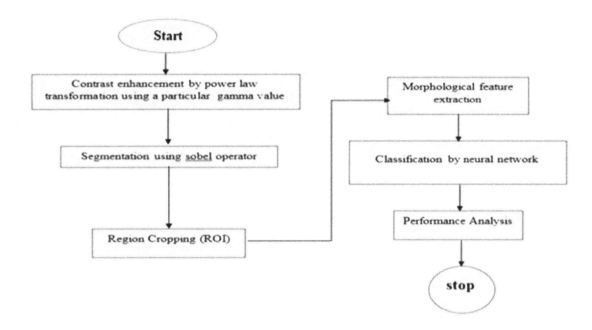

hancement of the suspected regions of interests (ROIs). Thus, image enhancement is an important step to improve the visual appearance of MRI.

Noise Removal

The first step of preprocessing is to convert the given image into a grayscale image. On procuring the grayscale image, the aim then is to filter for removing any noise, if present. In the proposed method, non-linear spatial filter (Median Filter) (Gonzalez & Woods, 2003) is applied in order to remove noise (Salt and Pepper noise).

Contrast Adjustment

In the proposed model, enhancement of suspicious regions is addressed by automated power-law transformation technique by employing some efficient contrast analyzing metrics. The enhanced brain MRI reduces the chance of misleading detection of lesions. A brief description of automated approach of power-law transformation is given below –

- Power law transformation: It is one of the frequently used image enhancement technique (Gonzalez & Woods, 2003),(Vimal & Thiruvikraman, 2012),(Li & Ray Liu, 1997)and represented by the following equation

$$s = cr^{\gamma} \tag{1}$$

Figure 2. (a) Plot of various Transformation Curves by varying γ; (b) Original Brain MRI; (c) Enhanced Brain MRI using automated approach of power-law transformation

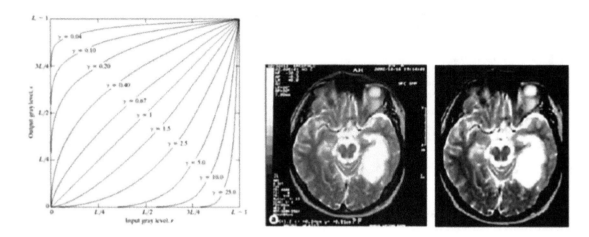

where r and s are the intensity variation of input and output images respectively, c is a constant generally kept at 1 and the value of γ is varied to achieve different level of enhancement,

Graphical representation of power-law transformation is described in Fig. 2, where we have found a family of curve for different variation of γ among which a particular γ produces the best enhancement in terms of visual inspection and clarity. However this choice of appropriate γ is subjective in nature. Proposed method is able to overcome this subjective ness and automate the enhancement procedure by analyzing following four quantitative measuring parameters (Vimal & Thiruvikraman, 2012).

- Average signal to noise ratio (ASNR): It is a conventional but important quantitative measuring parameter for analyzing the enhancement performance. ASNR can be formulated as

$$\text{ASNR} = \frac{f - b}{\sigma} \tag{2}$$

where f and b are the average brightness of the suspicious and its surrounding region (background) respectively; σ is the standard deviation of background region

- Peak signal to noise ratio (PSNR): It is another contrast evaluating parameter and getting larger value for better enhancement. PSNR is formulated as

$$\text{PSNR} = \frac{p - b}{\sigma} \tag{3}$$

where, p is the maximum gray-level value of the target region and σ is standard deviation of the background region.

- Distribution separation measure (DSM): It is evaluated based on probability distribution of suspicious region (target) and its surrounding background. Larger value of DSM provides better separation of target and its background region. DSM is expressed as

$$\text{DSM} = \left(|\mu_T^E - \mu_B^E| \right) - \left(|\mu_T^O - \mu_B^O| \right) \tag{4}$$

where,, are statistical mean of target and background region of enhanced image, are statistical mean of target and background region of original image respectively.

- Target to background contrast ratio (TBC): Objective of any enhancement procedure is highlighting the difference and homogeneity of target region in compare to its surrounding for better visualization. TBC is employed to measure this improvement and formulated as

$$\text{TBC} = \frac{\left(\mu_T^E \middle/ \mu_B^E \right) - \left(\mu_T^O \middle/ \mu_B^O \right)}{\sigma_T^E \middle/ \sigma_T^O} \tag{5}$$

where and are the standard deviation of target and background region of enhanced and original image respectively.

In the proposed approach, Brain MRI are examined by these four quantitative measuring parameters to achieve the best γ value for proper enhancement. Graphical representation of ASNR, PSNR, DSM and TBC with variation of γ value is shown in Fig 3.

Figure 3. (a) Highest value of ASNR, PSNR, TBC at γ =1.5 shows the best enhancement result; (b) Similarly highest value of DSM at γ =1.5 indicates the best enhancement achievement

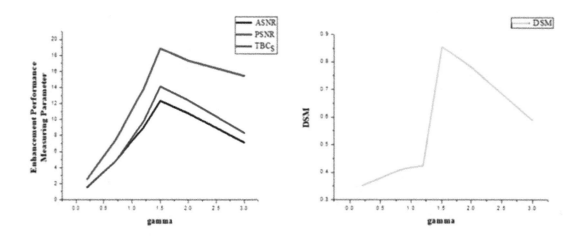

Segmentation

Followed by enhancement procedure, suspected regions must be extracted for analysis of benignancy/ malignancy of lesion and it is performed by segmentation technique. In case of difficult to diagnose brain MRIs, surrounding soft tissues, presence of cerebral cortex, ventricles etc., which may lead serious inaccuracies regarding the location and exact boundaries of tumors. Hence, computer assisted segmentation procedure is an important approach to yield the accurate categorization of masses.

Present study exploits a very simple and popular intensity based segmentation approach, known as K-means clustering technique (Abiwinanda et al., 2019). The algorithm of K-means approach partitions a collection of N number of pixels $[x_j, j = 1, 2, ..., N]$ into W number of groups $[w_i, i = 1, 2, ..., W]$ and finds a center in each group such that a cost function measure is minimized. When a distance metric is chosen as the similarity measure between a candidate pixel x_j in cluster w_i and the corresponding cluster center ci, the cost function is determined by

$$J = \sum_{i=1}^{W} J_i = \sum_{i=1}^{W} \left(\sum_{x_j \in w_i} \left\| x_j - c_i \right\| \right) \tag{6}$$

where the center of class w_i with size $|w_i|$ is computed by

Following K-means segmentation, morphological opening by reconstruction is applied to remove the unwanted glitches appeared in MRI due to heterogeneous nature of lesions. Now based on the segmented boundaries, feature of benignancy/malignancy of tumors are determined accordingly.

Figure 4. Stages of Preprocessing of Brain MRI, (a) Original Brain MRI, (b) Contaminated Brain MRI, (c) Filtered Brain MRI, (d) Contrast Enhanced Brain MRI using automated approach of power-law transformation

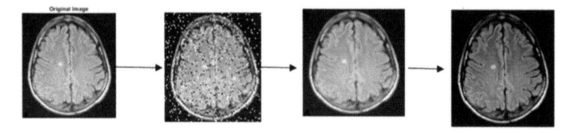

Morphological Feature Analysis

After segmenting the region of interests (ROIs), appropriate representation and description is required to classify them into benign or malignant group. This representation of characteristics is called features. Choosing a particular representation scheme is application specific.

An ideal feature extractor must yield a representation of characteristics that makes the task of classifier trivial. Hence, to analyze the tumors in MRI images, different features are captured and used to obtain

Figure 5. (a) Original Brain MRI; (b) Enhancement by automated power-law transformation; (c) segmentation by k-means algorithm; (d) Extracted tumor

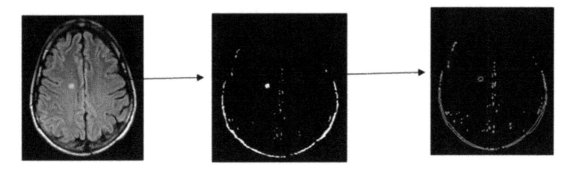

efficient classification results. From the reviews we have found that uncontrolled growth of malignant tumors introduces uneven shape irregularities and produces spiculated margin stellate shape lesion. Moreover, change of shape patterns from benign to malignant expresses the prognosis of cancer stages. Segmented ROIs are used directly to obtain those significant shape features.

These shape-based features play important role in classification. In the following sections, degree of spiculations and shape characterization are estimated using few conventional and self-explanatory features which are useful to characterize the tumors into different stages. These simple descriptors are as given below:

- **Compactness:** It is a numerical quantity representing the degree to which a shape is compact. Compactness meaning joined or packed together. It is closer to one for circular shaped object. Compactness of the brain tumor is defined as,

$$\text{Compactness} = \frac{P^2}{4\pi A} \tag{6}$$

- **Solidity:** Solidity is also known as convexity. The proportion of the pixels in the convex hull that are also in the object (Tumor). It is defined as,

$$\text{Solidity} = \frac{A}{CA} \tag{7}$$

Smallest bounding box

- **Eccentricity:** The number that characterizes how flat the ellipse looks is called the eccentricity

$$\text{Eccentricity} = \frac{W}{L} \tag{8}$$

- **Extent:** The proportion of the pixels in the bounding box that are also in the image object (Tumor).

$$\text{Extent} = \frac{A}{\textit{Smallest bounding box area}} \tag{9}$$

- **Modified Area (MA) Ratio:** This is a special kind of area where it is used to find the separation of features of the two classes. It is defined as,

$$\text{Modified area ratio} = \frac{|CA - A|}{A} \tag{10}$$

where CA is the convex area of masses

Classifier

The choice of classifier is determined by the choice of feature set and complexity of the problem. In this study, effective selection of morphological features leads the classification approach trivial and comfortable. In the present study, we have designed a conventional 3-layer feed-forward neural network (NN) structure for computation of benignancy/malignancy of tumor (Herzog et al., 2019),(Cheng & Cui, 2004). Initially NN is trained with well-defined samples and hence subsequently *test dataset* (a set of features with unknown classes) are examined to evaluate the discrimination accuracy.

Artificial neural networks (ANN)

Artificial neural networks (ANN) or connectionist systems are computing systems vaguely inspired by the biological neural networks that constitute animal brains.(Ricard et al., 2012)(Davies & Clarke, 2004) The neural network itself is not an algorithm, but rather a framework for many different machine learning algorithms to work together and process complex data inputs.

An ANN is based on a collection of connected units or nodes called artificial neurons, which loosely model the neurons in a biological brain. Each connection, like the synapses in a biological brain, can transmit a signal from one artificial neuron to another. An artificial neuron that receives a signal can process it and then signal additional artificial neurons connected to it.

The connections between artificial neurons are called 'edges'. Artificial neurons and edges typically have a weight that adjusts as learning proceeds. The weight increases or decreases the strength of the signal at a connection. Artificial neurons may have a threshold such that the signal is only sent if the aggregate signal crosses that threshold. Typically, artificial neurons are aggregated into layers. Different layers may perform different kinds of transformations on their inputs. Signals travel from the first layer (the input layer), to the last layer (the output layer), possibly after traversing the layers multiple times.

There are many types of neural network. Here we have used **fast forward backpropagation Neural Network.**

Figure 6.

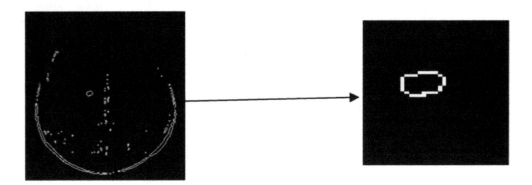

Fast Forward Backpropagation Neural Network

A feedforward neural network is an artificial neural network wherein connections between the nodes do *not* form a cycle. As such, it is different from recurrent neural networks.

The feedforward neural network was the first and simplest type of artificial neural network devised. In this network, the information moves in only one direction, forward, from the input nodes, through the hidden nodes (if any) and to the output nodes. There are no cycles or loops in the network.

Backpropagation algorithms are a family of methods used to efficiently train artificial neural networks (ANNs) following a gradient descent approach that exploits the chain rule. The main feature of backpropagation is its iterative, recursive and efficient method for calculating the weights updates to improve in the network until it is able to perform the task for which it is being trained.

Figure 7. Fast Forward Backpropagation Neural Network

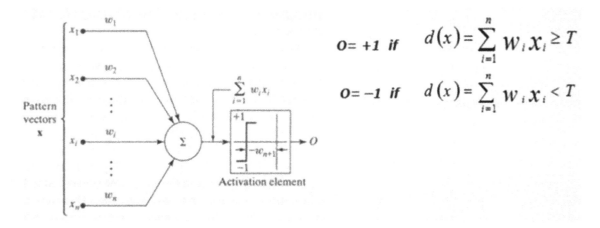

$$O = +1 \text{ if } \quad d(x) = \sum_{i=1}^{n} w_i x_i \geq T$$

$$O = -1 \text{ if } \quad d(x) = \sum_{i=1}^{n} w_i x_i < T$$

The output response of the network is a **linear function of inputs** with the coefficients w_i, where i=1,2,....n, called '**weights**'. The final output of the network denoted as '*O*' is called the **activation function**. If the decision function **d(x)** is greater than a **threshold value** T, then $O = +1$, else $O = -1$

NOTE- Testing samples are *different* samples than the training samples. The algorithm uses the parameters calculated with the training samples to predict the results on the testing samples and then compares the prediction to the target information to see how well the prediction went. It will make use of this information to decide how to re-calculate based upon the training samples.

There are two types of data which are feed to the neural network –

1. Training data
2. Test data

Design Steps

The neural network system is sketched in two things.

Ø Training of Neural Network

The model is initially fit on a **training dataset**, that is a set of examples used to fit the parameters (e.g. weights of connections between neurons in artificial neural networks) of the model. The model (e.g. a neural net or a naive Bayes classifier) is trained on the training dataset using a supervised learning method (e.g. gradient descent or stochastic gradient descent). In practice, the training dataset often consist of pairs of an input vector (or scalar) and the corresponding output vector (or scalar), which is commonly denoted as the *target* (or *label*). The targets for training are used to help the neural network understand that these are the outputs we're looking for. They are not used while testing. The current model is run with the training dataset and produces a result, which is then compared with the *target*, for each input vector in the training dataset. Based on the result of the comparison and the specific learning algorithm being used, the parameters of the model are adjusted.

Ø Testing of Neural network

Finally, the **test dataset** is a dataset used to provide an unbiased evaluation of a final model fit on the training dataset. Testing is done to check the correctness of the neural network. The output we get after testing is used to determine error rate and hence the accuracy of the neural network is achieved.

Performance Analysis

Effectiveness of the proposed AI based CAD system is estimated using several parameters such as overall classification accuracy, sensitivity, specificity, positive predictive value, negative predictive value (Kumar et al., 2019). Receiver operating characteristics (ROC) curve which is a trade off between sensitivity and specificity of the computer-based analysis system (Kumar et al., 2019)-(Kanadam & Chereddy, 2016) is also employed in the proposed study for describing the effectiveness of morphological feature analysis.

- **Sensitivity** – It is a measure of the proportion of actual positives that are correctly identified and is complementary to the false negative rate.

$$\frac{TP}{TP + FN} \tag{11}$$

- **Specificity** – It is a measure of the proportion of actual negatives that are correctly identified and is complementary to the false positive rate.

$$\frac{TN}{TN + FP} \tag{12}$$

- **Efficiency or Accuracy** of the classifiers for each texture analysis method is analyzed based on the error rate.

$$\frac{TP + TN}{TP + FP + TN + FN} \tag{13}$$

The exposition of true and false positive and true and false negative as follows:

table 1. exposition of true and false positive and true and false negative

Abbreviation	Exposition
TP- True Positive	Tumor is Malignant and classified as Malignant.
TN- True Negative	Tumor is Benign and classified as Benign.
FP- False Positive	Tumor is Benign and classified as Malignant.
FN- False Negative	Tumor is Malignant and classified as Benign.

Classification thresholding is a scalar-value criterion that is applied to a model's predicted score in order to separate the positive class from the negative class and it is used in binary classification.

EXPERIMENTAL RESULTS

Dataset: Our dataset for analysis of computer assisted diagnosis system consists of 100 numbers of randomly chosen brain MRI with either benign or malignant tumors from https://www.med.havard.edu/aanlib/home.html. Table -2 presents the statistics of training and test data samples.

As described above, automated power-law transformation enhances the visibility of brain MRI. Following this, segmentation of the suspicious region is achieved. Some of the enhanced and segmented results are described in Fig. 9.

In this proposed approach, initially classifier is trained with 22 numbers of brain MRI which include 11 number of benign tumor and 11 number of ill malignant tumors https://www.med.havard.edu/aanlib/home.html. Although there is a huge number of feature selection and optimization methods in the literature, our objective is to select simple morphological features for classification.

table 2. Statistics of training and test dataset

Training Samples		Test Samples	
Benign	Malignant	Benign	Malignant
11	11	45	33

Following figures draws the notion of scattered distribution of significant morphological features.

The most important part of computer assisted diagnosis system is to achieve the output results and its quality evaluation. Here, we have examined the accuracy of the proposed model by evaluating 88 numbers of test samples and then assessing the outcomes with Harvard University (https://www.med.havard.edu/aanlib/home.html). Some conventional performance indices such as sensitivity, specificity, true positive value, true negative value, false positive value, false negative value, overall classification accuracy is determined to estimate the effectiveness of the proposed model. Summary of these performance indices for different threshold value is shown in TABLE -3.

From the summary of TABLE -3, we have achieved encouraging value of accuracy and sensitivity for threshold value of 0.45. For this particular threshold value proposed model shows highest accuracy elsewhere it is degraded. ROC assessment of the proposed model is shown in Fig. 10.

In the following section, a comparison of experimental results with some other scientific research works using different approaches has been executed to compare the overall accuracy of the proposed model. TABLE -5 shows this summary.

FUTURE DIRECTION OF RESEARCH

In this study, we only focused on the design of simple CAD system to predict brain tumor prognosis. The accuracy obtained by the proposed model is 87.8%, which may be improved by incorporating more sophisticated segmentation approach, advanced feature extraction model and sensitive classifier.

Moreover, this prototype of CAD tool discriminates the benignancy/malignancy of brain tumor based on the morphological features. In future research, we may incorporate the textural contribution of tumors as significant feature set.

CONCLUSION

Proposed AI based Computer Aided Diagnosis system estimates the likelihood of a brain tumor in benign/malignant category. In this view, an automated contrast enhancement approach is proposed to enhance the visual clarity by considering four quantitative contrast enhancement matrices. Followed by enhancement, k-means clustering algorithm is used to segment the suspicious region of interest (ROI). Now based on the segmented boundaries five significant morphological features have been selected to improve the accuracy of ANN classifier.

Proposed approach also describes the 3D scatter distributions of different features for benign/malignant classes. Finally, benignancy/malignancy of brain tumor is examined and assessed by using well known receiver operating characteristic method of ANN classifier.

Figure 8. (a) Original brain MRI; (b) Enhancement by automated power-law transformation; (c) Segmented brain MRI using K-means clustering technique; (d) Extracted tumor

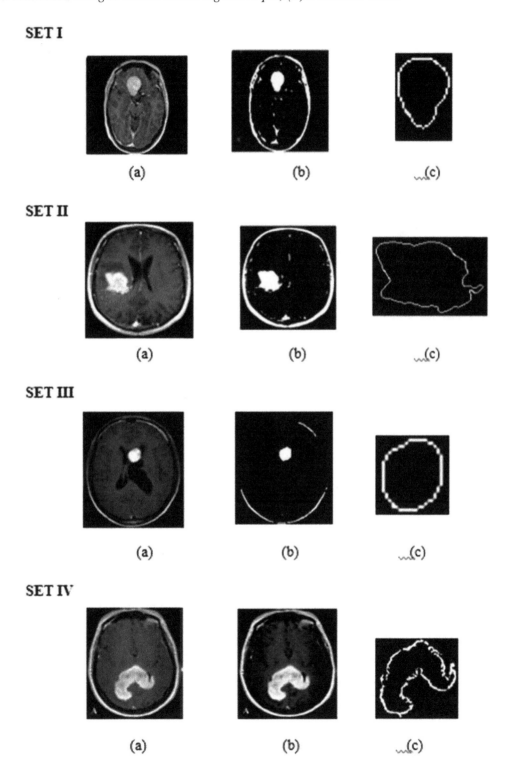

Figure 9. (a) 3D overlapping feature distribution of modified area, perimeter, compactness, solidity; (b) 3D feature distribution of eccentricity, compactness, extent; (blue bubbles are representing benign tumor and red bubbles are representing malignant tumor)

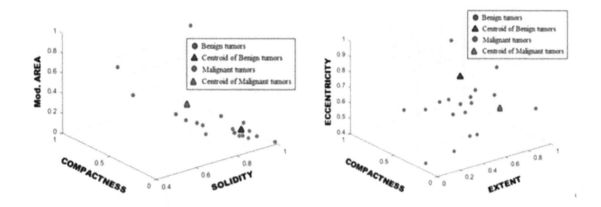

Table 3. Summary of performance indices for different threshold value of ANN classifier

Confidence threshold value	Sensitivity	1- Specificity	Accuracy
0.20	0.983	0.875	0.678
0.25	0.931	0.656	0.733
0.30	0.914	0.625	0.722
0.35	0.896	0.469	0.767
0.40	0.896	0.281	0.833
0.45	**0.879**	**0.156**	**0.878**
0.50	0.793	0.103	0.856
0.55	0.741	0.062	0.811
0.60	0.655	0.031	0.767
0.70	0.534	0.00	0.700

Table 4. Performance measure of proposed Computer Aided Diagnosis System

Sl. No.	Image	Classifier Result	Decision
1.	SET I	0.35	Benign
2.	SET II	0.72	Malignant
3.	SET III	0.23	Benign
4.	SET IV	0.8	Malignant

Figure 10. Graphical representation of Sensitivity vs 1 - Specificity (ROC curve)

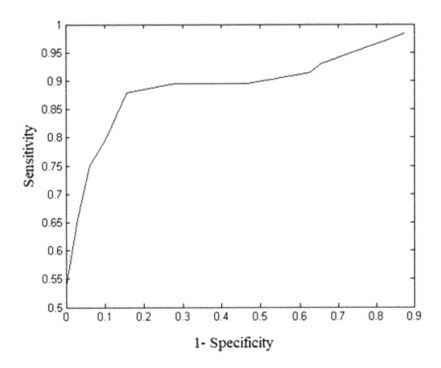

Table 5. Accuracy comparison among the proposed and state-of-the-art methods

S. No	Author	Year	Work	Accuracy
1.	*Vadivel et al. (Vadivel & Surendiran, 2013)*	2013	Construct a generalized fuzzy membership function for classifying the masses as round, oval, lobular and irregular	87.76%
2.	*Tustison et al. (Tustison et al., 2015)*	2015	Introduce a framework for supervised segmentation based on multiple modality intensity, geometry, and asymmetry feature sets.	87%
3.	*Abdel Nasser et al. (Abdel-Nasser et al., 2016)*	2016	Study the effect of factors such as pixel resolution, integration scale, preprocessing, and feature normalization on the performance of texture methods for mass classification	78%
4.	*Abiwinanda et al. (Abiwinanda et al., 2019)*	2019	Attempted to train a Convolutional Neural Network (CNN) to recognize the three most common types of brain tumors, i.e. the Glioma, Meningioma, and Pituitary.	84.19%
5.	**Proposed Method**	-----	Present study proposed AI based Computer Aided Diagnosis (CAD) system that refers to the process of automated contrast enhancement followed by identifying the region of interest (ROI) using k-means clustering technique and then classification of ROI into benignancy/ malignancy classes using five significant morphological feature selection.	87.8%

ROC assessment shows that sensitivity reaches its optimized value 87.9%. The result of the proposed method is enterprising with very low computational time and accuracy of 87.8%. Hence the proposed method of computer assisted detection procedure may encourage the medical practitioners to get alternative opinion.

ACKNOWLEDGMENT

This work is partially supported by the Center of Excellence (CoE) in Systems Biology and Biomedical Engineering, University of Calcutta funded by the World Bank, MHRD India. We would also like to thank to Dr. S. K. Sharma of EKO X-ray & Imagining Institute, Kolkata for providing us valuable comments on the subjective evaluation of the proposed classification scheme.

REFERENCES

34. Abdel-Nasser, M., Melendez, J., Moreno, A., & Puig, D. (2016). The impact of pixel resolution, integration scale, preprocessing, and feature normalization on texture analysis for mass classiðcation in mammograms. *International Journal of Optics, 2016*, 1–12. doi:10.1155/2016/1370259

35. Abiwinanda, N., Hanif, M., Hesaputra, S. T., Handayani, A., & Mengko, T. R. (2019). Brain tumor classification using convolutional neural network. In *World Congress on Medical Physics and Biomedical Engineering 2018*. Springer. 10.1007/978-981-10-9035-6_33

13. Adams, R., & Bischof, L. (1994). Seeded region growing. *IEEE Transactions on Pattern Analysis and Machine Intelligence, 16*(6), 641–647. doi:10.1109/34.295913

17. Adhikari, S. K., Sing, J. K., Basu, D. K., & Nasipuri, M. (2015). Conditional spatial fuzzy C-means clustering algorithm for segmentation of MRI images. *Applied Soft Computing, 34*, 758–769. doi:10.1016/j.asoc.2015.05.038

16. Alruwaili, M., Siddiqi, M. H., & Javed, M. A. (2019). *A robust clustering algorithm using spatial fuzzy C-means for brain MR images*. Egyptian Informatics Journal.

24. Bhaumik, H., Bhattacharyya, S., DasNath, M., & Chakraborty, S. (2016). Hybrid soft computing approaches to content based video retrieval: A brief review. *Applied Soft Computing, 46*, 1008–1029. doi:10.1016/j.asoc.2016.03.022

21. Bruce, L. M., & Adhami, R. R. (1999). Classifying Mammographic Mass Shapes using the Wavelet Transform Modulus-Maxima Method. *IEEE Transactions on Medical Imaging, 18*(12), 1170–1177. doi:10.1109/42.819326 PMID:10695529

19. Chandra, G. R., & Dr. Rao, K. R. H. (2016). Tumor Detection In Brain Using Genetic Algorithm. *Procedia Computer Science, 79*, 449–457. doi:10.1016/j.procs.2016.03.058

28. Cheng, H. D., & Cui, M. (2004). Mass lesion detection with a fuzzy neural network. *Pattern Recognition, 37*(6), 1189–1200. doi:10.1016/j.patcog.2003.11.002

12. Cheng, H. D., & Xu, H. (2002). A novel fuzzy logic approach to mammogram contrast enhancement. *Information Sciences*, *148*(1-4), 167–184. doi:10.1016/S0020-0255(02)00293-1

23. Dadabada, P. K., & Vadlamani, R. (2018). Soft computing hybrids for FOREX rate prediction: A comprehensive review. *Computers & Operations Research*, *99*, 262–284. doi:10.1016/j.cor.2018.05.020

18. Das, P., & Das, A. (2019). A fast and automated segmentation method for detection of masses using folded kernel based fuzzy c-means clustering algorithm. *Applied Soft Computing*, *85*, 105775. doi:10.1016/j.asoc.2019.105775

2. Davies, E., & Clarke, C. (2004). Early symptoms of brain tumours. *Journal of Neurology, Neurosurgery, and Psychiatry*, *75*(8), 1200–1207. doi:10.1136/jnnp.2003.033308 PMID:15258238

8. Gonzalez, R. C., & Woods, R. E. (2003). *Digital Image Processing* (2nd ed.). Pearson Education.

3. Herholz, K., Langen, K.-J., Schiepers, C., & Mountz, J. (2012). Brain Tumors. *Seminars in Nuclear Medicine*, *42*(6), 356–370. doi:10.1053/j.semnuclmed.2012.06.001 PMID:23026359

27. Herzog, S., Tetzlaff, C., & Worgotter, F. (2019). Evolving artificial neural network with feedback. *Neural Networks*. PMID:31874331

10. Kamil, D., & Ahmet, I. (2016). Effect of image enhancement on MRI brain images with neural networks. *Procedia Computer Science*, *102*, 39–44. doi:10.1016/j.procs.2016.09.367

30. Kanadam, K. P., & Chereddy, S. R. (2016). Mammogram Classiổcation using Sparse-ROI – A novel representation to arbitrary shaped masses. *Expert Systems with Applications*, *57*, 204–213. doi:10.1016/j.eswa.2016.03.037

9. Kim, Y., Kim, J. H., & Kim, C. S. (2014). VGEF: contrast enhancement of dark images using value gap expansion force and sorted histogram equalization. *Signal and Information Processing Association Annual Summit and Conference (APSIPA)*, 1-4.

29. Kumar, A., Ramachandran, M., Gandomi, A. H., Patan, R., Lukasik, S., & Soundarapandian, R. K. (2019). A deep neural network-based classifier for brain tumor diagnosis. *Applied Soft Computing*, *82*, 105528. doi:10.1016/j.asoc.2019.105528

26. Li, H., & Ray Liu, K. (1997). Fractal Modeling and Segmentation for the Enhancement of Microcalcifications in Digital Mammograms. *IEEE Transactions on Medical Imaging*, *16*(6), 785–798. doi:10.1109/42.650875 PMID:9533579

6. McVeigh, E. R., Bronskil, M. J., & Henkelman, R. M. (1986). Phase and sensitivity of receiver coils in magnetic resonance imaging. *Medical Physics*, *13*(6), 806–814. doi:10.1118/1.595967 PMID:3796476

14. Meenalosini, S., Janet, J., & Kannan, E. (2012). Segmentation of Cancer Cells in Mammogram Using Region Growing Method and Gabor Features. *International Journal of Engineering Research and Applications*, 1055–1062.

15. Qiao, J., Cai, X., Xio, Q., Chen, Z., Kulkarni, P., Ferris, C., Kamarthi, S., & Sridhar, S. (2019). Data on MRI brain lesion segmentation using K-means and Gaussian Mixture Model-Expectation Maximization. *Data in Brief*, *27*, 104628. doi:10.1016/j.dib.2019.104628 PMID:31687441

20. Rangayyan, R. M., El-Faramawy, N. M., Desautels, J. E. L., & Alim, O. A. (1997). Measures of acutance and shape for classification of breast tumors. *IEEE Transactions on Medical Imaging, 16*(6), 99–810. doi:10.1109/42.650876 PMID:9533580

1. Ricard, D., Idbaih, A., Ducray, F., Lahutte, M., Hoang-Xuan, K., & Delattre, J. Y. (2012). Primary brain tumours in adults. *Lancet, 379*(9830), 1984–1996. doi:10.1016/S0140-6736(11)61346-9 PMID:22510398

7. Rogosnitzky, M., & Branch, S. (2016). Gadolinium-based contrast agent toxicity: A review of known and proposed mechanisms. *Biometals, Springer, 29*(3), 365–376. doi:10.100710534-016-9931-7 PMID:27053146

4. Rogowska, J. (2000). Overview and fundamentals of medical image segmentation. In *Handbook of medical imaging*. Academic Press. doi:10.1016/B978-012077790-7/50009-6

5. Simmons, A., Tofts, P. S., Barker, G. J., & Arrdige, S. R. (1994). Sources of intensity nonuniformity in spin echo images at 1.5T. *Magnetic Resonance in Medicine, 32*(1), 121–128. doi:10.1002/mrm.1910320117 PMID:8084227

11. Tang, J., Liu, X., & Sun, Q. (2009). A Direct Image Contrast Enhancement Algorithm in the Wavelet Domain for Screening Mammograms. *IEEE Journal of Selected Topics in Signal Processing, 3*(1), 74–80. doi:10.1109/JSTSP.2008.2011108

33. Tustison, N. J., Shrinidhi, K. L., Wintermark, M., Durst, C. R., Kandel, B. M., Gee, J. C., Grossman, M. C., & Avants, B. B. (2015). Optimal symmetric multimodal templates and concatenated random forests for supervised brain tumor segmentation (simplified) with ANTsR. *Neuroinformatics, 13*(2), 209–225. doi:10.100712021-014-9245-2 PMID:25433513

32. Vadivel, A., & Surendiran, B. (2013). A fuzzy rule-based approach for characterization of mammogram masses into BI-RADS shape categories. *Computers in Biology and Medicine, 43*(4), 259–267. doi:10.1016/j.compbiomed.2013.01.004 PMID:23414779

25. Vimal, S. P., & Thiruvikraman, P. K. (2012). Automated image enhancement using power law transformations. *Sadhana, 37*(6), 239–245. doi:10.100712046-012-0110-4

22. Wanga, B., Liu, M., & Chenac, Z. (2019). Differential Diagnostic Value of Texture Feature Analysis of Magnetic Resonance T2 Weighted Imaging between Glioblastoma and Primary Central Neural System Lymphoma. *Chinese Medical Sciences Journal, 34*(1), 10–17. doi:10.24920/003548 PMID:30961775

31. Zhang, Y., Zhang, B., Coenen, F., & Lu, W. (2013). Breast cancer diagnosis from biopsy images with highly reliable random subspace classifier ensembles. *Machine Vision and Applications, 24*(7), 1405–1420. doi:10.100700138-012-0459-8

Chapter 11
Application of Machine Learning to Analyse Biomedical Signals for Medical Diagnosis

Upendra Kumar
Institute of Engineering and Technology, Lucknow, India

Shashank Yadav
Institute of Engineering and Technology, Lucknow, India

ABSTRACT

Interest in research involving health-medical information analysis based on artificial intelligence has recently been increasing. Most of the research in this field has been focused on searching for new knowledge for predicting and diagnosing disease by revealing the relation between disease and various information features of data. However, still needed are more research and interest in applying the latest advanced artificial intelligence-based data analysis techniques to bio-signal data, which are continuous physiological records, such as EEG (electroencephalography) and ECG (electrocardiogram). This study presents a survey of ECG classification into arrhythmia types. Early and accurate detection of arrhythmia types is important in detecting heart diseases and choosing appropriate treatment for a patient.

INTRODUCTION

The heart is a part of body, which task is to pump the blood with the help of the circulatory system of the body. The heart works like rhythmic contraction and dilation. Now-a-days many diseases have been common, that affect heart. The main reason of affecting heart by diseases is unhealthy and irregular lifestyle. There are many medical conditions like hypertension, diabetes which affect the heart. There are many types of heart diseases which can be categorised as

- Ischemic Heart Disease like Myocardial Infarction
- Arrhythmia

DOI: 10.4018/978-1-7998-2742-9.ch011

- Congenital Heart Disease
- Valvular Heart Disease
- Infections
- Inflammation

"Ischemic Heart Disease" is the most important heart disease. In the heart, there are three major arteries which supply blood to it; these arteries are called coronary arteries. The blockade in coronary arteries is the cause of Ischemic heart disease. The result of this blockade is shortage of nutrition to myocardial (heart muscle) cells. Blockage in one or more of these blood cells is the cause of Myocardial Infarction, i.e. Heart Attack. This medical condition can be end of life. If this condition is diagnosed at an early stage and medicated instantly, life can be survived (Roopa and Harish, 2017). Next category of heart disease is "Arrhythmia". It is a problem with the rate or rhythm of the heartbeat. The heart may beat too fast, too slow, too early, or irregularly. If this irregularity is not diagnosed and treated at an early stage, it can cause to death. Congenital Heart Diseases are by birth. Valvular Heart Diseases affect the heart valves. Some other conditions are Infections and Inflammation. These medical conditions can be diagnosed by interpreting biomedical signals like Electrocardiogram (ECG). Interpretation of ECG is done by biomedical expert, which can also be facilitated by automatic diagnostic systems.

BIOMEDICAL SIGNAL

Biomedical signal is generated from biological or medical source. The source of the signal can be from a cell level, molecular level, or an organ level. There are many types of such signals are usually used in hospital and research laboratory. Examples of such signals are the ECG i.e. Electrocardiogram which shows the electrical activity of the heart; EEG i.e. the Electroencephalogram which shows the brain activity; Evoked potentials like visual, auditory etc, which are brain's electrical replies to particular peripheral stimulation; speech signals; the electroneurogram which is related to the field potentials generated from local sections in the brain; the action potential signals generated from heart cells; the EMG i.e. Electromyogram which shows the muscle's electrical activity; the Electroretinogram generated from the eye; etc.

INTRODUCTION TO ECG (ELECTROCARDIOGRAM)

For investigations, ECG i.e. Electrocardiogram is one of the simple, relatively low in price, easily accessible, easily manageable, non-invasive process (Roopa and Harish, 2017). It is available at all places including rural areas with minimal infrastructure. Normally doctors can interpret an ECG with basic medical knowledge at remote places. Cardiac condition must be diagnosed properly at initial state. Time is the biggest factor during these medical conditions. Heart muscle is being damaged continuously in every minute in the absence of treatment. Therefore it is very important to recognize exactly and give treatment to these diseases.

Basically, ECG shows the electrical movement of the heart by time series signal. The signal involves a sequence of repetitive and stereotypes complex waveforms with a clear frequency of about 1 Hz. On different types of conditions, the heartbeat can be different across individuals and within individuals.

The first step is to develop an automated machine learning technique in ECG classification is to take out characteristic features from the waveform. Some features are examined first order and the features can be obtained directly from the ECG data such as RR time i.e. time between the largest peaks that comes in every heartbeat. Some other features are obtained from base signal. These features are taken out by using signal processing methods like Wavelets and Fourier Transforms (FTs). In a typical supervised classification scheme, the features are labelled with the decision outcome.

Figure 1. Normal ECG waveform

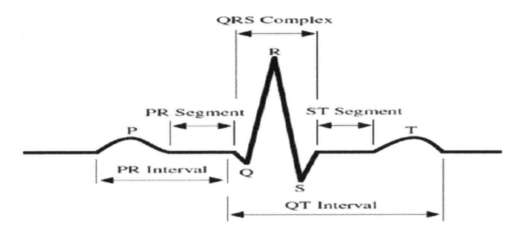

BACKGROUND KNOWLEDGE OF ECG

One signal of ECG includes of many ECG beats and every ECG beat comprises P wave, QRS complex, and the T wave. Every peak (P, Q, R, S, T, U), gaps (PR, RR, QRS, ST, and QT) and sections (PR and ST) of ECG signals have their regular amplitude or duration quantities. These peaks, intervals, and segments are assumed ECG characteristics or features. Figure 1 shows these characteristics for one ECG cardiac cycle, which are defined in Table I.

ECG FEATURES AND THEIR NORMAL DURATIONS

The Table I represents ECG characteristics along with their explanation and their periods (Jambukia et al., 2015).

Umer et al. (2014) proposed an algorithm which is based on windowing method for identification of different peaks and intervals used as feature points for classification system:

- R-peaks are the leading peaks in any ECG signal. R-peaks are discovered by forcing a threshold state on the amplitude of the ECG signal. This state is shown in following equation

$$T = (0.4) \times m \tag{1}$$

Table 1. ECG Features and their normal durations

Feature	Feature Details	Duration of feature (mille second)
Feature P	ECG first short upward motion	80 ms
Feature RR	Time duration between two consecutive R waves	0.6-1.2 s
Feature PR	It is computed from the starting of the P wave to the starting of the QRS complex	120-200 ms
Feature QRS	It is generally starts with a downward deflection Q, a greater upwards deflection R and finishes with a downward S wave	80-120 ms
Feature PR	It joins the P wave and QRS complex	50-120 ms
Feature ST	It attaches the QRS complex and the T wave	80-120 ms
Feature J-point	It is the point at which the QRS complex ends and the ST segment starts is called J-point	Not applicable
Feature T	It is generally a modest upward waveform	160 ms
Feature ST	It is computed from the J point to the finish of the T Wave	320 ms
Feature QT	It is computed from the starting of the QRS complex to the finish of the T wave	420 ms
Feature U	It is generally has low amplitude and often it is totally absent	Not declared

where T is the threshold value and m is the peak value of the ECG signal. The peaks with values larger than T may be considered as R-peaks of ECG.

- In an ECG signal, R-peaks are generated periodically. In each period, the threshold state will give different values for R-peaks. For that period, mean of the R values are calculated for R-peak selection.
- After the identification of R-peaks, RR interval (t_{rr}) is calculated as follows:

$$t_{rr}(i) = \frac{R_{loc}(i+1) - R_{loc}(i)}{f_s}$$

(2)

where f_s is sampling frequency (100 Hz) and for the P, Q, S, and T waves t_{rr} is used to form window in windowing method..

- Similarly other intervals like PR, QRS, QT can be calculated by some other equations available in various literature.

ECG CLASSIFICATION PROBLEM

Classifying the ECG signals is a main process in heart disease diagnosis. The difficulty in heart disorder diagnosis by using ECG is that for one disease, each person may have different ECG and two dissimilar diseases may have similar effects on normal signals of ECG (Jambukia et al., 2015).. These types of difficulties create complication in heart disorder diagnosis. The solution of these problems is to utilize the pattern classifier algorithms for improving the new patients ECG arrhythmia diagnosis. Problem of classifying the ECG is a type of multi-class classifying problem. It contains classes such as Normal, RBBB i.e. Right Bundle Branch Block, LBBB i.e. Left Bundle Branch Block.

NUMBER OF WAYS OF ECG CLASSIFICATION

There are two means by which ECG data can be categorised.

(i) Classifying the ECG signal
(ii) Classifying the ECG beat individually.

One cycle of cardiac includes P, Q, R, S, T, U wave which expresses one ECG beat. Thousands of such beats are included by one ECG signal.

STEPS OF ECG CLASSIFICATION

- Pre-processing
- Quantification of ECG wave
- Extraction of features
- Feature selection
- Classifying the ECG

Different types of pre-processing techniques for classifying ECG have been used by different researchers. Low pass linear phase filter and linear phase high pass filter are applied for noise removal. Methods like linear phase high pass filter, median filter, mean median filter are utilized for baseline adjustment.

For feature extraction CWT i.e. Continuous Wavelet Transform, DWT i.e. Discrete Wavelet Transform, ST i.e. S-Transform, DCT i.e. Discrete Cosine Transform, DFT i.e. Discrete Fourier Transform, PCA i.e. Principal Component Analysis, ICA i.e. Independent Component Analysis, Pan-Tompkins algorithm etc are used. To normalize the features, methods like Unity Standard Deviation (SD) and Z-score are applied.

For Classifying different methods are used such as FCM i.e. Fuzzy C-Means clustering, MLPNN i.e. Multilayer Perceptron Neural Network, ID3 decision tree, Feed forward neuro-fuzzy, QNN i.e. Quantum Neural Network, SVM i.e. Support Vector Machine, T2FCNN i.e. Type2 Fuzzy Clustering Neural Network, RBFNN i.e. Radial Basis Function Neural Network and PNN i.e. Probabilistic Neural Network classifier etc (Jambukia et al., 2015).

Example: Heartbeat Classification for Arrhythmia Detection

Figure 2 shows the automatic system for classifying the arrhythmia from ECG signals which are received by an equipment. This process can be divided into 4 sub-processes.

(1) Pre-processing of ECG signal (2) Segmentation of heartbeat (3) Extracting the features and (4) learning step/classification step. In every step, some action is performed and the final aim is the discrimination or identification of heartbeat type.

Figure 2. A diagram of the arrhythmia classification system

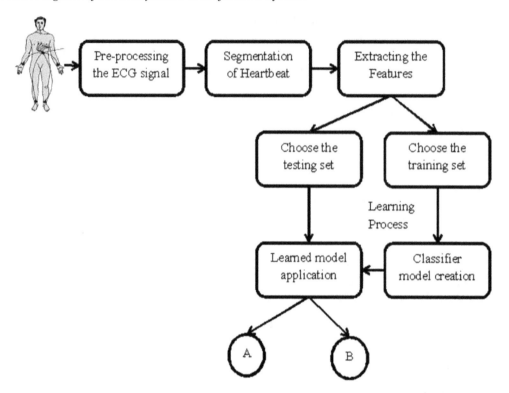

PRE-PROCESSING

For diagnosis the ECG signal preprocessing is the first step. Removal of Baseline wander (BW), removal of noise, and averaging of beat are some processes in pre-processing. Different pre-processing steps and the approach proposed by researchers for diagnosis are given below.

Baseline Wander Removal

Baseline wander is a disturbance due to breathing, movement in the body, and some changes in electrode impedance. Its frequency is very low (0-0.5Hz). The existence of baseline wander can complicate the ECG waveform assessment. It is therefore essential to remove this interference before proceeding with any additional functioning of the ECG signal. High-pass filtering is the most simple process to remove baseline wander (Ansari et al., 2017).

The Butterworth filter, for instance, was used by (Padhy et al., 2016), (Padhy and Dandapat, 2017) (cutoff=0.5Hz) and (Quesnel et al. 2014) (cutoff=0.67Hz) to remove BW, whereas (Garcia et al., 2003) applied a 3rd-order Butterworth filter whose frequency of cutoff based on the rate of heart (HR)(Sornmo, 1991). In addition, (Hadjem et al., 2016) and (Schmidt et al. 2014) applied high-pass filtering with 0.3 and 0.5Hz cutoff frequencies, respectively. Moreover (Murthy and Meenakshi, 2015) applied a derivative filter to eliminate less frequencies. As an alternative, (Bhoi et al., 2015), (Nidhyananthan et al., 2016), (Sharma et al., 2015), (Sharma and Dandapat, 2016) utilized average moving filtering (Rangayyan and Reddy, 2002) to eliminate BW. To estimate BW, other trials (Jaleel et al., 2016) applied median filtering.

For instance, (Lahiri et al., 2009) utilized a 100ms span median filter while (Jaleelet al., 2016) used a strategy that utilizes a mixture of curve fitting and average filtering to extract the baseline wander. The greatest benefit of baseline wander removal filtering algorithms is their simplicity, which requires computational requirements and minimal time for application.

Noise Removal

Typically, the ECG signal is contaminated with noise of high-frequency from power line interference (50/60Hz), electromyographic (EMG) noise from activity of muscle, movement artifact from movements of patient, and noise of radio frequency from other appliances (Ansari et al., 2017). In the literature, a range of techniques were used to decrease the noise impact in the signal of ECG. The low-pass filtering is the easiest and most popular method. (Minchole et al., 2005) and (Garcia et al., 2000), for instance, utilized a 25Hz cutoff frequency linear phase finite impulse response (FIR) filter. In addition, (Jager et al., 1992, 1998) applied a 6th-order Butterworth low-pass filter with a 55Hz cutoff frequency, while (Safdarian et al., 2014) and (Kora and Kalva, 2015) applied Butterworth and Sgolay filters without specifying the filter frequency and order, respectively. Applying moving average filters, (Safdarian et al., 2014), low-pass filtering can also be done. To remove high frequency noise, a 10-point moving average low-pass filter was introduced to the signal by (Murthy and Meenakshi, 2015). These techniques are attractive due to their simplicity and absence of high computational demands.

SadAbadi et al. (2007) used windowing concept to eliminate unwanted high frequency components i.e. noise from the ECG signal. The window's length is calculated using equation (3) which includes integer function of QRS dominant scale, a_{QRS}, and location of R-wave.

$$l_i(x) = 1 + (A.a_{QRS} - 1) \times \left(1 - e^{-\frac{1000B.(SI_i - x)^2}{fs.a_{QRS}}} \right) \tag{3}$$

Where, A and B are constant, SI_i denotes the sample index of ith detected R-wave, f_s is sample frequency, and x is the sample index. The sample index varies as per eqn. (4):

$$\frac{(SI_{i-1} + SI_i)}{2} \leq x \leq \frac{(SI_i + SI_{i+1})}{2} \tag{4}$$

The denoising window slides through the noisy signal in order to remove noises and the signal value at the centre of the window is fixed to the mean value throughout the window.

Ectopic Beats Removal

Ectopic beats (premature heartbeats) that are cause of irregular heart rhythm (Ansari et al., 2017). Premature ventricular contractions (PVC) and premature atrial contractions (PAC) are the most prevalent kinds of ectopic beats. Ectopic beats have a pattern that is clearly distinct from ordinary beats. Their occurrence can therefore confuse the ECG signal assessment. As a consequence, before the assessment, few studies have attempted to define and extract ectopic beats. For instance, (Jaleel et al., 2016) applied a QRS subtraction method that removes a template beat from the current beat (e.g. the median beat from the previous five beats) and utilizes the area under the residual signal to identify ectopic beats. As suggested in (Laciar et al., 2003), (Correa et al. 2014, 2016) utilized a model (visually low-noise ordinary beat) and multi-scale cross-correlation to align beats. The beats with a correlation level of less than 95 percentages were assumed ectopic and removed from the study.

QUANTIFICATION OF ECG WAVE

In most reviewed studies, features of the ECG, like the T wave, QRS complex, and isoelectric line, were recognized prior to the features selection. In order to accomplish this objective, a variety of algorithms were implemented in the literature.

Delineation of ECG

The delineation of the electrocardiogram is a basic stage in characterizing the wave ECG. There is a big range of suggested techniques in the ECG delineation literature survey. Pan and Tompkins are a common technique for detecting QRS complexes (Ansari et al., 2017). This algorithm differentiates squares and integrates the signal of ECG after band-pass filtering and uses rules set to the output signal to identify the difficulties of QRS. This technique has been commonly used (Murthy and Meenakshi, 2015) (Nidhyananthan et al., 2016) (Sharma et al., 2016) in the detection of MI and ischemic beat.

Isoelectric Line Detection

The amount of the ST-segment in MI and ischemia detection algorithms is often evaluated against the isoelectric level. The level is described as the average amplitude of the signal of ECG between the offset of the T wave and the onset of P wave during the period of electrical inactivity. Several techniques were used in the ischemia detection and MI literature to discover the isoelectric level. For instance, (Duskalov et al., 1998) examined a 100ms to 40ms window before the R wave to discover a 20ms interval with 5 Vms1 signal curve (2.5 Vms1 in some research) and applied the average quantity of the interval as the isoelectric stage. This technique has been applied in many studies e.g. (Goletsis et al., 2004), (Exarchos et al., 2006).

EXTRACTION OF FEATURES

If the ECG signal is pre-processed and segmented, different algorithms are used to obtain useful characteristics that enable MI or ischemia to be detected downstream (Ansari et al., 2017). Extraction techniques of characteristics vary from easy morphological characteristics calculated straight from the signal of ECG to metrics depends on complicated transformations and signal decomposition. Most of the literature reviewed that used signal processing algorithms to the signal of ECG did not use other contextual facts such as demographics of patients, manifestations, medical history, etc. For these techniques, this might be regarded as a significant limitation. The exceptions researches are (Goletsis et al., 2004), (Exarchos et al., 2006) that applied the age of the patient as a classifying function.

CLASSIFICATION

The ECG signals classification is a difficult issue because of classification procedure problems (Jambukia et al., 2015) existing in current literature survey. These challenges (Singh et al., 2012) in ECG classification process are due to absence of standardization of ECG characteristics, inconsistency among them, uniqueness of ECG models, non-existence of ideal ECG classifying rules, and inconsistency in patient ECG waveforms. It is also a problem in the classification of ECG arrhythmia to develop the most suitable classifier which are able to classify arrhythmia on real-time. ECG signal classification applications developed so for, are more accurate than manual in identifying irregularity type and to diagnose a new patient. It is also used in the diagnosis and therapy of patients with heart disease.

Figure 3. Complete diagram of ECG processing and classification of heartbeat

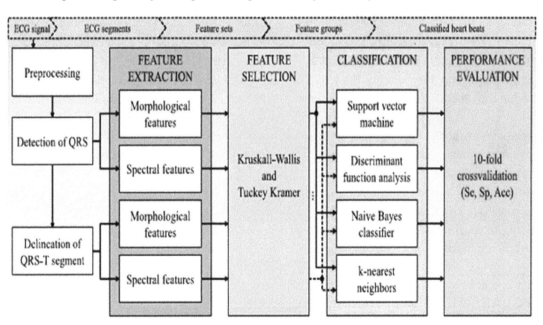

Figure 3 shows the complete process of ECG processing and classification of heartbeat used by Marsanova et al. (2017). After pre-processing ECG QRS complex and QRS-T segment have been used for feature exaction (morphological and spectral features). In this work, feature selection step is done by using Kruskall-Wallis and Tuckey Kramer techniques. Kruskal-Wallis (KW) statistical test (Bellotti T. et al. 2014) is a nonparametric technique for checking that the samples are created from the same distribution or not. This test will give the knowledge of medians of two or more clusters and further examines that they are different or not. In KW test, H statistic is considered as test statistic and the hypotheses are declared as:

H_0- Median of two populations is equal.
H_1- Median of two populations is different.

The different steps of the KW test are as follows.

i)   Sort the observations of the features in increasing order.
ii) Rank the sorted data points and if any bound values present then give an average rank.
iii) Add the different ranks of each output class.
iv) Calculate the H statistic using the equation (5)

$$H = \left[\frac{12}{N(N+1)} \sum_{k=1}^{c} \frac{T_k^2}{n_k} \right] - 3(N+1) \tag{5}$$

Where N is total number of observations across all output groups, c is number of output groups, T_k is sum of ranks of all observations in group k, n_k is number of observations in group k.

v)   Compute the critical chi-square value, $C_{\pm:k-1}^2$ with k-1 degrees of freedom and looking under the desired significance of alpha level.
vi) Finally the H value is compared with critical chi-square value. If H statistic is larger than critical chi-square value then discard the null hypothesis (H_0). If H statistic is not larger than chi-square value then there is not sufficient evidence to recommend that the means are unequal.

The above method is used to compare features from particular classes and helpful in discriminating various types of heartbeat. In this work, the extracted features with significance difference were selected among all pair of classes for further task of analysis.

Further, the classification is done by some other machine learning techniques like SVM i.e. Support Vector Machine, Discriminant function analysis, Naïve Bayes classifier, and k-nearest neighbours. For evaluating the performance (Se, Sp, Acc) which are (sensitivity, specificity and accuracy respectively) parameters are used.

ECG CLASSIFICATION PROBLEMS

1. **Deficiency of standardization of ECG features:** There is no generic or fixed in boundaries of ECG wave, amplitude domain and heuristically on time. The correctness of feature extraction methods depends on the temporally discovered features which are selected by these methods. Over bulky data sets, a little disparity in the quantities of the features may give an invalid classification.

2. **Inconsistency of the ECG features:** Individual heart rate changes according to physiological and mental circumstances. Depression, enthusiasm, workout, and other activities may alter the rate of heart. The heart rate changes consequently differs characteristics like interval of RR, interval of PR, and interval of QT. The characteristics required to be thoroughly altered, and the effect of the variable heart rate requires to be removed (Jambukia et al., 2015).

3. **Uniqueness of the ECG shapes:** Uniqueness of the ECG shape is related to the probability of intraclass resemblance and interclass irregularity of testing shapes detected in ECG dataset. It tells to what range the ECG shapes are scalable in satisfactorily greater database.

4. **Lack of ideal classifying instructions for ECG:** For classifying ECG, there is no any ideal classifying instructions that can support in classification procedure.

5. **Changed waveforms of Patients:** ECG records from many patients may have dissimilar signal slopes, amplitude, and timing that alter the ECG waveforms. That is why the classifying approach requires to cautiously classifying the signal of ECG.

6. **Single ECG Heart Beat disparities:** One ECG may have thousands of beats and there may be many types of these beats for example arrhythmia types. So classifying model requires to get qualified in such a manner that it generates minor faults on test database.

7. **Discovery of the best suitable classifier:** To find out the classifier that has the capability of classifying arrhythmia on real-time is a problem since classifying correctness depends on numerous arguments like variety in arrhythmia, kind of arrhythmia, chosen feature withdrawal technique, chosen arrhythmia dataset etc.

MACHINE LEARNING TECHNIQUES IN ECG ANALYSIS

Figure 4. Various Machine Learning Approaches

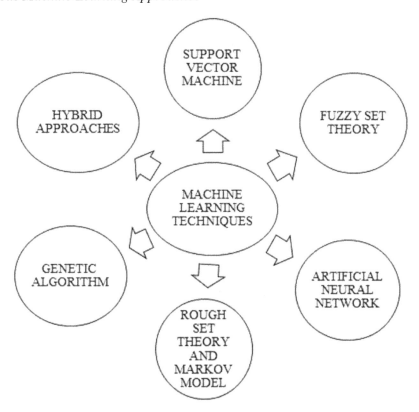

FUZZY BASED MACHINE LEARNING TECHNIQUES

Different types of algorithms have been proposed for implementing computerized ECG analysis and diagnosis. Fuzzy based machine learning is a process that is utilized by many authors for ECG analysis effectively. Smooth variables with membership functions are used by these algorithms in diagnosing diseases using ECG analysis (Lei et al., 2007). In addition, big quantities of information related to diseases such as coronary artery diseases are processed in modern medicines, for which various classifiers are used to evaluate the ECG (Pal et al., 2012).

Behadada and Chikh, (2013) performed a research on evaluating cardiac defects for this purpose by optimizing the classification of cardiac arrhythmias and detection of defects. Fuzzy decision tree was used by researchers as a methodology for diagnosing heart defects. They used the heartbeat information from the database of MIT-BIH. The suggested fuzzy tree can detect premature ventricular contraction anomalies where the false alarm rate is lowered to 19.76 percentage and the classifying rate is 71 percentage (Behadada and Chikh, 2013). Yet, the outcome is unsatisfactory compared to neural networks and some other methods. Lei et al. (2007) created an adaptive fuzzy ECG classifier to improve the efficiency of standard classifiers in alignment with this research. The classifier used the database for assessment of MIT-BIH arrhythmia. The advanced classifier is efficient as per the ECG signal inputs in terms of self-adaptation. The average right rate was 88.2%. However, in terms of understanding the distinct kinds of heart beats, both methods are lacking. In addition, the suggested approach's computational effectiveness (Lei et al., 2007) is considerably high.

ECG is commonly used in the diagnosis of heart disease where it is possible to use fuzzy inference schemes for efficient system evaluation (Goel et al., 2016). Research on fuzzy-based methods has evolved further by the inclusion of neural networks like fuzzy inference networks (Lei et al., 2007), integrating the advantages of neural networks for better learning and fuzzy sets for better knowledge of humans (Guler and Ubeyli, 2004). Similarly, Ceylan et al. (2009) utilized the Fuzzy Clustering Neural Network Algorithm for ECG assessment classification. The authors aimed to increase the level of accuracy for ECG beats for which 92 patient records are obtained from MIT-BIH databases. Also, back propagation 402 learning and type 2 fuzzy mean clustering algorithms are utilized. With the creation of high clustering efficiency, the suggested scheme led in a 99% precision. The analysis inferred that in this situation the training time was big, limiting the advantages. The result of fuzzy logic can be introduced in ECG assessment to knowledge-based systems (Jeyalakshmi and Robin, 2016).

The fuzzy decision tree offers some inferences and means of acquiring expertise to handle multi-varied information with complicated or missing values (Chen et al., 2009). For the reasons described above, it is commonly used as interference and expert systems to give the clarity. Pal et al. (2012) created a fuzzy expert system in the medical science stream for precise identification of coronary artery illnesses and removal from medical information uncertainties. The authors emphasized the tree representation rule organisation to obtain effective search from the Coronary Artery Disease (CAD) database. Therefore, it is concluded that fuzzy-based methods are efficient in computerized ECG assessment but require further inquiry to achieve a greater level of precision, particularly with respect to the localization of ST Elevation Myocardial Infarction (STEMI) culprit coronary artery.

NEURAL NETWORKS BASED MACHINE LEARNING TECHNIQUES

For classification Neural networks are applied after pre-processing, finding and withdrawal of feature from ECG signal. A diagnostic system for cardiac arrhythmias which was suggested by Gao et al. (2004) was based on an artificial neural network classifier. The Bayesian framework based classifier is composed with the backpropagation algorithm's application. A correctness of 90% was offered by the suggested system, which could be improved in the future. For the practical application the system is not acceptable.

An automated ANN i.e. Artificial Neural Network constructed classification was developed by Vishwa et al. (2011) for cardiac arrhythmia by applying multi-channel ECG records. 48 recordings from 1975 to 1979 are available in an MIT-BIH arrhythmia dataset which is used for classification. For validating the method, a Normal Sinus Rhythm (NSR) database is used. Some algorithms like the estimated feed forward ANN and the back propagation learning techniques are applied. The technique gives the accuracy of 96.77 percentages on MIT-BIH dataset and 96.21 percentage on NSR dataset but the study is not suitable to classify all 16 classes of arrhythmia.

Sao et al., (2015) also suggested ANN in the ECG for heart disorders diagnosed in the maximum sufficient manner. The ANN classifying technique was developed by the researchers for the same, in which the parameters such as Largest Lyapunov exponent, Spectral Entropy and Poincare plot geometry are measured along with utilizing the back propagation technique.

For improvement in the classifying of ECG signals, neural networks are broadly used according to Aruradha and Reddy (2008). For cardiac arrhythmia, the researchers developed an ANN-based classifier. To extract ECG information MIT-BIH databases are used. For the classification of cardiac arrhythmias from ECG data Artificial neural network (ANN) is used. A grouping of wavelets Back Propagation Algorithms (BPA) is used for classifiers. 90.56% effectiveness is obtained and the abnormal activities are identified by the classifiers. There are some drawbacks regarding proper validation against different databases.

To develop an ANN model for heart diseases diagnosis was the basic purpose of Jadhav et al., (2012). 12 lead ECG signal records information from UCI machine-learning source databases, was used by researchers for this aim. For classification momentum learning rule and static back propagation algorithms are applied. To calculate the performance of the suggested technique, Receiver Operating Characteristics (ROC), Mean Squared Error (MSE), and Area Under Curve (AUC) are the measurement methods. By these methods, 86.67% classification accuracy and the sensitivity 93.75% is achieved.

ECG assessment is extremely useful for the diagnosis of heart disease, according to Gupta and Chatur (2012). For ECG classification, the researchers used supervised artificial neural networks and data mining methods. the implementation of both methods is then compared, where the ANN use is made more efficient.

De Gaetano et al. (2009) created an algorithm based on supervised neural network to distinguish between ordinary beats in ECG signals and ischemic beats. Radial basis features and segments of R-wave (RRR interval) to identify the two kinds of beats, was used by the researchers. The scheme is subsequently validated on the European ST-T database. When identifying the ischemic beats from ECG information, the suggested classifier is assessed as accurate.

ROUGH SET THEORY AND HIDDEN MARKOV MODEL BASED MACHINE LEARNING TECHNIQUES

Rough Set Theory (RST) was established in the early 1980s and developed as a plan to reduce information uncertainty and ambiguity (Senthilkumaran and Rajesh, 2009). The issues solved by RST are linked to the decrease of redundant data, information dependency detection and information classification and information pattern evaluation (Deja and Paszek 2003). In addition, the benefit of using RST in ECG assessment is that it helps to formulate laws that are readily understood and lead to precise extraction of precious data from complicated databases (Tripathy et al., 2011).

Rough set theory is used to produce a robust model of classification (Barman et al., 2016). In computerized ECG assessment, several researchers in the current literature have used rough set theory in hopes of achieving maximum advantages.

One such Mitra et al. (2006) study showed an optimized rule-based rough set strategy for efficient diagnosis. A database of images formatted by TIFF was used in the research. Differentiation and syntactic techniques have been used by the authors, where automated feature extraction system from ECG is implemented. For the identification of diseases, a rule based rough set decision system is implemented. For Myocardial Infarction, the achieved accuracy is 100%. But the method is not proper for giving accuracy for untrained information set.

Barman et al. (2016) performed a survey using rough set theory and various classification systems to obtain accurate and correct data from the MIT-BIT arrhythmia database. Using the MATLAB tool, the information is first pre-processed and then RST is implemented for proper classification. The researchers also used pre-processing filtering techniques.

A rule selection algorithm for diagnosing Coronary Artery Disease (CAD) was developed by Setiawan et al. (2009). In this research, 920 patients records were collected from many hospitals in which CAD data was available. For applying Rough Set Theory, hybrid method of support filtering and RST rule importance selection are used. The suggested process is effective for selecting and identifying rules from a collection of rules, without compromising the classification quality. For future use, fuzzy reasoning can be applied to increase effectiveness.

A research by Huang and Zhang (2003) disclosed that RST implementation condenses the identification rules for determining the necessary information in ECG. On the same manner, Tripathy et al. (2011) performed an inquiry to identify features such as ECG, Blood Pressure and Maximum Heart Rate (MHR) affecting heart disease. For testing, a total of 250 patients were selected and distributed into 5 different categories according to heart diseases. In the study rough sets, Formal Concept Analysis (FCA) and decision rules are used. For identification of the heart diseases features, high effectiveness is achieved.

By assessing the ECG waveform, which can be achieved using Hidden Markov models (HMMs), the ECG signal is evaluated for knowledge acquisition. An HMM is commonly used for waveform segmentation of the ECG signal (Frénay et al., 2009). A study by Andreao et al. (2006) explored the use of HMM while performing heart beat detection and segmentation functionality in the classification of ECG. The researchers addressed various aspects such as modelling of waveforms, classification, unsupervised adaptation and segmentation. The research gave effective detection of heart beats with sensitivity of 99.79%.

GENETIC ALGORITHM BASED MACHINE LEARNING TECHNIQUES

By applying Genetic Algorithms (GA) to attain greater computing capabilities with less time used, ECG analysis has been commonly applied (Omran et al., 2009). However, to utilize maximum benefits, this strategy is incorporated with others. With ANN, SVM, and other techniques, various researchers have used GA. On the other side, there is a scarcity of methods for using GA alone in ECG assessment.

To improve the classification of Arrhythmia from ECG signals, Priyadarshini and Kumar (2015) applied a concept. MIT-BIH Arrhythmia database is used for implementing this concept. A temporary Genetic Algorithm (GA) is produced and for classification C4.5 and Naive Bayes algorithm are used in the research. As compared to C4.5 and Naive Bayes, the study found that the GA gives most stable accurate result. To find the most effective method, the research can be extended to other machine learning algorithms like SVM.

For ECG analysis and heart disease diagnosis, Omran et al. (2009) used GA with ANN. To identify the connection points in the ECG signal the ANN is used and GA is used to select the most accurate values to those points. It is best to use genetic algorithms to minimize error values and improve connection points. The error is minimized from 5.9487e-28 to 2.3116e-29 when GA is applied in the ANN model of identification and classification for 100 generations.

In the ECG assessment, El-Dahshan (2010) also used the genetic algorithm with another strategy. GA with wavelet transform (WT) has been integrated by the investigator to denoise ECG signals, using GA to determine the best parameters for appropriate wavelet denoising. The percentage root mean square and SNR are used to understand the approach's efficiency.

Silveira et al. (2007) developed a compression method using genetic algorithm to minimize ECG signal distortion in its analysis when considering the use of GA alone. To compare the efficiency of the suggested method, the classical wavelet Db3 is used. The experiment uses the MIT-BIH compression database. GA compression guarantees reduced values than the conventional Db3 technique of wavelet.

SUPPORT VECTOR BASED MACHINE LEARNING TECHNIQUES

There are many applications such as brain computer interfacing, ECG signal classification and diagnosis, image segmentation etc. in which Support vector classifiers are mostly used (Guler and Ubeyli, 2007).

Kampouraki et al., (2009) suggested a study in which classification of time series of heartbeat are done with the help of Support Vector Machines i.e. SVM. As compared to neural networks for classification the ECG signals with minimal signal to noise ratio, the SVM classifier gives a better performance.

For classification arrhythmia from ECG database, a technique is discovered by Polat et al. (2008). In this technique ECG databases are used which contains records of healthy as well as diseased persons with arrhythmia. For exact classification, a better technique is used i.e. Least Square Support Vector Machine (LSSVM). The technique is certified by classification effectiveness, sensitivity and ROC curves. 100% accuracy was achieved by the suggested technique while evaluating. But, the resulting accuracy is only suitable for atherosclerosis disease, and for others, the accuracy was not applicable.

The optimization of accuracy of identifying Arrhythmia by using ECG data set was the basic purpose of Batra and Jawa (2016). The dataset which contains 452 records was recovered from UCI Machine Learning Repository and the information related to Arrhythmia was mined. Machine learning algorithms and ECG diagnostic criteria were used by the researchers. For experiments many machine learning algorithms were used like random forest, neural networks, gradient boosting, decision trees, and support vector machines. However, researches were more focused to SVM. An accuracy of 83.04% was acquired by using the combined form of SVM and gradient boosting. The accuracy was amplified to 84.82% after using ECG criteria.

For actual classification and cardiac arrhythmias diagnosis, Wang and Chiang (2007) proposed a new technique which was based on SVM and Particle Swarm Optimization.

Nasiri et al. (2009) suggested a new technique for extracting features and ECG classification for cardiac arrhythmia disease. For improvement the process by identifying better feature subset, the SVM classifier was used, which gave the optimal classification of the signal. Genetic Algorithm was combined with SVM for utilization and enhancement the generalization performance, by many researchers. An accuracy of 93% was achieved by the technique suggested by the researchers.

HYBRID ALGORITHMS

In search of enhanced efficiency, hybrid methods for analyzing ECG signals have been widely researched. By applying the PCA i.e. Principal Component Analysis and the Neuro-Fuzzy classifier, Dalal and Birok (2016) created a hybrid classifier. With the use of a hybrid strategy, different heart functions are identified using the MIT-BIH database. The PCA method is used to obtain the necessary data from the database and then to evaluate and process the extracted data using ANN and Fuzzy logic-based classifier. The hybrid approach's effectiveness is estimated at 96%.

Another work by Bensujin et al. (2014) reviewed and defined a person's ECG signal for the ST Segment Elevation Myocardial Infarction (STEMI). 480 records of patients have been obtained from the MIT BIH database, divided into two sets. Database of Chinese Heart Disease is used to validate the technique. Methods of hybrid identification were used to detect heart rate, ischemic and STEMI extraction. For extraction of features, the K-means clustering algorithm is used. To identify STEMI from ECG signals, the Bacterial Foraging Optimization Algorithm (BFOA) is used. The assessment disclosed that 89% of the STEMI is recognized on the clustered information and 91% of the convergence rate. The suggested methodology is highly effective.

Finlay et al. (2015) determined the effect of electrode placement on the efficiency of defining occlusion of coronary arteries in order to gain higher efficiency. Selected 45 patients who were passing through Percutaneous Transluminal Coronary Angioplasty (PTCA) and contained 120 lead Body Surface Potential Maps (BSPMs) recording. BSPMs have been used to investigate the patients ' effect of electrode placement. To detect STEMI and non-STEMI, a computer algorithm is created. Researchers have found that the placement of lead electrodes has an important effect on STEMI and 12-lead ECG detection. However, it is noted that the suggested methodology's practical implementation is poor. Also, there was less patient number due to which the results could not be relied on.

The effectiveness of ECG localization of culprit vessel occlusion was examined by Ghosh et al. (2013) in acute STEMI. The research shortlisted 21 patients with acute myocardial infarction. In LAD i.e. Left Anterior Descending, RCA i.e. Right Coronary Artery and LCx i.e. Left Circumflex coronary arteries, the localization of the culprit vessel occlusion site was performed by dividing the patients into three groups. The outcomes reported that the ECG localization accuracy for LAD was 90.91%; for RCA it was 100%; and for LCx coronary arteries it was 90%. The sample size taken in the research, however, was small. The angiography was not processed instantly, which could have resulted in indeterminate results. Table 2 describes different machine learning methods used in ECG classification.

Table 2. Survey of ECG classification

Researcher (year)	Database	Aim	Algorithms	Performance	Remarks
Fuzzy Based Machine Learning Techniques					
Lei et al., (2007)	MIT-BIH arrhythmia.	To develop an adaptive fuzzy ECG classifying algorithm to increase the performance of predictable classifiers.	The fuzzy Sets	Average correct rate = 88.2%.	Computational efficiency is poor
Ceylan et al., (2009)	92 patient records from MIT-BIH Database	To increase the accuracy rate for ECG beats.	Fuzzy Clustering Neural Network Algorithm, Type 2 fuzzy Means clustering algorithm and back propagation 402 learning	Accuracy = 99%.	Less samples considered
Pal et al., (2012)	Coronary Artery Diseases (CAD) patient database	To develop screening expert system for detecting CAD	Fuzzy Tree and Rule Organization	Sensitivity= 95.85% Specificity= 83.33%	Methodology is not clear.
Behadada and Chikh, (2013)	MIT-BIH	To optimize the classification of cardiac Arrhythmias and detection Of abnormalities.	Fuzzy Decision Tree.	The False Alarm Rate Is 19.76%. Classification Rate is 71%.	Feature selection is not accurate.
Neural Networks Based Machine Learning Techniques					
Anuradha and Reddy, (2008)	MIT-BIH dataset	To develop an ANN-based classifier for cardiac arrhythmia.	Artificial Neural Network (ANN), Wavelets Back Propagation Algorithm	Accuracy =90.56%	Poor validation of methodology
De Gaetano et al., (2009)	European ST-T Database	To differentiate between the normal beats in ECG signals and ischemic beats	Radial basis functions and R- wave segments (RRR interval)	Provides high reliability.	Lack in Accuracy
Vishwa et al., (2011)	MIT-BIH arrhythmia database consisting of 48 recordings from 1975 and 1979	To improve an automated artificial neural network (ANN) based classifying system for cardiac arrhythmia by using multi-channel ECG recordings.	Estimated Feed Forward ANN and Back-Propagation learning algorithms	Accuracy=96.77% on MIT-BIH database Accuracy =96.21% on NSR database.	Unable to classify all 16 arrhythmia classes.
Jadhav et al., (2012)	UCI machine- learning Repository datasets	To develop an ANN model for diagnosing heart diseases.	Static Back Propagation algorithm, Momentum learning Rule	Accuracy =86.67% Sensitivity=93.75%.	Only binary classification
Gupta and Chatur, (2012)	Raw ECG signal	To improve ECG signal analysis	Artificial Neural Networks and Data Mining techniques	ANN approach is more productive than data mining.	Classification of only 4 types of heart beats

continues on following page

Table 2. Continued

Researcher (year)	Database	Aim	Algorithms	Performance	Remarks
Rough Set Theory and Hidden Markov Model Based Machine Learning Techniques					
Fuzzy Based Machine Learning Techniques					
Mitra et al., (2006)	TIFF formatted image database	To develop an optimized approach of rule based rough set for effective diagnosis.	Differentiation techniques and syntactic approaches.	100% Accuracy for Myocardial Infarction (MI).	Less accuracy for untrained sample.
Barman et al., (2016)	MIT-BIT arrhythmia database	To increase accuracy in ECG analysis.		Proposed mechanism is effective when compared to fuzzy classifiers.	Results are not well presented in terms of Accuracy evaluation.
Setiawan et al., (2009)	920 patients" data from different hospitals, having Coronary Artery Disease	To develop a rule selection method for diagnosing CAD.	Rough Set Theory (RST) with support filtering.	Proposed technique is efficient at selecting and extracting rules (27) from large number of rules (3881).	Accuracy of classification is increased.
Tripathy et al., (2011)	Testing data of 250 heart patients	To identify characteristics such as ECG, Blood Pressure and MHR that affect heart diseases.	Rough Sets, Decision Rules and Formal Concept Analysis (FCA).	High accuracy is obtained For determining the characteristic of heart diseases.	Validation can be further improved.
Andreao et al., (2006)	Two-channel QT Database	To increase heart beat detection and segmentation in ECG analysis	Hidden Markov Models	Sensitivity = 99.79%	High Accuracy
Genetic Algorithm Based Machine Learning Techniques					
Omran et al., (2009)	ECG Arrhythmia Database	To improve ECG classification and diagnosis	Genetic Algorithm with ANN	Error rate is reduced to 2.3116e-29 from 5.9487e-28 in 100 generations	Higher utilization is yet to be improved.
Dahshan et al., (2010)	MIT-BIH database	Denoising ECG signals effectively	GA with Wavelet Transform (WT)	The approach is successful in eliminating noise from ECG signal	Results are well demonstrated

continues on following page

Table 2. Continued

Researcher (year)	Database	Aim	Algorithms	Performance	Remarks
Fuzzy Based Machine Learning Techniques					
Priyadharshni and Kumar, (2015)	MIT-BIH Arrhythmia Database	To enhance the classification of Arrhythmia from ECG signals.	Improvised Genetic algorithm, C4.5 and Naïve Bayes classifier	Accuracy using GA= 90%, C4.5 = 72% and Naïve Bayes =50%	Genetic Algorithm have the most stable accuracy rate than Naïve bayes and C4.5 algorithm
Support Vector Based Machine Learning Techniques					
Polat et al., (2008)	ECG Arrhythmia dataset	To develop a technique for classifying arrhythmia from ECG dataset.	Least Square Support Vector Machine (LSSVM)	Accuracy =100%	Accuracy obtained is only for atherosclerosis disease.
Nasiri et al., (2009)	MIT-BIH arrhythmia database of 48 records	To improve feature extraction and ECG classification for cardiac arrhythmia disease.	SVM and Genetic Algorithm.	Accuracy = 93%	Accuracy can be further improved.
Batra and Jawa, (2016)	452 records from UCI Machine Learning Repository.	To optimize the accuracy of detecting Arrhythmia by using ECG.	SVM, Neural Networks, Decision Trees, Random Forest, Gradient Boosting. SVM was majorly emphasized.	With SVM, accuracy = 83.04% After applying ECG criteria, the accuracy = 84.82%.	Combined only gradient Boosting with SVM.
Hybrid Algorithm Based Machine Learning Techniques					
Ghosh et al., (2013)	21 patients With acute Myocardial Infarction	To examine the accuracy of ECG localization of culprit vessel occlusion in acute STEMI	Localization of culprit vessel occlusion site In LAD, RCA and LCx coronary arteries were performed by dividing the Patients into 3 groups.	Accuracy for LAD =90.91%, RCA =100%; and for LCx coronary arteries = 90%.	Sample size was small and Coronary Angiography was not done immediately
Bensujin et al., (2014)	480 patients' records from MIT BIH database	To examine and determine the STEMI in the ECG signal of a patient	Bacterial Foraging Optimization Algorithm (BFOA), K-means Clustering Technique	Identification rate = 89% and the convergence Rate = 91%	Pre-processing of data is not efficient
Finlay et al., (2015)	45 Patients undergoing angioplasty and had 120 lead BSPMs recording.	To determine the impact of electrode placement on the accuracy of identifying coronary artery occlusion.	Body Surface Potential Maps (BSPMs) and computerized Diagnostic Algorithm.	Sensitivity = 51.1% Specificity = 91.1%.	Poor practical applications.
Dalal and Birok, (2016)	MIT-BIH database	diagnosis via ECG analysis for improvement	Neuro-fuzzy and PCA classifying techniques	Correctness is 96%	Small sample size

ECG CLASSIFICATION

For classifying the ECG signals, many researchers have worked and applied to many types of pre-processing methods, many techniques for feature mining and many for classifying. For ECG classification, maximum researchers utilized the MIT-BIH arrhythmia dataset. Dallali et al. (2011) used DWT to extract RR interval and use Z score to normalize the RR interval. They utilized FCM to categorize beats from the ECG. They accomplished precision of 99.05 percentages. In (Dallali et al., 2011), the characteristics obtained by using DWT are the RR interval and the R point location. Pre-classification was performed utilizing the FCM and the ultimate classification was performed by utilizing the MLPNN 3-layer. The authors have attained 99.99 percentage precision.

DWT is utilized to mine R peak and RR intervals in (Ayub and Saini, 2011). MLPNN was used to classify the ECG. The error MSE i.e Mean Squared collected was approximately 0.00621. Khorrami et al. (2010) used DWT to extract the RR interval. MLPNN and SVM performance have been contrasted in this research. Patra et al. (2010) mined R peak and RR intervals from MIT-BIH arrhythmia dataset annotation file manually. Taking Zero mean, features are standardized and decreased utilizing FCM. As classifier, 3 layers of FFNN with the back propagation techniques are utilized. Naima et al. (2009) used Db4 discrete wavelet transform to extract R location and RR interval. FFNN trained with the algorithm of back propagation is applied. NN's sensitivity, specificity, and precision is 90%, 90%, and 95%, correspondingly. Khazaee (2013) calculated nxt_RR, prev_RR, and rat_RR from RR interval and standardized by means of zero and the standard unit deviation. The classifier PSO-SVM is applied to classify the ECG.

In (Moavenian and Khorrami, 2010), MITBIH arrhythmia database recordings calculate the RR interval. This paper compared MLPNN and SVM classifier. Result indicates that MLPNN is great for testing of performance while SVM demonstrates excellent performance in practice. Vishwa et al. (2011) used DWT to extract the RR interval and the R peak and standardized by the mean Zero. Band pass filter removed noise. The database of MIT-BIH arrhythmias and the database of normal sinus rhythm had been utilized. As a classifier, FFNN was applied with error propagation algorithm back. In[14], the chosen features were R peak, RRt interval (present timing RR interval at t time), RRt+1 interval (next t+1 time RR interval), QRSh (complex height QRS) and QRS width. Applying the Pan Tompkins algorithm, R peak and QRS complex are extracted. For noise removal, a low-pass linear phase filter is utilized and a median filter is applied to correct the baseline.

The sensitivity and the specificity attained were 96.251 percentage and 99.104 percentage respectively using the PSO-RBFNN classifier. Table 3 demonstrates the ECG classification study. It involves amount of characteristics, name characteristics, methods of pre-processing, database, methods of modelling, performance measurements used, and precision attained in every research.

CONCLUSION

Today the automated diagnostic systems are accepting the challenges of huge amount of problems of the patients suffering from variety of diseases. This challenge required medical experts in large amount with high skill. The automated diagnostic systems can assist medical experts to handle this challenge by building pre-diagnostic prediction tool. This scenario needs high accuracy of the systems which in turn requires better feature extraction and classification methods. The main purpose of this chapter is to present a detailed overview of the computational techniques that have been utilized in analysing biomedical

Table 3. ECG Classification Survey

Researchers Name	No. of Features used	ECG Features Used	Pre-processing Method	Database used	Modelling System	Performance Measures	Correctness (%)
Kannathal et al. (2003)	13	Heart rate, Heart rate changes, width of QRS, Standardised (ST wave, entropy QRS), Complexity features (QRS, ST), RR interval, Spectral entropy, ST segment length, ST angle of deviation, ST section deviation, ST section area	For extracting features: Tompkins algorithm (R) Elimination of noise: BVan Alste and schilder and Bandpass filter	Dataset MIT-BIH arrhythmia	FFNN 5 layer classifier which uses error back propagation technique, architecture of PNN, classifier SOM	Specificity, Sensitivity, Positive predictivity correctness	98.3 99.3 99.3
Acharya et al. (2004)	2	RR interval, R peak	For extracting features: Pan-Tompkins technique	Dataset MIT-BIH arrhythmia	FFNN 4 layer classifier and fuzzy classifier	Correctness	80-85%
Ozbay et al. (2006)	2	RR interval, R peak	Not declared by author	Dataset MIT-BIH arrhythmia	Methods for Pre-classification: Fuzzy clustering NN architecture Method for classification: MLPNN with back propagation	Average Testing error, training error, Training time,	0.22 0.28 196.95
Yu and Chou. (2008)	3	QRS segment, R peak, RR interval	Normalization: ICA, Zero mean & unity standard deviation	Dataset MIT-BIH arrhythmia	FFNN 3-layer classifier with back propagation algorithm, PNN	Specificity, Sensitivity, Correctness	99.906 98.508 98.710
Ceylan et al. (2009)	1	RR interval	For extracting Features: DWT	Dataset MIT-BIH arrhythmia	T2FCNN, 3-layered FFNN, fuzzy clustering neural network	Specificity, Sensitivity, Average detection rate	100 96.7 98.35
Naima and Timemy (2009)	2	RR interval, R location (max peak)	For extracting features: DWT, DFT, Db4, Haar	Dataset MIT-BIH arrhythmias	FFNN training algorithm Back propagation algorithm DFT-FFNN, DWT-FFNN	Specificity, Sensitivity, Correctness	90 90 95
Nasiri et al. (2009)	22	3 morphological features, 19 Temporal features, Intervals- PQ, RR, PT, PR, ST, TP	Removal of noise: DWT For reducing feature: meta-heuristic GA, PCA	Dataset MIT-BIH arrhythmias	Genetic algorithm-SVM	Correctness	93.46
Patra et al. (2010)	2	RR interval, R peak	For normalizing Features: Zero mean (reduce the effect of bias), Reducing the Data: PCA, FCM	Dataset MIT-BIH arrhythmias	FFNN 3 layer back propagation algorithm, PCA- FFNN, FCM-FFNN, FCM- PCA-FFNN, FCM-ICA-FFNN	Sum of square error Training time	3.99*10-40.13 656.42
Khorrami and Moavenian, (2010)	1	RR interval	Reduction of baseline, For extracting of features: CWT, DWT, DCT	Dataset MIT-BIH arrhythmias	FFNN 3 layer trained using back propagation algorithm, DWT-MLP, SVM, CWT-MLP	Mean square error (training and testing)	0.0349 0.0438 0.0056 0.1048

continues on following page

Table 3. Continued

continues on following page

Researchers Name	No. of Features used	ECG Features Used	Pre-processing Method	Database used	Modelling System	Performance Measures	Correctness (%)
Korurek and Dogan (2010)	5	RRt, RRt+1 interval, R peak, QRSh, QRS width	Removal of noise: Low pass linear phase filter Correction of baseline: median filter Extraction of feature: Pan Tompkins technique	Dataset MIT-BIH arrhythmias	RBFNN classifier: neuron centers. RBFNN Parameters: bandwidth of each neuron obtained by PSO PSO-RBFNN	Specificity, Sensitivity	99.104 96.251
Moavenian and Khorrami, (2010)	3	ratRR, nxtRR, prevRR	Normalizing technique: average of zero and standard deviation of unity, Cutting of signals by use of annotation file, Recognition of peaks and valleys	Dataset MIT-BIH arrhythmias	SVM kernel, PSO-SVM Optimize feature selection and parameters	Kernel function parameters r, Penalty parameter c, Best fitness	0.0086 28597.68 97.21
Dallali et al. (2011)	1	RR interval	Normalizing the features: Z score, Denoised: Baseline adjustment, Extracting the feature: DWT	Dataset MIT-BIH arrhythmias database	FCM and heart rate variability (HRV)	Accuracy	99.05
Dallali et al. (2011)	2	R point location RR interval	Extracting the features: DWT using Daubechies wavelet Of order 3	Dataset MIT-BIH arrhythmias	Pre-classifying techniques: FCM, Final classifying technique: MLPNN	Accuracy	99.99
Zeraatkar et al. (2011)	4	RR interval, R peak, QRS complex identification, T wave	Eliminating power line effect: Notch filter Baseline shift: median filter Reducing the effect of EMG noise: Discrete Butterworth filter	Dataset MIT-BIH arrhythmias, QT and T-wave alternans challenge, Normal sinus Rhythm	MLPNN classifier	Specificity, Sensitivity, Negative predictive value, Positive predictive value	88.50 96.77 90.16 96.18
Vishwa et al. (2011)	2	RR interval, R peak	Baseline noise reduction: segmentation of ECG beats Removal of low frequencies: FFT i.e. Fast Fourier transform, To restore ECG: Inverse FFT	MIT-BIH arrhythmia, QT and Normal sinus rhythm	Feed forward ANN with error back propagation	Index of Youden, Classifying correctness	0.9415 96.77
Ayub and Saini (2011)	2	RR interval, R peak	Not declared by author	Dataset MIT-BIH arrhythmia	Cascade forward neural network with back propagation technique	Averaged squared Error	0.00621
Daamouche et al. (2012)	6	RR interval, RR interval averaged over 10 last beats, QRS complex duration, 3 morphological features	QRS detection: ecgpuwave software (http://www.physiotools/ecguwave/src/), Wavelet filter,	Dataset MIT-BIH arrhythmia	SVM classifier	Specificity, Sensitivity, Positive predictivity	96.14 91.75 74.26

Table 3. Continued

Researchers Name	No. of Features used	ECG Features Used	Pre-processing Method	Database used	Modelling System	Performance Measures	Correctness (%)
Wang et al. (2012)	2	RR interval, R peak	Normalizing features techniques: Z score, Feature reduction: PCA and LDA	Dataset MIT-BIH arrhythmias	PNN classifier with probability density function	Specificity, Sensitivity, Accuracy	99.10 97.98 99.71
Jadhav et al. (2012)	1	RR interval	Extracting the feature: DWT	Dataset UCI arrhythmia	Generalized FFNN, MLPNN, Modular neural network	Specificity, Sensitivity, Accuracy	93.1 93.75 86.67
Sarkaleh and Shahbahrami (2012)	2	RR interval, R peak	Extracting the feature: DWT Up to 2 Level	Dataset MIT-BIH arrhythmia	MLPNN trained with error back propagation technique	Recognition Rate	Not declared by author
Kumari and Kumar, (2013)	1	RR interval	Extracting the feature: CWT, Symlets Reducing the feature: Symmetric uncertainty	Dataset UCI and MIT-BIH arrhythmia	Modular neural network–MLPNN	Recall, Precision, Root MSE	95.1 95.1 0.1765
Srivastava and Prasad (2013)	2	RR interval, QRS amplitude	Extracting feature: DWT	Dataset MIT-BIH arrhythmias	Combination of Fuzzy logic, Feed forward neuro fuzzy and MLPNN	Specificity, Sensitivity, Accuracy	90 80 85
Sadiq and Shukr, (2013)	10	Avg PR interval, avg QRS duration, avg RS amplitude, avg RT and max QS amplitude Peaks- R,P, Q,T,S	Extracting features: DWT, Low pass and High pass filter, Wavelet selection: Daubechies wavelet, Harr filter,	Dataset MIT-BIH arrhythmias	Db4-ID3, ID3 Decision tree Haar-ID3	Classification accuracy, Elapsed time	94 0.0046
Khazaee, (2013)	1	RR interval	RR interval identification and baseline reduction	Dataset MIT-BIH arrhythmias	SVM classifier with Kernel-Adatron (K-A) training algorithm, MLPNN with back propagation training algorithm,	Training time, MSE (Training and Testing error),	04:45 0.007656 0.1539
Joshi and Ghongade (2013)	1	QRS complex	Extracting feature: Pan Tompkins technique (QRS), Reducing feature: PCA, DWT	Dataset MIT-BIH arrhythmias	SVM, MLPNN, RBFNN classifier, PCA+SVM, PCA+RBF, DCT+RBF, DWT+RBF, DCT+SVM, DWT+SVM	Correctness	99.55
Muthuchudar and Baboo (2013)	6	QRS amplitude, QRS interval, P wave, PR interval, T wave, ST interval	Removal of noise: Wavelet transform (UWT)	Dataset MIT-BIH arrhythmia	Feed forward network with back propagation algorithm as training algorithm	Correctness	96

continues on following page

Table 3. Continued

Researchers Name	No. of Features used	ECG Features Used	Pre-processing Method	Database used	Modelling System	Performance Measures	Correctness (%)
Zidelmal et al. (2013)	2	QRS complex duration, RR interval	Extracting feature: Data normalization, DWT using db4, R peak detection- wavelet coefficient, Q, S peak- simple peak detection method	Dataset MIT-BIH arrhythmia	SVM with rejection	Minimal classifying cost, Average correctness with no rejection,	98.8 97.2
Vijayavanan et al. (2014)	12	Intervals- PR, RR, ST, QT, QRS duration, Segments- ST, PR, Peaks-R, Q, S, P, T	Extracting feature: DWT level-8, Remove baseline wander	Dataset MIT-BIH arrhythmias	Feed forward PNN classifier trained with extracted features	Correctness	96.5
Joshi and Topannavar, (2014)	2	RR interval (avg RR, local RR, previous RR, post RR), R peak (Pre-R segment, Pro-R segment)	Extracting Feature: ICA, Baseline wander correction: DWT, Reducing feature: PCA	Dataset MIT-BIH arrhythmias	SVM classifier	Subject oriented and class oriented evaluation	86 99
Tang and Shu, (2014)	27	Peaks-P, Q, R, S, T, 19 temporal features (distance between points), 3 angle features,	Extracting feature: DWT, Removal of baseline wanders and denoised: High pass and Low pass filter, Reducing feature: rough sets	Dataset MIT-BIH arrhythmias	QNN trained using gradient descent method	Correctness	91.7
Das and Ari (2014)	3	RR interval, QRS detection, R peak	Extracting feature: DWT level4, ST, Pan Tompkin's QRS detection algorithm, Normalization: Zero mean, Denoised and baseline wander removal: Band pass filter	Dataset MIT-BIH arrhythmias	MLPNN classifier, ST+WT+MLPNN, ST+MLPNN,	Correctness, Sensitivity	97.5 69.38

signals, especially ECG for detecting the heart diseases. Some common methods in biomedical signal analysis include some additional steps like pre-processing, biomedical signal wave characterization, feature extraction and classification. The chapter addressed different types of machine learning techniques that are used for ECG analysis to classify different heart diseases. These techniques are fuzzy logic, neural networks, rough set theory and hidden markov model, genetic algorithm, and support vector machines, etc. The validation techniques can be examined in order to evaluate the performance of these methods revealed that there is a need for comparative studies that use a uniform set of performance measures, consistent with the ones used in medical studies, and a robust validation strategy guaranteeing that the results are generalizable. Moreover, there is a growing need for new datasets especially ECG data of variety of diseases that contain a large number of patients with labels that are generated using recent medical guidelines for diagnosis of heart related diseases. Finally, the extracted features from the raw data should be assessed in the context of clinical factors before they can be adopted by medical expert or physicians in clinical practice. This technology has revolutionized the medical and healthcare industry.

REFERENCES

Acharya, R., Kumar, A., Bhat, P. S., Lim, C. M., Iyengar, S. S., Kannathal, N., & Krishnan, S. M. (2004). Classification of cardiac abnormalities using heart rate signals. *Medical & Biological Engineering & Computing*, *42*(3), 288–293. doi:10.1007/BF02344702 PMID:15191072

Andreao, R., Dorizzi, B., & Boudy, J. (2006). ECG signal analysis through hidden Markov models. *IEEE Transactions on Biomedical Engineering*, *53*(8), 1541–1549. doi:10.1109/TBME.2006.877103 PMID:16916088

Ansari, S., Duda, M., Horan, K., Andersson, H. B., Goldberger, Z. D., Nallamothu, B. K., & Najarian, K. (2015). A Review of Automated Methods for Detection of Myocardial Ischemia and Infarction using Electrocardiogram and Electronic Health Records. *IEEE Reviews in Biomedical Engineering*.

Anuradha, B., & Reddy, V. (2008). ANN classification of cardiac arrhythmias. *Journal of Engineering and Applied Sciences (Asian Research Publishing Network)*, *3*(3), 1–6.

Ayub, S., & Saini, J. P. (2011). ECG classification and abnormality detection using cascade forward neural network. *International Journal of Engineering Science and Technology*, *3*(3), 41–46. doi:10.4314/ijest.v3i3.68420

Barman, T., Ghongade, & Ratnaparkhi, A. (2016). Rough set based segmentation and classification model for ECG. *IEEE Conference on Advances in Signal Processing (CASP)*, 18-23. 10.1109/CASP.2016.7746130

Batra, A., & Jawa, V. (2016). Classification of Arrhythmia using Conjunction of Machine Learning Algorithms and ECG Diagnostic Criteria. *International Journal of Biology and Biomedicine*, *1*, 1–7.

Behadada, O., & Chikh, M. A. (2013). An interpretable classifier for detection of cardiac arrhythmias by using the fuzzy decision tree. *Artificial Intelligence Research*, *2*(3), 45–58. doi:10.5430/air.v2n3p45

Bellotti, T., Nouretdinov, I., Yang, M., & Gammerman, A. (2014). *Conformal Prediction for Reliable Machine Learning. Theory, Adaptations and Applications*. Morgan Kaufmann.

Bensujin, Vijila, C.K., & Hubert, C. (2014). Detection of ST Segment Elevation Myocardial Infarction (STEMI) Using Bacterial Foraging Optimization Technique. *International Journal of Engineering and Technology, 6*(2), 1212-1224.

Bhoi, A. K., Sherpa, K. S., & Khandelwal, B. (2015). Classification probabil-ity analysis for arrhythmia and ischemia using frequency domain fea-tures of QRS complex. *International Journal Bioautomation, 19*(4).

Ceylan, R., Ozbay, Y., & Karlik, B. (2009). A novel approach for classification of ECG arrhythmias: Type-2 fuzzy clustering neural network. *Expert Systems with Applications, 36*(3), 6721–6726. doi:10.1016/j.eswa.2008.08.028

Ceylan, R., Ozbay, Y., & Karlik, B. (2009). A novel approach for classification of ECG arrhythmias: Type-2 fuzzy clustering neural network. *Expert Systems with Applications, 36*(3), 6721–6726. doi:10.1016/j.eswa.2008.08.028

Chen, Y., Wang, T., Wang, B., & Li, Z. (2009). A survey of fuzzy decision tree classifier. *Fuzzy Information and Engineering, 1*(2), 149–159. doi:10.100712543-009-0012-2

Correa, R., Arini, P. D., Correa, L. S., Valentinuzzi, M., & Laciar, E. (2014). Novel technique for ST-T interval characterization in patients with acute myocardial ischemia. *Computers in Biology and Medicine, 50*, 49–55. doi:10.1016/j.compbiomed.2014.04.009 PMID:24832353

Correa, R., Arini, P. D., Correa, L. S., Valentinuzzi, M., Laciar, E., & ... (2016). Identification of patients with myocardial infarction. *Methods of Information in Medicine, 55*(3), 242–249. doi:10.3414/ME15-01-0101 PMID:27063981

Daamouche, A., Hamami, L., Alajlan, N., & Melgani, F. (2012). A wavelet optimization approach for ECG signal classification. *Biomedical Signal Processing and Control, 7*(4), 342–349. doi:10.1016/j.bspc.2011.07.001

Dalal, S., & Birok, R. (2016). Analysis of ECG Signals using Hybrid Classifier. *International Advanced Research Journal in Science. Engineering and Technology, 3*(7), 89–95.

Dallali, A., Kachouri, A., & Samet, M. (2011). Classification of Cardiac Arrhythmia Using WT, HRV, and Fuzzy C-Means Clustering. *Signal Processing: An Int. J., 5*(3), 101-109.

Dallali, A., Kachouri, A., & Samet, M. (2011). Fuzzy c-means clustering, Neural Network, wt, and Hrv for classification of cardiac arrhythmia. *ARPN J. of Eng. and Appl. Sci., 6*(10), 112–118.

Das, M. K., & Ari, S. (2014). ECG Beats Classification Using Mixture of Features. *International Scholarly Research Notices, 2014*, 1–12. doi:10.1155/2014/178436 PMID:27350985

De Gaetano, A., Panunzi, S., Rinaldi, F., Risi, A., & Sciandrone, M. (2009). A patient adaptable ECG beat classifier based on neural networks. *Applied Mathematics and Computation, 213*(1), 243–249. doi:10.1016/j.amc.2009.03.013

Deja, A. W., & Paszek, P. (2003). Applying rough set theory to Multi stage medical diagnosing. *Fundamenta Informaticae, 54*(4), 387–408.

Duskalov, I., Dotsinsky, I. A., & Christov, I. I. (1998). Developments in ECG acquisition, preprocessing, parameter measurement, and recording. *IEEE Engineering in Medicine and Biology Magazine, 17*(2), 50–58. doi:10.1109/51.664031 PMID:9548081

El-Dahshan, E. (2010). Genetic algorithm and wavelet hybrid scheme for ECG signal denoising. *Telecommunication Systems, 46*(3), 209–215. doi:10.100711235-010-9286-2

Exarchos, T. P., Papaloukas, C., Fotiadis, D. I., & Michalis, L. K. (2006). An association rule mining-based methodology for automated detection of ischemic ECG beats. *IEEE Transactions on Biomedical Engineering, 53*(8), 1531–1540. doi:10.1109/TBME.2006.873753 PMID:16916087

Finlay, D., Bond, R., Kennedy, A., Guldenring, D., Moran, K., & McLaughlin, J. (2015). The effects of electrode placement on an automated algorithm for detecting ST segment changes on the 12-lead ECG. *Computers in Cardiology, 42*, 1161–1164. doi:10.1109/CIC.2015.7411122

Gao, D., Madden, M., Schukat, M., Chambers, D., & Lyons, G. (2004). Arrhythmia Identification from ECG Signals with a Neural Network Classifier Based on a Bayesian Framework. *Twenty-fourth SGAI International Conference on Innovative Techniques and Applications of Artificial Intelligence*, 3(3), 390-409.

Garcia, J., Astrom, M., Mendive, J., Laguna, P., & Sornmo, L. (2003). ECG-based detection of body position changes in ischemia monitoring. *IEEE Transactions on Biomedical Engineering, 50*(6), 677–685. doi:10.1109/TBME.2003.812208 PMID:12814234

Garcia, J., Sornmo, L., Olmos, S., & Laguna, P. (2000). Automatic detection of ST-T complex changes on the ECG using filtered RMS difference series: Application to ambulatory ischemia monitoring. *IEEE Transactions on Biomedical Engineering, 47*(9), 1195–1201. doi:10.1109/10.867943 PMID:11008420

Ghosh, B., Indurkar, M., & Jain, M. K. (2013). ECG: A Simple Noninvasive Tool to Localize Culprit Vessel Occlusion Site in Acute STEMI. *Indian Journal of Clinical Practice, 23*(10), 590–595.

Goel, S., Tomar, P., & Kaur, G. (2016). A Fuzzy Based Approach for Denoising of ECG Signal using Wavelet Transform. *International Journal of Bio-Science and Bio-Technology, 8*(2), 143–156. doi:10.14257/ijbsbt.2016.8.2.13

Goletsis, Y., Papaloukas, C., Fotiadis, D. I., Likas, A., & Michalis, L. K. (2004). Automated ischemic beat classification using genetic algorithms and multicriteria decision analysis. *IEEE Transactions on Biomedical Engineering, 51*(10), 1717–1725. doi:10.1109/TBME.2004.828033 PMID:15490819

Guler, I., & Ubeyli, E. D. (2007). Multiclass support vector machines for EEG signals classification. *IEEE Transactions on Information Technology in Biomedicine, 11*(2), 117–126. doi:10.1109/TITB.2006.879600 PMID:17390982

Gupta, K. O., & Chatur, P. N. (2012). ECG Signal Analysis and Classification using Data Mining and Artificial Neural Networks. *International Journal of Emerging Technology and Advanced Engineering, 2*(1), 56–60.

Hadjem, M., Nait-Abdesselam, F., & Khokhar, A. (2016). ST-segment and T-wave anomalies prediction in an ECG data using RUSBoost. *IEEE 18th International Conference on e-Health Networking, Applications and Services (Healthcom)*, 1–6.

Huang, X. M., & Zhang, Y. H. (2003). A new application of rough set to ECG recognition. *Int. Conference on Machine Learning and Cybernetics*, *3*, 1729-1734.

Jadhav, S., Nalbalwar, S. L., & Ghatol, A. (2012). Artificial Neural Network Models based Cardiac Arrhythmia Disease Diagnosis from ECG Signal Data. *International Journal of Computers and Applications*, *44*(15), 8–13. doi:10.5120/6338-8532

Jager, F., Mark, R., Moody, G., & Divjak, S. (1992). *Analysis of transient ST segment changes during ambulatory monitoring using the Karhunen-Loeave transform. In Computers in Cardiology 1992, Proceedings of, IEEE. IEEE Comput.* Soc. Press.

Jager, F., Moody, G. B., & Mark, R. G. (1998). Detection of transient ST segment episodes during ambulatory ECG monitoring. *Computers and Biomedical Research, an International Journal*, *31*(5), 305–322. doi:10.1006/cbmr.1998.1483 PMID:9790738

Jaleel, A., Tafreshi, R., & Tafreshi, L. (2016). An expert system for differential diagnosis of myocardial infarction. *Journal of Dynamic Systems, Measurement, and Control*, *138*(11), 111012. doi:10.1115/1.4033838

Jambukia, S. H., Dabhi, V. K., & Prajapati, H. B. (2015). Classification of ECG signals using Machine Learning Techniques: A Survey. *International Conference on Advances in Computer Engineering and Applications*.

Jeyalakshmi, M. S., & Robin, C. (2016). Fuzzy based Expert system for sleep apnea diagnosis. *International Journal of Engineering Trends and Technology*, *35*(12), 555–558. doi:10.14445/22315381/IJETT-V35P312

Joshi, D., & Ghongade, R. (2013). Performance analysis of feature extraction schemes for ECG signal classification. *Int. J. of Elect. Electron. And Data Commun.*, *1*, 45–51.

Joshi, N. P., & Topannavar, P. S. (2014). Support vector machine based heartbeat classification. *Proc. of 4th IRF Int. Conf.*, 140-144.

Kampouraki, A., Manis, G., & Nikou, C. (2009). Heartbeat Time Series Classification with Support Vector Machines. *IEEE Transactions on Information Technology in Biomedicine*, *1*(4), 512–518. doi:10.1109/TITB.2008.2003323 PMID:19273030

Kannathal, N., Acharya, U. R., Lim, C. M., Sadasivan, P. K., & Krishnan, S. M. (2003). Classification of cardiac patient states using artificial neural networks. *Experimental and Clinical Cardiology*, *8*(4), 206–211. PMID:19649222

Khazaee, A. (2013). Heart Beat Classification Using Particle Swarm Optimization. *Int. J. of Intelligent Syst. and Applicat.*, *5*(6), 25–33. doi:10.5815/ijisa.2013.06.03

Khorrami, H., & Moavenian, M. (2010). A comparative study of DWT, CWT and DCT transformations in ECG arrhythmias classification. *Expert Systems with Applications*, *37*(8), 5751–5757. doi:10.1016/j.eswa.2010.02.033

Kora, P., & Kalva, S. R. (2015). Improved Bat algorithm for the detection of myocardial infarction. *SpringerPlus*, *4*(1), 666. doi:10.118640064-015-1379-7 PMID:26558169

Korurek, M., & Dogan, B. (2010). ECG beat classification using particle swarm optimization and radial basis function neural network. *Expert Systems with Applications*, *37*(12), 7563–7569. doi:10.1016/j.eswa.2010.04.087

Kumari, V. S. R., & Kumar, P. R. (2013). Cardiac Arrhythmia Prediction using improved Multilayer Perceptron Neural Network. *Research for Development*, *3*(4), 73–80.

Laciar, E., Jane, R., & Brooks, D. H. (2003). Improved alignment method for noisy high-resolution ECG and Holter records using multiscale cross-correlation. *IEEE Transactions on Biomedical Engineering*, *50*(3), 344–353. doi:10.1109/TBME.2003.808821 PMID:12669991

Lahiri, T., Kumar, U., Mishra, H., Sarkar, S., & Roy, A. D. (2009). Analysis of ECG signal by chaos principle to help automatic diagnosis of myocardial infarction. *Journal of Scientific and Industrial Research*, *68*(10), 866–870.

Lei, W. K., Li, B. N., Dong, M. C., & Vai, M. I. (2007). AFC-ECG: An Intelligent Fuzzy ECG Classifier. In book. *Soft Computing in Industrial Applications*, *39*, 189–199. doi:10.1007/978-3-540-70706-6_18

Luz E. J. S., Schwartz W. R., Chavez G. C., Menotti D. (2016). ECG-based heartbeat classification for arrhythmia detection: A survey. *Computer Methods and Programs in Biomedicine, 127*, 144–164.

Marsanova, L., Ronzhina, M., Smisek, R., Vitek, M., Nemcova, A., Smital, L., & Novakova, M. (2017). ECG features and methods for automatic classification of ventricular premature and ischemic heartbeats: A comprehensive experimental study. *Scientific Reports*, *7*(1), 11239. doi:10.103841598-017-10942-6 PMID:28894131

Minchole, A., Skarp, B., Jager, F., & Laguna, P. (2005). Evaluation of a root mean squared based ischemia detector on the long-term ST database with body position change cancellation. *Computers in Cardiology*, 853–856. doi:10.1109/CIC.2005.1588239

Mitra, S., Mitra, M., & Chaudhuri, B. B. (2006). An Approach to a Rough Set Based Disease Inference Engine for ECG Classification. *IEEE Transactions on Instrumentation and Measurement*, *55*(6), 2198–2206. doi:10.1109/TIM.2006.884279

Moavenian, M., & Khorrami, H. (2010). A qualitative comparison of artificial neural networks and support vector machines in ECG arrhythmias classification. *Expert Systems with Applications*, *37*(4), 3088–3093. doi:10.1016/j.eswa.2009.09.021

Murthy, H. N., & Meenakshi, M. (2015). ANN, SVM and KNN classifiers for prognosis of cardiac ischemia-a comparison. *Bonfring International Journal of Research in Communication Engineering*, *5*(2), 7. doi:10.9756/BIJRCE.8030

Muthuchudar, A., & Baboo, S. S. (2013). A Study of the Processes Involved in ECG Signal Analysis. *Int. J. of Scientific and Research Publications*, *3*(3), 1–5.

Naima, F. A., & Timemy, A. A. (2009). Neural network based classification of myocardial infarction: a comparative study of wavelet and fourier transforms. Academic Press.

Nasiri, J. A., Naghibzadeh, M., Yazdi, H. S., & Naghibzadeh, B. (2009). ECG Arrhythmia Classification with Support Vector Machines and Genetic Algorithm. *Third UKSim European Symposium on Computer Modeling and Simulation.*

Nidhyananthan, S. S., Saranya, S., & Kumari, R. S. S. (2016). Myocardial infarction detection and heart patient identity verification. *International Conference on Wireless Communications, Signal Processing and Networking (WiSPNET)*, 1107–1111. 10.1109/WiSPNET.2016.7566308

Omran, S. S., Taha, S. M. R., & Awadh, N. A. (2009). ECG Rhythm Analysis by Using Neuro-Genetic Algorithms. *Journal of Basic and Applied Sciences*, *1*(3), 522–530.

Ozbay, Y., Ceylan, R., & Karlik, B. (2006). A fuzzy clustering neural network architecture for classification of ECG arrhythmias. *Computers in Biology and Medicine*, *36*(4), 376–388. doi:10.1016/j.compbiomed.2005.01.006 PMID:15878480

Padhy, S., & Dandapat, S. (2017). Third-order tensor based analysis of multilead ECG for classification of myocardial infarction. *Biomedical Signal Processing and Control*, *31*, 71–78. doi:10.1016/j.bspc.2016.07.007

Padhy, S., Sharma, L., & Dandapat, S. (2016). Multilead ECG data compression using SVD in multiresolution domain. *Biomedical Signal Processing and Control*, *23*, 10–18. doi:10.1016/j.bspc.2015.06.012

Pal, D., Mandana, K., Pal, S., Sarkar, D., & Chakraborty, C. (2012). Fuzzy expert system approach for coronary artery disease screening using clinical parameters. *Knowledge-Based Systems*, *36*, 162–174. doi:10.1016/j.knosys.2012.06.013

Patra, D., Das, M. K., & Pradhan, S. (2010). Integration of FCM, PCA and neural networks for classification of ECG arrhythmias. *IAENG Int. J. of Comput. Sci.*, *36*(3), 24–62.

Polat, K., Akdemir, B., & Gune, S. (2008). Computer aided diagnosis of ECG data on the least square support vector machine. *Digital Signal Processing*, *18*(1), 25–32. doi:10.1016/j.dsp.2007.05.006

Priyadharshini, V., & Kumar, S. S. (2015). An Enhanced Approach on ECG Data Analysis using Improvised Genetic Algorithm. *International Research Journal of Engineering and Technology*, *2*(5), 1248–1256.

Quesnel, P. X., Chan, A. D. C., & Yang, H. (2014). Signal quality and false myocardial ischemia alarms in ambulatory electrocardiograms. *IEEE International Symposium on Medical Measurements and Applications (MeMeA)*, 1–5. 10.1109/MeMeA.2014.6860078

Rangayyan, R. M., & Reddy, N. P. (2002). Biomedical signal analysis: A case-study approach. *Annals of Biomedical Engineering*, *30*(7), 983–983. doi:10.1114/1.1509766

Roopa, C. K., & Harish, B. S. (2017). A Survey on various Machine Learning Approaches for ECG Analysis. *International Journal of Computers and Applications*, *163*(9).

SadAbadi, H., Ghasemi, M., & Ghaffari, A. (2007). A Mathematical Algorithm for ECG Signal Denoising Using Window Analysis. *Biomedical Papers of the Medical Faculty of the University Palacky, Olomouc, Czechoslovakia*, *151*(1), 73–78. doi:10.5507/bp.2007.013 PMID:17690744

Sadiq, A. T., & Shukr, N. H. (2013). Classification of Cardiac Arrhythmia using ID3 Classifier Based on Wavelet Transform. *Iraqi J. of Sci.*, *54*(4), 1167–1175.

Safdarian, N., Dabanloo, N. J., & Attarodi, G. (2014). A new pattern recog-nition method for detection and localization of myocardial infarction using T-wave integral and total integral as extracted features from one cycle of ECG signal. *Scientific Research Publishing, 7*, 818.

Sao, P., Hegadi, R., & Karmakar, S. (2015). ECG Signal Analysis Using Artificial Neural Network. *International Journal of Scientific Research (Ahmedabad, India)*, 82–86.

Sarkaleh, M. K., & Shahbahrami, A. (2012). Classification of ECG arrhythmias using Discrete Wavelet Transform and neural networks. *Int. J. of Comput. Sci. Eng. and Applicat., 2*(1), 1–13.

Schmidt, M., Baumert, M., Porta, A., Malberg, H., & Zaunseder, S. (2014). Two-dimensional warping for one-dimensional signals–conceptual framework and application to ECG processing. *IEEE Transactions on Signal Processing, 62*(21), 5577–5588. doi:10.1109/TSP.2014.2354313

Senthilkumaran, N., & Rajesh, R. (2009). A Study on Rough Set Theory for Medical Image Segmentation. *International Journal of Recent Trends in Engineering, 2*(2), 236–238.

Setiawan, N. A., Venkatachalam, P. A., & Fadzil, A. (2009). Rule Selection for Coronary Artery Disease Diagnosis Based on Rough Set. *International Journal of Recent Trends in Engineering, 2*(5), 198–202.

Sharma, L. N., & Dandapat, S. (2016). Detecting myocardial infarction by multivariate multiscale covariance analysis of multilead electrocardio-grams. *The International Congress on Information and Communication Technology, Springer Singapore, 439*, pp. 169–179.

Sharma, L. N., Tripathy, R. K., & Dandapat, S. (2015). Multiscale energy and eigenspace approach to detection and localization of myocardial infarction. *IEEE Transactions on Biomedical Engineering, 62*(7), 1827–1837. doi:10.1109/TBME.2015.2405134 PMID:26087076

Silveira, R. M., Agulhari, C. M., Bonatti, I. S., & Peres, P. D. L. (2007). A genetic algorithm to compress the electrocardiograms using parametrized wavelets. *IEEE International Symposium on Signal Processing and Information Technology.* 10.1109/ISSPIT.2007.4458092

Singh, Y. N., Singh, S. K., & Ray, A. K. (2012). Bioelectrical signals as emerging biometrics: Issues and challenges. *ISRN Signal Processing, 2012*, 1–13. doi:10.5402/2012/712032

Sornmo, L. (1991). *Time-varying filtering for removal of baseline wander in exercise ECGs. Computers in Cardiology, Proceedings.* doi:10.1109/CIC.1991.169066

Srivastava, V. K., & Prasad, D. (2013). Dwt-Based Feature Extraction from ECG Signal. *American J. of Eng. Research, 2*(3), 44–50.

Tang, X., & Shu, L. (2014). Classification of Electrocardiogram Signals with RS and Quantum Neural Networks. *Int. J. of Multimedia and Ubiquitous Eng., 9*(2), 363–372. doi:10.14257/ijmue.2014.9.2.37

Tripathy, B. K., Acharjya, D. P., & Cynthya, V. (2011). A Framework for Intelligent Medical Diagnosis Using Rough Set with Formal Concept Analysis. *International Journal of Artificial Intelligence & Applications, 2*(2), 45–66. doi:10.5121/ijaia.2011.2204

Umer, M., Bhatti, B. A., Tariq, M. H., Zia-ul-Hassan, M., Khan, M. Y., & Zaidi, T. (2014). Electrocardiogram Feature Extraction and Pattern Recognition Using a Novel Windowing Algorithm. *Scientific Research Advances in Bioscience and Biotechnology., 5*(11), 896–894. doi:10.4236/abb.2014.511103

Vijayavanan, M., Rathikarani, V., & Dhanalakshmi, P. (2014). Automatic Classification of ECG Signal for Heart Disease Diagnosis using morphological features. *International Journal of Computer Science and Engineering Technology, 5*(4), 449–455.

Vishwa, A., Lal, M., Dixit, S., & Vardwaj, P. (2011). Classification of Arrhythmic ECG Data Using Machine Learning Techniques. *International Journal of Interactive Multimedia and Artificial Intelligence, 1*(4), 67–70. doi:10.9781/ijimai.2011.1411

Vishwa, A., Lal, M. K., Dixit, S., & Vardwaj, P. (2011). Classification of arrhythmic ECG data using machine learning techniques. *Int. J. of Interactive Multimedia and Artificial Intell., 1*(4), 68–71.

Wang, J. S., Chiang, W. C., Yang, Y. T., & Hsu, Y. L. (2012). *An effective ECG arrhythmia classification algorithm.* Bio-Inspired Computing and Applications, Springer Berlin Heidelberg. doi:10.1007/978-3-642-24553-4_72

Wang, T. Y., & Chiang, H. M. (2007). Fuzzy support vector machine for multiclass categorization. *Information Processing & Management, 43*(4), 914–929. doi:10.1016/j.ipm.2006.09.011

Yu, S. N., & Chou, K. T. (2008). Integration of independent component analysis and neural networks for ECG beat classification. *Expert Systems with Applications, 34*(4), 2841–2846. doi:10.1016/j.eswa.2007.05.006

Zeraatkar, E., & … . (2011). Arrhythmia detection based on Morphological and time-frequency Features of t-wave in Electrocardiogram. *Journal of Medical Signals and Sensors, 1*(2), 99–106. doi:10.4103/2228-7477.95293 PMID:22606664

Zidelmal, Z., Amirou, A., Abdeslam, D. O., & Merckle, J. (2013). ECG beat classification using a cost sensitive classifier. *Computer Methods and Programs in Biomedicine, 111*(3), 570–577. doi:10.1016/j.cmpb.2013.05.011 PMID:23849928

Chapter 12
Artificial Bee Colony–Based Associative Classifier for Healthcare Data Diagnosis

M. Nandhini

ⓘ https://orcid.org/0000-0002-0542-8888

Department of Computer Science, Government Arts College, Udumalpet, India

S. N. Sivanandam

Department of Computer Science and Engineering, Karpagam College of Engineering, Coimbatore, India

S. Renugadevi

Department of Computer Science and Engineering, PSG College of Technology, Coimbatore, India

ABSTRACT

Data mining is likely to explore hidden patterns from the huge quantity of data and provides a way of analyzing and categorizing the data. Associative classification (AC) is an integration of two data mining tasks, association rule mining, and classification which is used to classify the unknown data. Though association rule mining techniques are successfully utilized to construct classifiers, it lacks in generating a small set of significant class association rules (CARs) to build an accurate associative classifier. In this work, an attempt is made to generate significant CARs using Artificial Bee Colony (ABC) algorithm, an optimization technique to construct an efficient associative classifier. Associative classifier, thus built using ABC discovered CARs achieve high prognostic accurateness and interestingness value. Promising results were provided by the ABC based AC when experiments were conducted using health care datasets from the UCI machine learning repository.

DOI: 10.4018/978-1-7998-2742-9.ch012

INTRODUCTION

Health care applications necessitate an efficient and accurate diagnostic system. Generally, physicians rely on the diagnostic system for providing treatments to the patients. An efficient diagnostic system provides a way to analyze and categorize the data. It helps in exploring interesting patterns/associations between the symptoms and diseases. It provides realistic decision-making in the disease diagnosis task. In recent times, it is proven that data mining techniques have gained significance in providing useful suggestions and predictions based on the existing data. Hence, data mining techniques are best suited to build an efficient diagnostic system. Broadly, data mining techniques are categorized into two, descriptive and predictive. Association rule mining is one of the descriptive data mining techniques, commonly used to find interesting patterns/associations in the form of If-then rules. The relationships/affinities among the attributes of the dataset are acquired from the generated rules. Classification is one of the predictive data mining techniques used to compute a model from the historical data to predict some response of interest. Thus, a health care diagnostic system using the knowledge of domain experts becomes essential for extracting interesting patterns and providing reasonable decision-making. In this work, an attempt is made to construct a health care diagnostic system by building a classification system using Class Association Rules (CARs) or simply class rules.

Associative Classification (AC) is one of the data mining techniques which integrate the concept of association and classification(Liu, Hsu, Ma, & Ma, 1998). The role of the association in AC is to extract a large number of interesting rules representing the relationship among the attributes whereas the classification is predefined with the class label for predicting the unknown data. Thus, the AC system is constructed using the generated CARs. Construction of AC involves two tasks, such as class rule generation and classification. In the 'rule generation' phase, all possible CARs i.e. class rules are discovered from the dataset and they are taken into classifier construction. AC is one of the classifiers extensively used in healthcare applications, because of its high precision classification. Inherently, healthcare data diagnosis desires high precision, so AC is more suitable for healthcare applications. Though AC is a competent classifier, its classification ability is often affected by the generation of many insignificant class rules in the 'rule generation' phase. Further, the number and significance of the generated class rules deteriorate the efficiency of the AC. To address this issue, in the literature, many evolutionary algorithms like (Shahzad & Baig, 2011), PSO(Mangat & Vig, 2014), Firefly algorithm (Nandhini, Rajalakshmi, & Sivanandam, 2017) are adopted within AC to generate significant class rules. A new approach has been proposed in this work to build an efficient classification system by generating a very few significant class rules using Artificial Bee Colony (ABC) algorithm within AC.

ABC is a meta-heuristic population-based algorithm motivated by the intelligent foraging behavior of honey bees(D Karaboga, 2005). It is highly used for optimizing solutions for mathematical problems. Three main components involved in this algorithm are employed bee, unemployed bee, and food sources. The foraging behavior aids to find the significant class rules among the generated rules. In this work, an attempt is made to generate very few significant Class Association Rules (CARs) using ABC algorithm to construct an efficient associative classifier. Incorporating ABC in AC considerably increases the performance of the classifier. ABC based AC (ABC-AC) achieves high prognostic accurateness and interestingness value. The generation of very few significant class rules using the ABC algorithm improves the interpretability of the result and provides more insight cognition into the classifier structure and the decision-making process. Promising results in terms of classifier accuracy are obtained by the ABC-AC when experiments were conducted using five health care datasets such as Breast cancer,

Cleve, heart, hepatitis and Pima from the UCI machine learning repository. Consecutively, to enhance the performance of the ABC-AC, T-test, a filter-based feature selection technique, is applied to retain significant and eliminate insignificant attributes from the dataset.

BACKGROUND

Associative Classification (AC)

AC is a supervised learning approach integrates association rule mining and classification techniques. Associative classification is slower than traditional classification but often ends up with higher accuracy. AC explores high confident association rules among multiple attributes of the dataset; and defeats the drawback of decision-tree induction, which it considers only one attribute at a time. Though AC achieves high classification accuracy, it generates a very large number of association rules resulting in high processing overhead. Sometimes, its confidence based rule evaluation measure may lead to overfitting. Classification Based on Association (CBA)(Liu et al., 1998) is the first Apriori based AC algorithm that generates all possible class rules satisfying the support and confidence threshold fixed by the user. It has two phases such as rule generator and classifier builder. All possible association rules using the Apriori algorithm (Agrawal & Srikant, 1994) are generated in the first phase. From the generated rules, a small set of class rules are taken to form the classifier. In the second phase, the first best class rule that satisfies the condition is selected to predict the class label of the test/unknown tuple. If no rule satisfies the test/unknown tuple condition, then it will come under the default class. Though the algorithm is elegant, it has its own disadvantages, as it generates rules in an iterative manner and picks only one best class rule for the test tuple classification. In the case of a larger dataset, data needs to be scanned many times which exponentially increases the time complexity and the number of rules. During classification, if more than one rules having equal confidence, it chooses a rule randomly, which may result in accuracy reduction. Classification Based on Multiple Association Rules (CMAR)(Li, Han, & Pei, 2001) is proposed to overpower the weakness of CBA. CMAR is FP Growth based AC algorithm, where FP Growth is one of the best substitutes of Apriori. CMAR classifies a tuple with more than one class rule. Though CMAR defers better classification accuracy than CBA, it commonly produces a large number of rules in the rule mining phase which requires more time and endeavor to select interesting rules among them. First Order Inductive Learner (FOIL) (Quinlan & Cameron-Jones, 1993), Predictive Rule Mining (PRM) and Classification based on Predictive Association Rule (CPAR) (Yin & Han, 2003) is further designed on the line to beat the problem of producing a small set of significant class rules without compromising time complexity. FOIL works better for binary class dataset; it uses FOIL's Information Gain measure to evaluate the gain value of each attribute and finally picks the best gain attribute to form the rule antecedent. Once the rule is formed, the class tuples which are satisfied by the generated rules are deleted and the procedure for finding the best gain attribute is followed. These steps are repeatedly performed until all the class tuples in the dataset are deleted. Though FOIL generates a small number of significant rules but fails to reach better accuracy than its predecessors. It also spends most of its time in evaluating the gain value of the attribute. In order to achieve better accuracy and efficiency, PRM is proposed, which is an improved version of FOIL. PRM uses the decay factor to reduce the weight of the tuple instead of deleting the tuples. It removes the tuple having a weight less than the specified gain threshold. CPAR, an extension of PRM uses a parameter called Gain_Similarity_Ratio(GSR) to find the close-to-the-best attributes in the rule generation phase. Instead of adding one best gain attribute in the rule antecedent, entire close-to-the-best attributes are included in the rule antecedent. Because of its inherent nature, CPAR outperforms the FOIL and PRM. Further CPAR is customized to enhance the accuracy by generating quality rules using Gain Ratio (CPAR-GR) (Nandhini & Sivanandam, 2015). Multi-label Multi-class Associative Classification (MMAC) (Thabtah, Cowling, & Peng, 2004) is an associative classification algorithm designed to handle the training data having multiple class. MMAC algorithm has three phases such as rule generation, recursive learning, and classification. In the rule generation phase, it scans the training data and generates all possible association rules. In the second phase, it proceeds to find more rules based on minimum support and minimum confidence from the unclassified instances. In the third phase, all the rules are merged together to form the final rule set and tested against test data. From the literature, it is found that the rule evaluation and selection tasks of AC are computationally expensive. Since AC generates a large number of rules during the 'rule generation' phase, heuristic approaches are typically used to evaluate and select the best ones among the generated rules. Hence, this proposed work motivates us to utilize a novel heuristic algorithm to optimize the 'rule generation' phase of traditional CPAR, an AC algorithm. It takes the essential inspiration of the ABC algorithm to customize the rule evaluation and selection tasks of the CPAR algorithm.

Heuristic Algorithm

In (Dervis Karaboga & Basturk, 2007), ABC is used for optimizing multivariable functions and the results are compared with Particle Swarm Intelligence (PSO) and Genetic algorithm (GA). It is identified that ABC works better than PSO and GA. It is found that, ABC does not trap up with local minimum and suitably used for multivariable, multimodal function optimization. Though, it is exploited to optimize the multivariable functions, the parameters affecting the performance and the convergence rate has to be explored.

Self-adaptive Position update in ABC (SPABC), in which three position update strategies are incorporated in the employed bee phase based on the fitness of the solutions. Each employed bee checks its fitness and accordingly adopts one of the position update strategies of standard ABC; Gbest guided ABC (GABC), and modified ABC (MABC).

ARTIFICIAL BEE COLONY ALGORITHM (ABC) BASED AC(ABC-AC)

The proposed methodology ABC-AC combines the concept of the ABC algorithm and CPAR in structuring the associative classifier. Generally, AC is a combination of association rule mining and classification tasks. In the proposed methodology, the ABC algorithm is used to extract CARs from the training dataset. The extracted CARs are used to form the classification model. In the classification phase, the test/unknown tuples are classified using the best k-CARs from the generated CARs. In general, the goal of an associative classifier is to build an efficient classification system using significant class rules (i.e. CARs). The intention of the ABC-AC is to generate a small set of significant CARs having maximum fitness value. Classifier thus built using significant CARs with maximum fitness value achieve better accuracy for test and unknown tuples. This section describes mathematically about associative classification and the steps of generating CARs using ABC algorithm.

Artificial Bee Colony Algorithm (ABC)

Algorithms such as Evolutionary algorithms (EA), Differential Evolution algorithm (DE), Genetic Algorithms (GA), Particle Swarm Optimization (PSO) are available for optimization purposes. Similarly, ABC is a meta-heuristic population based algorithm motivated by the foraging behavior of honey bees. It is highly used for optimizing numerical problems(Pham & Karaboga, 2000). It is one among the swarm intelligence algorithms, proposed by (D Karaboga, 2005). Swarm possesses intelligent behavior such as self-organizing, single agent failure tolerance. In this work, ABC is used to optimize the CAR generation process i.e. to generate significant CARs in less iteration. A CAR with the maximum fitness value is considered as significant. This optimization problem is formulated mathematically as follows:

A model $M = (S, f, C)$ has search space S defined over a finite set of CARs $(X_{ij} \rightarrow Y_c)$, where $X_{ij} \subseteq A_{ij}$, such that, $1 \leq i \leq n$, $1 \leq j \leq 10$, Y_c is the class attribute having 'c' values. In this work, only binary class datasets are considered, hence $c=0,1$.

- X_{ij} is the set of best gain attribute values, A_{ij} represent the jth value of the ith attribute of the dataset having 'n' attributes and each attribute has at most 10 values as each attribute is discretized using 10 bins [explained in Methodology section], 'c' represents the class of the dataset.
- An objective function is

$$Max\left(f\left(X_{ij} \rightarrow Y_c \right) \right)$$
$$= \pm * Cosine\left(\left(X_{ij} \rightarrow Y_c \right) + ^2 * All\ Confidence\left(X_{ij} \rightarrow Y_c \right) + ^3 * Coverage\left(X_{ij} \rightarrow Y_c \right) \right) \tag{1}$$

subject to $\alpha+\beta+\gamma=0$, $0\leq\alpha,\beta,\gamma\leq1$, where α, β and γ are user specified significance values for three measures i.e. Cosine similarity (2), AllConfidence (3) and Coverage(3). These values depend on the nature and domain value of the dataset and its attribute. Where,

$$Cosine\left(X_{ij} \rightarrow Y_c \right) = \frac{No.\ of\ tuples\ contain\ both\ X_{ij}\ and\ Y_c}{\sqrt{\left(No.\ of\ tuples\ contain\ X_{ij} * No.\ of\ tuples\ contain\ Y_c \right)}} \tag{2}$$

$$AllConf\left(X_{ij} \rightarrow Y_c \right)$$
$$= \min\left(\frac{No.\ of\ tuples\ contain\ both\ X_{ij}\ and\ Y_c}{No.\ of\ tuples\ contain\ X_{ij}}, \frac{No.\ of\ tuples\ contain\ both\ X_{ij}\ and\ Y_c}{No.\ of\ tuples\ contain\ Y_c} \right) \cdot \tag{3}$$

$$Coverage\left(X_{ij} \rightarrow Y_c \right) = \frac{No.\ of\ tuples\ contain\ X_{ij}}{Total\ no.\ of\ tuples} \tag{4}$$

- A set C of constraints among the CARs is

$$X_{ij} \cap Y_c = \varnothing, \ X_{ij} \neq \varnothing, \ Y_c \neq \varnothing$$

Three main components involved in the ABC algorithm are Food Source, Employed Bee, and Unemployed Bee.

Food Source

Food source generally represents the initial population. The value of food source can be determined by the factors such as distance from nest, amount of nectar, ease of extracting the energy, etc., In literature for many cases, quality of the food source is considered as a factor. The quality of the food source (i.e. CAR) is determined using customized fitness function (1) particularly designed for this work. In this work, the traditional ABC algorithm is customized to fit into the 'rule generation phase' of the CPAR algorithm. Initially, the attribute subset for each set (i.e. positive and negative set) is created using the minimum support threshold. From the attribute subset, all possible 1-attribute CARs i.e. antecedent length of the CAR is equal to one are generated. Generated 1-attribute CARs are taken as initial population (i.e. Food source).

Employed bee

Each employed bee is associated with one food source and vice versa. It collects information about the food source and shares it with unemployed bees. After sharing the information, it either abandons the food source or it continues its task. Whenever the bee abandons its food source it becomes the scout. ABC-AC intends to generate significant CARs by taking advantage of the objective function. Each 1-attribute CAR in the initial population is considered as a food source. In every iteration, the quality of the food source is determined using fitness function (1). With the maximum fitness value obtained in each iteration, neighborhood value for each 1-attribute CARs i.e. food source is calculated using (5). Neighborhood values are useful for finding new feasible solutions (i.e. CARs) in the population.

$$\boldsymbol{Neighborhood}\left(X_{ij} \rightarrow Y_c\right) = Max\left(f\left(X_{ij} \rightarrow Y_c\right)\right) - NSR * \left[Max\left(\boldsymbol{f}\left(X_{ij} \rightarrow Y_c\right)\right) - \boldsymbol{f}\left(X_{ij} \rightarrow Y_c\right)\right]$$

(5)

Where, $Max(f(X_{ij} \rightarrow Y_c))$ is the maximum fitness value obtained in the generation. $f(X_{ij} \rightarrow Y_c)$ is the fitness value of the $X_{ij} \rightarrow Y_c$. 'NSR' is the Neighborhood Similarity Ratio fixed by the user depends on nature and number of the attribute values of the dataset.

As an attempt, in this work, Neighborhood_Threshold (NT) (6) is calculated to produce a high number of feasible solutions (i.e. CARs) and to maintain optimum solutions in every iteration. Instead of choosing one CAR (i.e. food source) having the highest neighborhood value as the best source, CARs whose neighborhood values greater than equal to Neighborhood_Threshold (NT) are taken to the next iteration as best ones. Thus, ABC-AC selects more than one CAR (food source) as close-to-the-best CARs using NT. The CARs having neighborhood value greater than or equal to NT are considered as close-to-the-best CARs. All the close-to-the-best CARs are shared with unemployed bees and further taken to form higher attributes CARs in the next generation. I.e. 1-attribute CARs are taken to form 2-attributes CARs.

$$Neighborhood\_Threshold(NT) = NSR * Max\left(Neighborhood\left(X_{ij} \rightarrow Y_c\right)\right) \qquad (6)$$

Where, $Max(Neighborhood(X_{ij} \rightarrow Y_c))$ is the maximum neighborhood value obtained in each iteration. CARs that satisfy the 'NT' are considered as taken as best CARs and they are shared with unemployed bees. They are further taken to form the higher order attribute CARs. This process is repeated until the stopping condition (i.e. maximum number of generations) is met.

Unemployed Bee

There are two types of unemployed bees: onlooker bees and scouts. Onlooker bees collect information from the employed bee and select the best source based on the quality of the source i.e. CARs to explore the new ones around it. It gets the knowledge about the CARs and chooses the best CARs to occupy in the next generation using (7).

$$p_s = \frac{f\left(X_{ij} \rightarrow Y_c\right)}{\sum f\left(X_{ij} \rightarrow Y_c\right)} \qquad (7)$$

(7) is used to calculate the probability of selecting a CAR. The probability (p_s) of selecting a class rule increases with an increase in the fitness value of the CAR. Onlooker bees search for other CARs around the best one using neighborhood values (5). Scouts randomly search for the food source based on internal motivation. If the neighborhood value of the CAR is not improved after a fixed number of iterations i.e. stopping criteria, then the employed bee remove the CAR and become a scout. In the exploration process, local optima are searched by onlooker bees and in the exploitation process, local optima are evaluated by employed bees to find the global optima. Initial population and stopping criteria are two control parameters defined at the start of the algorithm. A number of onlooker and employed bees are considered in equal quantity and at each generation only one scout is going out to explore the search space. By comparing the food source positions, a new food source for the next iteration is determined. A greedy selection mechanism is used to decide the food source.

Feature Selection

Choosing promising features within a dataset for data modeling is difficult and needs more knowledge in the problem domain (Elisseeff & Guyon, 2003). Feature selection techniques are used to establish and remove extra, irrelevant and redundant attributes from the dataset which do not contribute to the classifier performance. Fewer attributes are desirable because it reduces the complexity of the classifier, and simpler to comprehend and elucidate. Feature selection is the process of choosing best attributes of the dataset that are most relevant to the predictive system. Feature selection methods are of two types, specifically, filter and wrapper. Filter methods select significant features based on their common characteristics towards the class label. With the help of the learning algorithm, wrapper methods choose significant features based on the performance of the classifier. Heuristic algorithms such as GA(Oluleye, Leisa, Leng, & Dean, 2014),PSO (Behjat, Mustapha, Nezamabadi-pour, Sulaiman, & Mustapha, 2013),ACO(Kanan, Faez, & Taheri, 2007) and ABC(Schiezaro & Pedrini, 2013) algorithms are used for feature selection to generate the most relevant subset of features by preserving the accuracy. In this work, filter based feature selection is performed as a pre-processing task prior to applying the ABC-AC algorithm. A T-test is a filter based approach which is employed to select the best features of the dataset (Yu & Liu, 2003). T-test computes t-score and p-value for each feature. Features having p-values higher than the user specified threshold are considered significant and they are used as predictors of the classification model.

METHODOLOGY

The proposed methodology incorporates three major phases such as the generation of Class Association Rules (CARs), rule evaluation, and ranking using Laplace accuracy and classification of the test tuple using the generated CARs. Similar to CPAR, ABC-AC is designed for binary class datasets. It needs input preprocessed dataset to be partitioned into a positive and negative set based on the class labels. In the first phase, with the help of minimum support, significant attribute values are selected to form an attribute subset. Using the attribute subset, all possible class association rules (CARs) are extracted using the ABC algorithm from the positive and negative sets separately. The rule based classifier is also built separately for the positive and negative sets. The second phase involves rule evaluation and ranking using Laplace accuracy to produce a reduced set of CARs. All the extracted rules are ordered and ranked using Laplace accuracy measure. Laplace accuracy is an error estimate measure used in FOIL, PRM, and CPAR to determine the significance of a CAR. In the final phase, k-best rules from each class/set that satisfies the given test tuple are selected. Average Laplace accuracy is calculated for each set and the class of the set having the highest value is assigned for the test tuple. Finally, the accuracy of the classifier is calculated by comparing the predicted and actual class labels. The activities involved in this methodology are outlined in the Figure 1.

Figure 1. Work flow of the proposed methodology

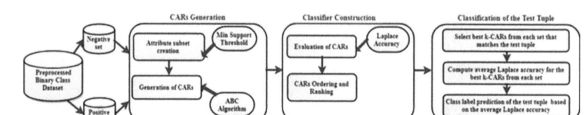

DATA PREPROCESSING

Health care datasets taken for experimentation need to be pre-processed as it consists of continuous valued attributes which cannot be directly taken for processing. Discretization is performed using Discretize filter in Weka 3.7. The missing values for nominal and numeric attributes in a dataset are also handled properly by substituting with its mode and mean values as per nature and attribute values. According to the requirement of the proposed methodology, the entire numeric attribute values are transformed into nominal attributes. Five health care datasets such as Breast cancer, Cleve, Heart, Hepatitis, and Pima are separately preprocessed using Weka 3.7 as per the requirements of the proposed methodology.

CARs GENERATION

The pre-processed dataset is taken as input for generating CARs. Based on the class label, the pre-processed dataset is partitioned into a positive and negative set. All the attributes except class attribute of the datasets are discretized for 10 levels of interval. These attributes have at most 10 discretized values which make the CAR generation process tiresome and time consuming. As an attempt, to simplify the rule generation process, the attribute subset is formed from the available set of attributes of the set and it is taken for the rule generation process, instead of taking all the attributes. An attribute subset is nothing but it contains a set of attribute values satisfying the user specified minimum support threshold. Using the attribute subset, 1-attribute CARs are generated. The fitness function of each CAR is calculated using the equation (1) and the neighborhood function is calculated using the equation (5) to determine the population for the next generation. This will get repeated until the terminating condition is met. The procedure involved in the generation of CARs using ABC is detailed in the following section.

ABC-AC Construction

Each 1-attribute CAR (i.e. food source) generated from the attribute subset is considered as the initial population. In every iteration, the quality of the food source is determined using fitness function (1). Actually, only a few CARs qualify the fitness function, but to generate more possible CARs in every iteration, neighborhood value is computed. The neighborhood value for each 1-attribute CARs i.e. food source is calculated using (5). In this work, Neighborhood_Threshold (NT) (6) is used to find the close-to-the-best CARs. Instead of choosing one CAR(i.e. food source) having the highest neighborhood value as the best source, CARs whose neighborhood values greater than equal to Neighborhood_Threshold (NT) is taken to next iteration as the best one. Thus, ABC-AC selects more than one CAR (food source) as close-to-the-best CARs using NT. The CARs having neighborhood value greater than or equal to NT are considered as close-to-the-best CARs. All the close-to-the-best CARs are shared with unemployed bees and further taken to form higher attributes CARs in the next iteration. i.e. 1-attribute CARs are taken to form 2-attributes CARs. This process is repeated until the stopping condition (i.e. maximum number of iteration) is met. Similarly, this procedure is repeated to generate all negative labeled CARs from the negative set.

CARs Evaluation and Ranking

Once the CARs are generated from positive and negative set, the error estimate of each CAR from the positive and negative set that matches the test tuple is calculated using (8). Based on the calculated Laplace values, CARs are arranged in the descending order.

$$Laplace\ Accuracy = \frac{(nc+1)}{(ntot+c)} \tag{8}$$

Where, 'c' represents the number of classes, '$ntot$' represents the total number of tuples satisfying class rule antecedent, 'nc' represents the total number of tuples satisfying both class rule antecedent and consequent.

Classification of the Test Tuple

The average Laplace accuracy of best k-matching rule from each set is calculated. The class/set having higher value is considered as the predicted class label of the given test tuple. Based on the predicted class, the actual class of the test tuple is compared to check whether ABC-AC is correctly classified or not. Evaluating a classifier is a major task in constructing a successful classifier model. The evaluation metrics help to discriminate the performance of the classifiers. Classification accuracy is one of the evaluation metrics commonly used to find the performance of the classification model (9). Table 1 explains the procedure of test tuple classification in detail. In this work, k is fixed as 5, i.e. the top 5 rules from each set that best match the test tuple are taken for classification.

$$Classification\ Accuracy = \frac{n_{correct}}{n_t} \tag{9}$$

Where '$n_{correct}$' is the number of correctly classified test tuples, 'n_t' is the total number of test tuples.

EXPERIMENTAL SETUP

The experiments are conducted using five health care datasets such as Breast cancer, Cleve, Heart, Hepatitis, Pima from the UCI machine learning repository. With respect to the class attribute, the pre-processed dataset is partitioned into a positive and negative set. To reduce the number of insignificant CARs and to generate significant ones, the attribute subset is formed using minimum support. As an initial step, attributes whose support value $>=$ the user specified minimum support (threshold) are taken as attribute subset and it is considered for the rule generation process. In this work, the minimum support threshold is set as 0.5. Using the attribute subset, all possible 1-attribute CARs are generated. The fitness and the neighborhood values are calculated for each generated 1-attribute CARs. For the varying values of NSR (i.e. 0.6 to 0.9), best 1-attribute CARs are selected to form the rule base for the next iteration. From the NSR value, NT is computed using (6). NT is used to find the close-to-the-best ones in

Table 1. Test tuple Classification

Test tuple classification:
Label: Predicted class label
$n_{correct}$: Number of correctly classified test tuple.
Input:

$T_{a_x \cup C_y}$ //Test tuple having attribute set 'a_x' and a class attribute 'C_y'

n_t //Number of test tuples
r_p //Set of positive class rules
r_n //Set of negative class rules
nr_p //Number of positive class rules
nr_n //Number of negative class rules
$Laplace_p$ //Laplace accuracy of positive class rules
$Laplace_n$ //Laplace accuracy of negative class rules
k //Top k CARs (i.e. $k=5$)from each set is taken for classification
Output: *Accuracy_per* // Classification accuracy in %
Method:
// Initialization of parameters
$k=0$
$Laplace_p =0$
$Laplace_n =0$
$n_{correct} =0$
for (i=1 to n_t)
for (j=1 to nr_p)

if ($a_x^{[T_i]} \subseteq Antecedent[r_{p^j}]$ & k<=5)

$Laplace_p$ += Laplace accuracy (r_{p^j})

$k+=1$
End if
End for
for (j=1 to nr_n)

if ($a_x^{[T_i]} \subseteq Antecedent[r_{n^j}]$] & k<=5)

$Laplace_n$ += Laplace accuracy (r_{n^j})

$k+=1$
End if
End for
if $Laplace_p >= Laplace_n$
$Label[T_i]= positive$
else
$Label[T_i]= negative$
End if

if $Predicted\_class[T_i] == c_y^{[T_i]}$)

$n_{correct} +=1$
End if
End for
*Accuracy_per = ($n_{correct} / n_t$)*100*

each iteration. Using the close-to-the-best ones, higher attribute CARs are generated. This procedure is repeated until it reaches the termination condition (i.e. maximum number of iteration=100). The above described procedure is performed for positive and negative set independently. When the test tuple is taken for classification, each generated CARs from both the positive and negative set is evaluated and ranked based on the Laplace accuracy (8). The best k-rules whose antecedent matches the test tuple are selected from both the set. In this work, k is set as 5, with respect to Laplace accuracy values, five top ranked matching CARs from each set are selected and their average Laplace accuracy of the set is computed. The class of the set having the highest average accuracy value is declared as the predicted class of the test tuple. Similarly, all the test tuples in the dataset are classified. At last, based on the number of correct test tuple classifications, the accuracy of the classifier is computed (9). Table 2 shows the accuracy of the ABC-AC obtained for five datasets with varying NSR values under 10-fold cross validation (10CV) and 50:50 test options.

Table 2. Accuracy (%) of the ABC-AC algorithm over five health care datasets

Dataset	Test options							
	10CV				50:50			
NSR	0.9	0.8	0.7	0.6	0.9	0.8	0.7	0.6
Breast Cancer	91.26	93.21	93.02	**94.25**	90.46	93.29	93.39	**94.25**
Cleve	79.08	**81.77**	81.50	75.57	80.76	**81.48**	80.22	78.06
Heart	77.32	**80.99**	76.31	72.07	82.12	**82.63**	80.52	75.64
Hepatitis	79.96	**86.04**	82.64	80.99	83.19	**83.89**	81.55	79.05
Pima	66.11	**66.55**	65.29	65.17	64.58	**68.97**	67.78	61.70
Average Accuracy(%)	78.75	**81.71**	79.75	77.61	80.22	**82.05**	80.69	77.74

From table 2, under two test options, it is inferred that for 0.8 NSR value, the ABC-AC algorithm yields good result in terms of classifier accuracy when compared to other NSR values. It is also identified that above mentioned NSR parameter setting (i.e. NSR=0.8) produce the highest accuracy for all datasets except Breast Cancer. On analyzing the factors, it is found that Breast Cancer has only 11 attributes with a class attribute. As the NSR is set high, the number of 1-attribute CARs generated from the 10 non-class attributes is less, which automatically reduces the number of higher attribute CARs in the next iteration. From the results, it is evident for the Breast Cancer dataset; the decrease of NSR value increases the classifier accuracy. Similarly, analyzing the performance of the ABC-AC classifier over the Cleve and Heart datasets, both has 14 attributes with one last class attribute produce roughly similar results under two test options for varying NSR values. Also, both the datasets produce good results for NSR=0.8 under two test options. A similar scenario appeared for the Hepatitis dataset having 20 attributes with a class attribute. ABC-AC classifier produces very poor accuracy for Pima when compared to other datasets. Even though, ABC-AC gives better accuracy for the NSR=0.8 value, it is unable to show a better result than it is obtained for other datasets. It is found that the Pima dataset has 29 attributes including a class attribute that maintains high dimensional attribute subset. The number of attributes considered for the rule generation process is high which leads to the generation of quite a lot of 1-attribute CARs thereby end up with messy and tedious CAR generation and ABC-AC classification. From the table 2, it is inferred that for NSR=0.8, the ABC-AC algorithm generates significant CARs. Thus classifiers built with significant CARs yield good results in terms classifier accuracy. Figures 2-5 represent the performance of the ABC-AC classifier for varying NSR values.

Consecutively, an effort is made to improve the performance of the ABC-AC classifier by performing feature selection using a T-test. T-test is a filter method commonly used to select the features having higher significance towards classification. Statistical T-test is performed to compute p-value and t-score for each attribute. Attributes with the p-value less than or equal to 0.05 are considered significant. The attributes which are less significant (i.e., greater than 0.05) are removed from the dataset.

From the table 3, it is inferred that for NSR=0.8, the ABC-AC using the T-test algorithm generates 1-attribute CARs with the top-ranked features. Under two test options, it is identified that for the NSR value=0.8, the ABC-AC algorithm with a reduced set of features produces good results in terms of classifier accuracy when compared to other NSR values. It is found that NSR=0.8 offers the highest accuracy for all datasets including Breast Cancer. On comparing with the performance of ABC-AC, it is found that ABC-AC with feature selection shows only considerable change in the classifier accuracy than ABC-AC without feature selection. Results prove that the classification model built over these datasets does not require any additional feature selection techniques to reduce the original set of features thereby retaining good ones.

Figure 2. Classifier Accuracy(%) of ABC-AC for NSR=0.9

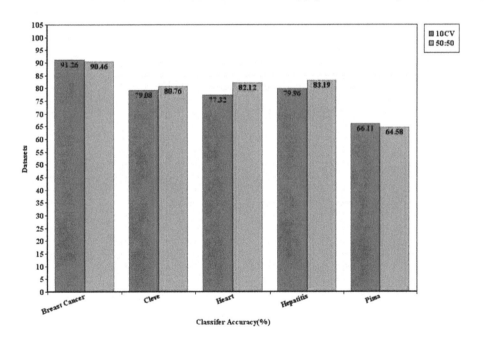

Performance of the ABC-AC in terms of Classifier Accuracy(%) under two test options for NSR=0.9

Figure 3. Classifier Accuracy(%) of ABC-AC for NSR=0.8

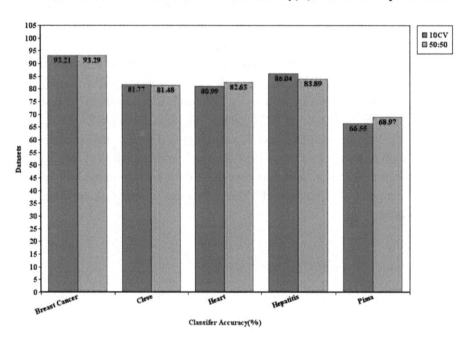

Figure 4. Classifier Accuracy(%) of ABC-AC for NSR=0.7

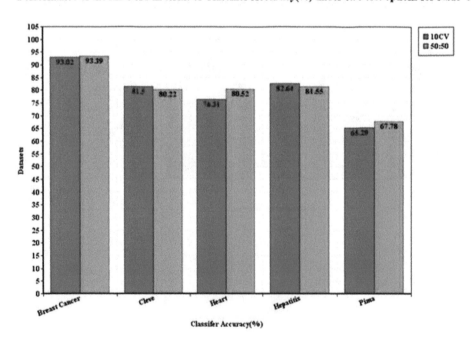

Figure 5. Classifier Accuracy(%) of ABC-AC for NSR=0.6

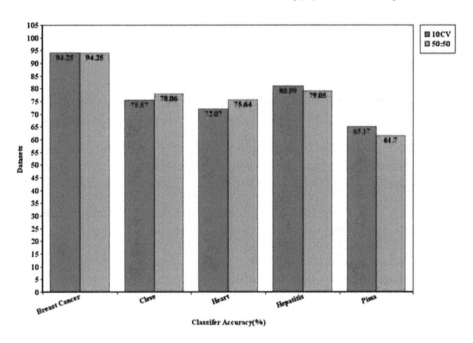

Table 3. Accuracy (%) of the ABC-AC algorithm over the attributes obtained using T-test

Dataset	Test options							
	10CV				50:50			
NSR	0.9	0.8	0.7	0.6	0.9	0.8	0.7	0.6
Breast Cancer	89.72	**94.4**	91.9	90.65	89.72	**93.39**	92.44	89.65
Cleve	78.09	**81.22**	74.46	76.72	76.51	**76.82**	76.3	71.28
Heart	78.86	**83.04**	78.68	77.87	77.32	**82.09**	77.48	73.18
Hepatitis	79.77	**81.58**	81.48	79.06	82.42	**80.69**	75.24	79.22
Pima	65.96	**68.4**	61.8	59.22	66.85	**70.18**	64.96	64.87
Average Accuracy(%)	78.48	**81.73**	78.16	59.22	78.56	**80.63**	77.39	64.87

CONCLUSION

Associative classification is one of the ubiquitous practices in data mining for commendable judgment. ABC-AC is the rule based classifier for the health care data diagnostic system implemented to generate eminent CARs for constructing an efficient classifier. The use of the ABC algorithm for CAR generation yields better accuracy for almost all datasets except Pima, a high dimensional dataset. To enhance the quality of the rule generation task and the classifier performance, feature selection techniques such as T-test is applied over five health care datasets to retain significant attributes by eliminating insignificant ones. From the results, it is evident that, ABC-AC with T-test does not achieve the classifier accuracy higher than ABC-AC. Use of feature selection shows the marginal change in the performance of the ABC-AC. In future other optimal feature selection techniques can be employed to improve the accuracy. Multi class datasets can also be focused in future.

REFERENCES

Agrawal, R., & Srikant, R. (1994). Fast Algorithms for Mining Association Rules. *Proc. of 20th International Conference on Very Large Data Bases,* 487–499. Retrieved from citeseer.ist.psu.edu/agrawal94fast.html

Behjat, A. R., Mustapha, A., Nezamabadi-pour, H., Sulaiman, M. N., & Mustapha, N. (2013). A PSO-Based Feature Subset Selection for Application of Spam /Non-spam Detection. *Communications in Computer and Information Science, 378 CCIS,* 183–193. doi:10.1007/978-3-642-40567-9_16

Elisseeff, A., & Guyon, I. (2003). An Introduction to Variable and Feature Selection. *Journal of Machine Learning Research,* 1157–1182. http://www.jmlr.org/papers/v3/guyon03a.html

Kanan, H. R., Faez, K., & Taheri, S. M. (2007). Feature selection using Ant Colony Optimization (ACO): A new method and comparative study in the application of face recognition system. Lecture Notes in Computer Science, 4597, 63–76. doi:10.1007/978-3-540-73435-2_6

Karaboga, D. (2005). An idea based on Honey Bee Swarm for Numerical Optimization. *Technical Report TR06, Erciyes University,* (TR06), 10.

Karaboga, D., & Basturk, B. (2007). A powerful and efficient algorithm for numerical function optimization: Artificial bee colony (ABC) algorithm. *Journal of Global Optimization, 39*(3), 459–471. doi:10.100710898-007-9149-x

Li, W., Han, J., & Pei, J. (2001). CMAR: Accurate and efficient classification based on multiple class-association rules. *Proceedings - IEEE International Conference on Data Mining, ICDM,* 369–376. 10.1109/icdm.2001.989541

Liu, B., Hsu, W., Ma, Y., & Ma, B. (1998). Integrating Classification and Association Rule Mining. *Data Mining and Knowledge Discovery,* 80–86.

Mangat, V., & Vig, R. (2014). Dynamic PSO-based associative classifier for medical datasets. *IETE Technical Review (Institution of Electronics and Telecommunication Engineers, India), 31*(4), 258–265. doi:10.1080/02564602.2014.942237

Nandhini, M., Rajalakshmi, M., & Sivanandam, S. N. (2017). Experimental and statistical analysis on the performance of firefly based predictive association rule classifier for health care data diagnosis. *Control Engineering and Applied Informatics, 19*(2), 101–110.

Nandhini, M., & Sivanandam, S. N. (2015). An improved predictive association rule based classifier using gain ratio and T-test for health care data diagnosis. *Sadhana - Academy Proceedings in Engineering Sciences, 40*(6), 1683–1699. doi:10.100712046-015-0410-6

Oluleye, B., Leisa, A., Leng, J., & Dean, D. (2014). A Genetic Algorithm-Based Feature Selection. *International Journal of Electronics Communication and Computer Engineering, 5*(4), 899–905.

Pham, D. T., & Karaboga, D. (2000). Intelligent Optimisation Techniques. Intelligent Optimisation Techniques. doi:10.1007/978-1-4471-0721-7

Quinlan, J. R., & Cameron-Jones, R. M. (1993). FOIL: A midterm report. Lecture Notes in Computer Science, 667, 3–20. doi:10.1007/3-540-56602-3_124

Schiezaro, M., & Pedrini, H. (2013). Data feature selection based on Artificial Bee Colony algorithm. *EURASIP Journal on Image and Video Processing, 2013*(1). doi:10.1186/1687-5281-2013-47

Shahzad, W., & Baig, A. R. (2011). Hybrid associative classification algorithm using ant colony optimization. *International Journal of Innovative Computing, Information, & Control, 7*(12), 6815–6826.

Thabtah, F. A., Cowling, P., & Peng, Y. (2004). MMAC: A new multi-class, multi-label associative classification approach. *Proceedings - Fourth IEEE International Conference on Data Mining, ICDM 2004*, 217–224. 10.1109/ICDM.2004.10117

Yin, X., & Han, J. (2003). *CPAR: Classification based on Predictive Association Rules*. doi:10.1137/1.9781611972733.40

Yu, L., & Liu, H. (2003). Feature Selection for High-Dimensional Data: A Fast Correlation-Based Filter Solution. *Proceedings, Twentieth International Conference on Machine Learning, 2*, 856–863. https://www.aaai.org/Papers/ICML/2003/ICML03-111.pdf

Chapter 13
Artificial Intelligence Approaches to Detect Neurodegenerative Disease From Medical Records:
A Perspective

Abhranil Gupta

Auctus Solutions, India

ABSTRACT

This chapter gives a brief overview of the state of the art of machine learning approaches in detection of the neurodegenerative disease from medical records (brain scans, etc.). It starts with an understanding of the sub-field of artificial intelligence, machine learning, then goes to understand neurodegenerative disease, with a focus on four major diseases and then goes on to giving an overview of how such diseases are detected using machine learning. In the end, it discusses the future areas of research that needs to be done in order to improve the field of research.

BACKGROUND

The application of artificial intelligence in the diagnosis of the disease is not at all new. But what is new is the approach that has been and is being regularly updated to be taken. The technologies that are taken like support vector machine and other technologies are of interest here. Basically these technologies are used to speed up the diagnosis process that is evident from the usage in the technologies and also remove the error in the process of diagnosis.

DOI: 10.4018/978-1-7998-2742-9.ch013

INTRODUCTION

Neurodegenerative disease is a condition of the humans where the Neurons or the brain cells are affected and hence the patient gets many kinds of symptoms like shaking, tremble etc. This condition is generally progressive in nature and is a disease of no perfect cure. This is the reason why

Introduction of Artificial Intelligence

A question that intrigued many philosophers and mathematicians alike is the fact that whether there is a mathematical description of what we call as learning and can that mathematical description be developed into a method which can be programmed in computer so that the computers can also think. We have tread a long way from the philosophical angle of computational machines that can think to what we call today as machine learning. Machine learning a part of artificial intelligence is the method by which the machines can also think in limited ways. To be able to make the computer learn and also think we have to take a multi-disciplinary way of thinking to be able to develop algorithms which can be converted into computer programs so that the machines can think Jordan, m. I., & Mitchell, t. M. (2015). Mathematical processes of learning is lying at the intersection of statistics, mathematics and computer technology. It is this multi-disciplinary approach that makes it possible for the computers to think in the ways that humans do but in limited domains. This field of research has a very unique and specific questions which it intends to answer:

1. Can we develop algorithms that it will make the computer think and reason?
2. How do humans reason and think?
3. Does the processes of human reason and thinking follow some specific laws which can be developed and denoted by mathematics?

These questions are rather philosophical than scientific one. To answer this questions we have to think in ways which is different from what people think about machine learning. The simple answer to this question lies in the fact that human thinking can be mathematically representable and be turned into a computer program so that it is possible for the computers to reason and think Murphy, k. P. (2012); Hastie, t., et al. (2005). Methods of artificial intelligence and machine learning are unique in nature in that they inculcate the various mathematical and statistical methods to learn but are also similar to how humans learn. Artificial intelligence and machine learning tries to emulate the way humans learn and it also so it's exceeds in doing it by the computational power in the speed of doing it. Most of the problems of artificial intelligence and its subset machine intelligence or what we called as machine learning is classification and regression. It is a requirement for the machine learning to classify the input data into various classes so that it may then worked upon the various classes of data so that it be able to make decisions and augmented for the human to make decisions. Mainly the methods of artificial intelligence is of finding the optimum solution to a problem devised by the humans for diverse requirements. This is a type of solution to a problem call the functional approximation. The accuracy of the functional approximation problem is to be increased by the learning that the machine is going through by online methods, reinforcement methods or other methods of machine learning. Machine learning which is a subset of artificial intelligence tries to emulate the problem into different classes of data and then trying to find out the one dimensional or multidimensional answer to the multi class data thus produced.

Talking about the starting of machine intelligence or artificial intelligence it started with Alan Turing work on whether the machines can think. The great Alan Turing also devised a test called the Turing test for building and actual thinking machine which can do all the reasoning the humans can solely depending upon the mathematical and other methods used in machine learning.

Methods of Artificial Intelligence

Although there are many methods of artificial intelligence we overhear restrict ourselves to some of them which are of interest in cad. Cad or computer aided diagnostics is a new field of research which tries to diagnose problems of medical importance why are computer learning methods like machine learning and others. The main issue in computer aided diagnostics is to further the methods of artificial intelligence and tailor it for the usage of medical purposes. The artificial intelligence techniques in use today are dependent upon the scientific breakthroughs in the fields of biology, science, mathematics and statistics. Mostly the methods of artificial intelligence are:

1. Ant colony optimization
2. Immune algorithm
3. Decision tree
4. Fuzzy algorithm
5. Particle swarm algorithm
6. Neural networks
7. Deep learning

Although all of them are not used in artificial intelligence algorithms many of them are of use in in AI algorithms, machine learning etc.

Ant Colony

Ant colony optimization or ant colony algorithm is a method of solving computationally complex problems where in finding the best route or path is very important in solving the problem. Examples of such problems are vehicle routing problem, travelling salesman problem and search problems where routing is an important part. Here the solution is to find out the best part available which not only decreases the cost but also increases the profit by the way a of determining the best path possible. This is a pheromone-based multi agent Probabilistic algorithm that uses artificial ants which can be considered as the multi agents to determine the best possible that the computational problem that is given. Basically this emulates the pheromone-based Communication of ants that is evident in the real life to determine optimum solution for the problem. The ants are experts in finding the best path for their foods and the method they use to do so is used here to determine the optimum path. The best way to the resources are communicated to the ants by a chemical laid down by other ants while exploring the surface. This exploration and communication of the resource of the ants are simulated in this type of algorithm. The algorithm not only communicates the candidate solution to other ants (simulated) but also the accuracy of the problem's solution is also remembered in the case. This way the best possible paths are found Parsons, S. (2005). In the animal world the ant's choice of choosing the path to the resource of their need is completely random. Let us suppose that there are two paths to the resource from the ant hill. There is a short path and there is a long path. The choice a particular ant upon which path it will take is entirely random. But it is also true that the short path that some ants take not only move the resource quickly to the ant hill but also travel more number of times. We can show that a simulated ant colony problem where the left part is the state from which the simulated ants start and the rightmost part is from where the ants learn about the fastest path. This algorithm was first proposed by Marco Dorigo in his PhD thesis where he not only articulated the full method of the ant colony optimization technique but also developed the simulated ant colony algorithm Dorigo, M. (1992). This methodology is since then diversified into many domains and solve a wider class of problems than was originally conceived by Dorigo. The cornerstone of the problem and its solution which was laid by Dorigo was that any optimization problem that is required to be solved by finding the best route can be solved by this method.

Fuzzy Algorithm

The main theory of the Boolean logic is that the truth value of any statement can be either true or false, either 0 or 1. In contrast, in the real life the statements cannot be said as entirely true or entirely false. This is the case of the fuzzy logic. The fuzzy logic can process and define statements that have partial truth values. This is fundamental of the fuzzy logic and any algorithm developed around it. In was introduced in its current form by Lofti Zadeh in the year 1965, Zadeh, L. A. (1965). The theory similar in nature called the infinite valued logic was studied by mathematicians as early as 1920's Jeffry, F. (2000). This logic is entirely based upon the observation that in real life the decisions are taken and observations are made in the imprecise fashion. In situations of reality we can show how imprecise information can lead to correct decisions but at some time precise information's turns up into catastrophic failures in decisions.

Overview of Learning Techniques

Although the above are a few examples of machine learning and Artificial Intelligence the main categories of the machine learning algorithms are

1. Supervised Learning
2. Semi supervised Learning
3. Reinforcement Learning
4. Online Learning

As the name of each of the categories suggest the main differentiating factor of these types of learning comes in the case of the mechanism by which it learns. The Supervises learning is done under the supervision of the Human operator, similarly semi supervised are the one where the learning is partially supervised. Reinforcement learning is an altogether different approach of learning where there is a method of rewards for learning correctly and the machine agents are programmed to maximize such rewards. The last one online learning is the way to learn when there is uncertain learning environment. Online learning of machine algorithms also helps the algorithm to learn about the existing knowledge coded in the software. Online learning is very important in the light of the new researches that is coming up in developing Computer aided Diagnostics and also in developing treatments for the diseases bye researches in medical fraternity. New treatments coming from the medical researchers takes a time like to come into the clinic due to the ignorance of the medical professionals and the medical researchers work. This type of medical IOT is of immense importance to reduce the time between the new treatments and coming from the medical researchers to the clinic. The day is not for away when everything from Diagnostics to new treatment to monitoring and prediction of the medical condition will be connected to one grid from which everybody can benefit. This is beneficial not only for the medical researchers and medical professionals but also for the patients who are the most important part of this whole new technology.

Learning via machines and computer aided diagnosis is the way forward in this time. We can make the machines learn and also uses its power of fast processing with high accuracy to our advantage in the diagnosis. This chapter deals with the diagnosis of the neurodegenerative disease using machine learning algorithm. The field of research is very important since early diagnosis of these types of disease will enable the patients and doctors to better manage the disease and also slow down the process of neuro-degeneration. From gait analysis to biomarker signals to bio-signals the research on the diagnosis of the neurodegenerative disease has come a long way but the important thing here that needs to mention is that the field of research has not reached saturation as of date. It is tried here to document the state of the art and also discuss some directions of research that may be useful in the coming years.

Overview of the Neurodegenerative Disease

The most important of the disease that is given here is

1. Alzheimer's Disease
2. Parkinson's Disease
3. Huntington's Disease
4. Amyotrophic Lateral Sclerosis Disease

These are the main four most important disease that causes serious damage in the life's of the patients.

Alzheimer's Disease

A serious decapitating disease that lets the person with cognitive, memory and other decline was first observed and described by Dr. Alois Alzheimer who was a German psychiatrist. This led to many observations and other features like hallucinations are later observed. Alzheimer disease is a neurological disorder that progresses with age and kills the brains cells which unfortunately cannot be recovered. This progressive disorder has no cure as of yet but there are researches which are still on to how to suppress and finally cure the disease. Alzheimer disease is also characterized by atrophy of the brain in very important center of the brain for learning and memory formation as can be seen in scans of patients. The atrophy of the brain (atrophy means shrinking) is not only limited to the domains of the hippocampus but is also observed in other areas of the brain. The most of the losses in such as the dendritic and the neuronal losses of the brain tissue. This loss as predicted by the volumetric scan of MRI is also been shown to be true in the autopsy neural counts. This progressive disease is also varies in its expression from patient to patient and also in inter regional basis in the same patient.

Parkinson's Disease

The disease is characterized by the motor dysfunction and other non-motor dysfunctions. The neurodegenerative disease also has other features that distinguish it into a neurodegenerative disease that affects the patient and his/her family. The term "parkinsonism" refers to a complex of disease symptoms. The symptoms are, but not limited to, resting tremor, bradykinesia, and muscular rigidity. The disease is often confused with diseases similar to it in features but are very different in pathological and other aspects. The motor aspect of the disease makes it a candidate to gait analysis.

Huntington Disease

What is known today as Huntington's disease or Huntington's chorea was not known until the lecture by George Huntington in the year 1872. This neurodegenerative disease like others has the characteristics of dementia and other effects like choreatic movements and other behavioral and other Psychiatric disturbance. This is a genetic disorder with the disease being transmitted from generation to generation P. J. Vinken and G. W. Bruyn 1968. Basically the symptoms of the disease is very varied and it affects the motor and cognitive domain with other psychiatric disturbance too. Other symptoms include, which are not very prevalent are weight loss (unwarranted), and circadian rhythm disturbance among others.

Amyotrophic Lateral Sclerosis

Amyotrophic lateral sclerosis is one of the most common neurodegenerative disease along with Parkinson's and Alzheimer's. This is the progressing disease that affects the motor neurons and leaves the patient in the vegetative state. This affects other areas of the brain but the motor neurons are the most affected. The disease progresses very rapidly with 50% of the disease dying within 3 years of onset Mitchell, J. D., & Borasio, G. D. (2007). The mechanism of the disease is poorly understood although there are many hypothesis proposed by researchers in the field Mitchell, J. D. (1987), Armon, C. (2003). Exotoxicity is the process by which some of the nerumodulators become toxic. These exotoxins cause neuronal death. However there are many other processes maybe involved but these are poorly understood.

The chapter here concentrates on the four main neurodegenerative disease like the ones listed and short descriptions given. These are the main disturbing disease that cause harm in the society. There are many other neurological disorders but these are the main disease that we are concentrating upon in this chapter. It is tried in this chapter to develop a framework, which if used can help save millions of lives in our society. The proposed framework could be an IOT (internet of things) based methodology in the global scale will not only help in the CAD (computer aided diagnostics) but also be of help to the doctors and other medical professionals who treat and give care to the patients of disorders like those mentioned and others. It is also tried to

1. Overview of the different methods of diagnosis of the disease like Neurodegenerative and others
2. Help in the treatment of the patients
3. Expert advice from expert medical professionals
4. Automated disease diagnosis and prediction of other features based upon the diagnosis

Machine Learning Used in Neurodegenerative Disease Diagnosis

Machine learning is a methodology using the concepts of Artificial Intelligence with its roots of in Artificial Intelligence. Artificial intelligence technique based machine learning and deep learning used as tool to diagnosis of the neurodegenerative disease or for that matter any other disease is better in one sense that it is fast and bias free. The other part of the diagnosis of the disease is that machine learning can produce results that are false positive. False positive is that the disease is not there but the program produces a result that there is disease. This types of errors cannot be totally eradicated from the machine learning algorithms as such errors are inherent to the algorithm. This is the reason why there is a requirement of human in the loop of the diagnosis of the disease. Although the humans (medical experts in this case) will have the final say in the diagnosis of the disease the machine learning code can only augment the decision making process and also expedite the process of diagnosis.

The machine learning algorithm can also improve itself and learn by its own from the experience it gathers from diagnosis decisions of the medical professionals. This way it may be of help to the common people who can expect a reasonably good predictor that the disease is present or not by using such medical diagnosis machine learning algorithm. These algorithms can be used for prediction purposes also. From the baseline scan or report of a patient and with the help of advance machine learning techniques we can predict the degradation of patients condition. This can be of help to the medical professionals too who can manage their treatment according to the prediction so made by the machine learning algorithm.

One of the methods of detecting neurodegenerative disorder is the gait analysis. The human gait is particularly affected in the presence of the neurodegenerative disease. The machine learning algorithms are also useful determining the medical test required and also improving upon the specification of the test learning from past experience. The main thing that is required is the data and the correct diagnosis to make the machine learn on its

Foremost importance of diagnosis with the help of computer and machine learning techniques in neurodegenerative diseases is the gathering of data and the early diagnosis of neurodegenerative diseases. The reason being very send these diseases are not curable as of yet and it can only restricted to some amount if the diagnosis is done early. This is the reason why machine learning techniques can be of help. Usage of machine learning techniques for diagnosis of neurodegenerative diseases is helpful in two records firstly it is very fast and secondly it is an augmentation of the diagnosis decision by medical professionals. The most important of all is data gathering. Data that is gathered from medical diagnosis records can be uploaded to a computer which then will be processed by a machine learning algorithm for learning processes or diagnosis of the disease. Flowchart is developed that will help in the formation of machine learning algorithms which will be of help for medical diagnostics. Here in the flowchart we can see that data gathering is at the top which is of foremost importance in machine learning algorithms. After the data is gathered a new patient data is to be uploaded into the machine learning algorithm for diagnostics and then and the diagnosis by the machine learning algorithm is to be done which will be rechecked by the medical professional whose decision is augmented by the machine learning algorithm and then the post processed data will be e again used for or relearning of the machine learning algorithm. The machine learning algorithm is developed to learn and relearn so that the accuracy of the algorithm increases and it helps medical professional more aptly for diagnosing medical situations correctly and in short time.

The System

Machine learning algorithms can not only be used for diagnosis of medical situations from pathological reports but also images of the brain can be used for diagnosis and prediction of disease degradation buy predictive analytics of machine learning. The most important of the machine learning algorithm usage for or brain diseases or other diseases is that the machine learning algorithm can use a large amount of data from which it can determine the reason behind that the disease and also it can do it very swiftly. The other reason why medical machine learning algorithms are used is that it can represent the knowledge of many medical expert professionals which can then be of help for the medical professionals and the patients alike. Algorithms of machine learning using image analysis can be of help for or diagnosis and predicting the amount of degradation of brain tissue in neurodegenerative diseases. There is no specific biological test for diseases like age related neurodegenerative diseases apart from the specific clinical features of the diseases which can only be recognized and diagnosed by careful examination of the medical records and break scans. This can be e a game changer if a medical diagnostics records be used in in development of machine learning algorithms which can accurately and very specifically zero into the specific features of the image of the brain scan which can then be used for diagnosis of the specific disease of patient Mckhann et al. 2011. This can be exemplified by the disease of age-related Alzheimer's there is impairment in the cognitive domain and also has other features like spatial disorientation and other such features Mckhann et al. 2011.

The data gathered and the diagnosis made can be used for disease modelling and helpful in finding out the reasons of the disease and also the cure of the disease via computational methods. The present approach of artificial intelligence based diagnosis on machine learning based diagnosis to the specific is to find out the specific features in the brain scan or the pathological report does received and try to collate it with the disease with which it is similar to the most.

Machine learning is used for diagnosis of neurodegenerative diseases like Parkinson's via pathological reports, brain scans and also via different methods and modalities of detecting the disease from handwritten notes to gait analysis. Handwritten notes and dynamic and static both has been used for the analysis for diseases like Parkinson's and Alzheimer's. The ink traces of the handwritten notes are used for checking and observation of tremble associated with many diseases like Parkinson's and Alzheimer's. The shaking of hands and the tremble are associated with diseases like Parkinson's due to the motor neurons are diseased and killed because of the disease Rosenblum, S et al. 2013. Some researchers have also tried to select the disease from healthy counterparts by enabling them to retrace pictures and spatial recognition tasks which are of utmost importance in recognizing diseases like Parkinson's and Alzheimer's Pereira, C. R et al 2016. Other diseases like that of amyotrophic lateral sclerosis and Huntington's disease do also show some kind of motor disease or motor neuron degeneration while the progression of the disease. All of these diseases has a specific feature and characteristic from which it can be recognized from other diseases. These specific feature can be extracted via machine learning techniques from drawings to brain scans and from pathological reports to human gait analysis.

In the Clinical Settings there is a huge amount of research that shows volumetric analysis of brain can be more useful for detection of diseases like Parkinson's and Alzheimer's multiple sclerosis and also brain lesion studies. Although the research indicates this to be e one of the major game changes in the detection of diseases like Parkinson's this is really done in clinical settings. The reason behind this is very simple, it requires trained personal and close inspection of the brain scans to actually detect the disease and what kind of disease the patient is having. In this regard machine learning software can be of great help. The software's scrutiny of the brain scans and detection of smallest of the deviations of brain tissue in areas of interest can actually be e helpful in detecting diseases early in their setting. This type of software's, machine learning algorithms, not only uses the image analysis as their primary tool but also uses other features of machine learning to detect the disease and also monitor the disease that can have effect in the patient. As discussed earlier machine learning algorithms can also be used for the help of the medical professional to predict if the disease can happen and also to predict the degeneration of the disease after their setting of the disease early Pohl, K. M. Et al, 2011; Chow, D. S. Et al, 2014.

Software's like Braim can be developed on the lines of machine learning and other technique to develop robust volumetric analysis of the brain from which we can infer the disease and also monitor the brain lesions in a patient for tumors that is occurring in the brain which is very slow in their growth. The slow growth tumors are also deadly for a particular person because of their position in the brain and also the pathology of it. To correctly detect the pathology of the brain tumor if first need to detect the position of it. This can be of help to the pathologists who can then use that information of the position of the tumor to do the tests required to detect type of the tumor. If such tumors and legends can be detected early on in the onset of it can in effect be helpful for the patient and the doctors for making the surgery for carrying out any other medical treatment for that particular disease. The Braim Software can be of help to the medical professionals due to its semi-automated and also automated feature which lets it segregate the brain scan MRI in two different regions of interest and also detect the pathology of the brain relation from its featured database it has about the brain Pathology. In this software we can also inculcate many features like pathology of the brain relation, pathology of other diseases like multiple sclerosis and Parkinson's and Alzheimer's with the help of which it can detect in a semi-automated or automated fashion the disease while the brain scan is ongoing.

In the research where the gait analysis is used it can be of help to use where we can use the data off of how the person walk, work or does anything in there day to day life can be of use to determine the disease very early e in its onset. Researches are still on with use of support vector machine, quadratic Bayesian classifier, quadratic normal Bayesian classifier, neural networks and other such approaches of machine learning to detect the disease from the day to day life chores. Support vector machine or neural network are all types of machine learning which are used for classification and the data presented to it. Here we try to develop not only classification methods but also using the data acquired from classification we can develop methods by which we can predict the degradation or improvement of disease due to certain types of medical treatment that is being given to the patient. This type of machine learning algorithms are not new. Research is still on and it continues to be a field of high importance since medical Diagnostics and computer-aided medical Diagnostics are the most important things that can be used today. Computer aided medical Diagnostics and the usage of it can be of great help to not only predict and detect the disease but also help in the research of how the disease is progressing in the patient and which type of medicines are making important progress in the patient. Machine learning algorithms in aid to Computer aided Diagnostics can help model diseases and model the response a particular medicine or a treatment is having on the disease of the patient. Here we try to develop a Framework more in the lines of internet of things in medical diagnostics where medical professionals, diagnostic centers, caregivers, machine learning experts and most importantly the patient can have a common platform where they can improve upon the disease and its treatment in a worldwide basis. Internet of things is making Rapid progress in many fields like manufacturing, supply chain etc. And it is also tried here to develop and platform internet of things can help the medical Diagnostics and medical profession in general. It is utmost importance we take help of Internet and internet of things to develop Technologies that will help medical profession in a positive manner.

To give a brief about the internet of things it is like the Internet of everything is connected to a specific kind of a cloud where all stakeholders are given importance according to their level of work and data can be shared and downloaded according to the importance of the person. All the data can be shared from anywhere and everywhere the question of data security and privacy comes into being. Here the sensors and other types of Data generating devices are all connected to a single network which transfer the data from the sensors and other data generating devices to the cloud and also transfers it to the stakeholders subscribe to it Zanella, A., et al, 2014.The applicability of such methods is huge as there are many features of the internet of things that can be of help to the patient and the medical professionals alike. The researches of the field can also take the help of this medical internet of things if we can say so to develop new methods and also model neurodegenerative diseases. The findings of the research can also be updated to this medical internet of things which can then be used by the medical professionals and the medical Diagnostics alike for the benefit of the patient. Where we try to develop a methodology as discussed earlier where the researcher medical professionals' patients and diagnostic centers can work coherently to develop new methodologies of treatment and classify the patients into groups according to the disease of the patient. This medical internet of things in a worldwide basis is the need of the hour.

The Framework proposed here is in the lines of the Framework that is being developed in the medical internet of things where the cloud will be automated on the full scale from Medical Diagnostics to the reporting of the disease to the treatment of it. This medical internet of things can be of help to the researchers who would like to model the medical condition of the patient who would then be available for new kinds of medicine which will be developed in the lines of the patient condition. The huge amount of data that will be gathered from this medical internet of things will be available and can be used for data mining to actually pinpoint the disease and from where the disease is emanating. This is also going to be helpful for the new or kinds of treatment that is coming up which can be simulated in the computer using the patient data so that the amount of time required for the treatment can be curtailed by a fraction.

In effect what we're trying to do via machine learning algorithms is to detect the neurodegenerative diseases and the specific of it from the symptoms that is available to ask and from the biological and pathological reports that that can be used for the diagnosis of the medical condition. Such software can be used scan through the Medical reports and other pathological reports to detect the medical condition which will otherwise have to be e done by the medical doctors who has to pinpoint the disease from the their experience and made take a little bit more time than the medical software. The medical software can augment the decision making process of the medical doctors and diagnostic centers by accurately and rapidly showing the relevant information to the medical professional. Machine learning algorithms and machine learning experts can also be of help developing new algorithms aid the process of medical diagnosis.

RESULTS

In general the diagnosis is a hypothetico – deductive process. In this process first a few observations are made and then based upon such observations some hypothesis is done. After the formation of the hypothesis new data is to be collected in accordance to the hypothesis made. In the light of the new data deductions are made. The deductions either gives a clear diagnosis or new hypothesis is created for be able to acquire more data for further investigation. In this regard many classical or advanced machine learning techniques can be used for diagnosis. The framework that is proposed here is to create a platform that takes in the data from the medical records to give a possible diagnosis of the disease. The platform so developed can be useful tool to the medical professional at an international level. The doctors from anywhere in the world can in effect use its benefits. The data acquired and the results obtained from the doctors can be stored in the cloud. This cloud based system will be accessible to other doctors. This will fasten the diagnosis process helping the medical and society at large. Many types of machine learning techniques like SVM (support vector Machine), or any other classifier can used to develop such a system.

The method of medical diagnosis via machine learning and other algorithms is very simple. First the data is gathered from the different sources like the Diagnosis Centre, the pathology center, the brain scans and the expert Advices from the doctor about the clinical observations that is made by the doctor which can aid in the process of diagnosis. The process of diagnosis from Medical scans is done by data acquisition methods followed by image preprocessing followed by feature extraction and feature classification. By this method the images of the brain scans are used to you first preprocess the medical scan from the noise in the image and then from the noise free image the feature extraction and feature classification is done. The feature extraction is done by the image analysis techniques of machine learning and feature classification is done by the machine learning classification algorithms with the help of the data required and stored in the software about the various features of a medical condition Singh, G et al, 2016. Even after such processes there can be false positive result can occur because of it a medical professional must be kept in the loop to actually decide whether the decisions taken by the machine learning algorithm is entirely correct or not. It is widely recognized that then size of each person is unique in nature with the uniqueness of different parts of the brain is also present. To standardize such of the brain sizes and the brain regions a different approach is taken to standardize it. After standardization only voxel based volumetric method is used to determine the volume of each of the regions of interest. It is only after this can there be test whether the person is having a medical condition or not. The total process of image preprocessing data acquisition and others are done in a very Swift manner by the machine learning algorithm of the computer. This this swiftness of working is helpful in trying to determine the medical condition fast and reliably so that the person can be treated early in the condition. The type of medical conditions determined by this type of software's are not A type of condition that can be e cured completely as of yet. This is the reason why and early diagnosis of the disease is very important.

DISCUSSION

There are many types of conditions in neurodegenerative diseases. We are concerned with only a few of them in this chapter. We tried to you elaborate upon the methods of new machine learning and also tried to show that a medical internet of things can be of immense help to the patients' caregivers and medical professionals. Such medical internet of things are coming up very fast. In this chapter we have given an overview about how this kind of things are coming up and how the diseases are recognized and pinpointed via Computer aided diagnostics. Although the field is very new but the field has immense strength of growth and also is not saturated. This makes the field very important for research of medical professionals and in machine algorithm researchers alike.

The aim in the chapter was to give up common platform for the medical professionals, diagnostic centers, machine learning algorithm professionals and the most importantly the patients. It is tried here to give the most up-to-date information about Computer aided Diagnostics and machine learning which is available in the market today. In the way forward it is an immense importance that all the searches from the field collaborate and Co create such kind of an ecosystem from which the medical professionals can take the help of the technology developed today to aid in the care of the patient. The type of neurodegenerative diseases discussed here are not curable and it is hence important to diagnose the medical condition as fast as possible and also manage the condition to the optimum so that the patient can be given the optimum care.

It is tried here to give an overview of the different methods of machine learning that is used to determine the diagnosis of the disease and the medical condition of the patient. Although this is the aim to do but an exhaustive list of all methods are not possible in this small chapter. It is tried here to give a glimpse of how the machine learning algorithms are used for medical diagnosis, what are the machine learning algorithms that are used and the basics of machine learning algorithms. Automation of the process of diagnosis is also a challenge to meet in the future. To meet the challenge and to mitigate the amount of time required to diagnose the neurodegenerative disease and classify it is tried to build a framework with the help of which this can be done. It is also tried here to explain how to use machine learning algorithms and let the doctors make use of it so that the patient care is at the optimum. The huge time lag between the diagnosis and the treatment of the disease has to come down so as to give optimum level of care to the patient. In this regard machine learning algorithms and other automated process which have been discussed can be of help. The most important of the all is the expert advice of the doctors who are kept in the loop of the Computer aided Diagnostics so that not only the machine learning can relearn about the condition of the patient but also the accuracy of the machine learning can be improved considerably.

It is tried with utmost sincerity to give the most relevant and latest information about medical professions and Machine learning algorithms. However it is important to note that a total exhaustive list of information about the Framework is not possible in a single chapter.

REFERENCES

Armon, C. (2003). An evidence-based medicine approach to the evaluation of the role of exogenous risk factors in sporadic amyotrophic lateral sclerosis. *Neuroepidemiology*, 22(4), 217–228. doi:10.1159/000070562 PMID:12792141

Chow, D. S., Qi, J., Guo, X., Miloushev, V. Z., Iwamoto, F. M., Bruce, J. N., Lassman, A. B., Schwartz, L. H., Lignelli, A., Zhao, B., & Filippi, C. G. (2014). Semiautomated volumetric measurement on post-contrast MR imaging for analysis of recurrent and residual disease in glioblastoma multiforme. *AJNR. American Journal of Neuroradiology*, 35(3), 498–503. doi:10.3174/ajnr.A3724 PMID:23988756

Dimitrov, D. V. (2016). Medical internet of things and big data in healthcare. *Healthcare Informatics Research*, 22(3), 156–163. doi:10.4258/hir.2016.22.3.156 PMID:27525156

Dorigo, M. (1992). *Optimization, learning and natural algorithms* (PhD Thesis). Politecnico di Milano.

Hastie, T., Tibshirani, R., Friedman, J., & Franklin, J. (2005). The elements of statistical learning: Data mining, inference and prediction. *The Mathematical Intelligencer*, 27(2), 83–85. doi:10.1007/BF02985802

Iram, S. (2014). *Early Detection of Neurodegenerative Diseases from Bio-Signals: A Machine Learning Approach* (Doctoral dissertation). Liverpool John Moores University.

Jeffry, F. (2000). Review of Metamathematics of fuzzy logics. *The Bulletin of Symbolic Logic*, 6(3), 342–346.

Johnson, K. A., Fox, N. C., Sperling, R. A., & Klunk, W. E. (2012). Brain imaging in Alzheimer disease. *Cold Spring Harbor Perspectives in Medicine*, 2(4), a006213. doi:10.1101/cshperspect.a006213 PMID:22474610

Jordan, M. I., & Mitchell, T. M. (2015). Machine learning: Trends, perspectives, and prospects. *Science*, 349(6245), 255–260. doi:10.1126cience.aaa8415 PMID:26185243

McKhann, G. M., Knopman, D. S., Chertkow, H., Hyman, B. T., Jack, C. R. Jr, Kawas, C. H., Klunk, W. E., Koroshetz, W. J., Manly, J. J., Mayeux, R., Mohs, R. C., Morris, J. C., Rossor, M. N., Scheltens, P., Carrillo, M. C., Thies, B., Weintraub, S., & Phelps, C. H. (2011). The diagnosis of dementia due to Alzheimer's disease: Recommendations from the National Institute on Aging-Alzheimer's Association workgroups on diagnostic guidelines for Alzheimer's disease. *Alzheimer's & Dementia*, 7(3), 263–269. doi:10.1016/j.jalz.2011.03.005 PMID:21514250

Mitchell, J. D. (1987). Heavy metals and trace elements in amyotrophic lateral sclerosis. *Neurologic Clinics*, 5(1), 43–60. doi:10.1016/S0733-8619(18)30934-4 PMID:3550416

Mitchell, J. D., & Borasio, G. D. (2007). Amyotrophic lateral sclerosis. *Lancet*, 369(9578), 2031–2041. doi:10.1016/S0140-6736(07)60944-1 PMID:17574095

Murphy, K. P. (2012). *Machine learning: a probabilistic perspective*. MIT Press.

Parsons, S. (2005). Ant Colony Optimization by Marco Dorigo and Thomas Stützle, MIT Press, 305 pp., $40.00, ISBN 0-262-04219-3. *The Knowledge Engineering Review*, 20(1), 92–93. doi:10.1017/S0269888905220386

Pereira, C. R., Pereira, D. R., Silva, F. A., Masieiro, J. P., Weber, S. A., Hook, C., & Papa, J. P. (2016). A new computer vision-based approach to aid the diagnosis of Parkinson's disease. *Computer Methods and Programs in Biomedicine*, 136, 79–88. doi:10.1016/j.cmpb.2016.08.005 PMID:27686705

Pohl, K. M., Konukoglu, E., Novellas, S., Ayache, N., Fedorov, A., Talos, I. F., ... & Black, P. M. (2011). A new metric for detecting change in slowly evolving brain tumors: validation in meningioma patients. *Operative Neurosurgery, 68*(suppl_1), ons225-ons233.

Rosenblum, S., Samuel, M., Zlotnik, S., Erikh, I., & Schlesinger, I. (2013). Handwriting as an objective tool for Parkinson's disease diagnosis. *Journal of Neurology*, 260(9), 2357–2361. doi:10.100700415-013-6996-x PMID:23771509

Singh, G., Vadera, M., Samavedham, L., & Lim, E. C. H. (2016). Machine Learning-Based Framework for Multi-Class Diagnosis of Neurodegenerative Diseases: A Study on Parkinson's Disease. *IFAC-PapersOnLine*, 49(7), 990–995. doi:10.1016/j.ifacol.2016.07.331

Summers, M. J., Madl, T., Vercelli, A. E., Aumayr, G., Bleier, D. M., & Ciferri, L. (2017). Deep machine learning application to the detection of preclinical neurodegenerative diseases of aging. *DigitCult-Scientific Journal on Digital Cultures*, 2(2), 9–24.

Vinken, P. J., & Bruyn, G. W. (Eds(1979*Handbook of clinical neurology*. North-Holland Publishing Company. doi:10.1002/ana.410060526

Waldner, J. B. (2007). *Nanocomputers and swarm intelligence*. ISTE.

Zadeh, L. A. (1965). Fuzzy sets. *Information and Control*, 8(3), 338–353. doi:10.1016/S0019-9958(65)90241-X

Zanella, A., Bui, N., Castellani, A., Vangelista, L., & Zorzi, M. (2014). Internet of things for smart cities. *IEEE Internet of Things Journal, 1*(1), 22-32.

Chapter 14
Clinical Decision Support Systems:
Decision-Making System for Clinical Data

Diviya Prabha V.
iD https://orcid.org/0000-0002-0956-7316
Periyar University, India

Rathipriya R.
iD https://orcid.org/0000-0002-3970-262X
Periyar University, India

ABSTRACT

Clinical data is increasing day-by-day mainly in hospitals by an ageing of the human population. Patients discharged from hospitals are readmitted due to health issues. As the number of patients increases, there are a smaller number of hospitals and an increase in healthcare costs. This results in ineffective decision making that minimizes the healthcare. Machine learning techniques score better for solving this kind of problem. The proposed work, minimum entropy feature selection with logistic regression (MELR), is performing better for the readmission rates. Decision cannot be based on the clinical knowledge and personal data about the patient. It must be precise in choosing the future patient outcomes. This chapter produces promising results for clinical data.

INTRODUCTION

Machine learning is involved to organize the data by making data fit into the model which predict the future outcomes. It helps to construct the model from the historical data available providing an efficient solution for the given problem. In last few years, various machine learning techniques, hybrid the two machine learning techniques to innovate new model to classify the data. Clinical data from hospitals and government health care sectors EHR (Electronic Heath Record) are maintained physically without any significant progress. These machine learning algorithm concepts integrate the future outcomes with

DOI: 10.4018/978-1-7998-2742-9.ch014

current historical data. As clinical data is increasing due to huge growth of population necessary model are required. Development of these algorithms is the foundation of machine learning concepts.

Traditional Strategy will lead to wide fluctuations in clinical data. Rather than collecting the diabetic data from mortality this study suggest that collecting the information about diabetic data from hospitals. This data help us to maintain level of blood glucose level. A model is recommended which makes the base for the diabetic patient to compare with the historical data to improve the healthcare. Now, the temporary analysis of this data states to reduce the readmission of diabetic patient.

Several machine learning algorithms executed to solve many problems. In analyzing the historical data feature selection is important to development the improvement of the model. This chapter paves a way to feature selection and machine learning techniques. The basic feature selection are carried out in previous paper that (Xing Yifan & Jai Sharma, 2016) does not give relevant solution to the problem. Some other best methods are needed to select the relevant features and reject the irrelevant features.

Entropy is the measure of uncertainty based on the target variable (Vimalkumar & Kalpesh, 2014). It shows the number of possible values (Lacson, R. C & Bowen Baker, 2019) to the target variable. In machine learning it also used to identify the maximum relation to the target variable. This chapter selects the features that are minimum uncertainty to the target variable. Finding the relevant features improves the accuracy of machine learning techniques.

The main objective of this paper is aimed to show the most significant features in dataset from the clinical data. The relevant features help to improve the accuracy level of the classification algorithms. The empirical results show that proposed works achieves remarkable dimensionality reduction from 50 features to 11 features for classification algorithms.

The chapter is organized as follows: The following sections describe the background study basic concepts of entropy-based feature selection are explained. The next section describes the proposed work of the chapter and finally concludes the paper

BACKGROUND STUDY:

In recent few decades, machine learning techniques are used in wide range to predict the disease based on the historical data. Many proposed algorithms are developed and studied from the researchers. In this section a few important works that are closely to the proposed work are discussed.

The prediction of readmission using big data tools based the drugs that are taken to the patient (Satish Boregowda, Rod Handy, 2016) .The care must be taken to the patient even after the discharge. The values of the patients are determined (Mingle Damian, 2017) by HbA1C results it is an important feature to control the glucose in in blood. Entropy is one of the important feature to select the (Yun Zheng, Chee Keong Kwoh, 2011) high dimensional features. High entropy alloy integrating with machine learning is doing better (Ziqing Zhou &Yeju Zhou, 2019). In this work the maximum entropy is used to optimize the objective solution of the proposed work (Rui Zhao & Xudong Sun, 2019). It also proposed three works based on the entropy. First, work is based on the weighted entropy second work is lower bound for optimization (Jayanthi, N & B. Vijaya Babu, 2017) and finally, prioritize framework on entropy. Differential entropy selecting the subset of features (Schulman & Chen, 2017) provides solution to the classification problem. The relevant features are selected it gives better accuracy. This entropy deals (Satish Boregowda & Rod Handy, 2016) nominal and real-valued data in the dataset. Neighborhood

(Yanpeng Qu, & Rong, 2019) Entropy to select the relevant features (Andrea Marcello & Roberto Battiti, 2018) using the neural network.

PROPOSED WORK:

This section discuss the data preprocessing and the proposed approach for feature selection .The dataset is from UCI repository Diabetes 130-US hospital dataset is taken. The dataset consist of 101768 patient records and which includes 50 features such as inpatient encounter, laboratory test, etc., These features are selected using Selecting K best feature, Decision Tree Classifier and results are compared with the proposed work.

For each variable, the entropy is calculated as the following formula the probability of the features with its log values. The features are selected based on the threshold value of the entropy it is fixed as 3 since this value is suitable for the dataset. The values that are <=3 are considered as the Features Selected (FS) and the values of entropy of features that are <3 are considered as rejected features (RS)

$$Entropy_{Selected}Features = \min\_threshold(\sum_{i=1}^{n} -P(Features_i)\log_2(P(Features_i))) \tag{1}$$

The decision making system is developed using minimum entropy features values. The hypothesis is subjected on the selection and rejection of the features.

Minimum Entropy Features = FS H ($Entropy_{Selected}Features$) <= 3

FR, H ($Entropy_{Selected}Features$) >3

The algorithm explains the proposed work MELR the patent data is loaded then data are preprocessed aggregating the label vector such as patient is readmitted or not instead of readmission in >30, readmission in <30 and not readmitted is the value of the target value. Likewise each and every feature is preprocessed.

Algorithm: MELR

```
START
F: All features from Dataset
F1: Selected Features
D= LOAD (Pateint_Data)
//Preprocessing
D= Preprocess (D)
D= String to Numerical (D)
//Select the Features (Proposed Work)
F1= D (Features through minimum entropy value)
D=Delete the features that have higher value
// Select the Best Model
```

```
T = Train and Test (F1)
T = Apply Machine Learning Algorithm (SVM, LR…)
// Calculate the Accuracy Measure
A= Precision, Recall F- Measure……
End
```

The table 1 exemplifies the values of the selected features. The mean, Standard Deviation (SD), Minimum and maximum value of the feature, variance, skewness and kurtosis are calculated, these values are increasing and decreasing based on the features.

Table 1. Selected Features Values

FEATURES	Mean	S.D	MIN	max	Variance	Skewness	KURTOSIS
F_1	66	16	5	95	254.1	0.63	0.28
F_2	3.71	5.2	1	28	27.8	2.56	6.0
F_3	1.3	1.7	0	6	2.90	1.31	0.85
F_4	0.63	1.26	0	21	1.59	3.61	20.71
F_5	1.74	2.19	0	8	4.80	2.34	3.63
F_6	0.46	0.49	0	1	0.24	0.15	-1.97
F_7	0.41	0.85	0	4	0.73	1.75	1.76
F_8	1.42	1.45	0	4	2.11	0.39	-1.22
F_9	16.02	8.12	1	81	66.05	1.32	3.46
F_10	0.22	0.68	0	4	0.47	2.96	8.14
F_11	4.39	2.98	1	14	8.91	1.1	0.85

Logistic Regression

It is one of the best statistical learning techniquies used to find the proabiblity of the features. Th output of the function is either a patient is readmitted or not. It works on logistic (DiviyaPrabha, V., & R. Ratthipriya, 2018)function as

$$p\left(\text{Readmitted}\right) = \frac{e^{F_1 + F_2 x \cdots}}{1 + e^{F_1 + F_2 x \cdots}} \tag{2}$$

The proability of each and individual feature is calculated using the above formula 2. Here p is the dependent variable and F1 and F2 are features. Each feature value is computed to predict the proabaility of patient readmission. The values are computed for the 11 features.

EXPERIMENTAL ANALYSIS

The experimental analysis of the proposed algorithms is tabulated in Table 2. The classification algorithm such as Decision Tree (DT), Random Forest (RF), Gradient Boosting Regression and Logistic Regression are used to classify patient readmission prediction. Comparatively the proposed work gives better results than the existing one.

Figure 1 depicts the classification accuracy of different algorithms. Figure 2 to figure 11 exemplifies the confidence interval of each feature the percentage of the interval diverges based on the value of the features. The study evaluates the features such as age, insulin, glyburide, A1Cresult, metformin, num_medications have the confidence interval greater than 90 per cent the other features are plotted based on the existing value. This plot concludes that these features support the prediction of readmission with the high confidence interval.

Table 2. Classification Accuracy

Classification Algorithm	Precision	Recall	F1-Score	Weighted Precision	Weighted Recall	Weighted F1-Score
DT	90%	89%	89%	92%	89%	91%
RF	90%	90%	90%	90%	86%	90%
GBT	90%	90%	90%	90%	90%	90%
MELR	92%	92%	91%	91%	92%	91%

Figure 1. Classification Accuracy

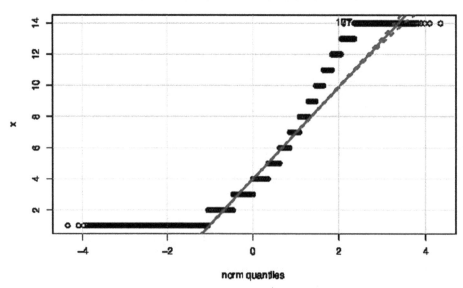

Table 3. Beta Coefficient Values

Iterations	F_1	F_2	F_3	F_4	F_5	F_6	F_7	F_8	F_9	F_10	F_11	Mean
1	0.1644	0.0019	0.0298	0.0056	-0.8389	-0.9206	0.0096	-1.4836	0.029	-0.8162	0.0026	0.346945
2	0.555	0.0232	0.0281	0.0223	-1.8177	-2.0176	0.0581	-3.2332	0.0481	-1.7911	0.0099	0.737718
3	0.5201	0.0194	0.0314	0.0205	-1.8231	-2.0568	0.0539	-3.2606	0.0501	-1.8335	0.009	0.751782
4	0.5447	0.0182	0.0339	0.0212	-2.0147	-2.3195	0.0581	-3.6263	0.056	-2.0784	0.0091	0.845245
5	0.6228	0.0186	0.034	0.024	-2.4189	-2.8595	0.0718	-4.3862	0.0659	-2.5801	2.5801	0.8025
6	0.6865	0.0179	0.0001	0.0273	-2.9416	-3.6366	0.1027	-5.37	0.067	-3.3348	0.0101	1.306491
7	0.6865	0.0179	0.01	0.0252	-3.001	-4.506	0.1058	-6.45	0.053	-3.3971	0.0587	1.490636
8	0.7034	0.012	0.1018	0.0234	-3.8932	-5.0146	0.1187	-7.0179	0.0468	-4.7281	0.0072	1.7855
9	0.7074	0.0101	0.11	0.0122	-4.4838	-5.7743	0.0506	-7.9094	0.0387	-5.5065	0.0062	2.067164
10	0.6227	0.0033	0.0935	0.0144	-5.3505	-6.7739	0.0461	-9.1104	0.0256	-6.5157	0.0051	2.449073
11	0.5485	0.0021	0.0623	0.0143	-6.2954	-7.8584	0.0203	-10.4189	0.0181	-7.6084	0.0043	2.864655
12	0.4873	0.0064	0.0312	0.0147	-7.3906	-9.1145	0.0052	-11.9622	0.0157	-8.8669	0.0034	3.342755
13	0.4343	0.0097	0.0349	0.0162	-8.4485	-10.2985	0.0029	-13.4445	0.027	-10.0487	0.0017	3.792136
14	0.3899	0.0144	0.0712	0.0134	-9.7915	-11.7968	0.0322	-15.3385	0.0468	-11.5428	0.0008	4.354627
15	0.3729	0.0149	0.0666	0.0154	-9.8052	-11.7987	0.0336	-15.3435	0.0515	-11.5428	0.0001	4.357745
16	0.3845	0.0141	0.0671	0.015	-9.6213	-11.5963	0.0314	-15.0891	0.049	-11.3411	0.0004	4.280564
17	0.3867	0.0141	0.0683	0.0166	-9.5999	-11.5729	0.0312	-15.0602	0.0491	-11.3178	0.0004	4.271455
18	0.3901	0.0149	0.0716	0.0166	-9.6735	-11.6571	0.0276	-15.1674	0.0503	-11.4015	0.0007	4.302518
19	0.3902	0.0145	0.0699	0.0161	-9.5901	-11.5634	0.0266	-15.0473	0.0489	-11.3084	0.0006	4.267445
20	0.3895	0.0145	0.0704	0.0159	-9.6192	-11.5959	0.028	-15.089	0.0494	-11.3407	0.0006	4.279664
30	0.3837	0.0146	0.0702	0.0159	-9.9777	-12.0717	0.027	-15.5337	0.0493	-11.8126	0.0006	4.439491
40	0.3905	0.0145	0.0705	0.0159	-12.990	-16.1097	0.0282	-19.2357	0.0494	-15.8163	0.0006	5.780245
50	0.3903	0.0145	0.0704	0.0159	-16.263	-20.4888	0.0281	-23.2633	0.0493	-20.1583	0.0006	7.236818
100	0.3903	0.0145	0.0704	0.0159	-19.575	-24.9194	0.0282	-27.3378	0.0493	-24.5513	0.0006	8.7104

Table 3 represents the beta co-efficient value for logistic regression model. For each iteration the features value increases and decreases. From F_1 to F_11 the values are not constant as i increase or decrease .The last column mean value represents the the increasing value of the feature it reaches to the value 8 from 0.3 goes in a positive way.

Figure 2. F_1

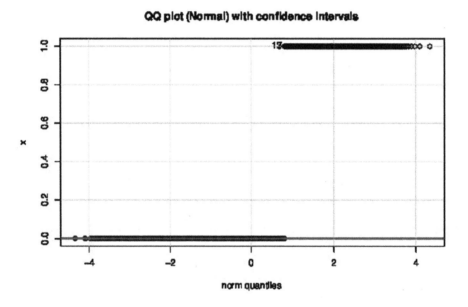

Figure 3. F_2

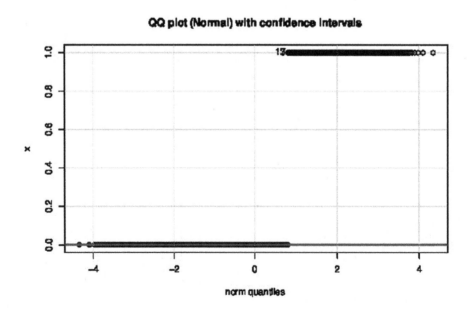

Figure 4. F_3

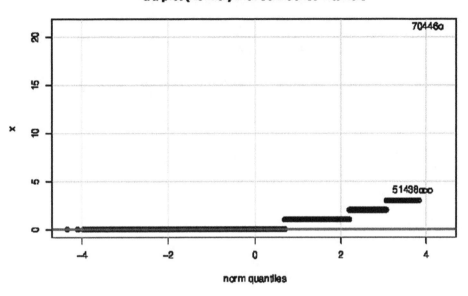

Figure 5. F_4

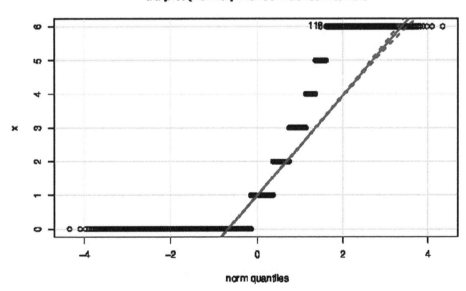

Figure 6. F_5

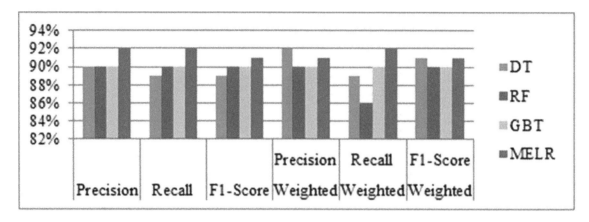

Figure 7. F_6

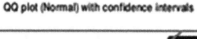

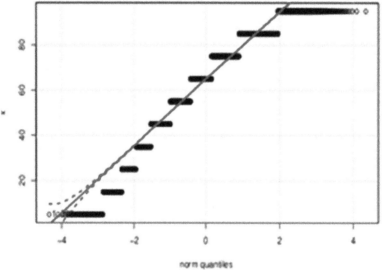

CONCLUSION

In this chapter provides a novel approach of minimum entropy feature selection is proposed to select the most significant features for clinical data. This method is efficient to select the features with high dimensional data. The logistic regression performs better than compared with the other classification algorithm. This algorithm takes the better decision making for predicting the patient is readmitted to the hospital or not form clinical data. This will siginifically reduce the risk of patients and hospitals.

Figure 8. F_7

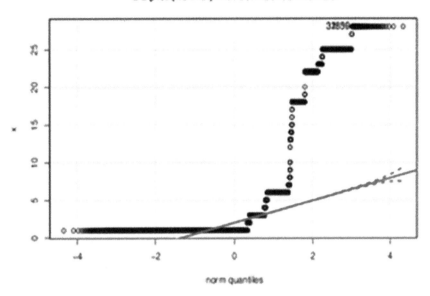

Figure 9. F_8

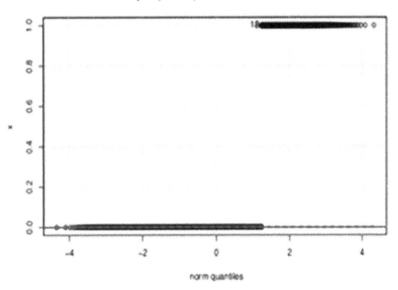

Figure 10. F_9

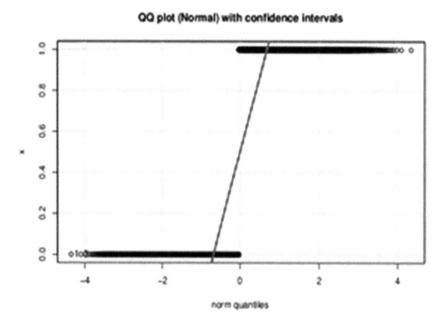

Figure 11. F_10

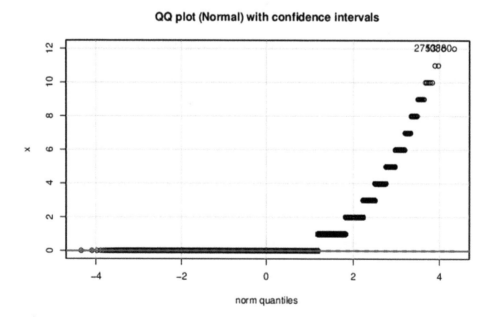

Figure 12. F_11

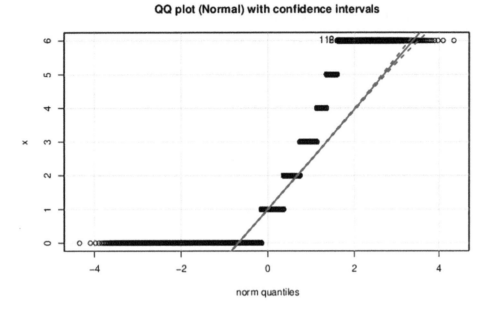

REFERENCES

Boregowda, S., Handy, R., Sleeth, D., & Merryweather, A. (2016). Measuring Entropy Change in a Human Physiological System. *Journal of Thermodynamics, 2016,* 1–8. doi:10.1155/2016/4932710

Damian. (2017). Predicting Diabetic Readmission Rates: Moving Beyond Hba1c. *Current Trends in Biomedical Engineering & Bioscience, 7*(3).

DiviyaPrabha & Ratthipriya. (2018). Prediction of Hyperglycemia using Binary Gravitational Logistic Regression (BGLR). *International Journal of Pure and Applied Mathematics, 118*(16).

Jayanthi, N., Vijaya Babu, B., & Sambasiva Rao, N. (2017). Survey on Clinical Prediction Models for Diabetes prediction. *Journal of Big Data, 4*(1), 26. doi:10.118640537-017-0082-7

Lacson, R. C., Baker, B., Suresh, H., Andriole, K., Szolovits, P., & Lacson, E. Jr. (2019). Use of machine-learning algorithms to determine features of systolic blood pressure variability that predict poor outcomes in hypertensive patients. *Clinical Kidney Journal, 12*(2), 206–212. doi:10.1093/ckjfy049 PMID:30976397

Schulman, J., Chen, X., & Abbeel, P. (2017). *Equivalence between policy gradients and soft q-learning.* arXiv preprint arXiv:1704.06440

Vimalkumar & Vandra. (2014). Entropy Based Feature Selection For MultiRelational Naïve Bayesian Classifier. *Journal of International Technology and Information Management, 23*(1). https://amethix.com/entropy-in-machine-learning/

Yanpeng, Q. R. (2019). Li Non-unique decision differential entropy-based feature selection. Elsevier.

Yifan& Sharma. (2016). *Diabetes patient Readmission Prediction using Big Data Analytics Tools.* Academic Press.

Zhao & Sun. (2019). *Maximum Entropy-Regularized Multi-Goal Reinforcement Learning.* Academic Press.

Zheng, Y., & Kwoh, C. K. (2011). A Feature Subset Selection Method Based On High-Dimensional Mutual Information. *Entropy (Basel, Switzerland), 13*(4), 2011. doi:10.3390/e13040860

Ziqing, Z., & Zhou, Y. (2019). *Machine learning guided appraisal and exploration of phase design for high entropy alloys.* Computational Materials, Nature.

Chapter 15
Diagnosis and Prognosis of Ultrasound Fetal Growth Analysis Using Neuro–Fuzzy Based on Genetic Algorithms

Parminder Kaur

 https://orcid.org/0000-0003-1954-3390
Guru Nanak Dev University, Amritsar, India

Prabhpreet Kaur

 https://orcid.org/0000-0001-8498-5940
Guru Nanak Dev University, Amritsar, India

Gurvinder Singh

Guru Nanak Dev University, Amritsar, India

ABSTRACT

Acquisition of the standard plane is the prerequisite of biometric measurement and diagnosis during the ultrasound (US) examination. Based upon the analysis of existing algorithms for the automatic fetal development measurement, a new algorithm known as neuro-fuzzy based on genetic algorithm is developed. Firstly, the fetal ultrasound benchmark image is auto-pre-processed using normal shrink homomorphic technique. Secondly, the features are extracted using gray level co-occurrence matrix (GLCM), grey level run length matrix (GLRLM), intensity histogram (IH), and rotation invariant moments (IM). Thirdly, neuro-fuzzy using genetic approach is used to distinguish among the fetus growth as abnormal or normal. Experimental results using benchmark and live dataset demonstrate that the developed method achieves an accuracy of 97% as compared to the state-of-the-art methods in terms of parameters such as sensitivity, specificity, recall, f-measure, and precision rate.

DOI: 10.4018/978-1-7998-2742-9.ch015

INTRODUCTION

There is a significant advancement in the analysis of ultrasound imaging and now use of modern machine learning into the medical image analysis field, this art is more challenging for the researchers (Maraci et al, 2017). Computer Aided Diagnosis (CAD) has become one of the major research subjects in medical imaging and diagnostic radiology. Ultrasound imaging modality is quite popular and most widely used modality for visualizing and studying the medical images for any disease conditions without causing any pain or discomfort to the patient (Ali *et al*, 2014; Jalalian *et al*, 2013; Cheng *et al*, 2010). Ultrasound imaging is widely used due to less costly and non-persistent nature as compared to other imaging modalities. The diagnosis is performed on various diseases based on image features such as the Echogenicity, Legion Shape, and Echo Texture (Kalyan *et al*, 2014). Accurate ultrasound-based fetal biometric measurements are important for delivery of high quality obstetrical health care. Common measurements include: the Bi-Parietal Diameter (BDP), Head Circumference (HC), Abdominal Circumference (AC), Femur Length (FL), Humerus Length (HL), and the Crown Rump Length (CRL). The American Institute of Ultrasound in Medicine (AIUM) publishes guidelines for measuring these values. These values help diagnose fetal pathology including growth restriction, microcephaly, and macrosomia. In addition, these are utilized to estimate the gestational age (GA) of the fetus (i.e., length of pregnancy in weeks and days). Accurate estimation of GA is important to determine the expected delivery date, assess the fetal size and monitor fetal growth as in Fig. 1 (Carneiro *et al*, 2017; Loughna *et al,* 2009; Hearn, 1995; Pramanik *et al*, 2013; Espinoza *et al*, 2013).

Figure 1. Fetal Ultrasound images of (a) head, (b) femur, (c) abdomen, (d) whole fetus of age 13 weeks

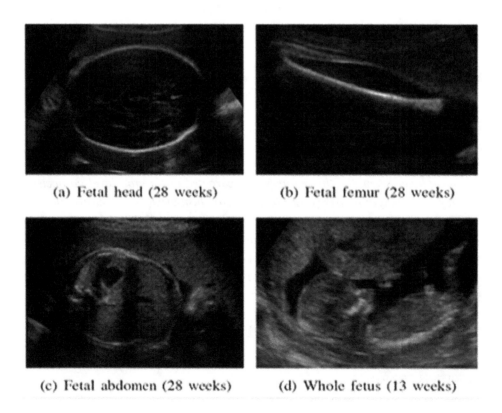

(a) Fetal head (28 weeks)   (b) Fetal femur (28 weeks)

(c) Fetal abdomen (28 weeks)   (d) Whole fetus (13 weeks)

The objective of this chapter is to perform Image enhancement using application of Ultrasound Fetus Development through the study of various Denoising Filtering, Feature Extraction and Machine Learning techniques. It also evaluates the quantitative denoising filtering techniques on the basis of Peak Signal-to-Noise Ratio (PSNR), Signal-to-Noise Ratio (SNR), Edge Preservation Index (EPI) and Coefficient-of-Correlation (CoC) measures. To achieve the desired objective, performance of Artificial Neural Network (ANN) based Ultrasound Fetus Development classification is assessed. Based upon outcome, hybrid Neuro-Fuzzy based Genetic approach on Ultrasound Fetus growth is proposed and compared with the existing technique (ANN) with respect to the parameters i.e. Kappa statistic, Mean absolute error, Root Mean Squared Error (RMSE), Relative absolute error, Root relative squared error, Accuracy, F-measure, Precision, Recall and Receiver Operating Characteristics (ROC) Area. 10 Fold Cross-Validation on the basis of Confusion Matrix and ROC in Classification Learner (MATLAB 2015b) has been applied to validate the results.

BACKGROUND

The ever increasing size of patient data in medical images imposes a research challenge during the scientific behavior for diagnosing, detecting and prediction of the diseases. Nowadays, the interests of the radiologists are attracted towards the medical data mining for patient care. Medical Image Denoising and Machine Learning is a great challenge for researchers. The detection and prediction of imaging is getting easier by the advancement in the technology. The quick development is an outcome of the requirement for faster, precise and less intrusive treatment. Advanced technology in radiology imaging equipment has additionally stimulated the use of imaging. As the numbers of patients are continuously expanding, the determination of researchers to achieve excellence in this field is increasing. The expanding number and poor quality of the images diminish radiologist's abilities to translate them. Machine Learning (ML) techniques are increasingly getting success in image based diagnosis, disease detection and disease prognosis. To reduce the operator dependency and achieve better diagnostic accuracy, CAD system is a valuable and beneficial means for fetal development detection and classification. Image denoising and ML Techniques plays an important role in the noise removal from Ultrasound Fetus Development Images. In this chapter, literature review of two categories of techniques such as Medical Denoising Techniques and Machine Learning Techniques is explained. Table 1 shows the review of image denoising filtering techniques along with the advantages of tools, techniques being used.

Most of the radiologists are interested in using Machine Learning methods due to the large amount of patient data. These methods help in time reduction, cost effectiveness and better and efficient results. Table 2 shows the review of medical denoising approach along with the relevant ML approach starting from the year 1992 till 2018.

Various types of noises and filtering techniques using transform methods are the inputs for the image processing step. Feature extraction and selection using machine learning are strongly needed in diagnosing the fetal development in ultrasound images. Such type of diagnosis is done as a comparative analysis of published work (Table 3). Eleven important specifications such as major contributions, application domain, G(Gray level co-occurrence matrices)/GL(Gray level run length matrices)/I(Invariant moments),F(Filtering),S(Speckle),WT(Wavelet Transform),GA(Genetic Algorithm),Fu(Fuzzy),ANN(Artificial Neural Network), DT(Decision Tree), SVM(Support Vector Machine), Ac(Accuracy) are used to perform comparison. Figure 2 schematically summarizes, how some of the state-of-the-art literature, in

Table 1. Review of Medical Denoising Approaches

Title, Author, Publication, Year	Classes	Tools/Techniques	Advantages
Title: Ideal spatial adaptation by wavelet shrinkage **Authors:** Donoho & Johnstone, 1994 **Publication:** Biometrika	Speckle reduction	Signal-dependent Multiplicative Speckle Noise Model, Discrete Wavelet Transform and Modeling of Wavelet Coefficients	Increases smoothness
Title: De-Noising by Soft-Thresholding **Authors:** Donoho,1995 **Publication:** IEEE Transaction On Information Theory	Image denoising	Abstract De-Noising Model	Increases statistical Inference
Title: Image Denoising using Wavelet Thresholding **Authors:** Kaur et.al, 2002 **Publication:** IEEE	Image denoising	Adaptive Threshold Estimation	Provide smoothness and Effective edge preservation
Title: A Wavelet Based Statistical Approach for, Speckle Reduction in Medical Ultrasound Images **Authors:** Gupta, 2003 **Publication:** IEEE	Speckle reduction	Novel Multiscale Nonlinear for Speckle reduction	Fast computation and better diagnosis
Title: Wavelet-based statistical approach for speckle reduction in medical ultrasound images **Authors:** Gupta et al., 2004 **Publication:** Medical & Biological Engineering & Computing	Speckle reduction	Novel Speckle-Reduction	Fast computation and Despeckling
Title: Homomorphic wavelet thresholding technique for denoising medical ultrasound images **Authors**: Gupta et al.,2005 **Publication:** Journal of Medical Engineering & Technology	Image denoising	Novel Homomorphic Wavelet Thresholding	Effective performance of wavelet based denoising
Title: A versatile technique for visual enhancement of medical ultrasound images **Authors:** Kaur et al., 2007 **Publication:** Science direct	Visual enhancement of image	Versatile Wavelet Domain despeckling	Provide better performance in speckle smoothing and edge preservation

fetal ultrasound images analysis maps between the interpretation and evaluation (using classification algorithms) with standard baseline validation point (Kaur et al., 2019).

CAD Fetus Development System

The development of CAD system for fetal development examination is depicted out in Figure 3. This work is directed at automatically locating abnormal signs of a disseminated textural nature found within fetal development. The primary contributions include the segmentation of the fetus picture based on multiple parameters, together with histogram and co-occurrence matrices in order to obtain characteristics from each and every sub image and the utility of Neuro-Fuzzy as a part of classification scheme into normal and abnormal cases. The scheme is initialized with the fetus image pre-processing using cropping and edge detection techniques. Then background subtraction is performed to eliminate the abnormalities from the pre-processed images. On the original and processed images, the histogram, GLCM features, GLRLM and the rotation invariant moments features are computed from each and every region.

Table 2. Explored Medical Denoising Techniques

Title, Author, Publication	Dataset	Features	Tools/Techniques Used	Classification Approach
Title: Image Coding Using Wavelet Transform **Author:** Antonini et al.,1992 **Publication:** IEEE Transactions On Image Processing	The intensity of each pixel is coded on 256 grey levels (8 bpp), 256 by 256 black and white images.	Entropy, PSNR	Wavelet Coefficients, Vector Quantization	Machine Learning
Title: Qualitative and Quantitative Evaluation of Image Denoising Techniques **Author:** Bedi & Goyal, 2010 **Publication:** International Journal of Computer Applications	Standardised Images	CoC, PSNR and S/MSE	Various Spatial filters like Median Filter, Lee Filter, Kuan Filter, Wiener Filter, Normal Shrink, Bayes Shrink	Image Denoising Using Spatial Filters
Title: Automated breast cancer detection and classification using ultrasound images: A survey **Author:** Cheng et al., 2010 **Publication:** Elsevier	Standardized Breast Images	Spiculation, Elipsoid Shape, Branch Pattern, Brightness of Nodule, Margin Echogenity	Filtering, Wavelet approaches, Histogram thresholding, Active Contor Model, MKF, Neural Network, Bayesian Neural Network, Decision Tree, SVM, Template Matching	CAD based System detection
Title: Digital Image Denoising in Medical Ultrasound Images: A Survey **Author:** Ragesh et al., 2011 **Publication:** ICGST AIML-11 Conference	Ultrasound images	Scatter density, Texture based contrast, MSE, RMSE, SNR, and PSNR	Multi-scale thresholding, Bayesian Estimation and Coefficient correlation, Application of Soft Computing like Artificial Neural Networks (ANN), Genetic Algorithms (GA) and Fuzzy Logic (FL)	Designing better algorithms correlating the Ultrasound image formation concepts and advanced digital image processing techniques
Title: A Novel Approach for Classifying Medical Images Using Data Mining Techniques **Author:** Mangai et al., 2013 **Publication:** International Journal of Computer Science and Electronics Engineering	Retinal fundus images of size 576x720 pixels.	Mean, Variance, Skewness and Kurtosis	Classifiers such as SVM, kNN, and NB	Machine Learning cl assifiers
Title: Image Denoising Method based on Threshold, Wavelet Transform and Genetic Algorithm **Author:** Liu, 2015 **Publication:** International Journal of Signal Processing	Images of Lena and Saturn Planet	Hard Threshold Function, Soft Threshold function	Wavelet Transform, Genetic Algorithm	Genetic Algorithm

Table 3. Related work of Medical Ultrasound Image Denoising with Data Mining Techniques

Author & Year	Major Contribution	Application Domain	G/GL/I	F	S	WT	GA	Fu	ANN	DT	SVM	Ac
Poonguzhali & Ravindran, 2008	Effective edge based statistics using GLCM	Liver Ultrasound	Yes	No	Yes	Yes	No	No	No	No	No	Yes
Suganya & Rajaram, 2012	Feature extraction algorithm on texture, shape, image color can't be associated to the detailed medical knowledge	Liver Ultrasound	No	Yes	No	No	No	No	No	No	Yes	No
Mitrea et al., 2012	Diagnosis and feature Recognition using Superior order GLCM	Liver Ultrasound	Yes	No	No	No	No	No	No	No	No	Yes
Rahmatullah et al., 2012	Anatomical features in Ultrasound images are detected.	Ultrasound Images	No	No	Yes	Yes	No	No	No	No	No	No
Kumar et al., 2013	Automatic segmentation using statistical features and Noise reduction	Liver Ultrasound	No	No	Yes	No	No	No	No	No	No	Yes
Kalyan et al., 2013	Combined feature recognition using GLCM, GLRLM, IH	Kidney Ultrasound	Yes	No	No	No	No	No	No	No	No	Yes
Singh et al., 2014	Textual analysis, Feature Extraction and Classification using LDA	Liver Ultrasound	Yes	Yes	Yes	No	No	No	No	No	No	Yes
Hiremath & Tegnoor, 2014	Contourlet and Fuzzy Transform for classification	Ovaries Ultrasound	No	No	No	No	No	Yes	No	No	No	Yes
Vardhan & Rao, 2014	GLCM architecture on image extraction	Gray level Image	Yes	No	Yes	No	No	No	No	No	No	No
Ali et al., 2014	Cancer progression and prediction in Liver Ultrasound	Liver Ultrasound (Cross house Hospital Kilmarnock United Kingdom)	No	Yes	Yes	No	No	No	No	No	Yes	Yes
Kalyan et al., 2014	Diagnosis of disease in Liver ultrasound using ANN	Liver Ultrasound(Jaslok Hospital and Research Centre, Mumbai)	Yes	No	Yes	No	No	No	No	No	No	No
Gonzalez et al., 2015	Optimal architecture of modular neural networks and fuzzy gravitational search algorithm for a pattern recognition application	Heart Disease	No	No	No	No	No	Yes	Yes	No	No	No
Ravishankar et al., 2016	Hybrid approach combining traditional texture analysis methods with for the automatic detection	Fetal Ultrasound (GE Healthcare, USA)	Yes	No	No	No	No	No	Yes	No	No	No
Proposed System	**Diagnosis and Prevention of Benchmark Images and Live Data Set Ultrasound Fetus Development using classification**	**Philips Ultrasound Images (Benchmark) and Civil Hospital Jalandher Ultrasound Fetus Development(Live Dataset)**	Yes	Yes	Yes	Yes	Yes	Yes	Yes	Yes	Yes	Yes

Figure 2. Baseline of Literature Review of Ultrasound Fetus Development from increasing automated image analysis on Y-axis from left to right along with the Ultrasound Detection Protocol on X-axis

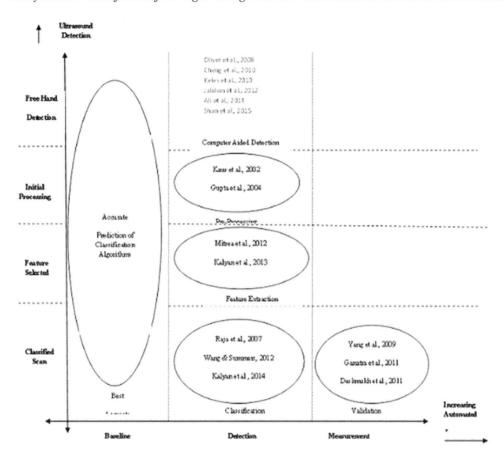

IMAGE ENHANCEMENT USING APPLICATION OF ULTRASOUND FETUS DEVELOPMENT

Ultrasonography is considered to be one of the most powerful techniques for imaging organs and soft tissue structures in human body. It is preferred over other medical imaging methods like Computed Tomography (CT) or Magnetic Resonance Imaging (MRI) because it is less expensive, non-invasive, versatile, portable, and does not use ionizing radiations. Despite their obvious advantages, Ultrasound images are contaminated with multiplicative noise called 'speckle' which is one of the major source of image quality degradation.

Since Ultrasound images are patient-specific, operator dependent and machine specific, the appearance of the image is closely associated with the patient's characteristics, the expertise of the clinician and the machine used. Because of the properties of image formation intrinsic to Ultrasound images, they might get affected by signal dropouts, missing boundaries, artifacts, attenuation, shadows or speckle. This makes ultrasound essentially the most challenging modality to operate with. In medical literature, speckle is treated as a distracting artifact as it tends to degrade the resolution and the object detectability. Moreover, in US images the speckle noise has a spatial correlation length on each axis, which is

Figure 3. Working of CAD Ultrasound Fetus Development System

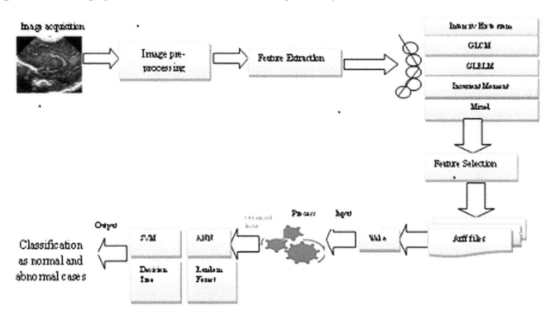

same as resolution cell size. This spatial correlation makes the speckle suppression a very difficult and delicate task, hence, a trade-off has to be made between the degree of speckle suppression and feature preservation [HYP].

Speckle is a form of multiplicative noise, which makes visual interpretation difficult (Gupta et al., 2004). Speckle significantly degrades the image quality and hence, makes it more difficult for the observer to discriminate the fine details of the images in diagnostic examinations (Gupta et al., 2005a). Image denoising is used to remove the noise while retaining the important signal features as much as possible (Gupta et al., 2007). The purpose of image denoising is to estimate the presence of noisy data in original image. Image denoising still remains a challenge for researchers because noise removal introduces artifacts and causes blurring of the images.

Protocols are developed to obtain the ideal images while retaining the features of region of interest e.g. shape and structures. Two dimensional fetal ultrasound images are commonly utilized to determine the gestational age of the baby, its weight and size as well as its growth patterns and abnormalities (Loughna et al., 2009). Normally, size of fetal is determined by employing two dimensional ultrasound measurements of head, abdomen, and femur, of about 20 week's fetal (Hearn-Stebbins, 1995), which is then compared to growth charts to identify normal and abnormal development. In order to minimize intra- and inter-observer variations, as well as produce better results, automated techniques for fetal biometric measurements are studied (Pramanik et.al, 2013; Gustavo et al., 2008). This also enhances the efficiency by minimizing the analysis time and the number of steps required for fetal measurement (Espinoza et al., 2013). Less experienced users are also benefitted from automated technique.

The automatic examination of Ultrasound images is a challenging field. The techniques applied to MRI or CT scan doesn't work with ultrasound images. The automated segmentation techniques earlier introduced in the fetal image area, concentrated on utilizing segmentation as a processing step to estimate biometric measurements. The methods which provide all fetal biometric measurements engaged in clinical practice are restricted. A healthy fetus changes its shape due to growth. Various organs which surround the region of interest create high variability in pose and shape for the similar structure of an appealing application of Picture Archiving and Communication Systems (PACS) environment together with CAD system.

IMAGE PRE-PROCESSING

Speckle noise diminishes the contrast of the image and causes ringing arti-facts on the edges of the image. Therefore, it diminishes the ability of humans to distinguish between the coarse and fine details of the image (Gupta et al., 2005)

There are multifarious filters to diminish the speckle noise. Each filter has its own statistical values. Different filters give different results for different images. Several state-of-the-art denoising filtering techniques namely Wiener, Median, Lee and Kuan are being analyzed by the researchers to improve the performance of these filters in terms of quality, reduction of run time and many more factors.

Speckle Noise Reduction Filtering Techniques

Median Filter

Median filter is a non-linear technique that works best with impulse noise (salt & pepper noise) while retaining sharp edges in the image. This filter types the encompassing pixels value in the window pane with an orderly collection and replaces the centre pixel within the defined window pane with the middle value in the collection.

$$\hat{i}(x, y) = \underset{(s,t) \in S_{xy}}{\text{median}} \{j(s, t)\}$$

{Where 'j(s, t)' = local window around the pixel (x, y) in the image to be processed and '$\hat{i}(x, y)$' = Resulting signal}

Lee Filter

Lee filter is dependent upon the variance of an area. If variance is low, smoothing will be performed. But if variance is high near edges, it will not be performed. Image can be approximated as given below:

Img (i,j) = I_m + W * (C_p − I_m)

{Where 'Img(i, j)'= Despeckled Image, 'I_m'= Mean Intensity Value, 'W' = Weighted Function, 'C_p'=Center Element in the Window}

Weighted function given as:Where 'σ^2' is the variance of the pixels values within the filter window i.e.

$$\sigma^2 = \left[1/N \sum_{i=0}^{N-1} (X_i)^2 \right]$$

{Where 'N' is the size of filter window, 'X_i' is the pixel value within the filter window at indices 'i'} and 'ρ^2' is the additive noise variance of the image given as:

$$\rho^2 = \left[1/M \sum_{i=0}^{N-1} (Y_i)^2 \right]$$

{Where 'M' is the size of the image, 'Y_i' is the value of each pixel in the image.}

Kuan Filter

The Kuan filter is considered more superior as compared to Lee filter. It does not make approximation on the noise variance within the filter window. It simply models the multiplicative noise i.e. speckle noise into an additive linear form, but it relies on the Equivalent Noise Look (ENL) from the image to determine a different weighted 'W' to perform the filtering (Gupta et al., 2004).

$W = (1 - C_u/C_i)(1 + C_u)$

The weighted function is computed from the estimated noise variation coefficient of the image, 'C_u' given as:

$C_u = \sqrt{1/ENL}$

And 'C_i' is the variation coefficient of the image given as:

$C_i = S/I_m$

Where 'S' is the standard deviation in filter window and 'I_m' is mean intensity value within the window.

Wiener Filter

Wiener is a low pass filter which is degraded by regular power additive noise. Wiener2 runs on the pixel wise adaptive Wiener method which is based on statistical information estimation from a local area neighborhood of every pixel. M = Wiener2(N,[i j], noise) filters the image where 'N' is pixel wise adaptive Wiener filtering, using neighborhoods of size i-by-j to calculate the local image mean and standard deviation. The default value for 'i' and 'j' is 3. The additive noise is assumed to be Gaussian White Noise. [M, noise] = Wiener2 (N, [i j]) also estimates the additive noise power before doing the filtering. Wiener2 returns this estimate in the form of noise. The Wiener2 function can be applied to a Wiener filter (a kind of linear filter) to an image adaptively, tailoring itself to the neighborhood image

Table 4. Comparison of diverse filtering techniques

Filters	Merits	Demerits	Properties
Median Filter	More robust, does not build any unrealistic pixel	More Computational Time	Edge preserves without blurring
Lee Filter	Speckle noise diminished	More computational time	Multiplicative filter
Kaun Filter	More efficient than lee filter	Noise still present on edges	ENL parameter needs to be computed
Wiener Filter	Superior for both noise removal and smoothing	Need to estimate power spectrum of original image	Trade off between inverse filtering and noise smoothing

variance. If the variance is large, Wiener2 performs little smoothness otherwise Wiener2 performs more smoothness (Kaur et al., 2016; Kaur et al., 2019).

FEATURE SELECTION

After all features are extracted from the image, the resultant data contains many redundant or irrelevant features. Features selection technique is used to remove those redundant and irrelevant features and to find the significant features, which are useful in further analysis. Feature selection is performed using Weka (Sharma et al., 2012) software of version 3.6.9. Weka is compatible with and recognizes only an '.arff' data files. Therefore, an '.arff' file is generated containing the value of extracted features including both normal and abnormal. In the feature extraction process, 16 features are extracted from each image but all of these features cannot be supplied to the neural network as the number of features is high. Although each feature is important in classification, only few of these features are very significant in classification and identification of the disease conditions. Therefore instead of using all of these features as input, only those features, which have high significance, are selected.

Classifier

In CAD system, classification among different domains is essential and its performance relies upon the effective performance of different characteristics and the classifier selection. Machine learning techniques in the field of medical imaging, computer vision, pattern recognition, etc can be used for classification. ANN is used for diagnosis of fetal development and acquiring substantial classification accuracy in daily activities. But it is presumed that ANN has definitely not revealed its advantage; therefore in this research work, ANN is enhanced with fuzzy logic and comparison of classification results is performed with ANN.

Artificial Neural Network (ANN)

A group of artificial neurons that are interconnected and utilize mathematical or computational models meant for processing the information based upon linked strategy is called as Neural Network (NN). ANN is a computational model that has the ability to map any kind of non-linear functional relationship between an input and an output to expected accuracy. This contains many processing units known as neurons and varies according to the linked information as well as the level of learning protocols used.

Multi-layer neural network is probably the most famous and straight-forward neural network. The neurons of the multi-layer feed forward NN are structured in 3 layers. In the first layer, the input nodes receive information from the outer world through a data file. In the second layer, the intermediate neurons found in several hidden layers enable non-linearity in the data processing. The third layer, i.e. the output layer, is actually utilized to give solution for any provided range of input values. In a fully connected ANN, every neuron inside a particular layer is actually linked to every neuron in the next layer by means of an associated weight "w(i,j)". Multi-Layer Perceptron (MLP) is commonly used like a classifier within the recognition involving patterns. The major disadvantage of MLP is that the back propagation algorithm utilizes a very long time throughout the training. The second issue is the network structure, i.e. there is no rule that enables a person to find the essential structure from a given application or training set. Figure 4 explains the working of ANN as a classifier, FC as Fuzzy Clustering Technique (Basheer & Hajmeer, 2000; Janghel et al., 2011).

Figure 4. A Schematic Diagram For A System Based On ANN

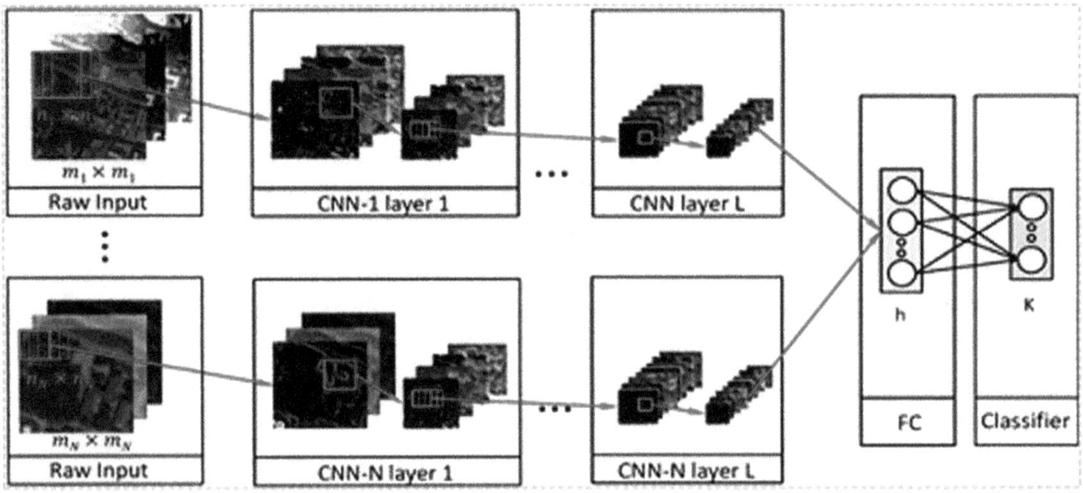

Neuro-Fuzzy

Integration of ANN with Fuzzy Inference System (FIS) has caught the attention of researchers from numerous scientific as well as engineering fields because smart systems can resolve real life issues. ANN learns from scratch through simply changing the interconnections among layers. Construction of FIS becomes easy when knowledge is conveyed within linguistic rules or with the help of fuzzy operators, fuzzy sets along with knowledge base. Likewise for building an ANN for an application the consumer must indicate the design as well as learning algorithm. The disadvantages associated with these methods appear complementary and hence it is obvious to think about developing an integrated system merging both the techniques. Though FIS offers the benefit of the ability to learn, the creation of linguistic rule is an advantage of ANN.

Neuro-fuzzy hybridization generates a hybrid smart system which synergizes both these methods by blending the human like reasoning ability of fuzzy systems with the learning and connectionist architecture of neural networks. Neuro-Fuzzy hybridization is referred as Fuzzy Neural Network (FNN) or Neuro-Fuzzy System (NFS). NFS includes the human like reasoning form of fuzzy systems by using fuzzy sets and a linguistic design composed of a set of IF-THEN fuzzy rules. The key strength of Neuro-Fuzzy systems is the universal approximates quality which has the capability to solicit interpretable IF-THEN rules. The effectiveness of Neuro-Fuzzy systems consists of two contradictory needs within fuzzy modeling, namely, interpretability versus accuracy, among which only one prevails. The Neuro-Fuzzy within fuzzy modeling study discipline is split among two areas: the Mamdani model, which is a linguistic fuzzy model centered on interpretability and the Takagi-Sugeno-Kang (TSK) model, which is a precise fuzzy model centered on accuracy (Janghel et al., 2011).

Proposed Methodology for Ultrasound Fetus Development

The proposed method is an extension of the algorithm given by (Kalyan et al., 2013) and includes a more extensive evaluation as well as a detailed feature analysis. The proposed methodology consists of four phases: A) Pre-Processing B) Feature Extraction and Selection C) Hybrid Approach Fuzzy-Neural-Genetic and D) Validation Result as shown in Figure 5.

In this application area, the acquisition of normal and abnormal fetal images is considered. Using MATLAB image processing toolbox, these images are then subjected to three different image pre-processing techniques, i.e. Denoising, Discrete Wavelet Transform, and Homomorphic NormalShrink Filtering Technique. The Region-of-Interest (ROI) from the acquired images is obtained. After image pre-processing, texture features like GLCM are extracted from the processed ultrasound images to compute the texture features. After extraction of features, feature selection method is used to obtain most significant and optimal features to depict the fetal characteristics. WEKA software is utilized within the feature selection phase to provide the selected significant features. These optimal features then act as an input to the Neuro-Fuzzy network for classification. Neuro-Fuzzy using genetic algorithm is employed for classifying the normal and abnormal fetal characteristics and also to determine which feature classifier is best for classification. The performance of the Neuro-Fuzzy based classifier is determined using Confusion Matrix (CM) and ROC curve analysis in Classification Learner (MATLAB).

Dataset

The experiment is performed on the online benchmark dataset available on http://www3.medical.philips.com and 12 real images collected from Civil Hospital, Jalandhar. Sample images are shown in the Figure 6.

IMAGE PRE-PROCESSING

The image pre-processing methods are used to get efficient results for further analysis. Three image pre-processing techniques such as Wavelet based Denoising, Homomorphic NormalShrink Filtering Technique based on 2-DWT (Two Discrete Wavelet Transform) are applied and then enhanced image cropping is applied. Cropping eliminates the undesirable parts of the image usually peripheral to the area of interest. The result is passed as an input to the feature extraction step.

Figure 5. Proposed Framework of Ultrasound Fetus Development

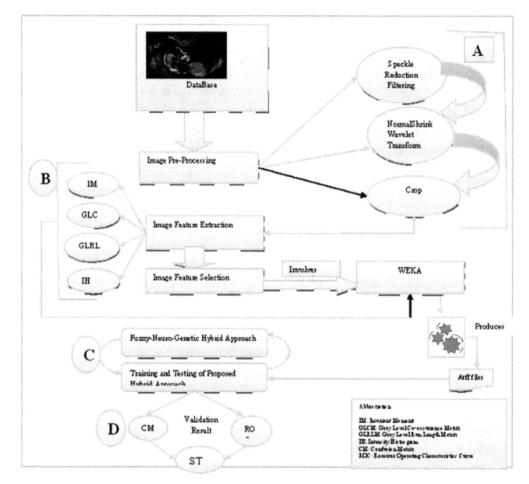

Wavelet Based Denoising

The steps explaining the Wavelet based Denosing of Medical Ultrasound fetal images as in Figure 7 are:

a)   Perform a suitable wavelet transform of the noisy data; (the wavelet basis may be chosen based on various factors including computational burden and ability to compress the Level 2 energy of the signal into a very few, very large coefficients).

b)   Perform a soft thresholding of the wavelet coefficients where the threshold depends on the noise variance (when the wavelet bases are chosen as in step 'a', thresholding kills the effect of the noise without killing the effect of the signal).

c)   The coefficients obtained from step 'b' are then padded with zeros to produce legitimate wavelet transform. These values are then inverted to obtain the signal estimate and the denoised output image (Gupta et al., 2007).

Figure 6. Database images (a) us_orig (b) us1 (c) us2 (d) us3

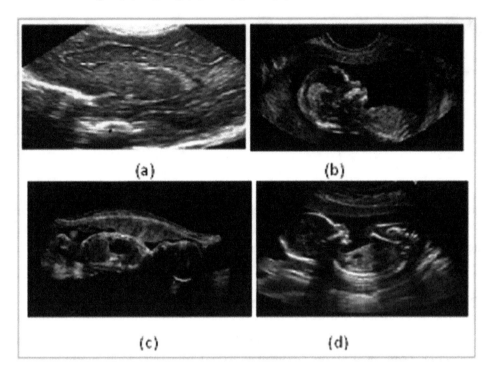

Figure 7. Wavelet Based Denoising

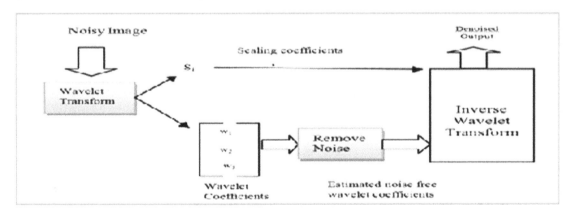

Implementation of 2d Wavelet Transform

The discrete wavelet transform (dwt) is identical to a hierarchical sub-band system where the sub- bands are logarithmically spaced in frequency and represent octave-band decomposition. By applying dwt, the image is actually divided i.e., decomposed into four sub-bands and critically sub-sampled as shown in figure 8:

Figure 8. Working Of 2dwt US Fetus Image

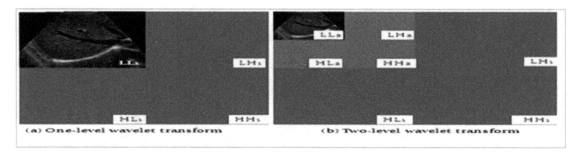

These sub-bands labeled LH1, HL1 and HH1 represent the finest scale wavelet coefficients i.e., detailed images while the sub-band LL1 corresponds to coarse level coefficients i.e., approximation image. To obtain the next coarse level of wavelet coefficients, the sub-band LL1 alone is further decomposed and critically sampled using similar filter bank.

Wavelet Based Homomorphic Normalshrink Technique

In the homomorphic techniques, the wavelet filtering is applied to the image-logarithm followed by an exponential operation. (Zong et al., 1996; Gupta et al., 2004) proposed a homomorphic wavelet shrinkage technique to separate the speckle noise from the original image.

NormalShrink is an adaptive threshold estimation method for image denoising in the wavelet domain based on the Generalized Gaussian Distribution (GGD) modelling of sub-band coefficients. It is computationally more efficient and adaptive because the parameters required for estimating the threshold depend on sub-band data.

The steps of NormalShrink for image denoising are as follows:

1) Take the logarithmic transform of the speckled image.
2) Perform multiscale decomposition of the image corrupted by Gaussian noise using wavelet transform.
3) Estimate the noise variance from subband HH1 using formula:

$$\hat{\sigma}^2 = \left[\frac{median\left(|Y_{ij}|\right)}{0.6745}\right]^2, \ 'Y_{ij}' \in subband \ HH_1 \quad \hat{\sigma}^2 = \left[\frac{median\left(|Y_{ij}|\right)}{0.6745}\right]^2, \ 'Y_{ij}' \in subband \ HH_1$$

4) For each level, compute the scale parameter 'β' using the equation:

$$\beta = \sqrt{\log\left(\frac{L_k}{J}\right)} \quad \beta = \sqrt{\log\left(\frac{L_k}{J}\right)}$$

5) For each sub-band (except the low pass residual):

   a)   Compute the standard deviation
   b)   Compute threshold T_N using equation
   c)   Apply soft thresholding to the noisy coefficients.
6)   Invert the multiscale decomposition to reconstruct denoised image
7)   Take the exponential of the reconstructed image obtained from step 6 (Gupta et al., 2007).

The image pre-processing work flow is analyzed in the Figure 9 which includes original benchmark image, ROI (Region of Interest) and the enhanced Normal Shrink Wavelet based filtered image.

Figure 9. Workflow of image preprocessing step, (a) original ultrasound image, (b) ROI image, (c) Enhanced NormalShrink Wavelet Cropped Image

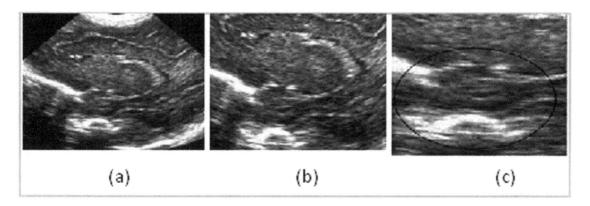

(a)　　　　　　(b)　　　　　　(c)

Feature Extraction Using Gray Level Co-Occurrence Matrix (GLCM)

GLCM is also referred as "Spatial Dependency". GLCM always accounts for the particular position of the pixel as compared to other pixel. Table 5 indicate the distinct combinations of pixel brightness values forms in medical images (Selvarajah & Kodituwakku, 2011; Poonguzhali & Ravindran, 2008).

Hybrid Neuro-Fuzzy-Genetic Approach

The detailed step-by-step methodology involved during the classification step using hybrid technique of Neuro-Fuzzy by Genetic approach is shown in Figure 10:

Training and Testing of Hybrid Approach

WEKA tool is used as a data mining process to make prediction on data. Neuro- Fuzzy using genetic algorithm is employed for classifying normal and abnormal fetal characteristics and also to determine which feature classifier is best for classification. Figure 11 determines the training, testing and predicted phases of the classification learner and the performance is validated in next phase using confusion matrix and ROC curve analysis.

Table 5. Features of GLCM

S.No	Name	Equation
1	Mean(μx,μy)	$\mu_x = \sum_{\hat{i}}\sum_{\Delta}\hat{i}.p_x\left(\hat{i},\Delta\right)$ $\mu_y = \sum_{\hat{i}}\sum_{\Delta}\Delta.p_x\left(\hat{i},\Delta\right)$
2	Standard Deviations	$\sigma_x = \sum_{\hat{i}}\sum_{\Delta}\left(\hat{i}-\mu\Delta\right)^2.p_x\left(\hat{i},\Delta\right)$ $\sigma_y = \sum_{\hat{i}}\sum_{\Delta}\left(\hat{i}-\mu y\right)^2.p_x\left(\hat{i},\Delta\right)$
3.	Autocorrelation	$f_1 = \sum_{\hat{i}}\sum_{\Delta}\left(\hat{i}\Delta\right).p_x\left(\hat{i},\Delta\right)$
4	Contrast	$f^2 = \sum_{n=0}^{N^9-1}n^2\{\sum_{\hat{i}=1}^{Ng}\sum_{\Delta=1}^{NG}p_x\left(\hat{i},\Delta\right)\mid\mid\hat{i}-\Delta\mid = n\}$
5	Correlation	$f_3 = \dfrac{\left[\sum\Delta\sum\Delta\left(\hat{i}\Delta\right)p_x\left(\hat{i},\Delta\right)-\mu x\mu y\right]}{\sigma x\sigma y}$
6	Cluster Shade	$f\Delta = \sum_{\hat{i}}\sum_{\Delta}\left(\hat{i}+\Delta-\mu x-\mu y\right)^3 p_x\left(\hat{i},\Delta\right)$
7	Dissimilarity	$f\Delta = \sum_{\hat{i}}\sum_{\Delta}\mid\hat{i}-l\mid.p_x\left(\hat{i},\Delta\right)$
8	Energy	$f\Delta = \sum_{\hat{i}}\sum_{\Delta}p_x\left(\hat{i},\Delta\right)^2$
9	Entropy	$f\Delta = \sum_{\hat{i}}\sum_{\Delta}p_x\left(\hat{i},\Delta\right)\log\left(p_x\left(\hat{i},\Delta\right)\right)$
10	Homogenecity	$f\Delta = \sum_{\hat{i}}\sum_{\Delta}\dfrac{1}{1+\left(\hat{i}+\Delta\right)^2}p_x\left(\hat{i},\Delta\right)$
11	Inverse Difference	Same as homogenecity

RESULTS AND FINDINGS RELATED TO ULTRASOUND FETUS DEVELOPMENT

The fetal development classification is carried out using WEKA. Four benchmark ultrasound images of human fetal available on http://www3.medical.philips.com as shown in (Figure 19) are used to carry out the pre-processing and feature extraction. Then, from the input, features extracted output perform the classification of fetal development. The proposed classification technique i.e. Hybrid (Neuro-Fuzzy using Genetic Algorithm) is compared with existing Artificial Neural Network (ANN) technique. The proposed system easily identifies the growth of fetal accurately.

Figure 10. Proposed Working of Hybrid Neuro-Fuzzy-Genetic Approach

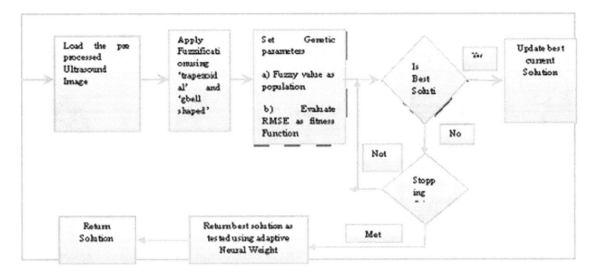

COMPARISON OF THE PROPOSED METHOD WITH EXISTING TECHNIQUE ON BENCHMARK IMAGES

The proposed method works using four benchmark fetal ultrasound images to obtain pre-processing results. Although, the number as well as dimensions of each image differs from the others, the proposed method effectively classifies abnormal and normal case. In the diagnosis of fetal development, accuracy of classification accuracy is essential because the consequences of an inappropriate diagnosis potentially result in health problems or even cause death. Table 6 shows the increase in average classification accuracy rate of different strategies. By utilizing only the shape features to differentiate fetal growth as normal or abnormal does not make classification accuracy more reliable. By integrating texture and shape characteristics or intensity and texture-shape characteristics maximum classification accuracy is achieved. The best rate of accuracy achieved during classification is 97% using Neuro-Fuzzy method. Hybrid technique provides maximum accuracy rate of classification, so it is most appropriate for CAD. To verify the efficiency of the proposed technique specificity, precision, sensitivity, recall, F-measure measures of all the techniques are computed as in Table 6. The values associated with sensitivity and specificity reveal one more way of the diagnosing accuracy that considers the variance in consequences of diagnostic. The performance of the system becomes better as the values of specificity and sensitivity becomes larger. The values of sensitivity and specificity represent that acquisition using proposed technique is larger among different methods. ROC curve is utilized for evaluating the accuracy which is shown in the Figure 12 and listed in Table 6. The superiority of proposed method over the existing ones is proved.

Analysis of the Proposed Method and Results of Existing Classifiers

The performance of the Neuro-Fuzzy is calculated by evaluating confusion matrix and ROC curve. The result shown in Table 7 represents the comparison in the performance of the proposed technique with existing one. The proposed technique extracts the abnormal cases accurately and more effectively along with the minimized False Positive (FP) rates information.

Figure 11. Working of Training, Testing and Prediction of Classification Learner

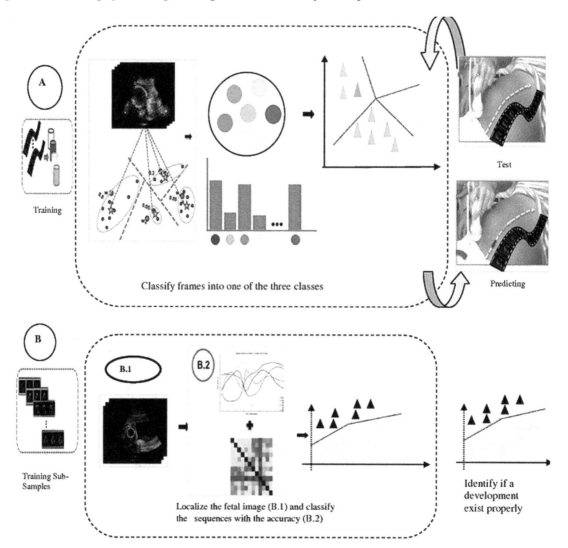

Assessment Measures

Matrix in Table 8 and Table 9 illustrates the actual versus the predicted class in classification problems represented in standard terms and for Benchmark Ultrasound Images respectively. Each column represents the instances in an actual class and rows represent the instances in a predicted class. True positives (TP) and true negatives (TN) show the number of samples correctly classified in the positive and negative classes, while false positives (FP) and false negatives (FN) represent the number of misclassified positive and negative examples respectively.

Table 6. Accuracy Evaluation Metrics of Existing ANN and Proposed (Hybrid) Technique of Benchmark Images

S.No	Image name	Accuracy (%)	TP Rate (%)	FP Rate (%)	Precision (%)	Recall (%)	F-Measure (%)	ROC Area (%)
\multicolumn{9}{c}{Existing ANN classification Technique}
1	Us_orig	85.38	0.853	0.073	0.898	0.853	0.846	0.89
2	Us1	89.30	0.893	0.053	0.907	0.893	0.892	0.92
3	Us2	86.7	0.867	0.067	0.879	0.867	0.865	0.9
4	Us3	89.3	0.893	0.053	0.919	0.893	0.891	0.92
\multicolumn{9}{c}{Proposed Hybrid (Neuro-Fuzzy using Genetic Approach) Classification Technique}
S.NO	Image name	Accuracy (%)	TP Rate (%)	FP Rate (%)	Precision (%)	Recall (%)	F-Measure (%)	ROC Area (%)
1	Us_orig	**97.30**	**0.973**	**0.013**	**0.975**	**0.973**	**0.973**	**0.999**
2	Us1	**90.70**	**0.907**	**0.047**	**0.917**	**0.907**	**0.906**	**0.99**
3	Us2	**93.3**	**0.933**	**0.033**	**0.934**	**0.933**	**0.933**	**0.994**
4	Us3	**94.7**	**0.947**	**0.027**	**0.947**	**0.947**	**0.947**	**0.995**

Table 7. Comparison of Classification Algorithm

Classifier Name	Artificial Neural Network (%)	Neuro- Fuzzy using Genetic (%)
Correctly classified instances	90.6667% 68	93.3333% 70
Incorrectly classified instances	9.3333% 7	6.6667 5

Table 8. Confusion Matrix

		Actual Class	
		Negative	Positive
Predicted Class	Negative	True Negative rate(TN)	False Negative Rate (FN)
	Positive	True positive rate(TP)	False Positive rate(FP)

Table 9. Confusion Matrix of Benchmark Ultrasound Images

		Actual Class	
		Negative	Positive
Predicted Class	Negative	68	70
	Positive	7	5

Accuracy

Accuracy represents how many predictions of the classifier are in fact correct, whereas the error rate is the percentage of misclassified examples in total. The accuracy or error might not be appropriate performance measure for imbalanced datasets where the class priors are very different because they will be strongly biased toward the majority class. The comparison in Figure 12 shows the accuracy of four benchmark images with the existing and the proposed technique.

$$\text{Accuracy} = \frac{TP + TN}{TP + TN + FP + FN}$$

Figure 12. Comparison graph depicting Accuracy of Benchmark Images

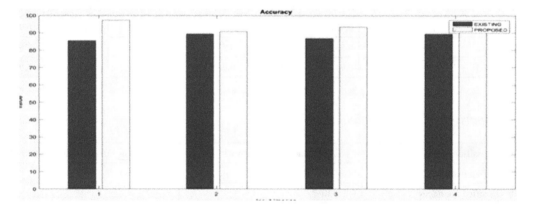

Recall or Sensitivity

Recall represents how many positive examples the classifier is able to correctly identify (in the recurrence problem, the percentage of patients with recurrence identified as such). Figure 13 and Figure 14 show the comparison between the existing and the proposed rate of sensitivity for different ultrasound images where as recall= sensitivity.

Specificity

Specificity represents how accurately the classifier behaves in terms of predicting the negative class (in the recurrence problem, this is the percentage of patients without recurrence identified as such)

$$\text{Specificity} = \frac{TN}{TN + FP}$$

Figure 13. Comparison Graph Depicting the Recall of Benchmark Images

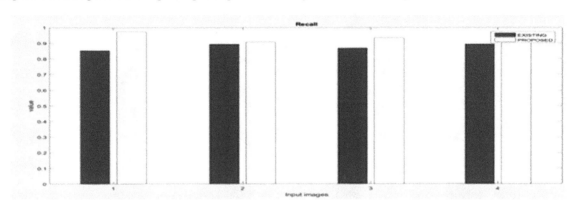

Figure 14. Comparison Graph Depicting the TPR of Benchmark Images

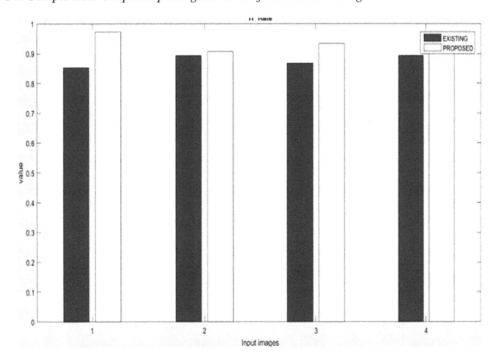

Precision

Precision shows the proportion of the correctly predicted positive cases relative to all the predicted positive ones (during the recurrence problem, this is the percentage of patients identified as actually being recur) as in Figure 15.

$$\text{Precision} = \frac{TP}{TP + FP}$$

Figure 15. Comparison graph depicting the Precision of Benchmark Images

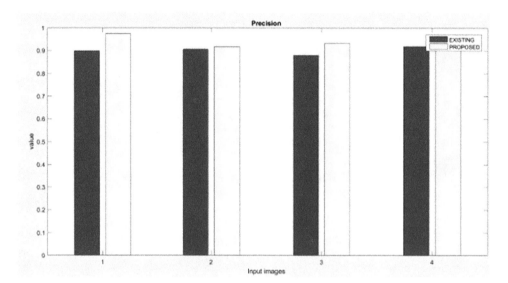

F-Measure

F-Measure is defined as the harmonic mean of precision and recall, providing a balance between both of them. It reflects the better performance of a classifier in the presence of an underrepresented class. Figure 16 shows the comparison of F-measure rate of benchmark fetal ultrasound images.

$$\textbf{F-measure} = \frac{\textbf{2TP}}{\textbf{2TP} + \textbf{FP} + \textbf{FN}}$$

Figure 16. Comparison graph depicting F-Measure of Benchmark Images

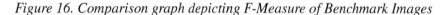

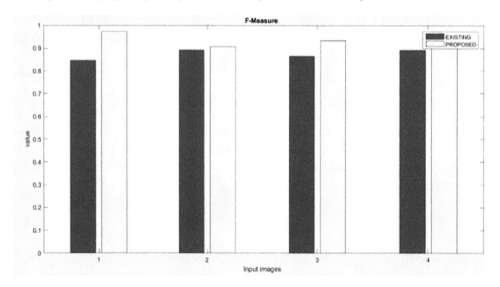

Fall Out or False Positive (FP) rate

FP rate is defined as the probability of falsely rejecting the null hypothesis for a particular test. Figure 17 shows the comparison between FP rate between existing and proposed technique.

Fall out= 1- specificity

Figure 17. Comparison graph depicting the FPR

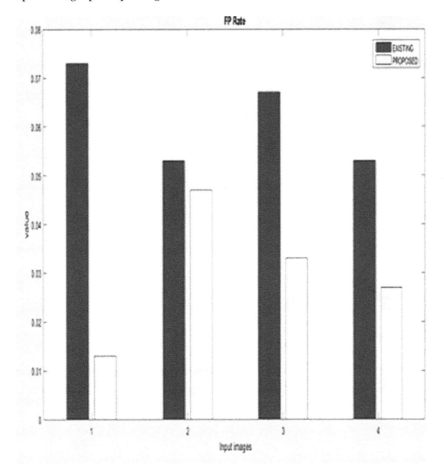

ROC Curve

The ROC curve is utilized in computing the predictive accuracy of the proposed model. This signifies the TP ratio as well as FP ratio. The region within the ROC curve is called Area Under Curve (AUC) i.e. the category among the finest techniques for comparing classifiers within two issues. The test outcomes perform better when the ROC curve goes up rapidly in the direction of upper left corner of the graph else when the value of AUC is greater. Region near 1 demonstrates the reliable examination while region near 0.5 indicates the unreliable evaluation. Figure 18 depicts the ROC area comparison between existing and proposed techniques.

Figure 18. Comparison graph depicting the ROC Area

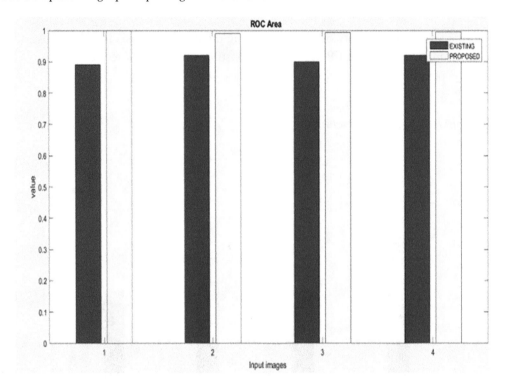

Experimental Setup and Performance Evaluation of Live Dataset

This section represents the experimental setup and discusses the performance evaluation of the proposed system. The dataset of benchmark fetal ultrasound is used publicly for experimental study and research. The live dataset is collected from **Civil Hospital, Jalandhar, Punjab** and 12 live fetal images are considered using the proposed scenario. Three live dataset results are included in the research work along with the online benchmark images. Experimental section includes sub-sections of datasets, pre-processed results and evaluation metrics, Feature extracted results (GLCM, GLRLM, Invariant Histrogram) out of which only GLCM results are shown using proposed and base result comparison. Validation result using Classification Learner is discussed in next section.

Dataset

All B-mode ultrasound images are collected from Civil Hospital Jalandhar. The patients' data report and their ultrasound images are initially analyzed and the images are shortlisted on the basis of the most prevalent fetal growth time period amongst the acquired data, age of the patient and time of pregnancy. Total of 12 fetal ultrasonic images selected (5 Normal cases and 5 Abnormal cases) of fetal growth. Figure 19 includes the four benchmark images and 12 real images.

Figure 19. Benchmark and Live Ultrasound Fetus Development Dataset

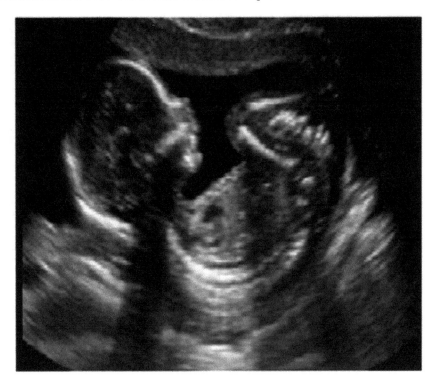

Pre-Processed State-of-Art Filtering Mechanism

The pre-processed mechanism includes the comparison of various basic filtering techniques i.e. Median, Wiener, Kuan with the Normal Shrink Filtering which is passed as input to the next step. Figure 20, Figure 21, Figure 22 and Figure 23 show the qualitative analysis between proposed NormalShrink Homomorphic and basic filtering techniques of benchmark images. The qualitative interpretation results in Figure 24, Figure 25 and Figure 26 predict that in real dataset the Normal Shrink Filtering Mechanism is better as compare to the basic Filtering Techniques Median, Wiener and Kuan Respectively.

Quantitative Result of Pre-Processing Parameter

The various quality metrics which can be used are as follow:

Peak Signal- to-Noise Ratio(PSNR)

This parameter computes the peak signal to rebuilt image called peak signal–to-noise. An input image, ' $\widehat{f}_n(a,b)$ ' provides n*m pixels along with rebuilt image ' $\widehat{F}_n(a,b)$ '. Where ' $\widehat{F}_n$ ' is a rebuilt through decoding the encoding type ' $\widehat{f}_n(a,b)$ ' error parameter computed for the luminance transmission simply therefore the pixels valuation range among black (0) as well as white (225). Mean Absolute Error (MAE) from the rebuilt image can be computed as defined as follows:

Figure 20. Benchmark Image of Different Filtering Mechanism As Compared To Normalshrink

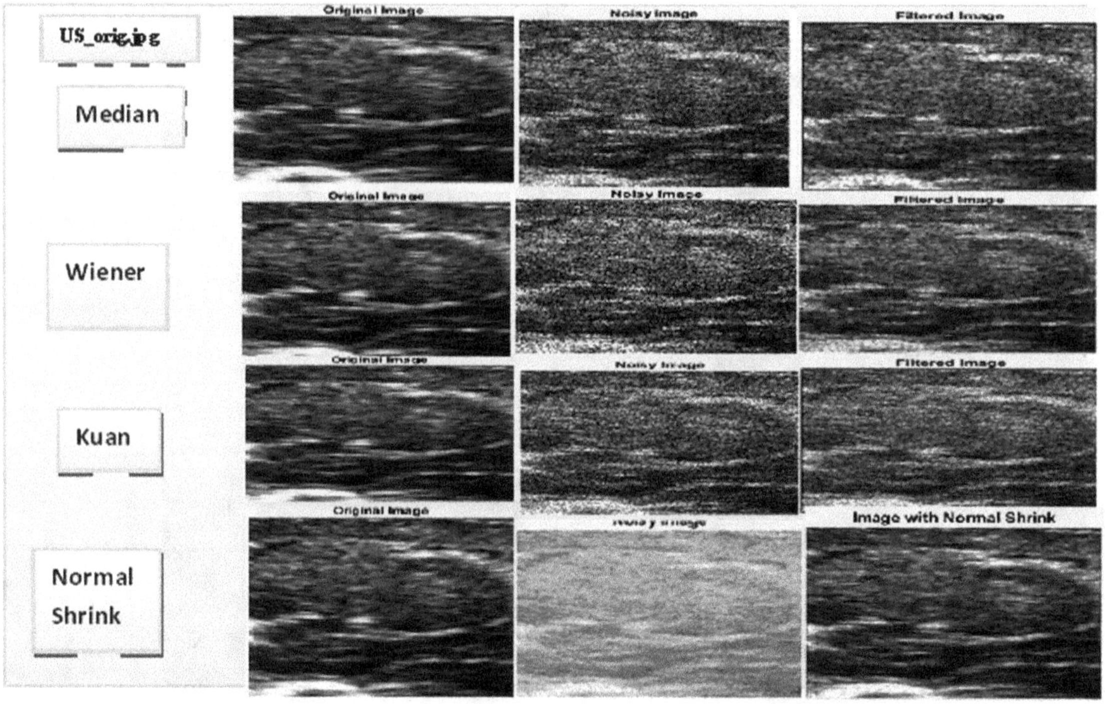

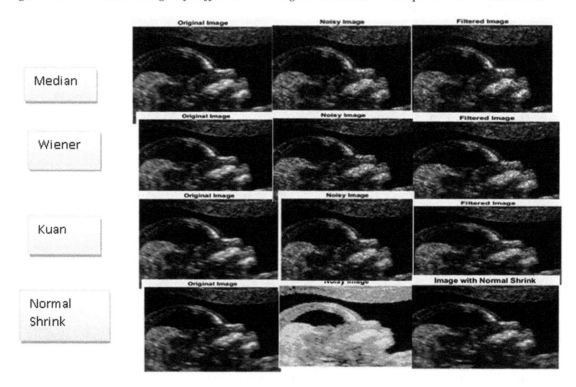

Figure 21. Benchmark Image Of Different Filtering Mechanism As Compared To Normalshrink

Figure 22. Benchmark Image Of Different Filtering Mechanism As Compared To Normalshrink

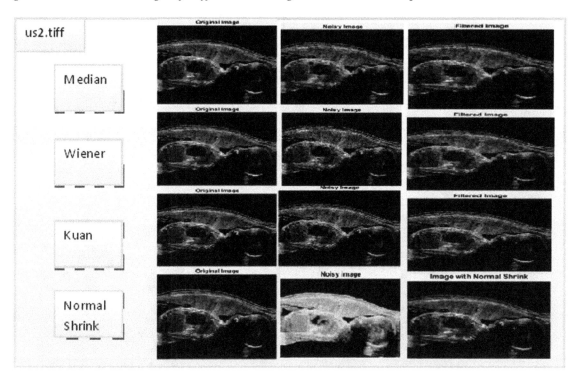

Figure 23. Benchmark Image Of Different Filtering Mechanism As Compared To Normalshrink

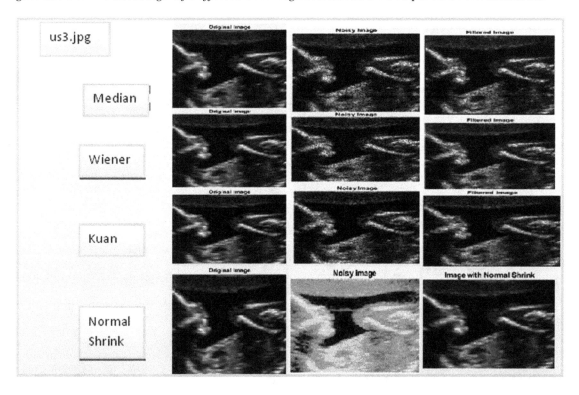

Figure 24. Live Dataset Image of different Filtering Mechanism as compared to NormalShrink

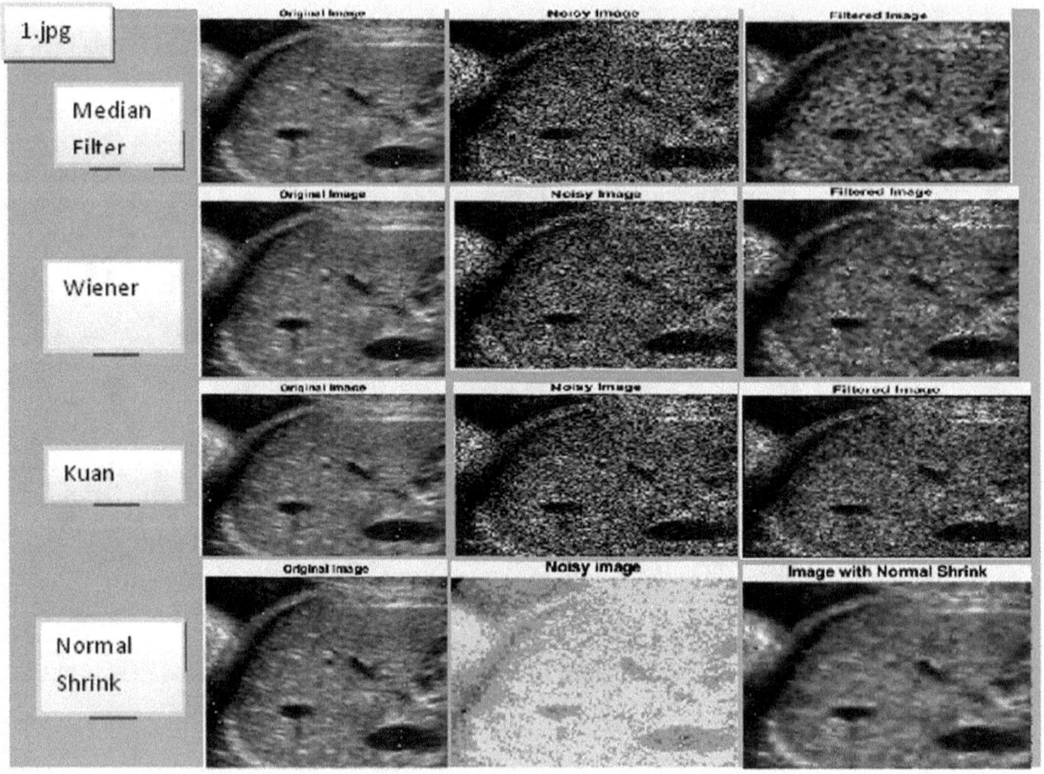

Figure 25. Live Dataset Image of different Filtering Mechanism as compared to NormalShrink

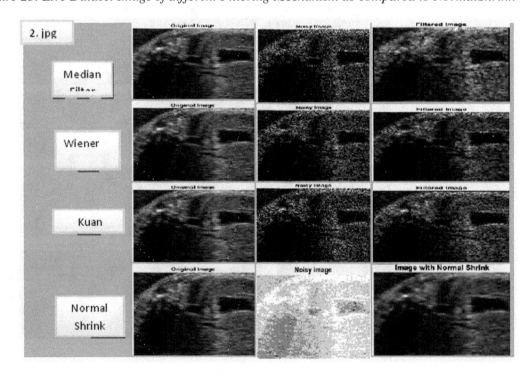

Figure 26. Live Dataset Image of different Filtering Mechanism as compared to NormalShrink

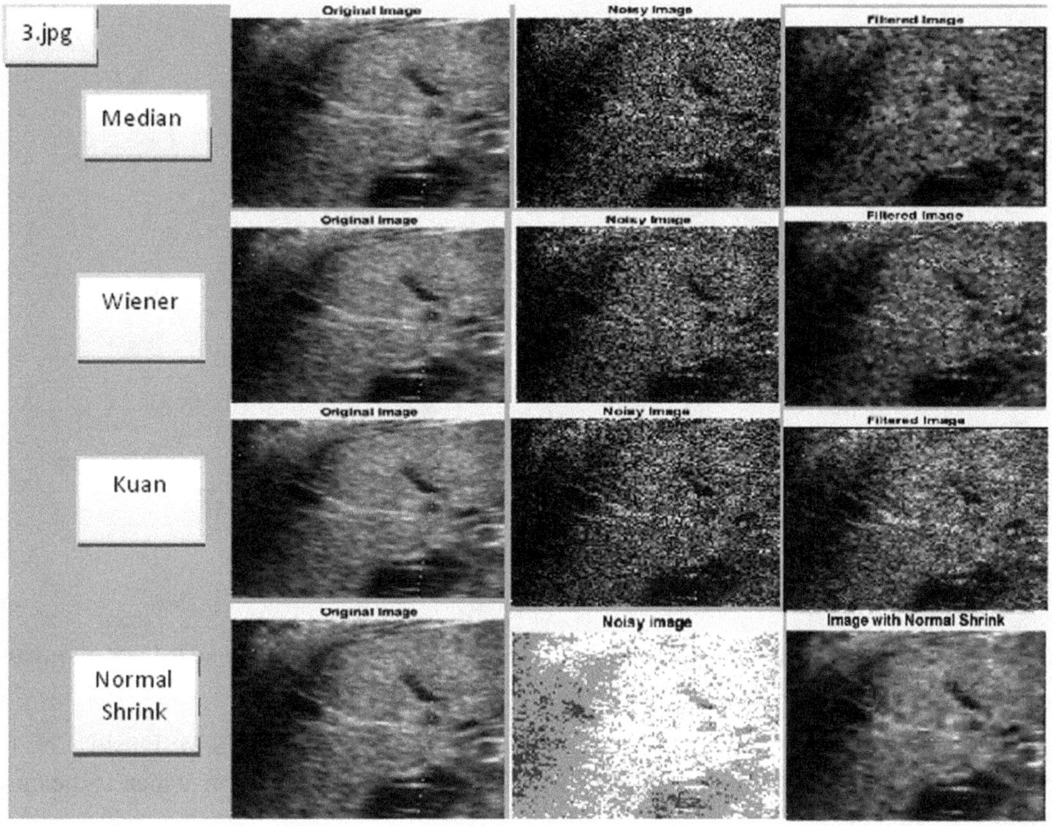

PSNR can be calculated using the following formula:

Signal-to-Noise Ratio(SNR)

$$SNR = 10\log 10\left(\frac{\sigma_g^2}{\sigma_e^2}\right)$$

Where 'σ_g^2' is variance of noise-free reference image, 'σ_e^2' is variance of error between the original and denoised image.

Mean Square Error (S/MSE)

$$MSE = \frac{1}{MN}\sum_{x=1}^{M}\sum_{y=1}^{N}\left[F(x,y)-I(x,y)\right]^2$$

Where 'I' is original image with dimensions M×N, 'N' is noisy image N and 'F' is denoised image.

Coefficient of Correlation(CoC)

$$CoC = \frac{\varepsilon\left(g - \bar{g}\right).\left(\hat{g} - \overline{\hat{g}}\right)}{\sqrt{\varepsilon\left(\Delta g - \overline{\Delta g}\right)^2 .\varepsilon\left(\Delta g - \overline{\Delta \hat{g}}\right)}}$$

Where ' $\bar{g}$ ' is mean of original image, ' $\overline{\hat{g}}$ ' is mean of denoised image.

Edge Preservation Index (EPI)

$$EPI = \frac{\varepsilon\left(\Delta g - \overline{\Delta g}\right).\left(\Delta \hat{g} - \overline{\Delta \hat{g}}\right)}{\sqrt{\varepsilon\left(\Delta g - \overline{\Delta g}\right)^2 .\varepsilon\left(\Delta g - \overline{\Delta \hat{g}}\right)}}$$

Where ' Δg ' is high pass filtered version of 'g' obtained with a 3*3 pixel standard approximation of Laplacian operator and ' $\overline{\Delta g}$ ', ' $\overline{\Delta \hat{g}}$ ' are mean of original and denoised image.

Table 10 analyses proves quantitatively using various metrics PSNR, SNR, S/MSE, EPI, CoC that in benchmark images and in live dataset, Normal Shrink is better than other filters which is the outcome of the pre-processed step.

Graphical Representation from Figures 27 to Figure 33 proves that PSNR is better in Normal Shrink than other filters. Greater the value of PSNR, better is the quality of the image as proved by Normal Shrink. As the value of SNR is larger, filter performance is better. The value of S/MSE should be low. The range of EPI and CoC lies between 0 and 1. Nearer to 1 proves better filter quality. In all the benchmark and live dataset, the value of SNR is more in case of Normal Shrink. S/MSE value is low whereas EPI and CoC value is nearer to 1 in NormalShrink as compared to other filtering technique i.e. proved quantitatively.

Feature Extraction (GLCM)

The feature extraction step includes four types i.e. GLCM, GLRLM, IH and IM. Only GLCM parametric results are included in this research work which is reflected in Table 11 and Table 12 for benchmark and live dataset respectively on the basis of existing method (ANN) and proposed method (Neuro-Fuzzy-Genetic).

The value in the variation is graphically proved from Figure 34 to Figure 40 using GLCM metrics in existing and proposed methods. The value of Root Mean Square Error (R/MSE) is decreased from existing ANN to proposed hybrid method, improvement in images are correctly instanced.

Table 10. Comparison of Spatial Filters with Homomorphic Filters

Filters \ Metrics	PSNR	SNR	S/MSE	EPI	CoC
US_Orig.jpg					
Median Filter	28.3459	4.2805	4.2805	-0.068695	0.797066
WienerFilter	29.2877	5.22234	5.22234	0.232257	0.840967
Kuan Filter	28.0519	3.98648	3.98648	0.126449	0.764639
NormalShrink	**30.9585**	**6.89313**	**6.89313**	**0.589181**	**0.941745**
Us1.jpg					
Median Filter	31.0319	5.41095	5.41095	0.0560177	0.949826
Wiener Filter	32.0089	6.38791	6.38791	0.153288	0.972189
Kuan Filter	31.4114	5.79046	5.79046	0.0817777	0.950076
NormalShrink	**34.6508**	**9.02986**	**9.02986**	**0.441993**	**0.986621**
US2.tiff					
Median Filter	32.2703	5.03807	5.03807	0.148425	0.978875
Wiener Filter	33.0217	5.78945	5.78945	0.226896	0.991976
Kuan Filter	33.224	5.99178	5.99178	0.278649	0.98501
NormalShrink	**34.7356**	**7.50337**	**7.50337**	**0.515596**	**0.991587**
US3.jpg					
Median Filter	30.5513	5.6013	5.6013	-0.107844	0.921417
Wiener Filter	31.763	6.81303	6.81303	0.195956	0.954831
Kuan Filter	30.6194	5.66935	5.66935	0.0842285	0.922236
NormalShrink	**34.3485**	**9.39854**	**9.39854**	**0.575885**	**0.983805**
1.jpg					
Median Filter	28.6272	4.54401	4.54401	-0.0867276	0.84789
Wiener Filter	29.5494	5.46615	5.46615	0.256514	0.856176
Kuan Filter	28.2915	4.2083	4.2083	0.104104	0.801264
NormalShrink	**31.1244**	**7.04117**	**7.04117**	**0.558952**	**0.941073**
2. jpg					
Median Filter	29.5463	5.45948	5.45948	-0.101541	0.890979
Wiener Filter	30.8996	6.81279	6.81279	0.322695	0.905894
Kuan Filter	29.2986	5.21177	5.21177	0.125384	0.85967
NormalShrink	**32.9776**	**8.89079**	**8.89079**	**0.633292**	**0.971189**
3.jpg					
Median Filter	28.9064	4.8403	4.8403	-0.12006	0.881449
Wiener Filter	29.9107	5.84462	5.84462	0.243092	0.894937
Kuan Filter	28.4418	4.37578	4.37578	0.0504628	0.832113
NormalShrink	**31.9488**	**7.88275**	**7.88275**	**0.58338**	**0.971514**

Figure 27. Graphical representation of pre-processing quantitative measure of benchmark image

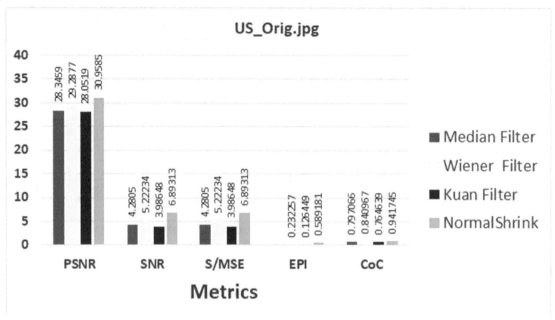

Figure 28. Graphical representation of pre-processing quantitative measure of benchmark image

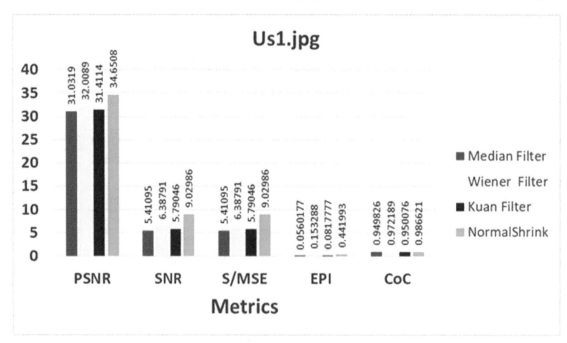

Figure 29. Graphical representation of pre-processing quantitative measure of benchmark image

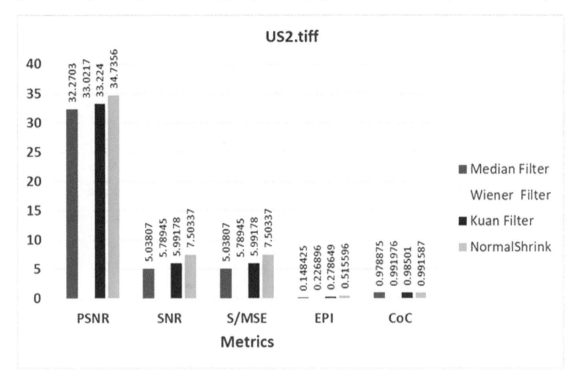

Figure 30. Graphical representation of pre-processing quantitative measure of benchmark image

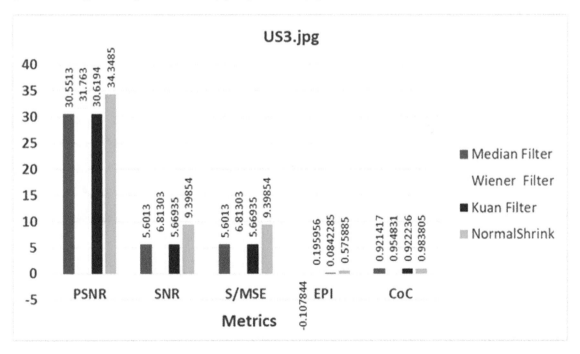

Figure 31. Graphical representation of pre-processing quantitative measure of live image

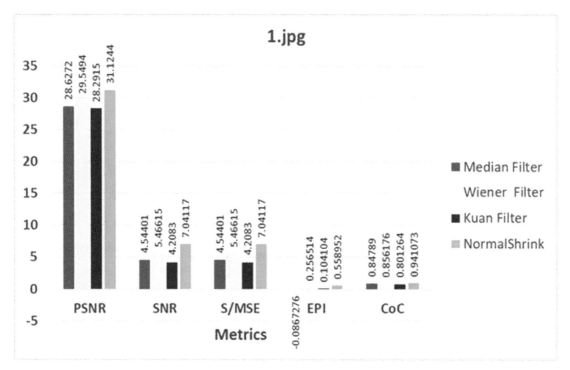

Figure 32. Graphical representation of pre-processing quantitative measure of live image

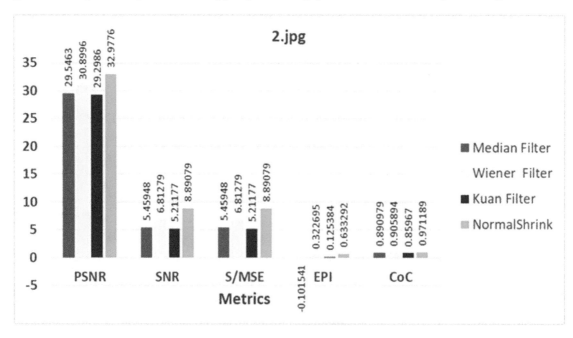

Figure 33. Graphical representation of pre-processing quantitative measure of live image

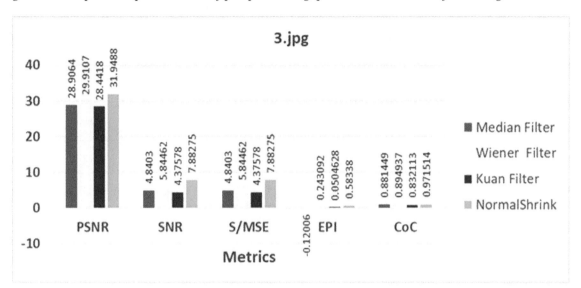

Table 11. Comparison of Existing ANN Technique with Proposed (Hybrid) Approach for Benchmark Dataset

Images	Correctly Classified Instances	Incorrectly Classified Instances	Kappa statistic	Mean absolute error	Root mean squared error	Relative absolute error	Root relative squared error	Coverage of cases (0.95 level)	Mean rel. region size (0.95 level)"
Benchmark ANN Existing Confusion Matrix Parameters									
Us_orig	70 93.3333%	5 6.6667%	0.9	0.0598	0.2075	13.4615%	44.0212%	93.3333%	33.3333%
Us1	70 93.3333%	5 6.6667%	0.9	0.0598	0.2075	13.4615%	44.0212%	93.3333%	33.3333%
Us2	64 85.3333%	11 14.6667%	0.78	0.1111	0.3072	25%	65.158%	85.3333%	85.3333%
Us3	70 93.3333%	5 6.6667%	0.9	0.0598	0.2075	13.4615%	44.0212%	93.3333%	33.3333%
Benchmark Proposed (Hybrid) Confusion Matrix Parameters									
Us_orig	72 96%	3 4%	0.94	0.0404	0.1558	9.0981%	33.0592%	97.3333%	36%
Us1	72 96%	3 4%	0.94	0.0404	0.1558	9.0981%	33.0592%	97.3333%	36%
Us2	68 90.6667%	7 9.3333%	0.86	0.0691	0.1971	15.5412%	41.8012%	100%	39.5556%
Us3	72 96%	3 4%	0.94	0.0404	0.1558	9.0981%	33.0592%	97.3333%	36%

Table 12. Comparison of Existing ANN Technique with Proposed (Hybrid) Approach for Live Dataset

Images	Correctly Classified Instances	Incorrectly Classified Instances	Kappa statistic	Mean absolute error	Root Mean Squared Error (R/MSE)	Relative absolute error	Root relative squared error	Coverage of cases (0.95 level)	Mean rel. region size (0.95 level)"
Live Dataset Existing ANN Confusion Matrix Parameters									
1.jpg	65 86.6667%	10 13.3333%	0.8	0.1026	0.2929	23.0769%	62.1365%	86.6667%	33.3333%
2.jpg	70 93.3333%	5 6.6667%	0.9	0.0598	0.2075	13.4615%	44.0212%	93.3333%	33.3333%
3.jpg	70 93.3333%	5 6.6667%	0.9	0.0598	0.2075	13.4615%	44.0212%	93.3333%	33.3333%
Live Dataset Proposed (Hybrid) Confusion Matrix Parameters									
1.jpg	68 90.6667%	7 9.3333%	0.86	0.0725	0.1925	16.3143%	40.8428%	98.6667%	41.7778%
2.jpg	72 96%	3 4%	0.94	0.0404	0.1558	9.0981%	33.0592%	97.3333%	36%
3.jpg	72 96%	3 4%	0.94	0.0404	0.1558	9.0981%	33.0592%	97.3333%	36%

Figure 34. Graphical Interpretation of the proposed method with existing ANN technique of Benchmark Image

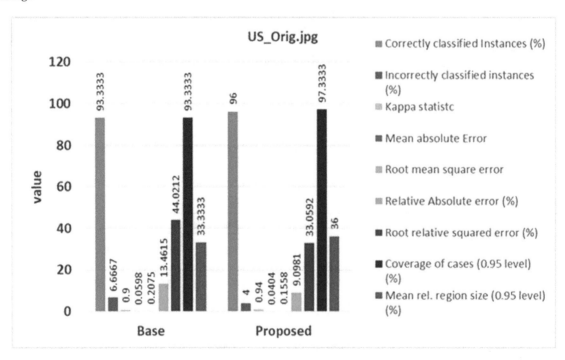

Figure 35. Graphical Interpretation of the proposed method with existing ANN technique of Benchmark Image

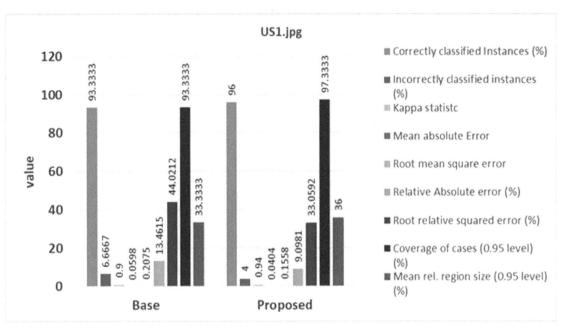

Figure 36. Graphical Interpretation of the proposed method with existing ANN technique of Benchmark Image

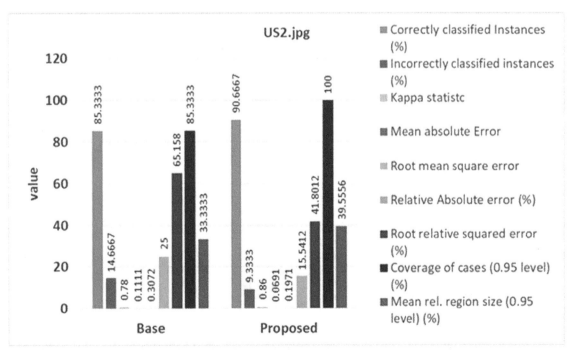

Figure 37. Graphical Interpretation of the proposed method with existing ANN technique of Benchmark Image

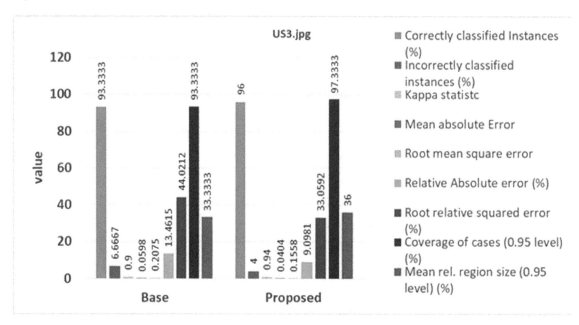

Figure 38. Graphical Interpretation of the proposed method with existing ANN Accuracy Parameters of Live Dataset

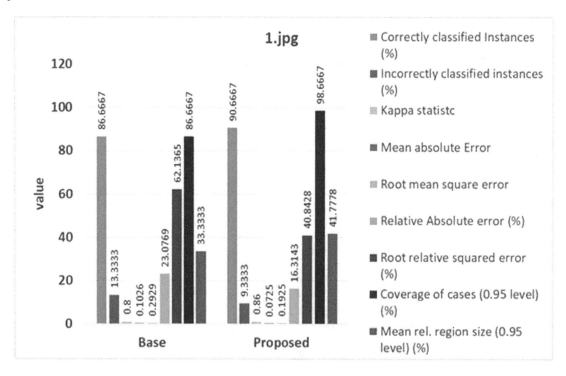

Figure 39. Graphical Interpretation of the proposed method with existing ANN Accuracy Parameters of Live Dataset

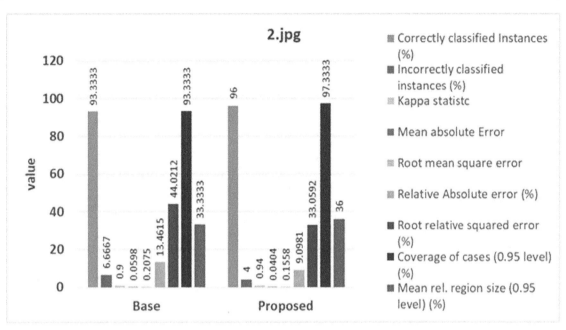

Figure 40. Graphical Interpretation of the proposed method with existing ANN Accuracy Parameters of Live Dataset

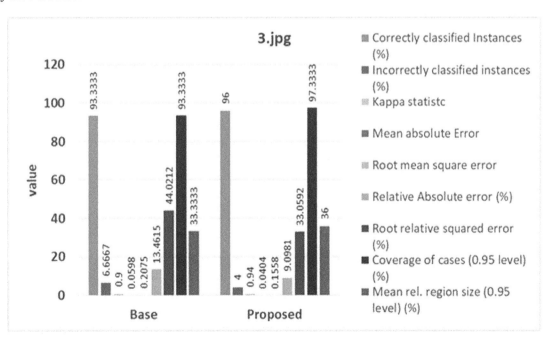

Confusion Matrix and ROC

The existing technique (ANN) and proposed (Neuro-Fuzzy-Genetic) approach results are compared using Confusion matrix, ROC curve and accuracy parameters TP, FP, Precision, Recall, F- Measure and ROC Area as described in Table 13 and Table 14 for benchmark and live dataset respectively. Table 15 represents the class instances result on correctly and incorrectly prediction.

Table 13. Comparison of Accuracy Evaluation of Existing and Proposed Method of benchmark images

Benchmark Existing ANN Accuracy						
Images	TP Rate	FP Rate	Precision	Recall	F-Measure	ROC Area
Us_orig	0.933	0.033	0.944	0.933	0.933	0.95
Us1	0.933	0.033	0.944	0.933	0.933	0.95
Us2	0.853	0.073	0.898	0.853	0.846	0.890
Us3	0.933	0.033	0.944	0.933	0.933	0.95
Benchmark Proposed(Hybrid) Accuracy						
Us_orig	**0.96**	**0.02**	**0.96**	**0.96**	**0.96**	**0.988**
Us1	**0.96**	**0.02**	**0.96**	**0.96**	**0.96**	**0.988**
Us2	**0.907**	**0.047**	**0.91**	**0.907**	**0.906**	**0.993**
Us3	**0.96**	**0.02**	**0.96**	**0.96**	**0.96**	**0.988**

Table 14. Comparison of Accuracy Evaluation of Existing and Proposed Method of live images

Live Dataset Existing ANN Accuracy						
Images	TP Rate	FP Rate	Precision	Recall	F-Measure	ROC Area
1.jpg	0.867	0.067	0.905	0.867	0.861	0.9
2.jpg	0.933	0.033	0.944	0.933	0.933	0.95
3.jpg	0.933	0.033	0.944	0.933	0.933	0.95
Live Dataset Proposed (Hybrid) Accuracy						
1.jpg	**0.907**	**0.047**	**0.927**	**0.907**	**0.905**	**0.997**
2.jpg	**0.96**	**0.02**	**0.96**	**0.96**	**0.96**	**0.988**
3.jpg	**0.96**	**0.02**	**0.96**	**0.96**	**0.96**	**0.988**

STATISTICAL ANALYSIS USING CLASSIFICATION LEARNER

Classification Learner is used to train the models using different classification algorithms such as decision tree, Support Vector Machine (SVM), Linear Discriminant Analysis (LDA), K- Nearest Neighbour (KNN), Naive Bayes (NB) and Ensemble Boosted Classification. These algorithms are used in this medical application area to validate the proposed workflow using 10 fold cross-validation methods (Kaur et al., 2019a). Let us have a brief discussion about these algorithms.

Table 15. Correctly and Incorrectly Instances in Confusion Matrix

	Base	Proposed
Us_orig.jpg	"a b c <-- classified as" 25 0 0 l a = 1 0 25 0 l b = 2 0 18 7 l c = 3	"a b c <-- classified as" 25 0 0 l a = 1 0 25 0 l b = 2 0 8 17 l c = 3
Us1.jpg	"a b c <-- classified as" 25 0 0 l a = 1 0 25 0 l b = 2 0 5 20 l c = 3	"a b c <-- classified as" 25 0 0 l a = 1 0 23 2 l b = 2 0 1 24 l c = 3
Us2.jpg	"a b c <-- classified as" 25 0 0 l a = 1 0 25 0 l b = 2 0 11 14 l c = 3	"a b c <-- classified as" 25 0 0 l a = 1 0 23 2 l b = 2 0 5 20 l c = 3
Us3.jpg	"a b c <-- classified as" 25 0 0 l a = 1 0 25 0 l b = 2 0 5 20 l c = 3	"a b c <-- classified as" 25 0 0 l a = 1 0 23 2 l b = 2 0 1 24 l c = 3
1.jpg	"a b c <-- classified as" 25 0 0 l a = 1 0 25 0 l b = 2 0 10 15 l c = 3	"a b c <-- classified as" 25 0 0 l a = 1 0 25 0 l b = 2 0 7 18 l c = 3
2.jpg	"a b c <-- classified as" 25 0 0 l a = 1 0 25 0 l b = 2 0 5 20 l c = 3	"a b c <-- classified as" 25 0 0 l a = 1 0 23 2 l b = 2 0 1 24 l c = 3
3.jpg	"a b c <-- classified as" 25 0 0 l a = 1 0 25 0 l b = 2 0 5 20 l c = 3	"a b c <-- classified as" 25 0 0 l a = 1 0 23 2 l b = 2 0 1 24 l c = 3

Figure 41. Graphical Interpretation of the proposed (Hybrid) Accuracy parameters with existing ANN technique of benchmark dataset

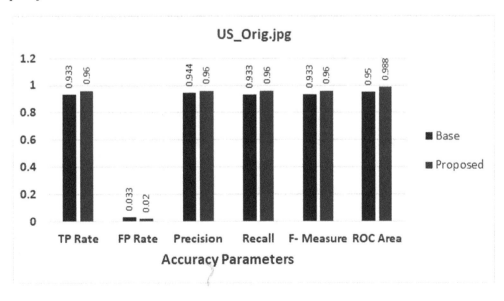

Figure 42. Graphical Interpretation of the proposed (Hybrid) Accuracy parameters with existing ANN technique of benchmark dataset

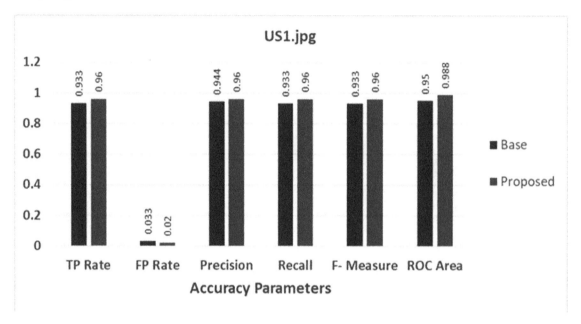

Figure 43. Graphical Interpretation of the proposed (Hybrid) Accuracy parameters with existing ANN technique of benchmark dataset

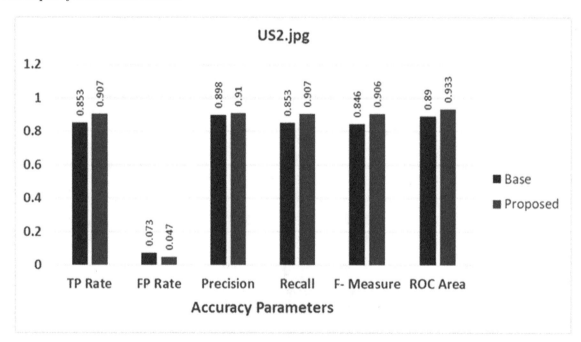

Figure 44. Graphical Interpretation of the proposed (Hybrid) Accuracy parameters with existing ANN technique of benchmark dataset

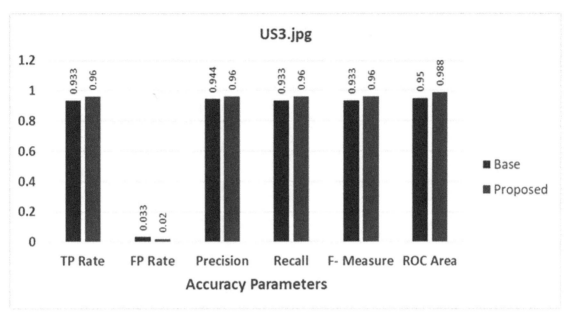

Figure 45. Graphical Interpretation of the proposed (Hybrid) Accuracy parameters with existing ANN technique of live dataset

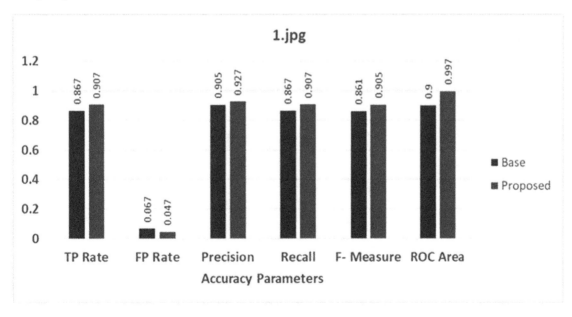

Figure 46. Graphical Interpretation of the proposed (Hybrid) Accuracy parameters with existing ANN technique of live dataset

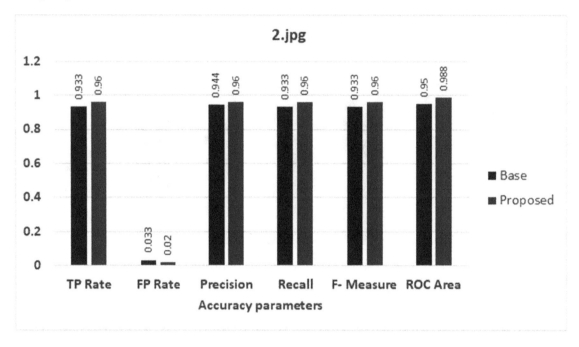

Figure 47. Graphical Interpretation of the proposed (Hybrid) Accuracy parameters with existing ANN technique of live dataset

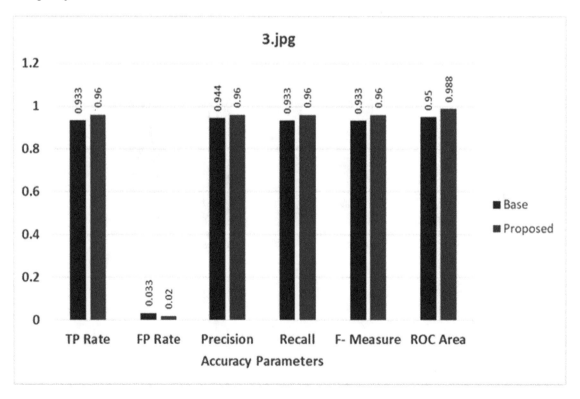

Classification Algorithms

Decision Tree

Decision tree is the predictive modelling approach used in machine learning, data mining and statistics. It is a supervised learning algorithm, that is, this algorithm consists of an outcome variable which is to be predicted from the given set of variables. Using these variables, a function is generated and mapped the input to the desired output. The population is divided into two or more homogeneous sets using the various distinct groups whenever possible. In a decision tree, the leaf nodes represent the target variables and the input variable is denoted by a path from parent node to children node (Sharma et al., 2012). Decision trees used in data mining are of two main types:

Classification tree

It is called a classification tree when the class to which the data belongs is predicted as the outcome or example in a medical test, suppose there are two classes. First class, is the blood test and second class, is for cancer detection consisting of various independent variables. If the blood test outcome is positive then cancer is detected, hence, a class is predicted for all the variables whose outcome is positive.

Regression tree

It is called a regression tree when the predicted outcome is a single value or a real number. Let us consider an example of a hotel. Suppose here there is two classes, first the number of bedrooms and second the house prices. Using this algorithm, the computer will anticipate the costs of the house in the light of the quantity of rooms; hence a value is predicted instead of a class.

The term which refers to both the above mentioned processes is called classification and regression tree analysis.

Advantages

- The key factor is the data preparation. The data preparation required for Decision trees is quite easy for the users and requires very little effort. If we have a dataset which measures cost in millions and loan age in years, then it will require some sort of normalization or scaling before we apply and implement a regression model and interpret correlation. In decision trees, the tree structure remains the same even if the transformation does not take place. Hence such transformations are unnecessary in this algorithm.
- Further, when a decision tree algorithm is applied on a training dataset, the top few nodes of the tree are essentially the most important variables in the dataset and feature selection is completely automated. Hence, decision tree performs feature selection implicitly.
- Another advantage is that the tree performance does not affected by the non-linear relationships between parameters, whereas simple regression models give out failing results because of highly nonlinear relationships between variables making such models invalid. But, decision trees do not need any assumptions of linearity in the data. Hence, they can be used in an environment where the parameters are nonlinearly related (Sharma et al., 2012).

Disadvantages

- But there are some limitations of a decision tree too, the more decisions there are in a tree, the less accurate any expected outcomes are likely to be. They are basically based on expectation than reality (Sharma et al., 2012).
- When actual decisions are made, the results may be different from those already planned. This may result in an unrealistic and bad decision.
- Also, Decision trees are also prone to indicate errors in classification, thus owing to diversity in perceptions and the constraints of applying statistical tools.
- To prepare a decision tree, advanced knowledge in statistical and quantitative analysis, is required. The probability of training people is raised. Hence the cost of training is rising.

Linear Discriminant Analysis (LDA)

LDA is a method used in statistics, pattern recognition and machine learning to find a linear combination of features that characterizes or separate two or more classes of objects or events. It's dimensionally reduction technique in the pre-processing step for pattern classification and machine learning applications.

Support Vector Machine (SVM)

SVM is one of the classification methods. This algorithm is used to "plot each data item as a point in n-dimensional space" where 'n' belongs to the "number of features" (Sharma et al., 2012).

The working of SVM is explained by the Maximal-Margin Classifier. The numeric input variable 'x' in the data forms an n-dimensional space. Suppose, there are two input variables, then it would form a two-dimensional space. A hyper-plane line in the graph splits the input variable space. The hyper-plane selected in SVM separates the points in the input variable space according to their class. The classes could be either class 0 or 1.Visualizing a line in the dimensional graph and according that all the input points are separated.

$$B0 + (B1 * X1) + (B2 * X2) = 0$$

Here the slope of the line is determined by the coefficients B1 and B2 and the intercept B0 is found by using the learning algorithm. X1 and X2 are the two input variables. Classification is made using this line. When the input values are plugged in the equation, we can determine whether a new point is above the line or below the line (Sah, R. D. & Sheetalani, 2017).

If the new point is above the line then the equation returns a value greater than 0 and it can be said that the point belongs to the (class 0) first class. If the new point is below the line then the equation returns a value less than 0 and then that the point belongs to the (class 1) second class. A value close to the line gives a value close to zero and it becomes difficult to classify the point. For larger magnitude values, the model has more confidence in the prediction. For training data that are linearly separable, select two parallel hyper-planes for prediction. They can be separated into two classes of data, and the distance between them is very large. The region bound by these two planes is called the "margin". The maximum-margin hyper-plane lies halfway between them. The SVM algorithm is implemented using a kernel. The equation for predicting a new input using the dot product of the input (x) and each support vector (xi) is as shown in the equation:

f(x) = B0 + sum(ai * (x,xi))

The coefficients 'B0' and 'ai' must be estimated from the training data by the learning algorithm for each input (Sharma et al., 2012).

Figure 48 includes several of red and green dots. The main advantage of SVM is data logistic regression. In logistic regression, it would become difficult to separate the red from the green dots, which can be easily done by SVM. Figure 49 includes SVM which includes over-fitting. It may form small bubble like boundaries which may harm the predictions.

Figure 48. SVM best case graph

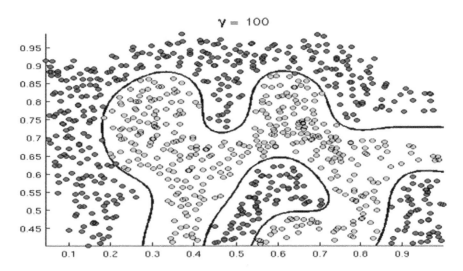

Figure 49. SVM over-fitting case

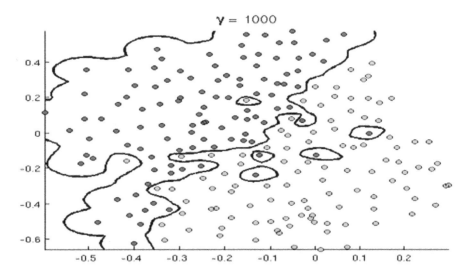

Fine KNN

KNN is one of the simplest algorithms and well understood when in practice. It is non-parametric lazy learning algorithm. Non parametric means it doesn't make any assumption on the underlying data distribution. And lazy means it doesn't use the training data points to do any generalization.

Ensemble Boosted

Ensemble learning is a machine learning concept in which the idea is to train multiple models (learners) to solve the machine problems. The main advantages of ensemble learning are reduced variance and reduced bias.

Statistical Analysis Based on Ultrasound Fetus Development Application

The result is validated using classification learner which includes confusion matrix and ROC based upon different classification algorithms i.e. Decision Tree, Linear Discriminant, SVM, KNN and Ensemble Boosted Trees as in Table 16.

Table 16. Standard Terms for Validating the Algorithms

Observations	Predictors	Response Variable	Response Classes	Size of Dataset	Validation
75	4	VarName5	3	5Kb	5-fold Cross Validation

Classification Algorithm using Confusion Matrix of Benchmark Images

Confusion Matrix is calculated using an algorithm to train the dataset such as Tree, LDA, SVM, Fine KNN and Ensemble Boosted. These all methods are applied on the four benchmark ultrasound fetus images as in Figure 50 to Figure 53.

Classification Algorithm using Confusion Matrix of Live Dataset

Confusion Matrix is used to train the different classifiers for live dataset. Out of 12 live dataset, only 3 images are validated using 10 fold cross-validation as in Figure 54, Figure 55 and Figure 56.

In this validation result, it is proved using confusion matrix that the value of SVM is higher than that of Fine KNN, Ensemble Boosted, tree & LDA, which means the improvement in images using classification algorithms is verified.

Classification Algorithm using ROC (Accuracy) of Benchmark Images

Figure 57 to 60 shows the validation of classification algorithms ROC for benchmark images.

Figure 50. Validation of Classification Algorithms using Confusion Matrix for benchmark image

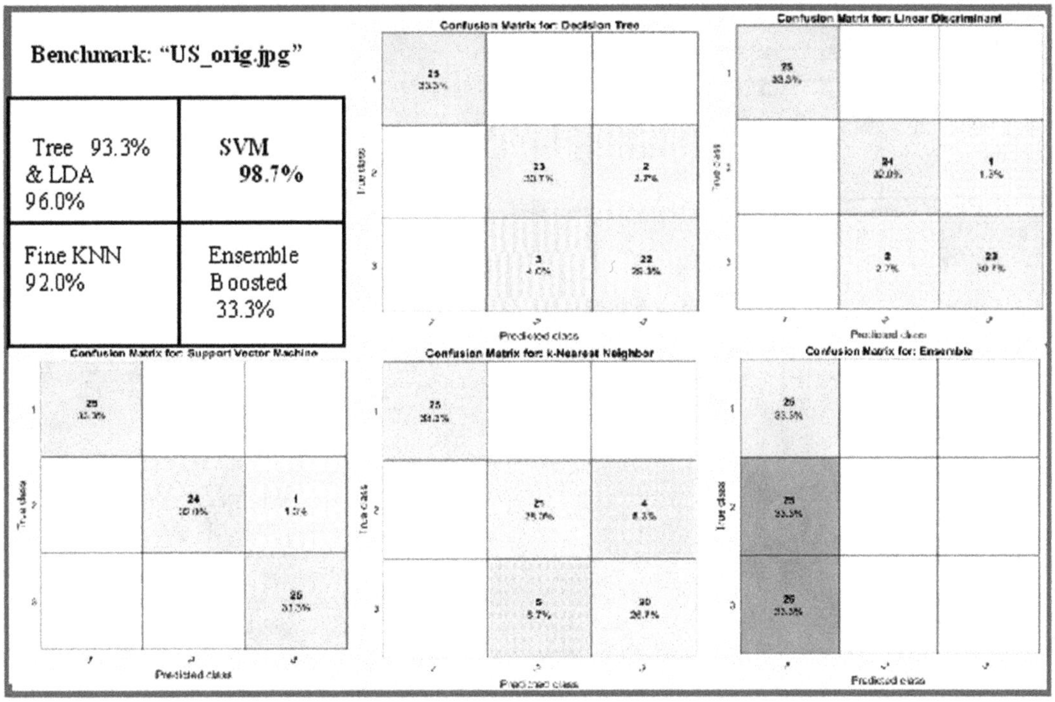

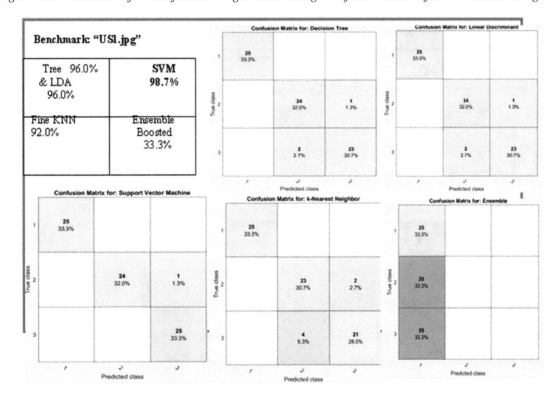

Figure 51. Validation of Classification Algorithms using Confusion Matrix for benchmark image

Figure 52. Validation of Classification Algorithms using Confusion Matrix for benchmark image

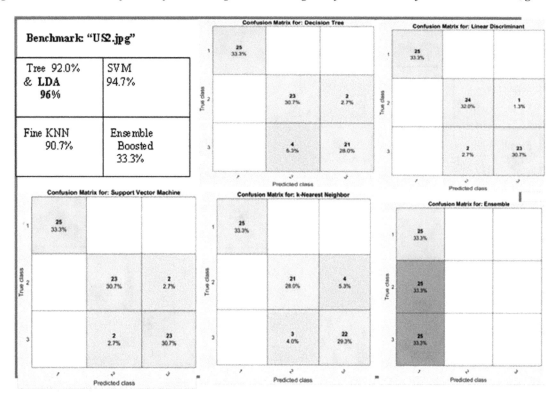

Figure 53. Validation of Classification Algorithms using Confusion Matrix for benchmark image

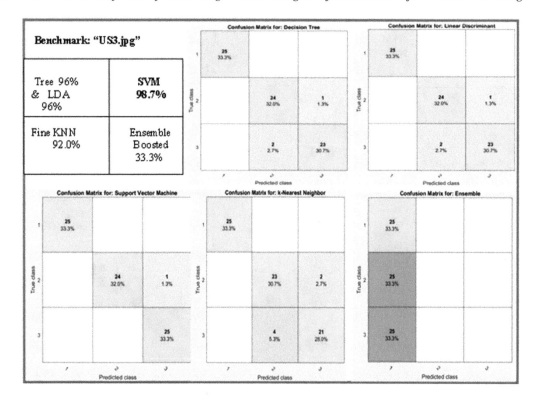

Figure 54. Validation of Classification Algorithms using Confusion Matrix for live image

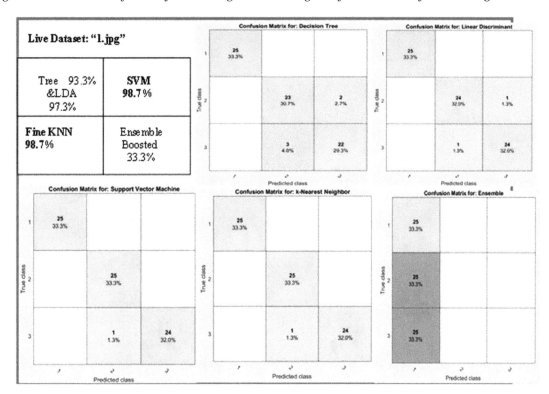

Figure 55. Validation of Classification Algorithms using Confusion Matrix for live image

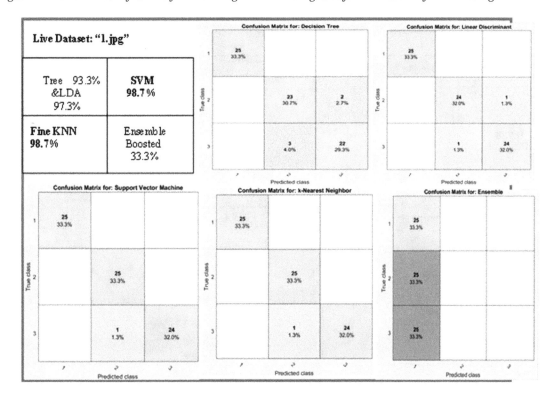

Figure 56. Validation of Classification Algorithms using Confusion Matrix for live image

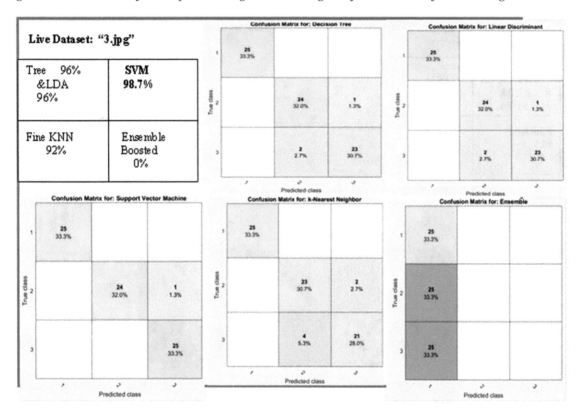

Figure 57. Validation of Classification Algorithms using ROC for benchmark image

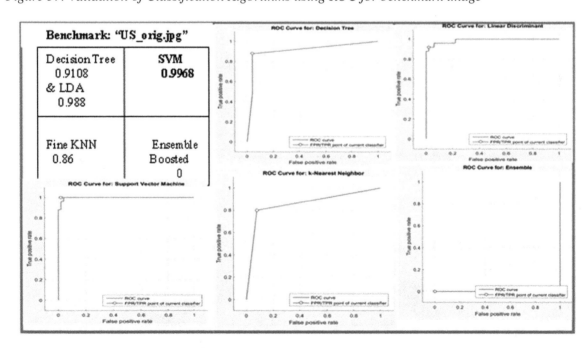

Figure 58. Validation of Classification Algorithms using ROC for benchmark image

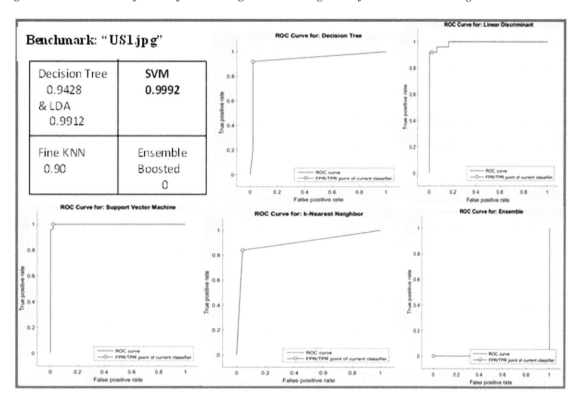

Figure 59. Validation of Classification Algorithms using ROC for benchmark image

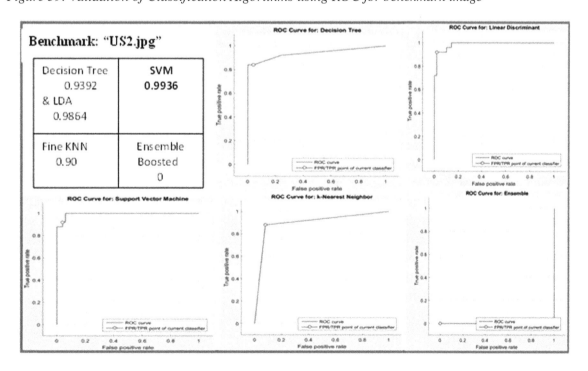

Figure 60. Validation of Classification Algorithms using ROC for benchmark image

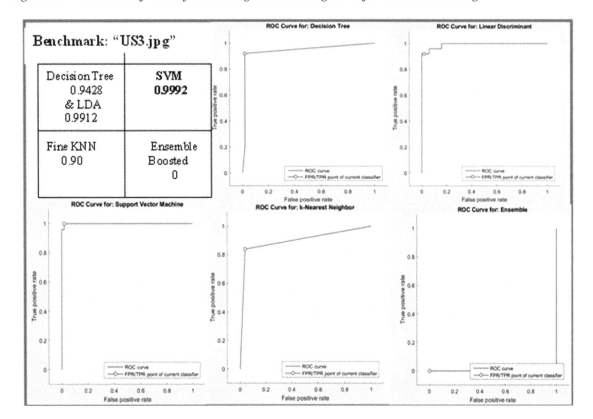

Classification Algorithm using ROC (Accuracy) of Live Dataset

Figure 61 to 63 shows the validation of classification algorithms using ROC for three live images.

FUTURE RESEARCH DIRECTIONS

The research work includes the benchmark and live dataset which is of limited size database. The future work is to create a larger fetal database. Data Augmentation to develop a CAD system for the early detection of the abnormal fetal growth and for other medical diagnosis problems will be developed. Future work will focus on assisting the radiologist in performing an in-depth exploration of the fetal growth and development within a short time and improve the accuracy of diagnosis of abnormal growth of fetal. An evaluation of multiple feature extraction techniques, which will provide a more accurate classification result, is to be achieved on live dataset in future consideration. Even the training and testing ratio should vary to check the working of the proposed work in a different perspective. The future consideration is to work on a large-scale network of deep learning internal layers and to help radiologists to accurately validate large datasets in less time.

Figure 61. Validation of Classification Algorithms using ROC for live image

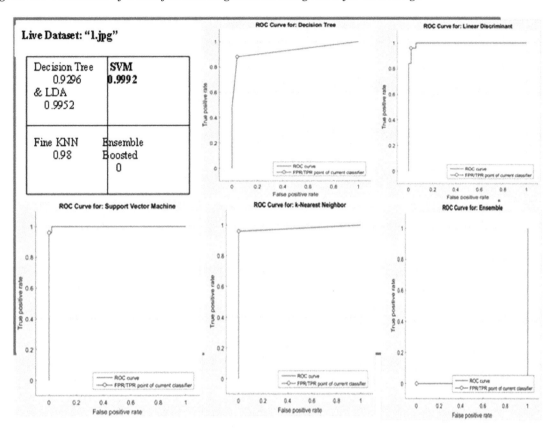

Figure 62. Validation of Classification Algorithms using ROC for live image

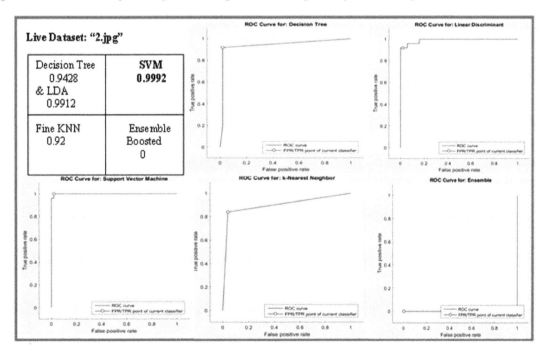

Figure 63. Validation of Classification Algorithms using ROC for live image

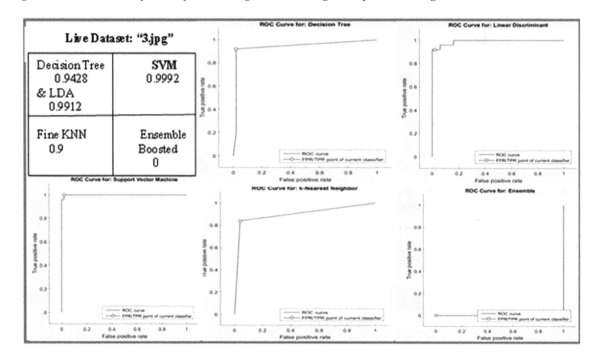

CONCLUSION

CAD plays an important role in predicting fetal growth. In this application area, an image enhancement filtering technique and classification method is used. The aim is to overcome the accuracy and sensitivity limitations of the current solutions in fetal growth and development identification. A comparison of different denoising filtering methods is performed with NormalShrink Homomorphic Filtering method in pre-processing step. Experimental evaluation results show a better performance of this method as compared to all other denoising filtering methods. The result reflects that both qualitatively and quantitatively Normal Shrink Homomorphic Filtering Methods outperform the spatial filters. Different classifier has been investigated for diagnosing the fetal development measurements. The accuracy of the classifier is predicted on the basis of the feature selection, training samples selected and the classifiers ability to learn from the training samples. The main objective, which is to find the better classifier for fetal diagnosis, is achieved in the results. The growth is distinguished as normal and abnormal using Neuro-Fuzzy classifier based on Genetic algorithm. The experiment is performed both on benchmark and live database. The proposed result proves to be more accurate and efficient as compared to Artificial Neural Network (ANN) which gives approximately 97% accuracy in training as well as testing. The values of sensitivity, specificity, precision and F-measure are better obtained from other methods. These promising results clearly demonstrate the great potential of the proposed approach in automatic image processing and classification of biomedical data. To evaluate the availability of the feature data and the classification accuracy, the AUC of ROC is used as assessment indicators. All of these measured indicators verify the effectiveness of the proposed method using Classification Learner on 10-fold cross-validation. SVM is the best validated approach in ROC as it covers 0.9998 area and Confusion Matrix accuracy rate is 97%.

REFERENCES

Ali, L., Hussain, A., Li, J., Zakir, U., & Yan, X. (2014). Intelligent image processing techniques for cancer progression detection, recognition and prediction in the human liver. Proceedings on Computational Intelligence in Healthcare and e-health. doi:10.1109/CICARE.2014.7007830

Antonini, M., Barlaud, M., Mathieu, P., & Daubechies, I. (1992). Image coding using wavelet transform. *IEEE Transactions on Image Processing*, *1*(2), 205–220. doi:10.1109/83.136597 PMID:18296155

Basheer, I. A., & Hajmeer, M. (2000). Artificial neural networks: Fundamentals, computing, design, and application. *Journal of Microbiological Methods*, *43*(1), 3–31. doi:10.1016/S0167-7012(00)00201-3 PMID:11084225

Bedi, C. S., & Goyal, H. (2010). Qualitative and Quantitative Evaluation of Image Denoising Techniques. *International Journal of Computers and Applications*, *8*(14), 31–34. doi:10.5120/1313-1775

Carneiro, G., Zheng, Y., Xing, F. & Yang, L. (2017). Review of Deep Learning Methods in Mammography, Cardiovascular, and Microscopy Image Analysis. *Springer Advances in Computer Vision and Pattern Recognition*, 11-32. doi:10.1007/978-3-319-42999-1_2

Cheng, H. D., Shan, J., Ju, W., Guo, Y., & Zhang, L. (2010). Automated breast cancer detection and classification using ultrasound images: A survey. *Journal of Pattern Recognition*, *43*(1), 299–317. doi:10.1016/j.patcog.2009.05.012

Donoho, D. L. (1995). Denoising by soft-thresholding. *IEEE Transactions on Information Theory*, *41*(3), 613–627. doi:10.1109/18.382009

Donoho, D. L., & Johnstone, I. M. (1994). Ideal spatial adaptation *via* wavelet shrinkage. *Biomefrika*, *81*(3), 425–455. doi:10.1093/biomet/81.3.425

Espinoza, J., Good, S., Russell, E., & Lee, W. (2013). Does the use of automated fetal biometry improve clinical work flow efficiency. *Journal of Ultrasound in Medicine*, *32*(5), 847–850. doi:10.7863/jum.2013.32.5.847 PMID:23620327

Gonzalez, B., Valdez, F., Melin, P., & Arechiga, G. P. (2015). Fuzzy logic in the gravitational search algorithm for the optimization of modular neural networks in pattern recognition. *Expert Systems with Applications*, *42*(14), 5839–5847. doi:10.1016/j.eswa.2015.03.034

Gupta, S., Chauhan, R. C., & Saxena, S. C. (2004). A wavelet based statistical approach for speckle reduction in medical ultrasound images. *Medical & Biological Engineering & Computing*, *42*(2), 189–192. doi:10.1007/BF02344630 PMID:15125148

Gupta, S., Chauhan, R. C., & Saxena, S. C. (2005). Locally adaptive wavelet domain Bayesian Processor for denoising medical ultrasound images using speckle modeling based on Rayleigh distribution. Proceeding on Vision, Image and Signal Processing, 152(1), 129-135.

Gupta, S., Kaur, L., Chauhan, R.C. & Saxena, S.C. (2003). A wavelet based statistical approach for speckle reduction in medical ultrasound images. *Proceedings on Convergent Technologies for Asia-Pacific Region*, 534-537. doi:10.1109/ TENCON.2003.1273218

Gupta, S., Kaur, L., Chauhan, R. C., & Saxena, S. C. (2007). A versatile technique for visual enhancement of medical ultrasound images. *Digital Signal Processing*, *17*(3), 542–560. doi:10.1016/j.dsp.2006.12.001

Gustavo, C., Georgescu, B. & Good, S. (2008). Knowledge-based automated fetal biometrics using syngo Auto OB measurements. *Siemens Medical Solutions*, 67.

Hearn-Stebbins, B. (1995). Normal fetal growth assessment: A review of literature and current practice. *Journal of Diagnostic Medical Sonography: JDMS*, *11*(4), 176–187. doi:10.1177/875647939501100403

Hiremath, P. S., & Tegnoor, J. R. (2014). Fuzzy inference system for follicle detection in ultrasound images of ovaries. *Soft Computing*, *18*(7), 1353–1362. doi:10.100700500-013-1148-x

Jalalian, A., Mashohor, S. B., Mahmud, H. R., Saripan, M. I., Ramli, A. R., & Karasfi, B. (2013). Computer-aided detection/diagnosis of breast cancer in mammography and ultrasound: A review. *Clinical Imaging*, *37*(3), 420–426. doi:10.1016/j.clinimag.2012.09.024 PMID:23153689

Janghel, R. R., Mehra, A., Shukla, A., & Tiwari, R. (2011). Intelligent Diagnostic System for the diagnosis and prognosis of Breast Cancer using ANN. *Journal of Computing*, *3*(3), 93–98.

Kalyan, K., Jain, S., Lele, R. D., Joshi, M., & Chowdhary, A. (2013). Application of artificial neural networks towards the determination of presence of disease conditions in ultrasound images of kidney. *International Journal of Computer Engineering & Technology*, *4*(5), 232–243.

Kalyan, K., Jakhia, B., Lele, R.D., Joshi, M. & Chowdhary, A. (2014). Artificial Neural Network Application in the Diagnosis of Disease Conditions with Liver Ultrasound Images. *Advances in Bioinformatics*, 1-14, doi: /708279 doi:10.1155/2014

Kaur, L., Gupta, S., & Chauhan, R. C. (2002). Image denoising using wavelet thresholding. *Proceedings of Indian conference on computer vision, graphics and image processing*, 1-4.

Kaur, L., Gupta, S., Chauhan, R. C., & Saxena, S. C. (2007). Medical ultrasound image compression using joint optimization of thresholding quantization and best-basis selection of wavelet packets. *Digital Signal Processing*, *17*(1), 189–198. doi:10.1016/j.dsp.2006.05.008

Kaur, P., Singh, G., & Kaur, P. (2016), Image Enhancement of Ultrasound Images using Multifarious Denoising Filters and GA. *IEEE International Conference on Advances in Computing, Communications and Informatics (ICACCI)*, 2375-2384.

Kaur, P., Singh, G. & Kaur, P. (2019). An Intelligent Validation system for diagnosis and prognosis of Ultrasound Fetal Growth Analysis using Neuro-Fuzzy based on Genetic Algorithm. *Egyptian Informatics Journal*, *20*(1), 55-87. doi:10.1016/j.eij.2018.10.002

Kumar, B. P., Prathap, C., & Dharshith, C. N. (2013). An Automatic Approach for Segmentation of Ultrasound Liver Images. *International Journal of Emerging Technology and Advanced Engineering*, *3*(1), 337–340.

Liu, Y. (2015). Image denoising method based on threshold, wavelet trans-form and genetic algorithm. International Journal of Signal Processing. *Image Processing and Pattern Recognition*, *8*(2), 29–40. doi:10.14257/ijsip.2015.8.2.04

Loughna, P., Chitty, L., Evans, T., & Chudleigh, T. (2009). Fetal size and dating: Charts recommended for clinical obstetric practice. *Ultrasound*, *17*(3), 160–166. doi:10.1179/174313409X448543

Mangai, J. A., Nayak, J., & Kumar, V. S. (2013). A novel approach for classifying medical images using data mining techniques. *International Journal of Computer Science & Electrical Engineering*, *1*(2), 188–192.

Maraci, M. A., Bridge, C. P., Napolitano, R., Papageorghiou, A., & Noble, J. A. (2017). A framework for analysis of linear ultrasound videos to detect fetal presentation and heartbeat. *J Med Image Anal*, *37*, 22–36. doi:10.1016/j.media.2017.01.003 PMID:28104551

Mitrea, D., Nedevschi, S., Socaciu, M., & Badea, R. (2012). The Role of the Superior Order GLCM in the Characterization and Recognition of the Liver Tumors from Ultrasound Images. *Wuxiandian Gongcheng*, *21*(1), 79–85.

Poonguzhali, S., & Ravindran, G. (2008). Automatic classification of focal lesions in ultrasound liver images using combined texture features. *Information Technology Journal*, *7*(1), 205–209. doi:10.3923/itj.2008.205.209

Pramanik, M., Gupta, M., & Krishnan, K. B. (2013). Enhancing reproducibility of ultrasonic measurements by new users. *SPIE Medical Imaging International Society for Optics and Photonics*, *8673*, 86730Q. Advance online publication. doi:10.1117/12.2008032

Ragesh, N. K., Anil, A. R., & Rajesh, R. (2011). Digital image denoising in medical ultrasound images: A Survey. *Proceeding on ICGST AIML-11 Conference*, 67-73.

Rahmatullah, B., Papageorghiou, A. T., & Noble, J. A. (2012). Image analysis using machine learning: anatomical landmarks detection in fetal ultrasound images. Proceeding on Computer Software and Applications, 354-355, doi:10.1109/COMPSAC.2012.52

Ravishankar, H., Prabhu, S. M., Vaidya, V., & Singhal, N. (2016). Hybrid approach for automatic segmentation of fetal abdomen from ultrasound images using deep learning. *IEEE Conference on Global Research*, 779-782, . 2016.7493382.10.1109/ISBI.2016.7493382

Sah, R. D., & Sheetalani, J. (2017). Review of Medical Disease Symptoms Prediction Using Data Mining Technique. *Journal of Computational Engineering*, *19*(3), 59–70.

Selvarajah, S., & Kodituwakku, S. R. (2011). Analysis and comparison of texture features for content based image retrieval. *International Journal of Latest Trends in Computing*, *2*(1).

Sharma, N., Bajpai, A., & Litoriya, R. (2012). Comparison the various clustering algorithms of weka tools. *International Journal of Emerging Technology and Advanced Engineering*, *2*(5), 73–80.

Singh, M., Singh, S., & Gupta, S. (2014). An information fusion based method for liver classification using texture analysis of ultrasound images. *Information Fusion*, *19*, 91–96. doi:10.1016/j.inffus.2013.05.007

Suganya, R., & Rajaram, S. (2012). Content based image retrieval of ultrasound liver diseases based on hybrid approach. *American Journal of Applied Sciences*, *9*(6), 938–945. doi:10.3844/ajassp.2012.938.945

Vardhan, M. H., & Rao, S. V. (2014). GLCM architecture for image extraction. *International Journal of Advanced Research in Electronics and Communication Engineering, 3*(1), 75–82.

HYP. (n.d.). www.mathworks.com/access/helpdesk/help/toolbox/images

Zong, X., Geiser, E. A., Laine, A. F., & Wilson, D. C. (1996). Homomorphic wavelet shrinkage and feature emphasis for speckle reduction and enhancement of echocardiographic images. *Medical Imaging: Image Processing, 2710*, 658–667. doi:10.1117/12.237969

Chapter 16
ECG Image Classification Using Deep Learning Approach

Pratik Kanani

https://orcid.org/0000-0002-6848-2507

Dwarkadas J. Sanghvi College of Engineering, India

Mamta Chandraprakash Padole

https://orcid.org/0000-0002-0695-5970

The Maharaja Sayajirao University of Baroda, India

ABSTRACT

Cardiovascular diseases are a major cause of death worldwide. Cardiologists detect arrhythmias (i.e., abnormal heart beat) with the help of an ECG graph, which serves as an important tool to recognize and detect any erratic heart activity along with important insights like skipping a beat, a flutter in a wave, and a fast beat. The proposed methodology does ECG arrhythmias classification by CNN, trained on grayscale images of R-R interval of ECG signals. Outputs are strictly in the terms of a label that classify the beat as normal or abnormal with which abnormality. For training purpose, around one lakh ECG signals are plotted for different categories, and out of these signal images, noisy signal images are removed, then deep learning model is trained. An image-based classification is done which makes the ECG arrhythmia system independent of recording device types and sampling frequency. A novel idea is proposed that helps cardiologists worldwide, although a lot of improvements can be done which would foster a "wearable ECG Arrhythmia Detection device" and can be used by a common man.

INTRODUCTION

With the current advancements and explosion of Artificial Intelligence in HealthCare Organizations, medical experts are constantly figuring out ways to narrow the gap between technology and healthcare so as to provide better services to patients.

DOI: 10.4018/978-1-7998-2742-9.ch016

Deep Learning in medical domain can unearth hidden opportunities and delve patterns from medical data, helping doctors to blend their expertise and technology to treat patients faster. Deep Learning is a vital subset of Machine Learning that uses neural networks to improve computational efficiency and accuracy and can solve problems where Machine Learning algorithms do not perform up to the mark.

Arrhythmias are classified into different types namely Atrial Fibrillations, supraventricular tachycardia, Premature Ventricular Contractions (PVCs), Atrial Premature Beat. Prolonged Atrial Fibrillations can increase the risk of getting a stroke. Continuous PVCs are major indications of a more dangerous heart behavior in the near future that may lead to heart failure. Patients having a paced ECG beat need to be precariously monitored as it may arrest the blood flow and cause serious life-threatening complications.

Before processing the ECG signal, one has to make sure that they obtain accurate ECG signal. The accurate signal means that the sampling frequency should be kept such that it should not miss out the natural ECG characteristics. For different sub waves in ECG the frequency ranges are different (Larisa & Mark, 2005), e.g., T wave ranges from 0–10 Hz, P wave 5-30 Hz and the QRS complex is within 8-50 Hz. The highest ECG frequency is around 50 Hz, so one has to keep it more than 100 Hz while sampling it, according to Nyquist rate (Mamta, 2014). The other aspect is that the obtained ECG signal should be noise free. As ECG signals are of low frequency, they include more low frequency corrupted signals. Noise suppresses the natural characteristics of ECG signal, which makes it more difficult to analyze in computing realm. To make an ECG signal noise free, there are many preprocessing techniques (Kanani, 2018). The pre-processing techniques are explained in further sections. The noised and pre-processed denoised (noise free) signals are presented in Figure 5 and Figure 6.

The main function of a Cardiologist is to master the analysis procedures, to analyze complex heart behavior, make accurate clinical decisions and that help treat patients for CVDs. As disease detection is of paramount importance, deep learning approach can help detect abnormalities faster, rather than sifting through large amounts of ECG datasets manually. Cardiologists can thus, focus on developing intensive care programs for patients. There is no definite assurance that these tools can completely supplant the expertise of cardiologists, but the aim is to facilitate cardiologists to take faster and better decisions.

Multiple numerical based mathematical techniques (Bilal et al., 2014) do exist to analyze the ECG signals and to get its standard PQRST point intervals. But as machine learning techniques outperform other techniques, Deep Learning Approach has been used to identify the ECG Arrhythmias. Currently five types of arrhythmias are being classified.

Firstly, ECG wave from the dataset are plotted and then converted to grayscale images. Two dimensional CNN is performed to achieve a workable accuracy. Then the ECG Heartbeat Categorization dataset is fed as training data and validated on testing data which is also collected from acclaimed MIT-BIH database and PhysioNet database. The trained model predicts whether the Wave rhythm is normal or abnormal and also it classifies the disease as defined in the standard database. The proposed model has also been tested for Mendeley ECG Signals (1000 fragments) and the model is able to successfully classify and label them.

Problem Definition

The concept of Deep Learning which is an important asset in the AI umbrella is of paramount importance in the Health Care sector. Deep Learning is a self-learning model which can learn from training data, improve quality, reduce response time and improve the ability to interpret results from clinical data. Given such a diagnosis problem especially in the field of Cardiology, deep learning and its high computational power is employed to improve the roadmap that starts with disease detection, classification and ends with patients getting treated. To summarize the entire process of Arrhythmia classification it starts with the prospective patient having symptoms like fluttering in the chest, fainting, dizziness, sudden pain in the chest and shortness of breath. If the symptoms are frequent enough and the heart rhythms continue to be erratic urgent medical care is needed. The cardiologist will suggest Electrocardiography to find an exact discrepancy in the patient's heart electrical system. ECG wave is basically the depiction of the heart's electrical activity on a 2-D graph where the Y-axis represents the amplitude in millivolt (mV) and the X-axis represents time. So, a continuous wave with a fixed sampled frequency is attained. The crux of the problem lies in identifying and classifying different waveforms from the graph and to label them as normal and abnormal. A normal ECG wave is shown in Figure 1 (Kovacs et al., 2012).

Figure 1. A normal ECG wave with PQRST reference points and its intervals

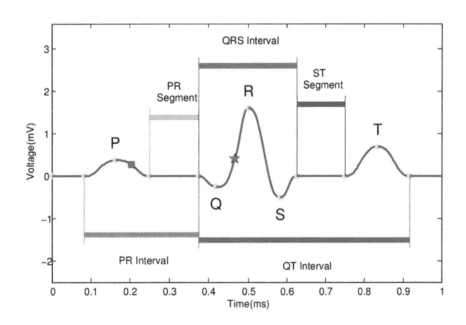

Due to the continuous nature of the wave, it becomes difficult sometimes to classify arrhythmias having similar electrical activity but are completely different. An improper diagnosis can take up more time which can prove fatal.

Such classifications can be aided with the help of a deep learning model that computes on grayscale images and learn via patterns formed by them. Instead of considering a number of features that are needed to train a machine learning model, proposed CNN model is trained on grayscale images. Once the training is done. All the patterns learned by layers of the model are finalized, validation data (testing images) is given as input that provides a classification label as the output. Once the classification is done, Cardiologists can take further steps depending on the severity of the problem and the degree of fluctuation from that of normal ECG waveform.

Literature Review

Authors Fulya Akdeniz and Temel Kayikcioglu in IEEE paper "Detection of ECG arrhythmia using Zhaos-Atlas Mark time-frequency distribution" the Signal Processing proposed Zhaos-Atlas Mark method used as a time-frequency distribution method to extract the feature from the ECG signals. Classification was used and seen that the best result was taken from K-Nearest Neighbor Classifier. Their System performance gave an accuracy, sensitivity, specificity, positive value 94.10%, 93.19%, 95.02%, 94.93% respectively.

Authors S. Celin and K. Vasanth in paper "Survey on the Methods for Detecting Arrhythmias Using Heart Rate Signals" has proposed a technique to characterize the electrocardiogram signal whether it is abnormal or normal, by applying different classification and feature techniques like linear and non-linear methods. The signals for the proposed process are obtained from the MIT-BIH database. It does basic artifacts and baseline wandering removal in its pre-processing phase. After that signals are given to thresholding window, spline window and hamming window to get QRS complexes.

Author R. Karthik et. al., in paper "Implementation of Neural Network and feature extraction to classify ECG signals" provides information regarding the use of ANN Classifiers and performance analysis of the same. They used the Pan-Tompkins Algorithm which consists of five steps to get a noise-free signal and feature extraction. They used ANN classifier to get a nonlinear mapping between the inputs and the outputs. Using Multilayer Perceptron Neural Network and improving accuracy by having hidden neurons it performs the adequate static mapping. Regular Perceptron Neural Network was used for a small set of data as they provided a better accuracy but were a bit redundant as the number of data samples increased.

Author Somsanuk Pathaoumvah, Kauzihiko Hamamoto and Phaumy Indahak in IEEE paper "Arrhythmias Detection and Classification base on a Single Beat ECG Analysis" provides information on novel features selection of Discrete Cosine Transform by analyzing frequency power spectrum. The database was MIT-BIH Arrhythmia database. In the process of feature extraction, five classes of ECG features are reduced by Fisher's Linear Discriminant Analysis. Discrete Fourier Transform was used and applied to each set of ECGs and with the energy compaction feature of DCT component features can be extracted and classified. The evaluation methods are a matrix of Sensitivity, Accuracy, Specificity.

Author Martin Kropf, Deiter Heyn and Gunter Schreeler in paper "ECG classification based on time and frequency domain features using random forests" provided information on disease classification using Random Forest Classifier. Data from the database was classified into four classes namely normal, suspicious to AF, Noise and another Arrhythmia. A total of 380 features were classified using bagged decision trees. The ECG signals were processed using MATLAB and MATLAB predictive modelling was used to test Multiple Random Forests. However, to avoid overfitting 10-fold cross validation was used. The results were evaluated by a MATLAB based Graphical user Interface into our existing model. For evaluation different key performance indicators were used including the Tailored F1 score for every class was calculated and the score was close to 94 percent.

Pre-Processing of ECG Signals

There exist multiple pre-processing techniques to denoise the ECG signals. They are mainly classified into hardware and software-based approaches. In hardware-based approach, one has to create different filters like band-pass and band-reject. These filters are the combinational circuits of L-C-R. These filters are mainly Adaptive Notch Filter, High pass IIR filter, Zero phase filter.

In software-based filter, concept of moving window is used. This window moves along the points and performs operations like averaging to smoothen the curve. One such popular filter is Savitzky-Golay filter. This filter is known for preserving ECG characteristics while removing the noise. One noised ECG signal is shown in Figure 2.

Figure 2. ECG signal with noise

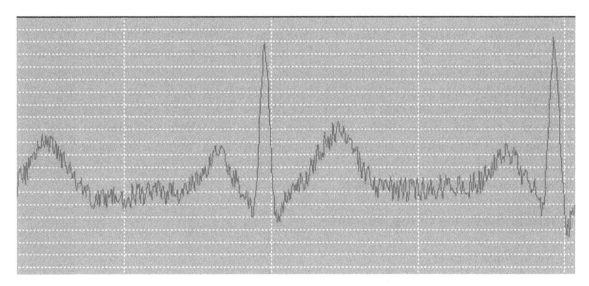

The above signal is taken from MIT ECG Simulator. After applying the Golay Filter the ECG signal is denoised which is shown in Figure 3. But while applying the Golay Filter, deciding its window size and the degree of polynomial is very important. If these parameters are chosen wrongly then it will affect the result performance. For current transformation of signals the polynomial degree is 3 and the window size is 21.

Figure 3. Denoised ECG signal After Appling Savitzky-Golay Filtering

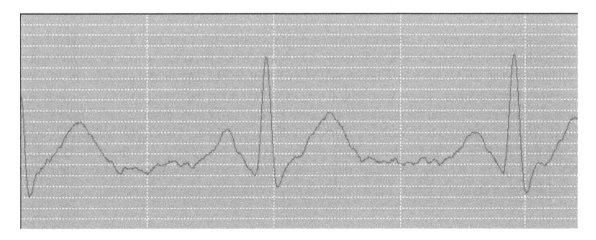

WORKING WITH DATASET

This section explains the whole procedure of our study. It illustriously delineates information about the dataset used, the method applied and techniques used.

Description of the Dataset

The dataset for our study was taken from Kaggle (Shayan Fazeli, 2018) which is composed of two fundamental datasets. The heartbeat signals are derived from MIT-BIH Arrhythmia dataset and The PTB Diagnostic ECG database. The source dataset takes into account a large number of samples as it is the natural prerequisite for training a deep learning model. The downloadable source files contain illustrious CSV files which indicate the reading of ECG signals sampled at 125 Hz. The matrix representation of CSV files clearly states that each row contains a portion of the heart's electric signal. The signals correspond to the shape of Heartbeats which are normal and also which are affected by some sort of Arrhythmias. The important characteristic of the dataset is that it is a "well-labelled dataset" and the last element of each row represents the class to which that row belongs to. All the signals are pre-processed and padded with zeroes wherever required.

Numerical Statistics of the Dataset

- **Arrhythmia Dataset**
  - The total number of ECG samples - 109446.
  - Number of Categories for Classification – 5
  - Sampling Frequency of the ECG recordings - 125 Hz
  - Labelled Classes: ['Normal': 0, 'Atrial Premature Beat': 1,'Premature Ventricular Contraction': 2, 'Fusion of Paced and Normal Beat':3, 'Paced beat':4]
- **The PTB Diagnostic ECG Database**
  - The total number of ECG samples - 14552.
  - Number of Categories - 2
  - Sampling frequency of the ECG recordings - 125 Hz

Building the Training Data set

Every wave whether normal or abnormal forms a definite pattern between their R-peaks and the model is trained based on these fixed definite patterns. The MIT BIH database has been used for building our training dataset which would be fed as an input to our CNN classifier. The database consists of a CSV file wherein each row depicts a single heartbeat. Every ECG beat in the database contains some part of the signal from the previous and the next beat. A cropping algorithm, which removes this additional signal from the beat resulting in a beat depicting a single cardiac cycle is used. The cropping algorithm detects the two R-peaks from the beat and then slices the beat between these two points. Since the input to our CNN model is a two-dimensional image, the resulting signal obtained from our cropping algorithm is plotted to form a grayscale image. Figure 4 shows how the cropping algorithm works.

Figure 4. Cropping Algorithm Crops R-R interval

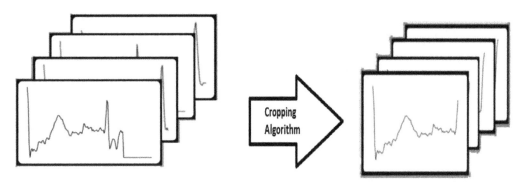

As a result, each individual ECG beat from the dataset is transformed into a grayscale image (128 X 128 pixels) which is one of the five labelled types as mentioned above. Figure 5 shows samples of each of the 5 types of ECG beats.

Figure 5. Samples of ECG beats and their Labels

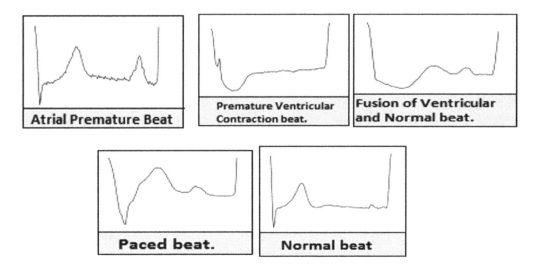

Removing Noisy Images

Initially when Label wise dataset is plotted, it is found that it has a particular labelled beat which is very clear and noise free, but it has bit noisy and noisier beats as well. Some noisy images are shown in Figure 6.

In order to filter the dataset and to feed our CNN model a definite pattern for training, some noisy images from the dataset are removed whereas some of them are still kept intact in order to introduce some forced errors. Doing this will help our model learn better. Table 1 shows total number of images present before and after the pre-processing dataset.

Figure 6. Noisy Beats in each Category

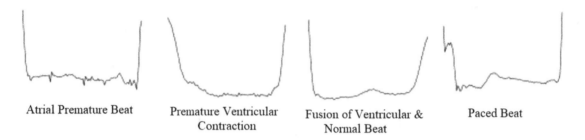

Atrial Premature Beat   Premature Ventricular   Fusion of Ventricular &   Paced Beat
                                    Contraction   Normal Beat

Data Augmentation

One of the main perks of using an image as input is Data Augmentation. In the field of Medical data analysis, Data Augmentation plays a very important role because the majority of the medical data is normal. For better classification, it is essential that all the classes (labels) have a balanced distribution of samples or data points. Specificity and Sensitivity can be increased and overfitting can be reduced by balancing the input data through data augmentation. Three ECG arrhythmia beats (APB, PVC, PB) have been augmented with the help of an inbuilt class in Keras called ImageDataGenerator. It takes different parameters which are required for augmentation like zoom_range, shear_range, height_shift_range, width_shift_range, rotation_range, horizontal_flip etc .The different parameters that were given to the ImageDataGenerator class were shear_range = 10, height_shift_range = 0.05, width_shift_range = 0.015, so this results in three different augmented images of a single ECG data. Figure 7 shows example of data augmentation.

Table 1. Dataset Size for and after pre-processing

Category	Total images before pre-processing	Total images after pre-processing
Atrial Premature Beat	7019	780
Premature Ventricular Contraction	4748	1035
Fusion of Ventricular and Normal Beat	606	563
Paced Beat	5539	2677
Normal PTB Dataset	4005	1030 (Normal Categories are combined together)
Normal MIT_BIH Dataset	6071	

SYSTEM ARCHITECTURE AND PROPOSED METHODOLOGY

Each individual ECG recordings from the Kaggle database which consisted of frequently used MIT-BIH dataset were transformed into grayscale images having dimension of 128*128 pixels. Proposed deep learning-based solution for the ECG arrhythmia classification consists of different phases which are as follows: Building the training data set, removing images containing noise, Data Augmentation, CNN classifier, validation set.

These final pre-processed, augmented images were used as an input data for training our CNN model. To enlarge the training dataset and to ensure even distribution of classes, Data Augmentation was done on the database. To validate our CNN model and to demonstrate the practical use case, Mendeley's dataset was considered which comprised of full ECG recordings. The entire ECG recording is cropped between R-R interval and converted to grayscale images. Whenever ECG wave forms come, the system should separate each waveform to get different R-R interval waves. After that each R-R interval wave is fed to the pre trained machine learning model. This model will carry out the classification for each and every wave. Normally the batch of minimum 6-7 waves are taken and each wave is classified for its label. If all wave turns out to be normal then entire ECG waveform is normal and if few wave forms are normal and any of is abnormally labelled, let say "x" then the ECG waveforms are having 'x' arrhythmia in that. In this method, all training (80%) and testing (20%) images are stored in numpy and this numpy is used to train and test the model.

Figure 7. Data Augmentation

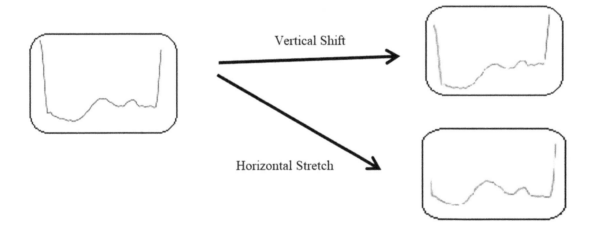

MODEL DESCRIPTION AND DIFFERENT OPTIMIZERS

The CNN model has optimized the various hyper-parameters to increase the classification accuracy and to curtail overfitting. Figure 9 contains detailed information about the different layers in the CNN model. Different classes like softmax, dense, dropout, Activation, flatten, normalization, convolution and max-pooling have been used. The model is trained in the sequential fashion starting from input layer till output layer. Image size taken for the input is 128x128 and the total 20 epochs are done. The layer sequence and ordering are shown in Figure 9 and different terminologies with their necessity is explained further.

The various optimisations performed to improve classification accuracy are:

Figure 8. System Architecture

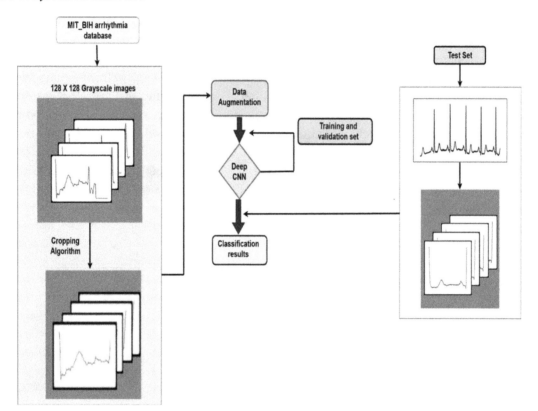

Figure 9. Model Description

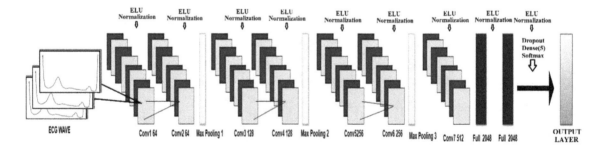

Kernel Initializations

For proper functioning of the deep learning model, proper initialization of weights, to achieve convergence, weights have to be initialised smartly. Xavier initialization is used in our proposed CNN model. The main motivation for using Xavier initialization is that it initializes the weights in such a way that the neuron activation functions are not starting out in saturated or dead regions. In other words, the weights have to be initialized with random values that are not "too small" and not "too large.

Activation Function

Not all of the information is useful, some of it is just noise, hence it becomes extremely important to select an appropriate activation function which helps the network to use the useful information and suppress the irrelevant data points. Non-linear activation functions like Rectified Linear Units (ReLU), Leakage Rectified Linear Units (LReLU), and Exponential Linear Units (ELU) are the most widely used ones.

$$ReLU(x) = max(0, x)$$
$$LReLU(x) = max(0, x) + \alpha min(0, x)$$
$$ELU(x) = x \text{ if } x \; ^3 \; 0 \; \gamma(exp(x) - 1) \text{ if } x < 0$$

Where the value of leakage coefficient (α) is 0.3 and the value of the hyper parameter(γ) is 1.0. Although ReLU is used as an activation function in most of the CNN models, LReLU and ELU are also effective in some cases because they do produce certain negative values, while ReLU considers negative values to be zero which deactivates some nodes and they no longer contribute to the learning. All the three functions are experimented and found ELU to be most effective for the image-based ECG arrhythmia classification.

Regularization/Normalization

Batch Normalisation has been used as a technique to reduce overfitting and to improve the performance and stability of the network. The idea is that, instead of just normalizing the inputs to the network, the inputs to all the layers within the network have to be normalized. Though, Batch Normalisation is applied normally between the Convolution layer and the activation function, it was more effective by applying it after the ELU activation function.

Dropout

A fully connected layer occupies most of the parameters, and hence, during training, the neurons develop a co-dependency amongst themselves, which curbs the individual power of each neuron leading to over-fitting of training data. Hence, to avert overfitting, the dependency is reduced by using Dropout. Dropout has been applied after the Batch Normalisation is applied to the fully-connected dense layers. Convolutional blocks have not been dropped because the number of free parameters it contains is not sufficient and co-adaptation has to be given more priority than reducing overfitting.

TEST CASE

The data source for ECG wave which is not used in proposed learning model either in testing or training is taken from Mendeley ECG dataset. This dataset has 1000 ECG fragments. Mendeley's dataset consisting of files containing labelled data for various arrhythmias. On plotting the Matlab files for any disease one can get an entire wave as shown in the Figure 10.

Now after applying cropping algorithm on this wave, so as one can ponder upon the specific pattern formed between R-R peaks.

Figure 10. ECG Wave form for Atrial Premature Beat from Mendeley's Dataset

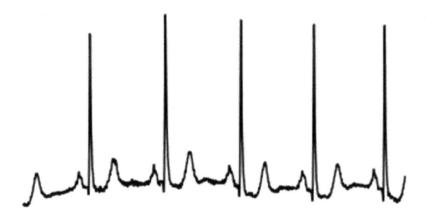

The output of the cropping algorithm is also a grayscale image with fixed dimensions of 128x128. When this cropped wave of Atrial Premature Beat is given to the proposed system. System classifies it correctly and the output is as shown in Figure 11.

Figure 11. Input images from Mendeley's dataset and output as Atrial Premature Beat

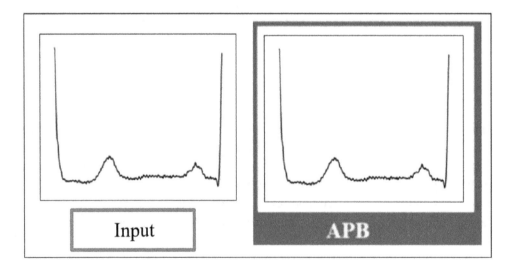

RESULTS AND CONCLUSIONS

Our proposed study aims to help cardiologists worldwide and with the developments of AI in the health care sector, our study will add value in this domain. This chapter proposes to help refine the vast clinical data, find patterns amongst them and to improve the accuracy parameter which is of paramount importance to serve a patient well. By implementing classification using Deep Learning, certain Machine Learning tasks like feature extraction and noise filtering have been avoided. Using the intense computational power to learn from data, workable accuracy has been achieved. The proposed model is achieving the accuracy level of 97.78%. This chapter does not wish to supplant the brilliance of cardiologists and their expertise but through our tool wish to add value to their work. So, this chapter is to use technology as to augment expertise in a health monitoring system in the proposed case-Cardiology.

FUTURE SCOPE

Heart failure or a sudden Stroke is something that cannot be foreseen. It comes unforeseen and takes away lives of people, thus, shattering many families forever. Arrhythmias and irregular heart's electrical system do provide us with important information of what may be coming next. Many people living in remote areas do not have cardiologists available when something uncertain happens, so a wearable ECG analysing device which constantly monitors and raises alarm if it detects something abnormal is proposed. This device is conceptualised to be cost effective so no common man suffers from untimely cardiac arrests. Another application can be Health Monitoring Robot in hospitals in which the data from our tool is fed and the robot will take care of patient's diet, exercise according to how healthy the patient's heart is. This Deep Learning approach and proposed system model can be applied for Recognizing Identical Reads from DNA Sequencing (Mamta et al., 2013) after necessary modifications to make it more efficient.

REFERENCES

Activation functions in Neural Networks. (n.d.). https://www.geeksforgeeks.org/activation-functions-neural-networks/

Akdeniz, F., & Kayikcioglu, T. (2018). Detection of ECG arrhythmia using Zhao-Atlas Mark time-frequency distribution. *26th Signal Processing and Communications Applications Conference (SIU)*, Izmir, Turkey. 10.1109/SIU.2018.8404585

Bilal, M. U., & Ahmed, B. (2014). Electrogram feature extraction and pattern recognition using a novel windowing algorithm. *Advances in Bioscience and Biotechnology*, 5(11), 886–894. doi:10.4236/abb.2014.511103

Celin, S., & Vasanth, K. (2017). Survey on the Methods for Detecting Arrhythmias Using Heart Rate Signals. *Journal of Pharmaceutical Sciences and Research.*, 9(2), 183–189.

Comparison of non-linear activation functions for deep neural networks on MNIST classification task. (n.d.). https://arxiv.org/pdf/1804.02763.pdf

Data Augmentation | How to use Deep Learning when you have Limited Data — Part 2. (n.d.). https://medium.com/nanonets/how-to-use-deep-learning-when-you-have-limited-data-part-2-data-augmentation-c26971dc8ced

Dropout in (Deep) Machine learning. (n.d.). https://medium.com/@amarbudhiraja/https-medium-com-amarbudhiraja-learning-less-to-learn-better-dropout-in-deep-machine-learning-74334da4bfc5

Dropout Regularization in Deep Learning Models With Keras. (n.d.). https://machinelearningmastery.com/dropout-regularization-deep-learning-models-keras/

ECG signals (1000 fragments). (n.d.). https://data.mendeley.com/datasets/7dybx7wyfn/3

ELU-Networks. (n.d.). *Fast and Accurate CNN Learning on ImageNet*. http://image-net.org/challenges/posters/JKU_EN_RGB_Schwarz_poster.pdf

FunctionsA. (n.d.). https://ml-cheatsheet.readthedocs.io/en/latest/activation_functions.html

Heartbeat Categorization DatasetE. C. G. (n.d.). https://www.kaggle.com/shayanfazeli/heartbeat

How to Accelerate Learning of Deep Neural Networks With Batch Normalization. (n.d.). https://machine-learningmastery.com/how-to-accelerate-learning-of-deep-neural-networks-with-batch-normalization/

Kanani, P., & Padole, M. (2018). Recognizing Real Time ECG Anomalies Using Arduino, AD8232 and Java. In M. Singh, P. Gupta, V. Tyagi, J. Flusser, & T. Ören (Eds.), *Advances in Computing and Data Sciences. ICACDS 2018. Communications in Computer and Information Science* (Vol. 905). Springer. doi:10.1007/978-981-13-1810-8_6

Karthik, Tyagi, Raut, Saxena, & Kumar. (n.d.). *Implementation of Neural Network and feature extraction to classify ECG signals*. https://arxiv.org/ftp/arxiv/papers/1802/1802.06288.pdf

Keras: The Python Deep Learning library. (n.d.). https://keras.io/

Kovács, P. (2012). ECG signal generator based on geometrical features. *Annales Universitatis Scientiarum Budapestinensis de Rolando Eötvös Nominatae. Sectio Computatorica. 37.*

Kropf, M., Heyn, D., & Schreeler, G. (2017). ECG Classification Based on Time and Frequency Domain Features Using Random Forests. *Computers in Cardiology, 44*, 1–4. doi:10.22489/CinC.2017.168-168

Padole, M. (2014). Distributed approach to pattern matching in genomics. Dept. of Computer Science and Engineering, The M.S University of Baroda. Available http://14.139.121.106/pdf/2014/oct14/1.pdf

Padole, Parekh, & Patel. (2013). Signal Processing Approach for Recognizing Identical Reads From DNA Sequencing of Bacillus Strains. *IOSR Journal of Computer Engineering, 10*(1), 19-24.

Pathoumvanh, S., Hamamoto, K., & Indahak, P. (2014). Arrhythmias Detection and Classification base on Single Beeat ECG Analysis. *The 4th International Conference on Information and Communication Technology, Electronics and Electrical Engineering (IJCTEE-2014).*

PreprocessingI. (n.d.). https://keras.io/preprocessing/image/

Savitzky-golay-filter. (n.d.a). https://github.com/swallez/savitzky-golay-filter/blob/master/src/mr/go/sgfilter/SGFilter.java

Savitzky-Golay Filter. (n.d.b). http://www.statistics4u.com/fundstat_eng/cc_filter_savgolay.html

Savitzky–Golay filter. (n.d.). https://en.wikipedia.org/wiki/Savitzky%E2%80%93Golay_filter

SimulatorE. C. G. (n.d.). http://www.mit.edu/~gari/CODE/ECGSYN/JAVA/APPLET2/ecgsyn/ecg-java/source.html

Tereshchenko, L. G., & Josephson, M. E. (2015). Frequency Content and Characteristics of Ventricular Conduction. *Journal of Electrocardiology*, *48*(6), 933–937. doi:10.1016/j.jelectrocard.2015.08.034 PMID:26364232

Understanding Xavier Initialization In Deep Neural Networks. (n.d.). https://prateekvjoshi.com/2016/03/29/understanding-xavier-initialization-in-deep-neural-networks/

What is an intuitive explanation of the Xavier Initialization for Deep Neural Networks? (n.d.). https://www.quora.com/What-is-an-intuitive-explanation-of-the-Xavier-Initialization-for-Deep-Neural-Networks

Chapter 17
Genetic Data Analysis

M. Shamila

ⓘ https://orcid.org/0000-0001-9105-9531
Malla Reddy Engineering College, India

Amit Kumar Tyagi

ⓘ https://orcid.org/0000-0003-2657-8700
Vellore Institute of Technology, Chennai, India

ABSTRACT

Genome-wide association studies (GWAS) or genetic data analysis is used to discover common genetic factors which influence the health of human beings and become a part of a disease. The concept of using genomics has increased in recent years, especially in e-healthcare. Today there is huge improvement required in this field or genomics. Note that the terms genomics and genetics are not similar terms here. Basically, the human genome is made up of DNA, which consists of four different chemical building blocks (called bases and abbreviated A, T, C, and G). Based on this, we differentiate each and every human being living on earth. The term 'genetics' originated from the Greek word 'genetikos'. It means 'origin'. In simple terms, genetics can be defined as a branch of biology, which deals with the study of the functionalities and composition of a single gene in an organism. There are mainly three branches of genetics, which include classical genetics, molecular genetics, and population genetics.

INTRODUCTION

Genetics (WHO, 2002) is the investigation of genes, genetic variety and heredity in living organism. Genetics is the basic of heredity. Heredity is the transmission of genetically based characteristics from ancestor to descendant. Any form of heritable feature is known as a character. Some examples for this type of characters are eye color, hair color, height etc. DNA (deoxyribo nucleic acid) is the main genetic substance of all living organism. DNA of Human being consists of 23 pairs of chromosomes. For example, chimpanzees consist of 24 pair of chromosomes. This means only 2% difference between human and chimpanzee in DNA structure. That is the main reason because humans are said to genetically evolved from ape like creature especially chimpanzee. Genetic studies were carried out since the

DOI: 10.4018/978-1-7998-2742-9.ch017

classical era where the scientist like Aristotle and Hypocrites put forward some theories like how the parental characteristics are passed to the offspring. However, breakthrough was achieved in 19th century when Gregor Mendal experiments with pea plants and discovered the fundamental laws of inheritance.

In cells gene is part of DNA. Genes can be defined as instruction manual to create a living being. Every gene has two alternative forms. And this alternative form is known as alleles. The four nitrogen bases present in the DNA are adenine (A), thymine (T), guanine (G) and cytosine (C). A pair with T and C with G. Thus, in the double stranded form, each strand contains all the necessary information, redundant with its partner strand. Genes are arranged linearly along the DNA sequence. Human DNA consists of 3billion bases. According to the U.S. National Library of Medicine (NLM) more than 99 percent of these bases are identical in all people.

Genetic analysis is the general procedure of contemplating and looking into in fields of science that include hereditary qualities and molecular biology. There are various applications that are created from this exploration, and these are likewise viewed as parts of the procedure. Genetic analysis can be utilized for the most part to depict strategies both utilized in and coming about because of the sciences of hereditary qualities and molecular biology, or to applications coming about because of this research. The process of genetic analysis began in the primitive days itself. Early people found that they could use selective breeding to improve yields and creatures. They additionally distinguished acquired qualities in people that were dispensed with throughout the years. The numerous hereditary investigations step by step advanced after some time.

As we mentioned above genetics is the study of hereditary, which emphasis on the study of limited number of genes with specific function whereas genomics (WHO, 2002; WHA, 2004)is a new term which focus on study of whole organism gene set called as genome. Genomics become popular in the last couple of decades due to the advancement of technologies. But most of the time these two terms are often used interchangeably. We can consider genetics as a subset of genomics. The table 1 shown below give insight to distinction between these two terms.

Algorithm

Genetic algorithm: Genetic algorithm works based on the principle of genetics and natural science. It is commonly used to solve optimization problems, in research, and in machine learning.

Table 1. Difference between Genetics and Genomics

Genetics	Genomics
It focuses on study of functionalities of a single gene	It includes study of whole gene and the inter relationships among them
Gene refers to particular DNA sequence of a single chromosome	Genome is complete hereditary information of an organism
Father of genetics is Gregor Mendal	Introduced by Tom Roderick
Biochemistry and biology help to explore this field	Can be explored with the help of bioinformatics and molecular biology
It emphasis on single gene behaviour	It emphasis entire genome of an organism

Figure 1. Basic Genetic Terminology (Vijini, 2017)

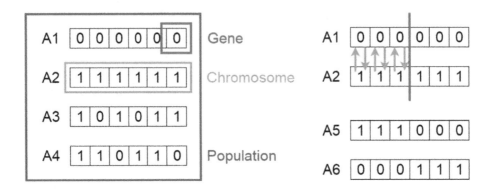

As shown in figure 2 the process begins with an initial population (which may be generated either using random method or using some heuristics), choose parents from this population for mating. Crossover and Mutation operators are applied on the parents to generate new off-springs. And finally, these off-springs replace the existing individuals in the population and the process repeats. In this way genetic algorithms actually try to mimic the human evolution to some extent.

Figure 2. Procedure of a Genetic Algorithm (Amin & Raja Azlina, 2013)

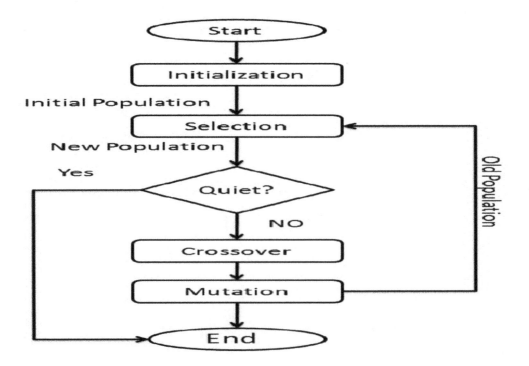

The genetic data appear in the form of numerical values. The general numerical data analysis methods such as statistical method (Weir, 1990) will not suite for genetic genomic data analysis due to its huge size and the amount of information it holds. The data retrieved from genetic analysis can be used for multiple applications like estimating frequencies for example likelihood estimation, measures of gene diversity, population structure which including genetic distance, analyses between generations, molecular data such as DNA sequence comparisons etc. Genomic data analysis technique includes hamming distance algorithm and approximate edit distance algorithm (Wagner & Fischer, 1974). Hence most of the algorithm support to respective data but, no algorithm support both of the data. Hence a unique type of algorithm/tool is required for such type of data [which contains DNA, RNA, and chromosome information].

Hence, the organization (remaining part) of this chapter is followed as: Section 2 discusses work related to genetic modelling or analysis. Further, importance of genetic data and genetic analytics is being discussed in section 3. Some existing tools are being discussed (with respect to analysing genetic data) in section 4. Further, section 5 discusses some real time application for genetic data and genetic analytics. Section 6 discusses some critical issues and open challenges. Further, section 7 discusses/ provides several opportunities with respect to genetic analytics (including research gaps, for future work) In last, this is being concluded in section 8 with notifying some essential future enhancement required in genetic analytics from research communities (in brief).

RELATED WORK

During the late 19th century Gregar Mentel concluded from his experiment that heredity is a static thing and is passed onto offspring's. In this era Haeckel identified that heredity material is present in nucleus. In the same duration chromosomes are identified as carrier of genetic information. In 20thcentaury the rediscovery of Mendelian principles was done. The study of chromosomal abnormalities like duplication, deletion etc. is done during this period. Structure of DNA identification is also being done during this time period. In the early 21st century human genome sequence was published. The makeover in genomic analytics field happened by Human genome project (Abecasis et al., 2012; Auton et al., 2015). Further, figure 3 describe the main inventions in the field of genetics.

Most of the researcher has done impressive work with respect to analysis of genomic data and genetic data. Some projects or studies (completed/ ongoing) based on genomic data are included in table 2.

Most of the researcher has tried to utilize genetic and genomic data to make prediction and to generate decisions (based on the efficient analytical process). Hence, this section discusses work related to evolution of genetic data, genetic analytics, etc., in brief. Now, next section discusses importance of genetic data and genetic analytics in various applications (via discussing a use case).

Importance of Genetic Data/Genetic Analytics

Genes give instruction to our body to produce different types of proteins, which are essential to grow and survive. Minor changes in genes cause changes in protein production which affect the working of the body. Damage in some genes may leads to rare genetic disease. By studying the functionalities of genes or its interaction with other substances helps the scientist to identify some diseases like cancer, diabetes, and heart diseases in the earlier stages. In the future the scientist may use genetic data to predict,

Figure 3. Timeline of Genomic History (Efthymioua et al., 2016)

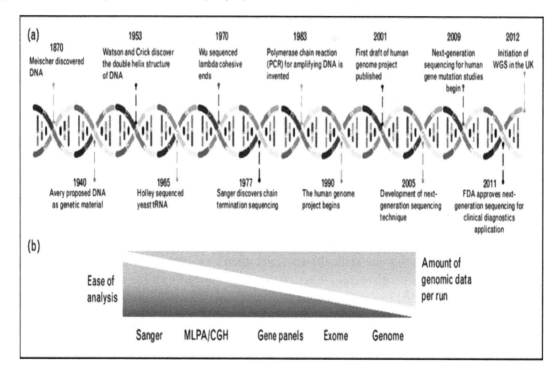

identify, and treat or to prevent some chronic diseases. This study also leads to the invention of personalized medicines. To conduct pilot studies on incorporating genomic data into clinical care, a number of healthcare systems have developed bioinformatics infrastructures to process NGS data through a group of databases supplementary to the EHRs (Hornoch et al., 2013).Due to advancement in technology the cost of genetic test is less and we can include this test in our regular medical care for better treatment. The companies like 23andme, anscestor.com collect blood samples or saliva as sample and they retrieve genetic information from these samples. Other than identification of relationship between diseases and genetics, these tests can also use in paternity test, legal and forensic etc. With the help of genetic analytics scientist are able to identify new genes that cause illness or threat to human life. The genetic analytics help to create a genetics-based healthcare platform. Genetic data can be used in human applications like

- Testing for genetic disorders.
- Using genome editing in patients.
- Using genetic technologies for extending life.
- Using genome editing for cosmetic reasons.

In case of animals, this data can be recommended for the following purposes

- Using genetic technologies in animals in order to of prevent and cure human disease.
- Using genetic technologies in animals for food.

Table 2. Available Projects based on Genomic Data

Project	Purpose
Human Genome project	Goal was to identify the sequence of nucleotide base pairs that make DNA, and also to identify and map different gene functional activities.
deCODE (Gulcher et al., 1997)	Used genomic data and e-healthcare records to study hereditary cause of common diseases.
PMRP (McCarty et al., 2007)	More than 20,000 participants enrolled to form a resource enabling researchers to investigate which genes cause diseases, which genes predict reactions to medicine, and how environment and genes work together to cause diseases.
I2B2 (Butte & Kohane, 2006)	Helps the researchers to utilize existing clinical data and genomic data for research inventions and also facilitate the design of targeted treatment for individual patients with diseases having genetic origins.
CKB (Chen et al., 2005)	To identify the complex, inter relationship among genes and environmental factors on the risks of common genetic disorders.
eMERGE (Rasmussen-Torvik et al., 2014)	To evolve methods and techniques for utilizing EHRs for genomic research to produce genomic medicine.
UK biobank (Munoz et al., 2016)	To upgrade the prevention, diagnosis, and therapies of a wide range of serious and life-threatening sickness through a collection of 500,000 volunteers' bio samples and health data.
GANI_MED (Grabe, 2014)	To develop targeted strategies for the prevention, diagnosis, and treatment of diseases, causes the specific characteristics of an individual patient or a well-defined patient group.
KPRPGEH (Hoffmann et al., 2011)	To identify the hereditary and environmental factors that influence common disease.
SCAN_B initiative (Saal et al., 2015)	To enhance survival and quality of life for breast cancer patients with the help of gene expression and genomic tumour profiling into the clinical routine for breast cancer.
PGPop (Postmus et al., 2014)	To identify a person's genetic make-up affects with respect to drugs.
MVP (Reiber & LaCroix, 2016)	To participate one million members and use their clinical and genetic record to enhance health care for veterans.
Cancer 2015 study (Wong et al., 2015)	To categorize cancers molecularly using MPS to promote more targeted therapies of cancer patients and improve patient survival and outcomes.
Precision medicine initiative (Collins & Varmus, 2015)	To achieve better insights into the biological, environmental, and behavioural influences for medical treatment and preventive methods that takes into account individual variability in genes, environment, and lifestyle by using the genomic and clinical data of a million Americans.

This data has also impact on plants as well. They are

- Using genetic technologies to develop new medicines in less cost, for example use of tobacco plants to produce biopharmaceuticals for treatment of disease like HIV
- Preventing crop damage, for example use of genome editing to reduce the risk of fungal disease in plants.
- Supplementing poor diets, Example, genome editing of rice to golden rice which provide more dietary Vitamin A.

Different methods of genetic study are as follows

- Pedigree analysis
- Karyotyping
- Breeding

- Twin study
- Statistical analysis

Hence, this section discusses importance of genetic data and genetic analytic with explaining a use case in popular sector like healthcare. Now, next section will discuss about some (available) existing tools to analyse genetic data.

Existing Tools or Algorithm to Analyse the Genetic Data

Genetics and genomics are two different scenarios of healthcare application. A lot of data (genetic and genomic) is being collected in medical care. For each data different type of analytic tool and prediction mechanism are being used to make effective decisions and prediction results. For example, some tools or algorithm are being used in (with respect to) providing privacy for genomic data, which are illustrated here as follows:

a) Controlled Access: Researchers who are in need of data from the Controlled Access tier (Controlled Data) for their work should obtain an approved Data Access Request through the Database of Genotypes and Phenotypes (dbGaP) (National Center for Biotechnology Information, 2016) and agree with all the data use and publication policy. Controlled data access includes unique individual information such as primary sequencing data (like DNA, RNA), Raw and processed Exon array data etc.

b) Differential privacy (Dwork, 2006): Query or output privacy is preserved using differential privacy. The protect strength is measured with the help of privacy budget, where a smaller budget provides a stronger protection, and vice versa. Perturbation-based techniques are generally used to achieve differential privacy.

c) Encrypted solution: One method for cryptographic privacy is homomorphic encryption (Frederick, 2015). Here arithmetic operations are performed in encrypted data itself rather than in plain text. It comes mainly in three flavours. They are partial homomorphic encryption, full homomorphic encryption and qasi homomorphic encryption.

Baldi et al., (2011) proposed a cryptographic protocol to determine whether there exists a biological parent-child relationship between two individuals. Ayday et al., (2013) recently conducted privacy-preserving computation of disease risk based on genomic and non-genomic data. Moreover this, two important tools in genetic engineering are: Restriction Enzymes (used to cut DNA) and Small DNA vectors (helpful for transferring the pasted DNA). Hence, some of the existing tools for genetic data analysis are included in the below table.

Genomic data can be analysed statically in two ways. They are family-based analysis (Karen et al., 2017) and population-based analysis (Karen et al., 2017). Genomics techniques are mainly focused on DNA sequencing, DNA structure analysis, genome editing, population genomics, DNA-protein interactions, phylogenomic, or synthetic biology. High-throughput DNA sequencing technologies and bioinformatics have transformed genome analysis by mapping and decrypting coding and non-coding DNA sequences, their evolution and inter-relationships. Some of the tools are explained below

(i)   DNA sequencing tool: They provide base calling, chromatogram display and high-quality sequence region evaluation. For example, EGassember, CAP3, DCA, QUAST.

(ii)   Sequencing errors: Tools help to identify errors in case of mismatched protein sequences. For example, frameD, AMIgene.

(iii) Genome visualization: Tools which allow genomic sequence to be visualized during sequence analysis. For example, CGView Server, DNA plotter.

(iv)   Synthetic gene: This tool helps to synthesis new genes with specific functionalities. For example, Gene Design.

(v)   Genome Comparison: Tools help to make comparative studies among different sequences. For example, SyntTax, AutoGRAPH.

Table 3. Tools Available for Genetic Data Analysis with Description

Tools	Description
Avadis	It is proprietary software used for analysis and visualization of gene expression data.
CLASSIFI(Cluster Assignment for Biological Inference)	It is data mining tool for identifying cluster of similar genes.
DAVID(Database for Annotation, Visualization and Integrated Discovery)	Web based tool used to provide integrated solutions for the analysis of genome scale data sets.
EASE	It is used for summarizing the given gene list.
EGAN (Exploratory Gene Association Networks)	Software tool used to visualize and interpret gene interaction, metadata coincidence etc.
EGOn V2.0 (explore Gene Ontology)	It is a web-based tool for mapping microarray data on to the Gene Ontology structure.
FunCluster	It is a genomic data analysis tool indented for functional analysis of gene data.
GENECODIS	It is a web-based tool for the functional analysis of gene lists.
STEM (Short Time-series Expression Miner)	It is a Java program for clustering, comparing, and visualizing short time series gene expression data.
THEA (Tools for High-throughput Experiments Analysis)	It is an integrated information processing system dedicated to the analysis of post-genomic data.
GENES	software package used for data analysis and processing with different biometric models and is useful in genetic studies applied to plant and animal breeding

As we can see that both data have essential role in identifying the effect of prediction and decision analysis (with respect to many applications). Same prediction mechanism can be useful for an individual patient for care or for different patients based on the quality of predicted data. More over some general tools or algorithm are available in healthcare application (Raghupathi & Raghupathi, 2014) for making better informed decisions or to perform prediction, which are mentioned in the table below:

The data set available for our discussed tools are mentioned at the end of this chapter (refer: after bibliography). Hence, this section discusses about several available tools for analysing genetic data and genomic data as well. Now, next section will discuss about one popular application where genetic data is most popular and genetic analytics is being used frequently (to make some decision/ prediction).

Table 4. Tools/Platform Available for medical Data Analysis with Description

Platform/tool	Description
The Hadoop Distributed File System (HDFS)	Open source distributed data processing platform, which aggregate data in unique way. It adapts divide and conquer technology. It has a capability to process large amount of data by portioning the data set in to different servers. And finally, it merges the results (Borkar et al., 2012; Ohlhorst, 2012) from all the nodes.
MapReduce	It acts as an interface between sub tasks and gather the outputs from all the nodes.
Hive	This support structured query language (SQL) with Hadoop platform. It also helps to create Hive query language.
Zookeeper	It works on the principle of centralized architecture. It supports various services, which can be used by big data application parallel.
Jaql	It facilitates functional declarative query language which helps to process huge data set. It supports parallel processing by converting "high level" queries into "low level "queries
Avro	It provides data serialization services. Other additional features include versioning and version control

Real Time Application of Genetic Data and Genetic Analytics

Genetic data play an important role in the area of biological study. Its importance also spread in other areas like medical care in terms of curing diseases or in view of personalized medicine. Combination of DNA sequences of two different species are used to manufacture antibiotic, hormones or other disease preventive materials. Vaccines likewise have been hereditarily re-designed to trigger an insusceptible reaction that will ensure against explicit diseases. Gene therapy is another invention of genetics. In this a specific gene is introduced into the body which either corrects the genetic disorder or helps the body to resist against the disease and repair by own. The human genome project is another development in the world of genetics which brings out the importance of genome. Genome is the complete set of genetic material present in a cell. This project succeeded in mapping location and function of all genes present in human body. This in turn helps the researchers to study particular gene in detail, damage to specific gene causes what effect in human body? How can we overcome that?

Genetics analytics is popular in the field of forensic also in terms of finding the criminals. In forensic science the role of genetics come into existence because the culprit always leaves some material like hair, skin, blood, fingerprint etc., in the spot. The thorough examination of these substances helps to identify the exact criminal or sometime it helps to save wrongly accused person. Mark Twain published a book named "The Tragedy of Pudd'nhead Wilson, and the Comedy of Those Extraordinary Twins", in this he narrated a story of a murder committed by one person and blamed on his twin. The fingerprint evidence helped the twin to save his life because Fingerprints are unique to the individual; even identical twins have the same DNA but different fingerprints. Sometimes these types of evidence may not visible. To overcome this, new technologies arrived to analyse the invisible prints.

Apart from the above-mentioned applications genetic factors play an important role in identifying hair texture (Fujimoto et al., 2008), eye color (Sturm & Larsson, 2009) intelligence (Deary et al., 2009) etc. Genetic data can also use to the likelihood of conceiving twins (Hoekstra et al., 2008), athletic performance (Ahmetov & Fedotovskaya, 2015). Hence, this section discusses one real time application (including a problem) with respect to genetic data and uses of genetic analytics. Now, next section will discuss several critical issues and challenges required to be focus in near future by research communities.

Issues and Challenges in Genetic Analytics

Although more than 6000 Mendelian disorders have been analysed at the genetic level so far, we still do not have a clear idea of the most of their impact in health and diseases (Rehm et al., 2015). Even though technologies are growing, the people in the rural area are unaware of the advantages of genetics test. The hindrance to utilize these services includes lack of knowledge regarding the requirement of genetics referral, insufficient number of genetic providers, insufficient protection inclusion, and misguided judgments regarding genetic tests. Analysing genomic data is computationally difficult and combining them with other clinical data increases the complexity (Priyanka et al., 2014) Due to advancement in science the genome sequencing expense is less compare to olden days. This advancement helps to include this in normal health test. This help to predict the diseases, especially chronic diseases like tumour in advance before they actually occur. Potential advancements in genomic sequencing helped healthcare and life sciences organizations to generate petabytes of data around medical research (with respect to patient data), but very few organizations can fully utilize their genomic data for meaningful predictions because the data is disordered and they lack access to analytics at large scale.

As we mentioned in the introduction part, genetic analytics helps to peep into our future, still some issues are associated with the study of genetics. They are mentioned below as:

i.   Self-governance: Each new hereditary test causes significant issues for prescription, general wellbeing, and social arrangement with respect to the conditions under which the test ought to be utilized, how the test is executed, and what utilizations are made of its outcomes. Concern for autonomy refers to the privilege of people to control the future utilization of hereditary material used the study of particular reason. People those who have under gone genetic test also have rights to decide whether their data can be shared to a third party, either in terms of insurance or in case of research.

ii. Privacy: Privacy can be defined as authorized access to private data. When a person undergoes genetic test, privacy can be defining as privilege of a person to take decision about to whom all they can share their genome information. The third party can be insurance team, family members, and researcher etc. The two federal laws which provide security for genetic data are GINA (Genetic Information Non-Discrimination Act) and HIPAA (Health Insurance Portability and Accountability Act). These laws help to restrict the use of personal genome data but no guarantee that data will not be miss used once it is in hands of outsider. Some encryption techniques are also implemented to achieve the same. But these methods also did not provide results up to the mark in case of genetic data analysis The Fair Information Practices Principles (FIPPs) offer a framework for enabling data sharing and usage based on the guidelines adopted by the U.S. Department of Health and Human Services (Baker et al., 2016). These principles consist of: individual access, data correction, data transparency, individual choice, data collection and disclosure barrier, data quality and integrity, safeguards, and accountability.

iii. Confidentiality: Some parts on the genetic result include more sensitive data, which has to be completely protected from an outsider. Privacy ensures authorized use of data but confidentiality refers to how far a person can access to the available genetic data. Regarding people includes respecting their zone of protection and tolerating their choices to control access to data about them. The infringement of rights to confidentiality occurs either through breaches or via carelessness. Confidentiality of health care information especially genetic information has to be protected because disclosure of a person's medical condition not only cause harm to him or her but also for their family members.

Hence, this section discusses several open issues and challenges (in detail) related to genetic analytics. Now, next section will discuss several opportunities towards tools required for genetic analytic in near future for better prediction or making useful decision. Also, next section will discuss several research gaps in genetic analytics which will be more helpful for future researchers.

Opportunities for Future in Genetic Analytics

The study of massive amount of genetic data helps to revolutionize the field of healthcare, pharmaceutical and agricultural industries. Genome sequencing and re-sequencing method help to develop modern plant breeding techniques. There are new methods that enable DNA to be modified more precisely. One example is CRISPR-Cas9, essentially a molecule that can find a particular point in a genome and snip out or insert chunks of DNA in a precisely targeted way. Another example goes by the name of ZFNs, and progress here is further forward, i.e., it is the basis of a technique to attack HIV that is currently in phase 2 clinical trials.

Compare to olden days the cost of genetic engineering is coming down, once if it is cheap and easy it is going to use more widely. So, we can achieve innovative invention in the field of genetics. This in turn helps to keep the population healthy and safe. The genomic data analytics plays a vital role in predictive analytics. The medical care solutions of the future combine an individual's DNA and other information to produce personalized treatments for each patient, identify chronic disorders causing different cancers, and develop targeted treatments that wipe out harmful / defective cells while keeping the healthy ones intact. Next-generation genomic sequencing is revolutionizing medicine. This helps to save life by providing more efficient care. Medical imaging data is a type of Big Data in health research. Imaging genomics is a quickly growing field derived from recent advancement in multimodal imaging data and high-throughput omics data (Karen et al., 2017).

With the help of genetic engineering, we can change each and every aspect of an unborn child. The main cause of Diabetics is hereditary and life style. If a person has a history of diabetic for his/her ancestor then he/she is more susceptible to diabetic, but with genetic engineering everything seems to be flexible.

Hence, this section discusses several opportunities which require as must (mandatory) in near future for providing effective decision and productive results. Now, this work will be concluded with some future enhancement in next section.

SUMMARY

Genetics is a branch of biology concerned with the study of genes, genetic variation, and heredity in organisms. Due to recent development in technology and medical care, we have moved to the use of internet of things devices in several applications (Amit & Shamila, 2019; Shamila et al., 2019) like medical, transportation, etc., where such smart device is collecting a lot of data (related to patient) from medical devices. This data is highly useful in making some decision for same treatment for different people. With respect to that, in medical care application genetic analysis and genetic testing is being done. Note that Genetic analysis totally differs from Genetic testing. Genetic analytics is being done with genes, or proteins, etc., in simple words, genetic analysis means "the study of a sample of DNA to look for mutations (changes) that may increase risk of disease or affect the way a person responds to treatment". Genetic analytics (on Big data) is growing phase, require lot of attention from research communities to solve many critical problems like having not skilled people for analysis this genetic data, lack of standard tool, non-efficient algorithm, etc. Hence, keeping such things (concerns/ facts) in our mind, we try to incorporate all required information (related to genetic analytics) in this chapter. This chapter has included several interesting things/ facts related to genetic analytics such as role of genetic analytic in healthcare care, tools available in current for analysing genetic data, critical issues and challenges, etc. As future, we can try to make (build) some efficient tools and algorithms for genetic analytics or to analysis genomic data.

REFERENCES

Abecasis, G. R., Auton, A., Brooks, L. D., DePristo, M. A., Durbin, R. M., Handsaker, R. E., … McVean, G. A. (2012). An integrated map of genetic variation from 1,092 human genomes. *Nature*, *491*(7422), 56–65. doi:10.1038/nature11632 PMID:23128226

Ahmetov, I. I., & Fedotovskaya, O. N. (2015). Current Progress in Sports Genomics. *Advances in Clinical Chemistry*, *70*, 247–314. doi:10.1016/bs.acc.2015.03.003 PMID:26231489

Amin, D., & Raja Azlina, R.M. (2013). Feature Selection Based on Genetic Algorithm and Support Vector Machine for Intrusion Detection System. *SDIWC*.

Auton, A., Brooks, L. D., Durbin, R. M., Garrison, E. P., Kang, H. M., Korbel, J. O., … Abecasis, G. R. (2015). A global reference for human genetic variation. *Nature*, *526*(7571), 68–74. doi:10.1038/nature15393 PMID:26432245

Ayday, E., Raisaro, J. L., McLaren, P. J., Fellay, J., & Hubaux, J. P. (2013). Privacy-preserving Computation of Disease Risk by Using Genomic, Clinical, and Environmental Data. *USENIX Workshop on Health Information Technologies*.

Baker, D. B., Kaye, J., & Terry, S. F. (2016). Governance through privacy, fairness, and respect for individuals. *EGEMS (Washington, DC)*, *4*(2), 1207. doi:10.13063/2327-9214.1207 PMID:27141520

Baldi, P., Baronio, R., & Cristofaro, E. D. (2011). Countering GATTACA: efficient and secure testing of fully-sequenced human genomes, *Proceedings of the 18th ACM Conference on Computer and Communications Security*. 691-702. 10.1145/2046707.2046785

Borkar, V. R., Carey, M. J., & Chen, L. (2012). Big data platforms: What's next? *ACM Crossroads*, *19*(1), 44–49. doi:10.1145/2331042.2331057

Butte, A. J., & Kohane, I. S. (2006). Creation and implications of a phenome-genome network. *Nature Biotechnology*, *24*(1), 55–62. doi:10.1038/nbt1150 PMID:16404398

Chen, Z., Lee, L., Chen, J., Collins, R., Wu, F., Guo, Y., Linksted, P., & Peto, R. (2005). Cohort profile: The Kadoorie Study of Chronic Disease in China (KSCDC). *International Journal of Epidemiology*, *34*(6), 1243–1249. doi:10.1093/ije/dyi174 PMID:16131516

Collins, F. S., & Varmus, H. (2015). A new initiative on precision medicine. *The New England Journal of Medicine*, *372*(9), 793–795. doi:10.1056/NEJMp1500523 PMID:25635347

Cynthia, D. (2006). Differential privacy. *International Colloquium on Automata, Languages and Programming*, *4052*, 1–12.

Deary, I. J., Johnson, W., & Houlihan, L. M. (2009). Genetic foundations of human intelligence. *Human Genetics*, *126*(1), 215–232. doi:10.100700439-009-0655-4 PMID:19294424

Efthymioua, S., Manolea, A., & Houlden, H. (2016). Next-generation sequencing in neuromuscular diseases. *Current Opinion in Neurology*, *29*(5), 527–536. doi:10.1097/WCO.0000000000000374 PMID:27588584

Fujimoto, A., Kimura, R., Ohashi, J., Omi, K., Yuliwulandari, R., Batubara, L., Mustofa, M. S., Samakkarn, U., Settheetham-Ishida, W., Ishida, T., Morishita, Y., Furusawa, T., Nakazawa, M., Ohtsuka, R., & Tokunaga, K. (2008). A scan for genetic determinants of human hair morphology: EDAR is associated with Asian hair thickness. *Human Molecular Genetics*, *17*(6), 835–843. doi:10.1093/hmg/ddm355 PMID:18065779

Grabe, H. J., Assel, H., Bahls, T., Dorr, M., Endlich, K., Endlich, N., ... Fiene, B. (2014). Cohort profile: Greifswald approach to individualized medicine (GANI_MED). *Journal of Translational Medicine*, *12*(1), 144. doi:10.1186/1479-5876-12-144 PMID:24886498

Gulcher, J. R., Jonsson, P., Kong, A., Kristjansson, K., Frigge, M. L., Karason, A., ... Sigurthoardottir, S. (1997). Mapping of a familial essential tremor gene, FET1, to chromosome 3q13. *Nature Genetics*, *17*(1), 84–87. doi:10.1038/ng0997-84 PMID:9288103

Hoekstra, C., Zhao, Z. Z., Lambalk, C. B., Willemsen, G., Martin, N. G., Boomsma, D. I., & Montgomery, G. W. (2008). Dizygotic twinning. *Human Reproduction Update*, *14*(1), 37–47. doi:10.1093/humupd/dmm036 PMID:18024802

Hoffmann, T. J., Kvale, M. N., Hesselson, S. E., Zhan, Y., Aquino, C., Cao, Y., Cawley, S., Chung, E., Connell, S., Eshragh, J., Ewing, M., Gollub, J., Henderson, M., Hubbell, E., Iribarren, C., Kaufman, J., Lao, R. Z., Lu, Y., Ludwig, D., ... Risch, N. (2011). Next generation genome-wide association tool: Design and coverage of a high-throughput European-optimized SNP array. *Genomics*, *98*(2), 79–89. doi:10.1016/j.ygeno.2011.04.005 PMID:21565264

Hornoch, T. P. (2013). A survey of informatics approaches to whole-exome and whole-genome clinical reporting in the electronic health record. *Genetics in Medicine*, *15*(10), 824–832. doi:10.1038/gim.2013.120 PMID:24071794

Karen, Y. (2017). Big Data analytics for genomic medicine. *International Journal of Molecular Sciences*, *18*(2), 412. doi:10.3390/ijms18020412 PMID:28212287

Kumar Tyagi, & Shamila. (2019). *Spy in the Crowd: How User's Privacy is getting affected with the Integration of Internet of Thing's Devices.* Elsevier.

McCarty, C. A., Nair, A., Austin, D. M., & Giampietro, P. F. (2007). Informed consent and subject motivation to participate in a large, population-based genomics study: The marshfield clinic personalized medicine research project. *Community Genetics*, *10*(1), 2–9. doi:10.1159/000096274 PMID:17167244

Munoz, M., Pong-Wong, R., Canela-Xandri, O., Rawlik, K., Haley, C. S., & Tenesa, A. (2016). Evaluating the contribution of genetics and familial shared environment to common disease using the UK biobank. *Nature Genetics*, *48*(9), 980–983. doi:10.1038/ng.3618 PMID:27428752

National Center for Biotechnology Information. (2016). *The Database of Genotypes and Phenotypes (dbGaP)*. Author.

Ohlhorst, F. (2012). *Big Data Analytics: Turning Big Data into Big Money*. John Wiley & Sons. doi:10.1002/9781119205005

Postmus, I., Trompet, S., Deshmukh, H. A., Barnes, M. R., Li, X., Warren, H. R., ... Donnelly, L. A. (2014). Pharmacogenetic meta-analysis of genome-wide association studies of LDL cholesterol response to statins. *Nature Communications*, *5*(1), 5068. doi:10.1038/ncomms6068 PMID:25350695

Priyanka, K. (2014). A Survey on Big Data Analytics in Health Care. *International Journal of Computer Science and Information Technologies*, *5*(4), 5865–5868.

Raghupathi, W., & Raghupathi, V. (2014). Big data analytics in healthcare: Promise and potential. *Health Information Science and Systems*, *2*(1), 3. doi:10.1186/2047-2501-2-3 PMID:25825667

Rasmussen-Torvik, L. J., Stallings, S. C., Gordon, A. S., Almoguera, B., Basford, M. A., Bielinski, S. J., ... Connolly, J. J. (2014). Design and anticipated outcomes of the eMERGE-PGx project: A multicenter pilot for preemptive pharmacogenomics in electronic health record systems. *Clinical Pharmacology and Therapeutics*, *96*(4), 482–489. doi:10.1038/clpt.2014.137 PMID:24960519

Rehm, H. L., Berg, J. S., Brooks, L. D., Bustamante, C. D., Evans, J. P., Landrum, M. J., ... Nussbaum, R. L. (2015). Clingen—The clinical genome resource. *The New England Journal of Medicine*, *372*(23), 2235–2242. doi:10.1056/NEJMsr1406261 PMID:26014595

Reiber, G. E., & LaCroix, A. Z. (2016). Older women veterans in the women's health initiative. *The Gerontologist*, *56*(Suppl. 1), S1–S5. doi:10.1093/geront/gnv673 PMID:26768382

Robert, F. (2015). Core Concept: Homomorphic encryption. *Proceedings of the National Academy of Sciences of the United States of America*, *112*(28), 8515–8516. doi:10.1073/pnas.1507452112 PMID:26174872

Saal, L. H., Vallon-Christersson, J., Hakkinen, J., Hegardt, C., Grabau, D., Winter, C., ... Schulz, R. (2015). The Sweden Cancerome Analysis Network—Breast (SCAN-B) initiative: A large-scale multicenter infrastructure towards implementation of breast cancer genomic analyses in the clinical routine. *Genome Medicine*, *7*(1), 20. doi:10.118613073-015-0131-9 PMID:25722745

Shamila, M., & Vinuthna, K. (2019). A Review on Several Critical Issues and Challenges in IoT based e-Healthcare System. IEEE.

Sturm, R. A., & Larsson, M. (2009). Genetics of human iris color and patterns. *Pigment Cell & Melanoma Research*, *22*(5), 544–562. doi:10.1111/j.1755-148X.2009.00606.x PMID:19619260

Vijini, M. (2017). *Towards data science-blog*. Academic Press.

Wagner, R. A., & Fischer, M. J. (1974). The string to string correction problem. *Journal of the Association for Computing Machinery*, *21*(1), 168–173. doi:10.1145/321796.321811

Weir, B. S. (1990). Genetic data analysis. Methods for discrete population genetic data. Academic Press.

WHA 57.13. (2004). *Genomics and World Health.* Fifty Seventh World Health Assembly Resolution.

WHO. (2002). Genomics and World Health: Report of the Advisory Committee on Health research. Geneva: WHO.

Wong, S. Q., Fellowes, A., Doig, K., Ellul, J., Bosma, T. J., Irwin, D., ... Chan, K. S. (2015). Assessing the clinical value of targeted massively parallel sequencing in a longitudinal, prospective population-based study of cancer patients. *British Journal of Cancer*, *112*(8), 1411–1420. doi:10.1038/bjc.2015.80 PMID:25742471

KEY TERMS AND DEFINITIONS

Chromosome: a strand of DNA tightly wrapped around proteins called histones. Chromosomes are the way DNA is organized in a cell.

DNA: It stands for deoxyribonucleic acid. The carrier of heredity composed of nucleotides. It carries genetic information within a cell that is transmitted from generation to generation.

Gene: The basic unit of heredity. Typically, a gene is a segment of DNA that occupies a particular location on a chromosome, and encodes for a protein.

Genetics: It focuses on study of functionalities of a single gene.

Genome: The complete set of genes in an organism. The total genetic content in one set of chromosomes.

Genomics: It includes study of whole gene and the inter relationships among them.

Chapter 18
Heart Disease Prediction Using Machine Learning

Shiva Shanta Mani B.
Indian Institute of Information Technology, Kottayam, India

Manikandan V. M.
SRM University AP, Andhra Pradesh, India

ABSTRACT

Heart disease is one of the most common and serious health issues in all the age groups. The food habits, mental stress, smoking, etc. are a few reasons for heart diseases. Diagnosing heart issues at an early stage is very much important to take proper treatment. The treatment of heart disease at the later stage is very expensive and risky. In this chapter, the authors discuss machine learning approaches to predict heart disease from a set of health parameters collected from a person. The heart disease dataset from the UCI machine learning repository is used for the study. This chapter discusses the heart disease prediction capability of four well-known machine learning approaches: naive Bayes classifier, KNN classifier, decision tree classifier, random forest classifier.

INTRODUCTION

Nowadays heart disease is one of the leading causes of death in middle-aged people. Heart diseases such as coronary heart disease, heart attack, congestive heart failure, and congenital heart disease are very common in both men and women. As per the study conducted by centers for disease control (CDC), heart disease is a major reason for death in countries like United States, United Kingdom, Australia, and Canada. It is surprising that one in every four deaths in the United States as a result of some kind of serious heart disease. There are different reasons for heart diseases such as smoking habits, eating foods with high-fat content, lack of exercise, etc. The precaution for heart disease includes quitting smoking, controlling the blood pressure, maintaining proper body mass index, and regular exercising.

DOI: 10.4018/978-1-7998-2742-9.ch018

There are two approaches to treat heart diseases: medication and surgery. The heart diseases in its initial stage can be cured using the medication, but the same disease in later stages may need surgical treatment. The heart disease treatment at the later stage is expensive and there is a huge risk even though the advanced surgical technologies are available for treatment. So it will be useful if there is an automated system to predict heart disease. In this paper, we discuss a set of machine learning approaches for heart disease prediction. The experimental study has been carried out using the UCI machine learning repository for heart diseases.

The rest of this chapter is discussing the related work, the proposed scheme, the future research directions, and the conclusion.

BACKGROUND

This paper aims at analyzing the various machine learning approaches for heart disease prediction. A few relevant works in this area are discussed in this section. Heart disease is a term that assigns to a large number of medical conditions related to the heart. These medical conditions describe the abnormal health conditions that directly influence the heart and all its parts. Heart disease is a major health problem. A recent statistics about heart diseases are reported in (Go, 2014).Some preventive mechanisms for heart diseases are discussed in (Shepherd, et al., 1995). A neural network-based heart disease prediction system is discussed in (Singh, Singh, & Pandi-Jain, 2018) and the authors used 15 medical parameters of the patient. A multilayer perceptron neural network with back propagation is used to develop a trained model. A KNN based approach for remote patient monitoring is discussed in (Enriko, Suryanegara, & Gunawan, 2018). A firefly algorithm based heart prediction technique is discussed in (Long, Meesad, & Unger, 2015).

In this manuscript, we used a set of machine learning approaches for heart disease prediction. Four well-known machine learning approaches are used in this study and those are discussed in this section.

1. **Naive Bayes Classifier:** Naive Bayes classifier is based on Bayes theorem. It makes strong independent assumptions between features, which means every pair of features is independent compared to every other feature (Rish, 2019). In this study, the Gaussian Naive Bayes classifier is used. If the training dataset contains null values for some specific parameter then it is better to use naive Bayes classifier. The major advantages of naive Bayes classifier are listed below:
   ◦ Simple and fast
   ◦ Possible to make probabilistic prediction
   ◦ Strong independent attribute assumptions
2. **KNN Classifier:** The KNN stands for K-nearest neighbor and it can be used for both in classification and regression problems (Goldberger & Hinton, 2005). It is widely disposable in real-life scenarios since it is non-parametric, which means it does not make any underlying assumptions about the distribution of data. A given test data is classified by the majority vote of its neighbors. We can choose the value of K where K is the number of nearest neighbors of an object for which we wish to vote.
3. **Decision Tree Classifier:** The decision tree is in the form of a tree structure. It is a simple and widely used classification technique. It breaks the data into subparts, makes decisions, and at the same time decision tree is incrementally developed (Du & Zhan, 2002).

The main advantages of decision tree approaches are listed below:

- Decision trees implicitly perform feature selection.
- Non-linear relationships between parameters do not affect tree performance.

The major limitations of decision tree approach are the following:

- Working with continuous attributes (binning).
- Avoiding over fitting.
- Super Attributes (attributes with many unique values).

4. **Random Forest classifier:** The random forest can be used for both regression and classification. It is also known as random decision forest. Basically, a collection of trees is known as a forest. This method is used to build predictive models. The random forest searches for the important (best) feature among the random subset of features while splitting (Liaw & Wiener, 2002). The importance of each feature can be known easily by seeing how many tree nodes uses that feature and reduces the impurity. It is something like a group of dull students together can be equal to a clever student. In the same way, the group of decision trees is combined to build a random forest. Hence, it can give a better prediction accuracy.

The advantages of using random forest classifier is given below:

- It can be used for both classification and regression models.
- It is easy to use because its default hyper parameters use good predictive results.

The limitations of random classifier is listed below:

- Large number of trees can make algorithm slow.
- Random forest is fast to train the model but slow in prediction.

In this book chapter, we have analyze the capability of above-mentioned machine learning approaches in the prediction of heart disease.

SOLUTIONS AND RECOMMENDATIONS

There are so many classification and regression techniques are available for prediction. In this study, we have used four well-known classification techniques: naive Bayes classifier, KNN classifier, decision tree, and random forests. The overview of the proposed scheme is shown in **Algorithm 1: Proposed system**

```
Step 1: Load the dataset
Step 2: Pre-process (data cleaning) the dataset. During pre-processing remove
the null values with some valid information.
Step 3: Split the dataset into training and testing data.
```

```
Step 4: Develop a trained model using training data and a specific machine
learning approach (naive Bayes/KNN classifier/decision tree/random forests).
Step 5: Find the confusion matrix by analyzing the predicted output from the
trained model while feeding the test data.
Step 6: Compute the classification accuracy, precision, and recall.
Step 7: Compare the results from various machine learning approaches and pick
the best approach.
```

In most of the cases, it is difficult to say which classification technique will give better classification accuracy. Therefore, we have considered all four machine learning approaches and find heart disease prediction capability. The selection of training data also influences the prediction capability, therefore we have adopted the following strategies:

- 75%, 80% and 90% of the data from the dataset are used for training, and the remaining 25%, 20% and 10% respectively is used for testing purpose.
- Changed the random state value in the classification algorithm while splitting the dataset into training data and testing data.
- We have done data cleaning by removing samples with null values.

The classification results from the experimental study can be analyzed to select the best technique for heart disease prediction and the same can be used for the practical purpose. The heart disease dataset contains 14 attributes. The attributes are listed in Table 1.

Table 1. Attributes of heart disease dataset

Sl. No.	Attribute
1	Age in years
2	Sex
3	Chest pain type
4	Resting blood pressure
5	Serum cholesterol in mg/dl
6	Fasting blood sugar
7	Resting electrocardiographic results
8	Maximum heart rate achieved
9	Exercise induced angina
10	Depression induced by exercise relative to rest
11	The slope of the peak exercise ST segment
12	Number of major vessels (0-3) colored by fluoroscopy
13	Thalassemia: 3 = normal; 6 = fixed defect; 7 = reversible defect
14	The predicted output

Figure 1. Overview of the proposed system

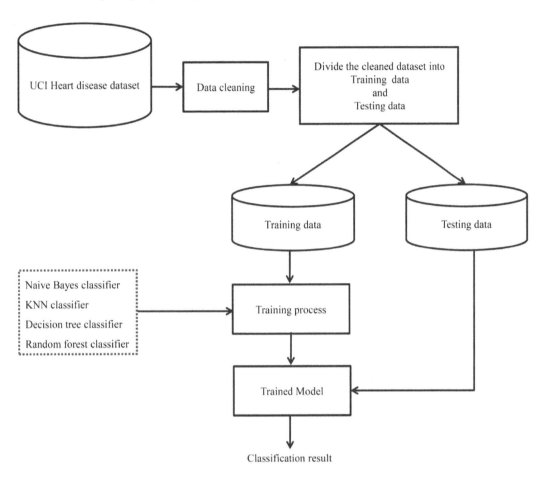

The experimental study has been carried out on a machine with the Intel Core i3 processor with 4GB RAM. The algorithms are implemented using Python3. During the experimental study, we have used the heart disease dataset which is publicly available in UCI machine learning repository (Dua & Taniskidou).

The classification scheme can be evaluated using three efficiency parameters: detection accuracy (DA), recall (RE), and precision (PR) (Powers, 2011). These are briefly described below:

$$DA = \frac{TP}{\left(TP + FP\right)}$$

where,

- TP: Number of testing samples with heart disease are declared as heart disease
- FP: Number of testing samples without heart disease is declared as heart disease
- TN: Number of testing samples without heart disease is declared as without heart disease
- FN: Number of testing samples with heart disease is declared as without heart disease

During result analysis, we have considered detection accuracy, precision, recall, training time (in seconds), and testing time (in seconds). During the experimental study the training has been carried out with 90% of data, 80% of data, and 75% data to observe the efficiency accuracy. Table 2 shows the results while 90% of data has been used for training, Table 3 shows the results while 80% of data has been used for training, and Table 4 shows the results while 75% of data has been used for training. The graphical representation of detection accuracy, precision, and recall for all the three different training process are depicted in Figure 2, Figure 3, and Figure 4.

Table 2. 90% of the data used for training

Classifier	AC	PR	RE	Training Time (in Seconds)	Testing Time (in Seconds)
Naive Bayes	0.700	0.830	0.700	0.00216699	0.00082278
KNN	0.800	0.640	0.800	0.00102639	0.00140381
Decision tree	0.767	0.829	0.767	0.00099659	0.00040197
Random forest	0.833	0.786	0.833	0.0119205	0.00114417

Table 3. 80% of the data used for training

Classifier	AC	PR	RE	Training Time (in Seconds)	Testing Time (in Seconds)
Naive Bayes	0.667	0.672	0.667	0.002833	0.000899
KNN	0.667	0.460	0.667	0.000605	0.001741
Decision tree	0.733	0.705	0.733	0.002133	0.000591
Random forest	0.717	0.628	0.717	0.019505	0.001106

Table 4. 75% of the data used for training

Classifier	AC	PR	RE	Training Time (in Seconds)	Testing Time (in Seconds)
Naive Bayes	0.527	0.500	0.527	0.00354	0.00354
KNN	0.514	0.264	0.514	0.000517	0.00268
Decision tree	0.514	0.264	0.514	0.00169	0.000397
Random forest	0.559	0.415	0.559	0.0165	0.001229

From the experimental results, it can be observed that all the four schemes are giving good detection accuracy, precision, and recall while training with 90% of data. The random forest classifier able to predict heart disease with an accuracy of 0.833 without losing the precision and recall values. In general, the training process is an offline process therefore we are not concerned about the training time. Once the trained model is ready, it can be used by any number of users, and hence training time does not influence much in heart disease prediction. But testing time is very much important since it may be a real-time process. The naive Bayes classifier and decision tree classifier is efficient in terms of testing time. From all these observations, the KNN classifier and random forest classifier are doing good prediction but testing time is comparatively high as compared to the testing time for naive Bayes classifier and decision tree classifier. Since the health care applications are more concerned about the prediction accuracy as compared to the processing time, we suggest KNN classifier or random forest classifier for heart disease prediction.

Figure 2. 90% of data has been used for training

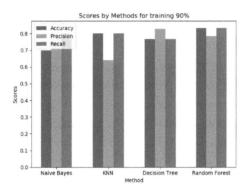

Figure 3. 80% of data has been used for training

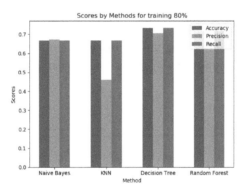

Figure 4. 75% of data has been used for training

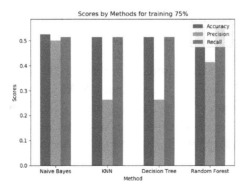

FUTURE RESEARCH DIRECTIONS

There are lots of scopes to work further in this domain. The researchers can try to improve the efficiency of heart disease prediction through hybrid machine learning approaches in which we will use the combinations of various machine learning approaches. The people can work to identify the crucial attributes in the heart disease dataset so that training and testing can be carried out by considering only the crucial attributes instead of all the 14 attributes.

CONCLUSION

The early detection of heart diseases is very crucial and we have discussed the use of machine learning for heart disease prediction. We have considered four well-known machine learning techniques: naive Bayes classifier, KNN classifier, decision tree classifier, and random forest classier for heart disease prediction. The standard heart disease dataset from the UCI machine learning library with 14 attributes are used in this study. We have analyzed and compared the heart prediction capability and processing time from various schemes and concluded that KNN classifier or random forest classifier is suited for heart disease prediction. Future works can be carried to find a minimal set of attributes from the heart disease dataset which may give better prediction capability.

ACKNOWLEDGMENT

We thank the host institutions for providing the facility to complete the research project. This research received no specific grant from any funding agency in the public, commercial, or not-for-profit sectors.

REFERENCES

Du, W., & Zhan, Z. (2002). Building decision tree classifier on private data. In *International conference on Privacy, security and data mining* (pp. 1-8). IEEE.

Dua, D., & Taniskidou, E. K. (n.d.). *UCI Machine Learning Repository*. Retrieved March 2018, from http://archive. ics. uci. edu/ml

Enriko, I. K., Suryanegara, M., & Gunawan, D. (2018). Heart Disease Diagnosis System with k-Nearest Neighbors Method Using Real Clinical Medical Records. In *International Conference on Frontiers of Educational Technologies*, (pp. 127-131). 10.1145/3233347.3233386

Go, A., Mozaffarian, D., Roger, V. L., Benjamin, E. J., Berry, J. D., Blaha, M. J., Dai, S., Ford, E. S., Fox, C. S., Franco, S., Fullerton, H. J., Gillespie, C., Hailpern, S. M., Heit, J. A., Howard, V. J., Huffman, M. D., Judd, S. E., Kissela, B. M., Kittner, S. J., ... Turner, M. B. (2014). Executive summary: heart disease and stroke statistics—2014 update: a report from the American Heart Association. *Circulation*, *129*(3), 399–410. doi:10.1161/01.cir.0000442015.53336.12 PMID:24446411

Goldberger, J., & Hinton, G. E. (2005). Neighbourhood components analysis. *Advances in Neural Information Processing Systems*, ●●●, 513–520.

Liaw, A., & Wiener, M. (2002). Classification and regression by random Forest. *R News*, ●●●, 18–22.

Long, N. C., Meesad, P., & Unger, H. (2015). A highly accurate firefly based algorithm for heart disease prediction. *Expert Systems with Applications*, *42*(21), 8221–8231. doi:10.1016/j.eswa.2015.06.024

Powers, D. M. (2011). Evaluation: From precision, recall and F-measure to ROC, informedness, markedness and correlation. *Journal of Machine Learning Technologies*, 37–63.

Rish, I. (2019). An empirical study of the naive Bayes classifier. In Workshop on Empirical Methods in Artificial Intelligence, (pp. 41-46). Academic Press.

Shepherd, J., Cobbe, S. M., Ford, I., Isles, C. G., Lorimer, A. R., Macfarlane, P. W., McKillop, J. H., & Packard, C. J. (1995). Prevention of coronary heart disease with pravastatin in men with hypercholesterolemia. *The New England Journal of Medicine*, *333*(20), 1301–1308. doi:10.1056/NEJM199511163332001 PMID:7566020

Singh, P., Singh, S., & Pandi-Jain, G. S. (2018). Effective heart disease prediction system using data mining techniques. *International Journal of Nanomedicine*, *13*, 121–124. doi:10.2147/IJN.S124998 PMID:29593409

Chapter 19
Heuristic Approach Performances for Artificial Neural Networks Training

Kerim Kürşat Çevik

ⓘ https://orcid.org/0000-0002-2921-506X

Akdeniz University, Turkey

ABSTRACT

This chapter aimed to evaluate heuristic approach performances for artificial neural networks (ANN) training. For this purpose, software that can perform ANN training application was developed using four different algorithms. First of all, training system was developed via back propagation (BP) algorithm, which is the most commonly used method for ANN training in the literature. Then, in order to compare the performance of this method with the heuristic methods, software that performs ANN training with genetic algorithm (GA), particle swarm optimization (PSO), and artificial immunity (AI) methods were designed. These designed software programs were tested on the breast cancer dataset taken from UCI (University of California, Irvine) database. When the test results were evaluated, it was seen that the most important difference between heuristic algorithms and BP algorithm occurred during the training period. When the training-test durations and performance rates were examined, the optimal algorithm for ANN training was determined as GA.

INTRODUCTION

The term Artificial Intelligence (AI), which is based on imitation of human processes of thinking and acting as the starting point, was first introduced to the literature by McCarthy at a conference on the subject in Dartmouth, USA in 1956 (McCarthy, Minsky, Rochester, & Shannon, 2006). The purpose of the AI is to implement human behavior in machines. The sub-branch that applies AI algorithms to machines is called Machine Learning. Artificial Neural Network (ANN) is a field of study in machine learning. ANN approaches that try to create a new system inspired by the neurons in our brain are used in classification problems (Öztemel, 2003).

DOI: 10.4018/978-1-7998-2742-9.ch019

ANNs are computer systems that can learn events using data determined by people and determine the response to unlearned events. They are successfully applied in areas that human brain can easily realize such as learning, classification, association, optimization, feature determination and generalization (Öztemel, 2003).

ANNs are currently used to solve a variety of problems. ANNs are successfully applied in areas as classification, estimation and modeling. ANN can be used to process or analyze all kinds of data. They are successfully applied in business life, finance, industry, education and scientific areas with complex problems, in solving problems that cannot be solved by fuzzy or simple methods, and in nonlinear systems (Çetin, 2007).

BACKGROUND

Various methods have been used for training of ANNs. These methods are widely classified into two sets as supervised and unsupervised learning. In training ANNs with supervised learning, both the input data and the output data are provided. In unsupervised learning, only the input data are provided in training ANNs and it is expected to estimate outputs (Nabiyev, 2003). The Backpropagation training algorithm (or generalized delta rule) technique, which is a gradient-descent method, is one of the most popular training algorithms in the domain of neural networks (Rumelhart, Hinton, & Williams, 1988). The back propagation algorithm is a family of methods used to efficiently train artificial neural networks by following a gradient-based optimization algorithm using the chain rule (Kahramanli & Allahverdi, 2008). As ANNs generate complex error surfaces with multiple local minima, BP tends to converging into local minima rather than global minima (Gupta & Sexton, 1999; Valian, Mohanna, & Tavakoli, 2011). Many advanced learning algorithms have been proposed in recent years in order to overcome the shortcomings of gradient based techniques (Valian et al., 2011). These algorithms include direct optimization method using a polytope algorithm (Curry & Morgan, 1997), Evolutionary Algorithms (EA), a class of general search technique (Salchenberger, Cinar, & Lash, 1992) and genetic algorithm (GA) (Sexton, Dorsey, & Johnson, 1998). Other techniques, such as EA, have been applied to the ANN problem in the past (Cantú-Paz, 2003; Cotta, Alba, Sagarna, & Larrañaga, 2002) and they have tried to avoid the local minima in the error that usually occurs in complex problems.

Many researchers have preferred meta-heuristic optimization algorithm since conventional numerical methods have some computational drawbacks in solving complex optimization problems. In recent years, various meta-heuristic algorithms have been successfully applied to various engineering optimization problems. When compared to conventional numerical methods, EA has provided better solutions for most complicated real-world optimization problems (Valian et al., 2011). In meta-heuristic algorithms, many rules and randomness are combined to imitate natural phenomena. These phenomena include the biological evolutionary processes such as the Genetic Algorithm (GA) (Goldberg & Holland, 1988; Holland, 1992), Evolutionary Algorithm (EA) (Fogel, 1998), Artificial Immunity (Hofmeyr & Forrest, 2000) and Differential Evolution (DE) (Storn, 1996) animal behavior such as Ant Colony Algorithm (ACA) (Dorigo & Di Caro, 1999) and Particle Swarm Optimization (PSO) (Shi & Eberhart, 1999), human's intuition such as Tabu Search Algorithm (Glover, 1977); and physical annealing processes, such as simulated annealing (SA) (Valian et al., 2011).

There are various academic and commercial software programs developed for ANN training. The most widely used commercial software are as Matlab, GoldenGem, EasyNN-Plus, Harbinger, SprinN Lite, TradingSolutions, LTF- Cimulator, BrainCom, EasyNN, Alyuda NeuroIntelligence, Neuro Solutions, Statistica, Mathematica, Netmaker, JOONE, Fuzzy COPE and so on (Tosun, 2018).

When the academic studies in this field are examined, it is seen that the software is realized and tested in many different programming languages. In their study conducted in 2008, Bayındır and Sesveren (2008) presented computer based an artificial neural network (ANN) software to learning and understanding of artificial neural networks. They developed four different training algorithms by changing the momentum factor of BP and provided the use of these algorithms. It was concluded that the developed software was used by 10 different graduate students and it contributed to comprehend the artificial intelligence (Bayindir & Sesveren, 2008). In his thesis study conducted in 2010 Kose developed ANN and fuzzy logic based software via C# programming language. In the study, ANN training was performed using the back propagation algorithm and the hyper parameters determined by the user; and the system was compared with Matlab commercial software (Köse, 2010). In their study conducted in 20012 Çevik and Dandıl presented software for ANN training by using BP algorithm. The software was developed via C#. NET programming language and enabled a standard user modeling using ANN. The developed ANN training software was implemented in the example of image classifications of the numbers of and successful results were obtained (Çevik & Dandıl, 2012). In their study Tuncay et al., designed web based ANN training software. The designed software provides object-oriented programming, XML and AJAX technologies and allows the user to model ANN with remote access. It was stated that 95% of the students in the school that the programme was tested were helpful in understanding the ANN correctly (Yiğit, Işık, & Bilen, 2014). In 2017, Arı and Berberler tried to develop visual and flexible software in which learning, generalization features of ANN could be easily seen and estimation and classification problems could be applied by using C#.NET programming language. In this study, the training was performed by using back propagation algorithm for single and multi-layer networks. The authors concluded that they have implemented user-friendly Turkish software (Arı & Berberler, 2017).

MAIN FOCUS OF THE CHAPTER

The chapter is organized as follows. In this section, information about artificial neural cells and ANNs are provided. GY, GA, PSO and IC algorithms used in ANN training are explained. The visual design tool developed in this study is explained in section 3. In addition, tests conducted with the data set used are mentioned in this section. In section 4, the results obtained from the test of the system are presented. The paper is ended with discussion section.

Artificial Neural Networks (ANN)

Artificial Neural Networks (ANN) is one of the machine learning algorithms. They are named as 'artificial' neural networks because they are inspired by the structure and the function of the human brain (Nabiyev, 2003). ANN is a method frequently used in classification problems and in which successful results are obtained (Öz, Köker, & Çakar, 2002).

Back Propagation Algorithm

The back propagation algorithm is a regularly used algorithm for multilayer ANN structures (Kahramanli & Allahverdi, 2008). The learning rule of this algorithm aims to reach the optimal values for the weights of the network by calculating the total error at the lowest level. The output of the network is calculated against the inputs presented to the network. The expected output value is compared with the calculated output values, and therefore the error is calculated. These errors are then propagated backward through the respective components. In the next iteration, the error is reduced. The error is calculated as "error=expected-output". Network weights between the output layer and the intermediate layer are updated. Then, the outputs between the intermediate layers and finally the weights between the input layer and the hidden layer are updated. In Figure 1, BP algorithm is expressed with pseudo-codes.

Figure 1. Expression of back propagation algorithm with pseudo codes (Dandıl & Gürgen, 2019)

1:	Training pattern is defined.
2:	Neural network structure is defined.
	The number of the neurons, number of the hidden layer neurons, the output layer neurons, learning rate n and momentum rate are determined.
3:	Random connection weights (Wi) and bias weights of θ_1 and θ_2 are determined.
	Minimum error value is determined. E_{min}
4:	By applying 1 set of input patterns each time, the error is spread out over the layers and the general error is calculated.
	Error$<E_{min}$ controlled
5:	The errors calculated in the output are back propagated in the direction of hidden error layer and input layer, and the weights are updated.
6:	The steps 4 to 5 are repeated until the conditions are achieved.

Particle Swarm Optimization Algorithm

Particle swarm optimization (PSO), which was developed by R.C. Eberhart and J. Kennedy in 1995, is a population based optimization technique inspired by social behavior of bird flocking (Kennedy, 1995). It is designed to solve nonlinear problems. It is used to find solutions to multi-parameter and multivariate optimization problems (Xiaohui, 2006).

There are many similarities between PSO and evolutionary computational techniques such as genetic algorithms. The system is initialized with a population of random solutions and then it searches for the optima by updating generations. In PSO, potential solutions are called as particles. These particles fly through the problem space by tracking the current optimum particle. The most important difference of PSO from classical optimization techniques is that it does not need derivative information. This reduces the complex processing load required for the solution of various problems. In addition, PSO algorithm is easy to implement because of the small number of parameters that need to be set. PSO can be applied successfully in many areas such as function optimization, fuzzy system control, and artificial neural network training (Awad, 2006; Ghoshal, 2004; Juang & Lu, 2006; Zhao, Ren, Yu, & Yang, 2005).

PSO simulates the behavior of bird flocking. The birds' randomly searching food in the space that they do not know where the food is resemble to seeking a solution for a problem. While searching the food, the birds follow the bird which is nearest to the food. Each single solution called as "particle" is a bird in the search space. When the particle moves, it sends its coordinates to a function, so that the fitness value of the particle is measured. (So, how far the particle is away from the food is measured). A particle must remember its coordinates, its velocity (how quickly it travels in every dimension in the solution space), the best fitness value that it has achieved so far, and the coordinates it obtains. How the particle's velocity and direction in each dimension of the solution space will change each time is directly proportional to the combination of the best coordinates of its neighbors and its own best coordinates. Individuals will act according to their own experiences and the experiences of their neighbors. In other words, information sharing among individuals will be provided (Çevik & Koçer, 2013).

All of particles have fitness values that are evaluated by the fitness function to be optimized, and have velocities that direct the flying of the particles. The particles fly through the problem space by tracking the current optimum particles.

In PSO, the solution space of the problem can be multidimensional depending on the number of variables or unknowns.

For example the solution space of $5x^2+2y^3-(z/w)^2+4$ function is 4 dimensional due to x,y,z and w unknowns. The position of a particle defined in the solution space is determined as $P=[x,y,z,w]$ four coordinates.

For example, a solution can be found by setting the function equal to zero. A particle as $P=[3,3,8,1]$ represents the fitness function for $x=3$, $y=3$, $z=8$ and $w=1$ coordinates. There are no difficulties for PSO to work on complex problems of 4 or more dimensions that people cannot visualize (Awad, 2006).

PSO is initialized with a group of solutions (random particles) and then optimum solution is searched by updating. In each iteration, each particle is updated by following two best values. The first one is the best position of the particle that it has achieved so far. This value is called as pbest and it must be stored. The other best value is the coordinates that have been achieved so far by all the particles in the population and provide the best solution. This best value is a global best value and called as gbest. Suppose that there are n number particles with D number parameters. In this case, the population particle matrix equation is as in Equation (1) (Awad, 2006)

$$X=\begin{bmatrix} x_{11} & x_{12} & \cdots & \cdots & x_{1D} \\ x_{21} & x_{22} & \cdots & \cdots & x_{2D} \\ \cdots & \cdots & \cdots & \cdots & \cdots \\ \cdots & \cdots & \cdots & \cdots & \cdots \\ x_{n1} & x_{n2} & \cdots & \cdots & x_{nD} \end{bmatrix} \qquad (1)$$

The i-th particle in the particle flock matrix is expressed as follows.

$$x_i = \begin{bmatrix} x_{i1}, & x_{i2}, \ldots, x_{iD} \end{bmatrix} \qquad (2)$$

The position of the i-th particle (pbesti) which gives the previous best-fit value is expressed as follows:

$$pbest_i = \begin{bmatrix} p_{i1}, & p_{i2}, ..., p_{iD} \end{bmatrix}$$

(3)

gbest is single in each iteration for all particles and expressed as follows:

$$gbest_i = \begin{bmatrix} p_1, & p_2, ..., p_D \end{bmatrix}$$

(4)

The velocity of the i-th particle (the change amount of the position in each dimension) is expressed as follows:

$$v_i = \begin{bmatrix} v_{i1}, & v_{i2}, ..., v_{iD} \end{bmatrix}$$

(5)

The particle velocity and the particle position are updated according to the following equations after the ideal value is obtained.

$$v_i^{k+1} = v_i^k + c_1 \Delta rand_1^k \Delta \left(pbest_i^k - x_i^k \right) + c_2 \Delta rand_2^k \Delta \left(gbest^k - x_i^k \right)$$

(6)

$$x_i^{k+1} = x_i^k + v_i^{k+1}$$

(7)

In equation (6) c1 and c2 are learning factors. c1 and c2 are positive acceleration constants which change the velocity of each particle towards pbest and gbest positions. c1 allows the particle to move according to its own experience, and c2 allows it to move according to the experience of other particles in the flock.rand1 and rand2 are random numbers ranged between [0,1] that are distributed uniformly. k represents the iteration number, i represents the particle indices (Juang & Lu, 2006).

Low values for c1 and c2 allow particles to wander far from target regions before being pulled back towards target regions. However, it may take longer to reach the target region. On the other hand, high values may cause with abrupt movement towards or past target regions while it accelerates reaching the target. It was stated in the experiments of researchers on this algorithm that the best results were obtained when c1= c2=2 gives good results (Li-Ping, Huan-Jun, & Shang-Xu, 2005; Shi & Eberhart, 1998; Xiaohui, 2006).

The procedure required for the PSO algorithm is summarized in Figure 2 (Çavuşlu, Karakuzu, & Şahin, 2010).

Genetic Algorithm

GA is a computer program that enables the solution of problems that are difficult or impossible to solve by deterministic methods through evolutionary stages. Optimization problems which are complex, with large number of constrains, whose objective function cannot be solved and do not have exact solution is related to GA. GAs have the ability to find an approximate solution in a short time, even if there is not a definite solution for difficult optimization problems (Paksoy, 2007).

Figure 2. Code structure of PSO algorithm

```
For     each particle
        {Initialization conditions}
End
Do      {
        For     each particle
                {Calculate fitness value, If the fitness value is better than the best fitness
                value (pBest) set current value as the new pBest}
        End
        Choose the particle with the best fitness value of all the particles as the gBest
        For     each particle
        {Calculate particle velocity according equation (6)
        Update particle position according equation (7)}
        End
While {iteration number < maximum iteration number or training criteria < target training
        criteria}
```

Genetic Algorithm (GA) is a method which was introduced by John Holland in 1975 and it's a nature-inspired evolutionary algorithm (Chen, Tiong, & Chen, 2019). Genetic Algorithm starts with a population of candidate solutions to an optimization problem and ay applies iteratively different operators for generating better solutions. These operators are based on random processes and they allow Genetic algorithms to explore the search space in different directions. Genetic Algorithms evaluate each individual of the population by using a "fitness" function. In this step, most of the fitted individuals are selected for reproduction to get better feasible solutions. The reproduction process consists of crossover and mutation operators. The evaluation, selection and reproduction are repeated until some stopping conditions are achieved (Kaabi & Harrath, 2019).

Genotype and Phenotype

According to genetics, each individual has a genotype (hereditary structure) and a phenotype (hereditary appearance) that results from these hereditary (genetic) characteristics. The genotype of an individual encodes the phenotype of that individual. During reproduction, the child inherits the genotype from the parents (both mother and father). Therefore, while the development of individuals occurs at the phenotype level, genetic operators occur at the genotype level.

Allele

They are the smallest units on a chromosome. In nature, alleles consist of two symbols, such as XY. In genetic algorithm applications, it is usually expressed with a single symbol (it can take the value of 0 or 1).

Gene

It is an allele or a sequence of alleles representing a particular phenotype characteristic within a chromosome (individual). That is, an external phenotypic characteristic of an individual is represented by genes formed by the combination of one or more alleles.

Chromosome

It is a series of alleles representing a solution in GA, of a certain length and containing all the genetic information of the individual. All possible solutions to the optimization problem are represented by a chromosome. Although there is more than one chromosome in nature, most GA applications use one chromosome (Aksakal, 2014).

Figure 3. Allele-Gene-Chromosome Relationship

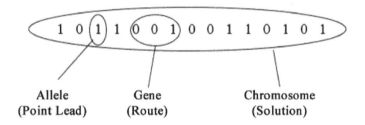

Allele   Gene   Chromosome
(Point Lead)   (Route)   (Solution)

Population

It is a set of solutions formed by a certain number of points in the solution space, that is, it consists of a certain number of chromosomes. In the start of GA, these solutions are randomly created and generally the size of this population is kept constant throughout the algorithm. In the start of the algorithm, the most important point to be determined is the size of this population and which individuals will be selected for reproduction. The size of the solution set must be determined for the effective and efficient operation of the algorithm (Aksakal, 2014).

Smaller population will not enable GA to search different parts of the solution space at the same time, but very large population will reduce the efficiency of the algorithm by reducing the convergence speed of the algorithm The GA stages are given in Figure 4.

The process of GA is as follows (Figure 2) respectively: Selection, initial population, crossover, mutation, calculation of fitness function, generating of offspring, stopping the cycle (Güleç, 2014).

Figure 4. Genetic Algorithm Flow Chart (Bentley, 1999)

- **Generate initial random population**
→ • **Evaluate all individuals to determine their fitness**
- **Reproduce individuals according to their fitness into "mating pool". (Higher ←**
  fitness=more copies of an individual)
- **Randomly take two individuals from the mating pool**
- **Use random crossover to generate two offspring**
- **Randomly mutate offspring**
- **Place offspring into population**
- **Has population been filled with new offspring? No**

                       Yes

Is there an acceptable solution? (Or have x generation been produced?
No   Yes

FINISHED

Encoding solutions

The primary requirement for GA development is that each individual is defined as a sequence of bits of the same size. Each of these sequences represents any point in the solution space of the problem (Yeniay, 2001).

Generation of initial population

A solution group is generated in which possible solutions are coded. In the chromosomes indicated by the binary coding method, a random number generator can be used to generate the initial population (Emel & Taşkın, 2002; Yeo & Agyei, 1998).

Calculation of the fitness function

In the solution, a fitness function is determined for the desired result and the entire population is evaluated according to this value. With this method, it is ensured that individuals in each generation approach the value of fitness function, and individuals who do not meet this condition are eliminated. Increasing the fitness value of a solution increases the chances of survival and growth and the chance to be represented in the next generation (Yeniay, 2001).

Selection

In this phase, the fittest individuals are selected and they will pass their genes to the next generation. The selected individuals are gathers in a mating pool (Fığlalı, 2002). There are different selection techniques in GA such as elite selection, rank selection, roulette wheel, tournament selection.

Crossover: In GAs, crossover is provided with some operations. Crossover is based on the ability of parents to change gene combinations and produce new individuals from a certain point (Figure 5).

Figure 5. Schematic crossover representation between two parents with a regional variation of genetic information (Jo & Gero, 1998)

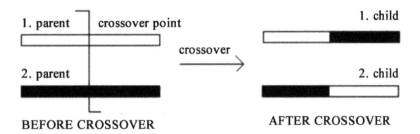

Mutation process

The mutation process, which is performed to ensure and maintain genetic diversity (Bräysy, 2001), is conducted to produce new chromosomes from existing chromosomes. If the existing gene combination does not contain all the necessary information, the desired solutions can be produced by mutation.

Generation of offspring and stopping the cycle

If the population of individuals with the desired fitness function is reached after the cycle is repeated, the cycle is stopped. The cycle can be stopped if the predetermined number of strings is achieved (Yeo & Agyei, 1998), a target is achieved, a certain number of iterations are achieved, or a fitness function is provided (Fung, Tang, & Wang, 2002).

Artificial Immune Algorithm

The clonal selection algorithm is an artificial immune optimization algorithm that is used by the natural immune system to define the basic features of an immune response to an antigenic stimulus (Glover, 1977). According to this principle, only those cells that recognize antigens proliferate. The selected cells undergo affinity maturation process. With this process, the selected cells have improved similarity to antigens (Kirkpatrick, Gelatt, & Vecchi, 1983). Figure 6 shows the flowchart and process steps of the clonal selection algorithm.

The processing steps of the clonal selection algorithm can be described as follows. Ag represents antigen set and Ab represents antibody set;

1. The affinity measure (attraction) between N number Ab in the Ab set and Ag set is determined. The fit indices matrix (fi) calculated depending on the affinity is determined.
2. The n highest affinity Ab is selected and Abn is generated.

Figure 6. AI clonal selection algorithm flow diagram

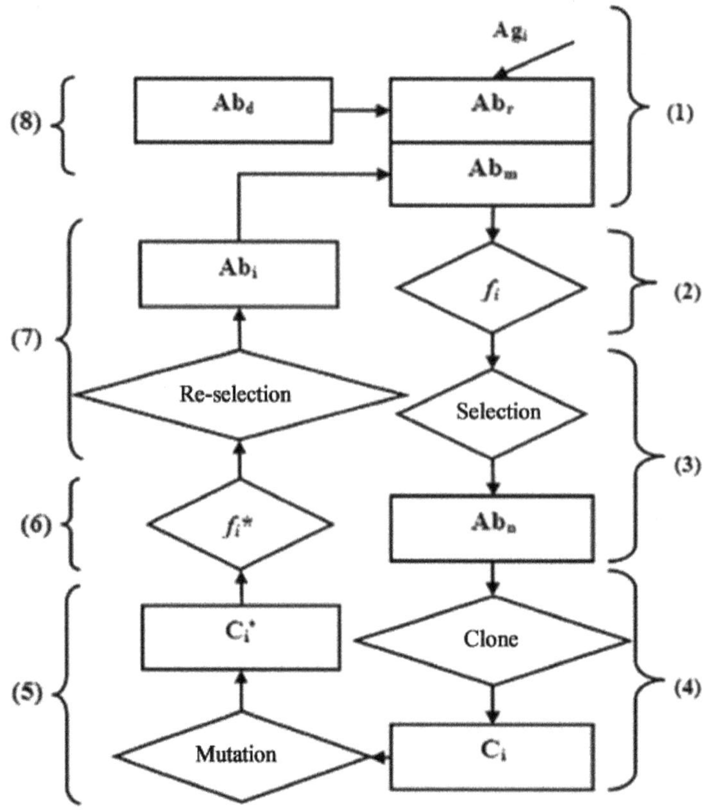

3.   The selected n number Ab is cloned independently according to their affinity to the antigens and Ci set including the cloned cells is generated. The cell with the highest antigenic affinity is further cloned. Equation 8 is used for cloning. In this equation Nc represents the total number of clones for each antigen, β represents cloning factor, and N represents total antibodies. (If the multiplication of the cloning factor and antibody number is not an integer, the round function is used to determine the number of antibodies to be cloned).

$$N_C = \sum_{i=1}^{N} round\left(\beta.N\right) \tag{8}$$

4.   Cells in the cloned Ci set are mutated inversely proportional to their antigenic affinity and (Ci *) set in which the mutated cells are included is generated. The cell with the highest affinity has the smallest mutation rate. Thus, this cell is the least mutated cell. Each cell mutates according to the expression in Equation 9. In this expression α is mutation rate, ρ is mutation factor and f is affinity measurements (exp in the equation refers to the number of natural logarithms)

$$\alpha = \exp(-\rho.f) \tag{9}$$

5. The affinity values (fi*) of each cell in the Ci* cloned cells set with the cells in Ag antibodies set are calculated.
6. Ab with the highest affinity in maturated Ci* set is reselected. If the affinity of this cell is higher than its respective Ab memory cell, this cell will replace this memory Ab.

Finally, d number lowest affinity cell in Abr will replace the d number Abd cell and therefore diversity is provided (Dandıl & Gürgen, 2019).

SOLUTIONS AND RECOMMENDATIONS

In this chapter it was aimed to evaluate heuristic approach performances for artificial neural networks training. For this purpose software which can perform ANN training was developed using four different algorithms. The software was developed via C#.NET and Visual Studio, which are among the most powerful programming languages, and implemented. The welcome screen image of the software that will provide training and testing of data via ANN with four different training algorithms from a single menu is given in Figure 7.

Figure 7. Welcome screen image of the designed ANN training software

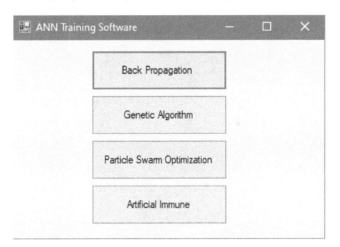

In order to make the software designed to be user-friendly, the designs of the software, which works in four different structures, are designed as similar to each other as possible. Only minor design differences have emerged with respect to the algorithm parameters (Hyper Parameter). The screen images of this developed software are shown in Figures 8, 9, 10 and 11.

A common data set was used to test the designed software. While determining this data set, attention was paid to the classification problems in which ANN is used most. In addition, a relatively easy-to-train dataset was selected since the time to reach a certain error amount or number of steps was also tested in addition to the training error performance.

Figure 8. ANN training with Back Propagation Algorithm

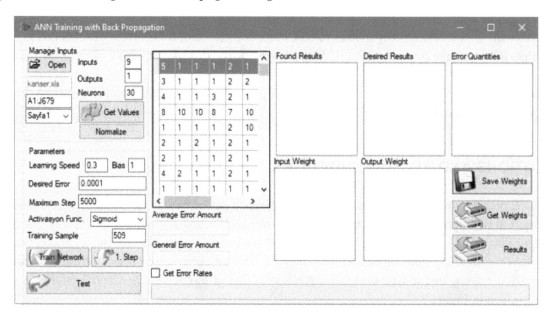

Figure 9. ANN training with Genetic Algorithm

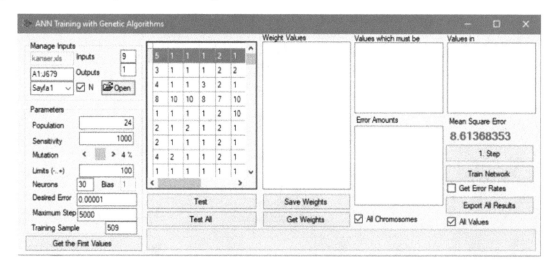

The breast cancer data set used in the study was taken from UCI (University of California, Irvine) database (H, 1992).

In order to determine whether breast cancer is benign or malignant, nine characteristics are examined in the cells taken from the sick people. These nine cell properties that will be used for the input data of ANN are as Clump Thickness, Uniformity of cell Size, Uniformity of cell Shape, Marginal Adhesion, Single epithelial Cell Size, Bare nuclei, Bland Chomatin, Normal nucleoli and Mitoses. The classification output that can be obtained according to these nine types of input data was selected as "2" or "4". If the result is "2", it is a benign cancer cell and if the result is "4", it is a malignant cancer cell. There are 679 data in total. Values and classification data for these properties are shown in Table 1 (H, 1992).

Figure 10. ANN training with Particle Swarm Optimization Algorithm

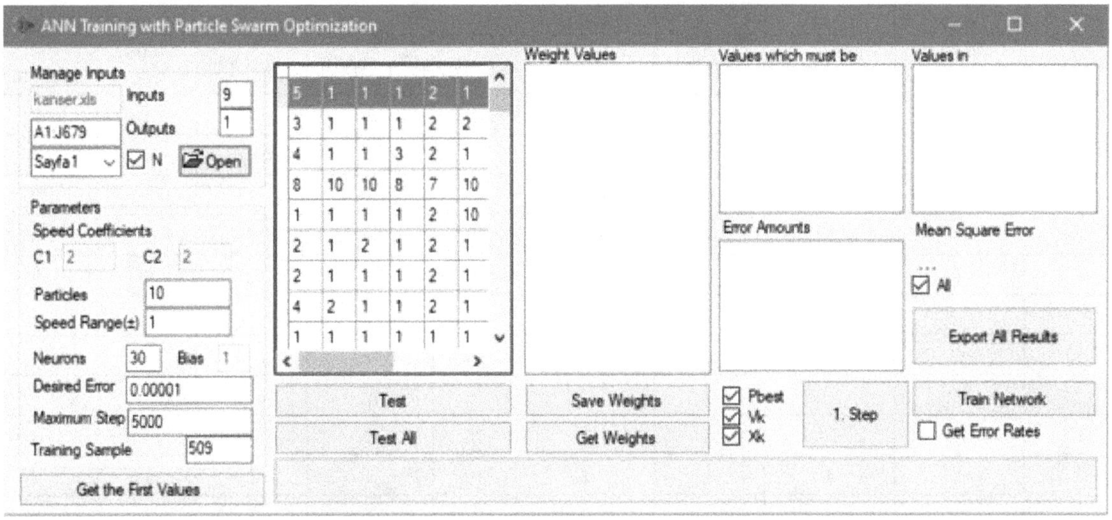

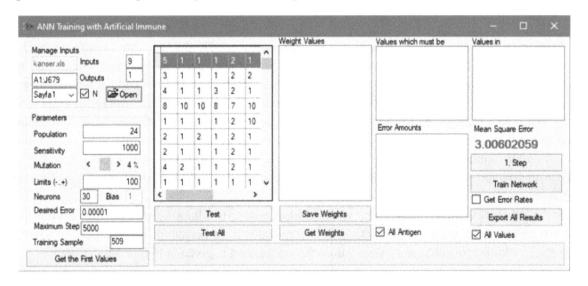

Figure 11. ANN training with Artificial Immune Algorithm

RESULTS

The software, which includes four different methods designed for the training of ANN, has been tested on the breast cancer dataset. The same ANN design was used in the testing of all algorithms. Since there were 9 data in the input layer, there were 9 neurons, the number of hidden layers was single and it included 30 neurons, and the output layer was a single neuron. The designed ANN model is shown in Figure 12. The parameters of ANN were taken as Learning Coefficient 0.1 and Bias 1 and all parameters were constant in all algorithms. In total, 679 data records were divided into two as 75% (509 data) training and 25% (170 data) test. The distribution of the selected data was homogeneous.

Table 1. Breast Cancer Data Set

Cluster Thickness	Cell Uniformity Size	Cell Uniformity Shape	Marginal Adhesion	Single Epithelial Cell Size	Lean Core	Bland Chromatin	Normal Nucleol	Mitosis	2 Bening 4 Malignant
5	1	1	1	2	1	3	1	1	2
5	3	3	3	2	3	4	4	1	4
3	1	1	1	2	2	3	1	1	2
7	4	6	4	6	1	4	3	1	4
4	1	1	3	2	1	3	1	1	2
...	....	....	...	...	...	...	...	...	...
...	....	....	...	...	...	...	...	...	...
...	....	....	...	...	...	...	...	...	...
8	10	10	8	7	10	9	7	1	4
1	1	1	1	2	10	3	1	1	2
2	1	2	1	2	1	3	1	1	2
10	7	7	6	4	10	4	1	2	4
4	2	1	1	2	1	2	1	1	2

In addition, K Fold Cross Validation, which is frequently used in the literature to evaluate machine learning models on a limited data sample, was applied in order to accurately measure the overall performance of the system. According to the data set, it was determined as K=4 and the operations were repeated 4 times and training and test data were replaced at each step. Then, the average of these values was taken. The mean square error (MSE), which is frequently used in the literature besides its training time and classification success, was used for performance analysis. In addition the personal computer (PC) used for running the software had Intel Core i5-3337U 1.8 GHz processor, 8 GB RAM, 128 GB SSD with 500/500 MB read and write speed, Nvidia Geforce GT 630M 2 GB (128Bit) Graphics card and Windows 10 operating system.

In the test process, all algorithms were run for 500 steps or up to 0.00001 errors; average training time, test and training MSE values and classification success rates were measured. These values are shown in Table 2. In addition, the change in MSE values during training is given in Figure 13.

FUTURE RESEARCH DIRECTIONS

For the following studies, other heuristic algorithms can be added to these algorithms, and therefore Training-test times can be further reduced and the desired success rate can be achieved.

Figure 12. ANN structure designed for test operations

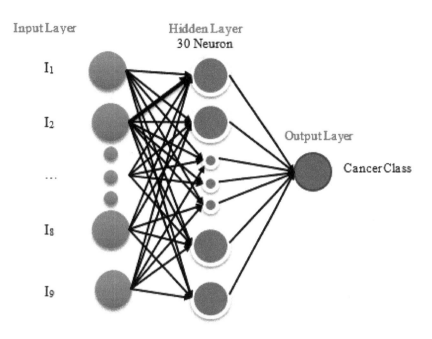

Figure 13. Change in MSE value during training

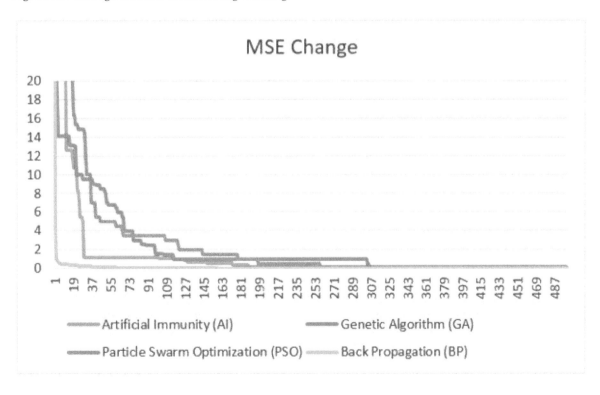

Table 2. System Results

Algorithm	Duration	Step Number	Training Error	Test Error	Test Classification Success
Back Propagation (BP)	10 min 57 sec	500	0.00073	0.00026	100
Particle Swarm Optimization (PSO)	3 min 44 sec	377	0.00001	0.00072	100
Genetic Algorithm (GA)	1 min 1 sec	500	0.00001	0.00001	100
Artificial Immunity (AI)	55 sec	500	0.00423	0.00089	100

CONCLUSION

In this chapter, three heuristic algorithms (Particle Swarm Optimization-PSO, Genetic Algorithm-GA, and Artificial Immune-AI) performance, which can be used as an alternative to Back Propagation (BP) Algorithm, which is frequently used in the literature for the training of Neural Networks, were tested. Software was designed by using C#.Net in order to make these operations and then present them to the users. In the test process, in order to measure algorithm performance, breast cancer dataset which was obtained from UCI (University of California, Irvine) database was used. In particular, an easy-to-identify dataset was selected

According to the performance tests, the most important difference between the heuristic algorithms and BP algorithm was observed during the training time. Considering the increase in the data size, training time can increase to large amounts. Therefore, the use of heuristic algorithms in ANN training has significantly reduced training time. Training time varies depending on the heuristic type of algorithm; however it was found that it was certainly shorter than the BP algorithm. The AI algorithm reached the minimum value in terms of time, however it was found that AI was not at the desired level in terms of training and test success. For this reason, when the training-test time and success rates were examined, the most optimal algorithm was determined as GA.

REFERENCES

Aksakal, B. (2014). Solving vehicle routing problem with time windows and spesific demands of a company by using genetic algorithm (Msc). Istanbul Technical University, İstanbul.

Arı, A., & Berberler, M. E. (2017). Interface Design for Prediction and Classification Problems with Artificial Neural Networks. *Acta INFOLOGICA*, *1*(2), 55–73.

Awad, H. A. (2006). *A novel particle swarm-based fuzzy control scheme.* Paper presented at the 2006 IEEE International Conference on Fuzzy Systems. 10.1109/FUZZY.2006.1681969

Bayindir, R., & Sesveren, Ö. (2008). Design of a visual interface for ANN based systems. *Pamukkale University Journal of Engineering Sciences*, *14*(1), 101–109.

Bentley, P. (1999). An introduction to evolutionary design by computers. *Evolutionary Design by Computers*, 1-73.

Bräysy, O. (2001). *Local search and variable neighborhood search algorithms for the vehicle routing problem with time windows*. Vaasan yliopisto.

Cantú-Paz, E. (2003). *Pruning neural networks with distribution estimation algorithms*. Paper presented at the Genetic and Evolutionary Computation Conference. 10.1007/3-540-45105-6_93

Çavuşlu, M. A., Karakuzu, C., & Şahin, S. (2010). Hardware Implementation of Artificial Neural Network Training Using Particle Swarm Optimization on FPGA. *Journal of Polytechnic, 13*(2), 83–92.

Çetin, E. (2007). *Artificial Intelligence Applications*. Seçkin Publishing.

Çevik, K. K., & Dandıl, E. (2012). Development of Visual Educational Software for Artificial Neural Networks on. Net Platform. *Journal of Information Technology, 5*(1), 19–28.

Çevik, K. K., & Koçer, H. E. (2013). A Soft Computing Application Based On Artificial Neural Networks Training by Particle Swarm Optimization. *Suleyman Demirel University Journal of Natural and Applied Science, 17*(2), 39–45.

Chen, C., Tiong, L. K., & Chen, I.-M. (2019). Using a genetic algorithm to schedule the space-constrained AGV-based prefabricated bathroom units manufacturing system. *International Journal of Production Research, 57*(10), 3003–3019.

Cotta, C., Alba, E., Sagarna, R., & Larrañaga, P. (2002). Adjusting weights in artificial neural networks using evolutionary algorithms. In *Estimation of distribution algorithms* (pp. 361–377). Springer. doi:10.1007/978-1-4615-1539-5_18

Curry, B., & Morgan, P. (1997). Neural networks: A need for caution. *Omega, 25*(1), 123–133. doi:10.1016/S0305-0483(96)00052-7

Dandıl, E., & Gürgen, E. (2019). Prediction of Photovoltaic Panel Power Outputs using Artificial Neural Networks and Comparison with Heuristic Algorithms. *European Journal of Science and Technology,* (16), 146-158.

Dorigo, M., & Di Caro, G. (1999). *Ant colony optimization: a new meta-heuristic*. Paper presented at the Proceedings of the 1999 congress on evolutionary computation-CEC99 (Cat. No. 99TH8406). 10.1109/CEC.1999.782657

Emel, G. G., & Taşkın, Ç. (2002). Genetic Algorithms and Applications. *Uludağ University Journal of Faculty of Economics and Administrative Sciences, 21*(1), 129–152.

Fığlalı, A. E. O. (2002). Reproduction operator optimization of Genetic Algorithms in flowshop scheduling problems *ITU. Engineering Journal (New York), 1*(1), 1–6.

Fogel, D. B. (1998). *Artificial intelligence through simulated evolution*. Wiley-IEEE Press.

Fung, R. Y., Tang, J., & Wang, D. (2002). Extension of a hybrid genetic algorithm for nonlinear programming problems with equality and inequality constraints. *Computers & Operations Research, 29*(3), 261–274. doi:10.1016/S0305-0548(00)00068-X

Ghoshal, S. P. (2004). Optimizations of PID gains by particle swarm optimizations in fuzzy based automatic generation control. *Electric Power Systems Research, 72*(3), 203–212. doi:10.1016/j.epsr.2004.04.004

Glover, F. (1977). Heuristics for integer programming using surrogate constraints. *Decision Sciences*, *8*(1), 156–166. doi:10.1111/j.1540-5915.1977.tb01074.x

Goldberg, D. E., & Holland, J. H. (1988). Genetic algorithms and machine learning. *Machine Learning*, *3*(2), 95–99. doi:10.1023/A:1022602019183

Güleç, D. (2014). *Optimization of user accessibility in architectural design using genetic algorithm-aDA:Case study on health campuses* (PhD). Istanbul Technical University. Retrieved from http://archive.ics.uci.edu/ml/datasets/Breast+Cancer

Gupta, J. N., & Sexton, R. S. (1999). Comparing backpropagation with a genetic algorithm for neural network training. *Omega*, *27*(6), 679–684. doi:10.1016/S0305-0483(99)00027-4

Hofmeyr, S. A., & Forrest, S. (2000). Architecture for an artificial immune system. *Evolutionary Computation*, *8*(4), 443–473. doi:10.1162/106365600568257 PMID:11130924

Holland, J. H. (1992). *Adaptation in natural and artificial systems: an introductory analysis with applications to biology, control, and artificial intelligence*. MIT Press. doi:10.7551/mitpress/1090.001.0001

Jo, J. H., & Gero, J. S. (1998). Space layout planning using an evolutionary approach. *Artificial Intelligence in Engineering*, *12*(3), 149–162. doi:10.1016/S0954-1810(97)00037-X

Juang, C.-F., & Lu, C.-F. (2006). Load-frequency control by hybrid evolutionary fuzzy PI controller. *IEE Proceedings. Generation, Transmission and Distribution*, *153*(2), 196–204. doi:10.1049/ip-gtd:20050176

Kaabi, J., & Harrath, Y. (2019). Permutation rules and genetic algorithm to solve the traveling salesman problem. *Arab Journal of Basic and Applied Sciences*, *26*(1), 283–291. doi:10.1080/25765299.2019.1615172

Kahramanli, H., & Allahverdi, N. (2008). Design of a hybrid system for the diabetes and heart diseases. *Expert Systems with Applications*, *35*(1-2), 82–89. doi:10.1016/j.eswa.2007.06.004

Kennedy, J. E. R. (1995). Particle swarm optimization. *Proceedings of IEEE International Conference on Neural Networks IV*. 10.1109/ICNN.1995.488968

Kirkpatrick, S., Gelatt, C. D., & Vecchi, M. P. (1983). Optimization by simulated annealing. *Science*, *220*(4598), 671-680.

Köse, U. (2010). *Developing Education Software For Fuzzy Logic And Artificial Neural Networks* (Msc). Afyon Kocatepe University, Afyon.

Li-Ping, Z., Huan-Jun, Y., & Shang-Xu, H. (2005). Optimal choice of parameters for particle swarm optimization. *Journal of Zhejiang University. Science A*, *6*(6), 528–534. doi:10.1631/jzus.2005.A0528

McCarthy, J., Minsky, M. L., Rochester, N., & Shannon, C. E. (2006). A proposal for the dartmouth summer research project on artificial intelligence, august 31, 1955. *AI Magazine*, *27*(4), 12–12.

Nabiyev, V. (2003). *Artificial Intelligence: Problems, Methods, Algorithms* (Vol. 724). Seçkin Publishing.

Öz, C., Köker, R., & Çakar, S. (2002). *Character-based plate recognition with artificial neural networks.* Paper presented at the Electrical, Electronics and Computer Engineering Symposium (ELECO 2002), Bursa.

Öztemel, E. (2003). *Artificial neural networks.* Papatya Publishing.

Paksoy, S. (2007). A genetic algorithm for project scheduling (PhD). Cukurova University, Adana.

Rumelhart, D. E., Hinton, G. E., & Williams, R. J. (1988). Learning representations by back-propagating errors. *Cognitive Modeling, 5*(3), 1.

Salchenberger, L. M., Cinar, E. M., & Lash, N. A. (1992). Neural networks: A new tool for predicting thrift failures. *Decision Sciences, 23*(4), 899–916. doi:10.1111/j.1540-5915.1992.tb00425.x

Sexton, R. S., Dorsey, R. E., & Johnson, J. D. (1998). Toward global optimization of neural networks: A comparison of the genetic algorithm and backpropagation. *Decision Support Systems, 22*(2), 171–185. doi:10.1016/S0167-9236(97)00040-7

Shi, Y., & Eberhart, R. C. (1998). *Parameter selection in particle swarm optimization.* Paper presented at the International conference on evolutionary programming.

Shi, Y., & Eberhart, R. C. (1999). *Empirical study of particle swarm optimization.* Paper presented at the Proceedings of the 1999 Congress on Evolutionary Computation-CEC99 (Cat. No. 99TH8406). 10.1109/CEC.1999.785511

Storn, R. (1996). Differential evolution design of an IIR-filter. *Proceedings of IEEE international conference on evolutionary computation.* 10.1109/ICEC.1996.542373

Tosun, S. (2018). *Software Used in Artificial Neural Networks.* Retrieved from http://www.suleymantosun.com/yapay-sinir-aglari-uygulamasinda-kullanilan-yazilimlar/

Valian, E., Mohanna, S., & Tavakoli, S. (2011). Improved cuckoo search algorithm for feedforward neural network training. *International Journal of Artificial Intelligence & Applications, 2*(3), 36–43. doi:10.5121/ijaia.2011.2304

XiaohuiH. (2006). *PSO Tutorial.* Retrieved from http://www.swarmintelligence.org/tutorials.php

Yeniay, Ö. (2001). An Overview of Genetic Algorithms. *Anadolu University Journal of Science and Technology, 2*(1), 37–49.

Yeo, M. F., & Agyei, E. O. (1998). Optimising engineering problems using genetic algorithms. *Engineering Computations, 15*(2), 268–280. doi:10.1108/02644409810202684

Yiğit, T., Işık, A. H., & Bilen, M. (2014). Web based educational software for artificial neural networks. *The Eurasia Proceedings of Educational & Social Sciences, 1*, 276–279.

Zhao, F., Ren, Z., Yu, D., & Yang, Y. (2005). *Application of an improved particle swarm optimization algorithm for neural network training.* Paper presented at the 2005 International Conference on Neural Networks and Brain.

Chapter 20
Mental Health Through Biofeedback Is Important to Analyze:
An App and Analysis

Rohit Rastogi
iD https://orcid.org/0000-0002-6402-7638
ABES Engineering College, India

Devendra Kumar Chaturvedi
iD https://orcid.org/0000-0002-4837-2570
Dayalbagh Educational Institute, Agra, India

Mayank Gupta
Tata Consultancy Services, India

ABSTRACT

Many apps and analyzers based on machine learning have been designed to help and cure the stress issue. This chapter is based on an experiment that the authors performed at Research Labs and Scientific Spirituality Centers of Dev Sanskriti VishwaVidyalaya, Haridwar and Patanjali Research Foundations, Uttarakhand. In the research work, the correctness and accuracy have been studied and compared for two biofeedback devices named as electromyography (EMG) and galvanic skin response (GSR), which can operate in three modes: audio, visual and audio-visual with the help of data set of tension type headache (TTH) patients. The authors used some data visualization techniques that EMG (electromyography) in audio mode is best among all other modes, and in this experiment, they have used a data set of SF-36 and successfully clustered them into three clusters (i.e., low, medium, and high) using K-means algorithm. After clustering, they used classification algorithm to classify a user (depending upon the sum of all the weights of questions he had answered) into one of these three class. They have also implemented various algorithms for classifications and compared their accuracy out of which decision tree algorithm has given the best accuracy.

DOI: 10.4018/978-1-7998-2742-9.ch020

INTRODUCTION

As we can see that almost everyone is suffering from many kind of stress and we all get some indicators which shows that we are suffering from stress rather it be physical, emotional, personal, sleep or behavioral. But manually the level of stress is difficult to calculate and also the people are much more reliable on medication for getting relief. Many times, the individual is lost in physical pleasure, accumulation of facilities and due to lack of right understanding about the self, one bears the ignorance about one's own being. Due to which they suffer from stress most of the time. These consist of pharmacological treatment, physical therapy, acupuncture, relaxation therapy or alternative medicine. So main focus of our project is to check the stress level of a person and give remedies to them accordingly. We are more focused on giving remedies to people which do not include any kind of medications.(PyCharm, n.d.; Rastogi, Chaturvedi, Satya, Arora, & Chauhan, 2018)

Motivation

The experimental research work done by us has motivated us to use our knowledge and make an effort to reduce the stress level of people. Automation and mechanization is rapidly increasing with intelligent machines. Science has done miracles and almost in all walks of life, most works are being done by scientific gadgets and it has no doubt made the human life simpler. It has helped to handle complex issues but contrary to this, there is a dark side of the picture that it has created some negative aspects and challenging situations too. The present crisis of science to human life is that the stress, tension, depression, anxiety, hatred, headache, frustration, suicidal tendency and violence is increasing in our world day by day. The happiness index has been reduced rapidly everywhere. The Human personality is degraded in terms of value system.(Arora et al., 2017; Chaturvedi et al., 2018; Rastogi, Chaturvedi, Satya, Arora, Yadav et al, 2018)

OBJECTIVE OF RESEARCH

1. To study and compare the correctness and accuracy of Electromyography(EMG) and Galvanic Skin Response(GSR) biofeedback in three modes: audio, visual and audio-visual.
2. Our project is to check the stress level of a person and give remedies to them accordingly, by classifying them into one of the three categories: low, medium & high stress level.
3. Comparing the efficiency of different algorithms used for classification.

SCOPE OF THE RESEARCH WORK

Measuring the effect of various indicators like physical, sleep, behavioral, personal and emotional parameters are indicators of stress on different levels of stress. The purpose is to reduce the use of medication to lower the level of stress. Measuring the accuracy of the range decided to track the level of stress of a person. A runnable system which checks the stress level of a person. The main objective is to develop a system which gives the remedies which do not involve any kind of medication to a person according to their stress level.(Chaturvedi et al., 2017; Satya et al., 2019)

RELATED PREVIOUS WORK

1. MoodKit a popular app based on IOS which uses the foundation of Cognitive Behavioral Therapy (CBT) and provides different mood improvement activities to different users which are more than 200 in number. Developed by two clinical psychologists, MoodKit helps one to change the thinking pattern and method, to develop self confidence, awareness, creativity, situation handling and problem solving and wise healthy attitude(List of best 25 mobile apps used for mental and physical health, n.d.).

2. Another very good mental health helping app is Mind Shift which has been developed to facilitate teen agers and adults to face the challenges of depression and frustration along with anxiety. The app Mind Shift focuses the sight of users about their thought process for(List of best 25 mobile apps used for mental and physical health, n.d.).

3. Khanna A, Paul M, Sandhu JS. exhibited a detailed research work and in depth study to check accuracy and comparison of efficiency of GSR and EMG biofeedback training process and consequently progressive muscle relaxation process for decreasing the blood pressure and respiratory rate for those subjects who were suffering heavily from acute level of headache(What is biofeedback?, 2008).

4. Biofeedback is getting popular now as an alternate therapy and informs the subject and experimenter both about the current status of headache. It also helps to avoid the excessive use of medications and anti-oxidants for muscle relaxation. It helps the subjects from shifting the dependency on costly medications and consecutive side effects(Chauhan et al., 2018d).

5. Chronic TTH was found as the most common problem in all subjects of every type of gender, age, rural-urban sector of any demographical regions. Since most of the problems are psycho somatic so psycho and psychosocial factors are in consideration to study it (Kikuchi et al., 2012).

REQUIREMENT SPECIFICATION

Experimental Perspective

The Proposed experimentation and analysis is totally based on our earlier research work named "Chronic TTH analysis by EMG and GSR biofeedback on various modes and various medical symptoms" (Arora et al., 2019) and on "Analytical Comparison of Efficacy for Electromyography and Galvanic Skin Resistance Biofeedback on Audio-Visual Mode for Chronic TTH on Various Attributes" (Chauhan et al., 2018d). These work have been well published and cited by many in the same domain of research.

In this work, we created a website which comprises Short Form of Health Survey popularly known as SF-36 as the initial survey for the mental status of the subject. Each participants was required to answer the questions and based on their reponses, their individual different scores on various parameters were calculated. Some set of questions were giving one kind of score and other set of questions were giving other kind of responses. The scores were clear indicators for the current status of mental, social, physical and inner health of an individual and high score alays indicate that one posses good health and he/ she should maintain it. Average score is indicator of precautions and related guidelines and advisory are issued to him/ her. The low score is alarming bell and immediately subject is warned to visit psychiatrist and nearby mental hospital. Since the extreme situation can be panic and worst to be as suicidal tendency. This app is analyzer, a guide for those who want immediate and online relaxation in some critical circumstances.(Rastogi, Chaturvedi, Satya, Arora, Singhal et al, 2018; Satya et al., 2018; Sharma et al., 2018)

SYSTEM INTERFACES

1. Anguler6, CSS, JavaScript and Bootstrap are used for front end of web portal.
2. Node Js and Express Js are widely used in web platform as back end.
3. Mongo Db is applied for data storage and database creation purposes.
4. Jupyter is used to implement Machine Learning Algorithm in Python.
5. Visual Studio Code platform is used to develop the website.(Rastogi, Chaturvedi, Satya, Arora, Sirohi et al, 2018; Vyas et al., 2018)

HARDWARE INTERFACES

The project occurred in different configurations of system as below:

1. Operating System: Linux, Unix, Windows
2. x86 - 64 processor
3. 8 GB RAM
4. Web Server: local host provided by Angular CLI and NPM server
5. For Mongo Db version 4.0 installed in OS
6. NPM packages should be installed. (Rastogi, Chaturvedi, Satya, Arora, Sirohi et al, 2018; Vyas et al., 2018)

SOFTWARE INTERFACES

a. Python 3.6
b. Angular 6
c. Node 10.0.0
d. Mongo db 4.0
e. **PyCharm Platform:** Very popular now a days as an Integrated Development Environment (IDE). Python specially uses it for computer programming. Designed by the Czech company Jet Brains. Provides end users the code analysis, a graphical debugger, an integrated unit tester, integration with version control systems (VCSes), and supports web development with Django[PyCharm, n.d.].
f. **Machine Learning with Python language:** Machine Learning uses Data Mining techniques and other learning algorithms to build models of what is happening behind some data so that it can predict future outcomes. It's a particular approach to AI.
g. **Deep Learning**: It is one type of Machine Learning that achieves great power and flexibility by learning to represent the world as nested hierarchy of concepts, with each concept defined in relation to simpler concepts, and more abstract representations computed in terms of less abstract ones.

h. **Artificial Intelligence:** It uses models built by Machine Learning and other ways to reason about the world and give rise to intelligent behavior whether this is playing a game or driving a robot/car. Artificial Intelligence has some goal to achieve by predicting how actions will affect the model of the world and chooses the actions that will best achieve that goal. It is very much programming based.(Saini et al., 2018)

Machine Learning is the name given to generalizable algorithms that enable a computer to carry out a task by examining data rather than hard programming. It's a subfield of computer science and Artificial intelligence that focuses on developing systems that learn from data and help in making decisions and predictions based on that learning. ML enables computers to make data-driven decisions rather than being explicitly programmed to carry out a certain task. Math provides models; understand their relationships and apply them to real-world objects.(Bansal et al., 2018)

i. **Supervised Learning:** These are "predictive" in nature. The purpose is to predict the value of a particular variable (target variable) based on values of some other variables or explanatory variables). Classification and Regression are examples of predictive tasks. Classification is used to predict the value of a discrete target variable while regression is used to predict the value of a continuous target variable. To predict whether an email is spam or not is a Classification task while to predict the future price of a stock is a regression task. They are called supervised because we are telling the algorithm what to predict. Methods are Linear Regression, Logistic Regression, Decision Trees, Random Forests, Naïve Bayes Classifier, Bayesian Statistics and Inference, K-Nearest Neighbor. (Yadav et al., 2018)

j. **Unsupervised Learning:** These are "descriptive" in nature. The purpose is to derive patterns that summarize the underlying relationships in data. Association Analysis, Cluster Analysis and Anomaly detection are examples of Unsupervised Learning. They are called unsupervised because in such cases, the final outcome is not known beforehand. With unsupervised learning there is no feedback based on the prediction results. Methods are K-Means Clustering, Hierarchal Clustering, Clustering using DBSCAN, Feature Selection and Transformation, Principal Components Analysis (PCA).(Gupta et al., 2019)

MEMORY CONSTRAINTS

To run data on python programs, 2 GB memory space will be required and for both to run the node local host server and angular frontend local host, 1 GB space will be used.

OPERATIONS

Operations that will be done by user on our product are:

1. An user can do registration if they are new user.
2. After successful registration, user will be able to login to our site any time.

3. All those registered users, if don't have given any test then they will be redirected to test page as soon as they will login.
4. All those users who have successfully registered, if they have responded to questionnaire earlier they will be redirected to their dashboard.
5. On their dashboard they will find displayed stress level along with three options: given a re-questionnaire responses, remedies and statics.
6. He can go to any of the options.
7. All the users will get some remedies to follow and practice in their daily life.
8. After few days they can go through the retest.

The time duration for whole experiment was 6 months which included stress recognition through biofeedback devices and providing its remedy through app. For stress level measurements, Short form of health Survey SF-36 questionnaire was used questionnaire and Biofeedback therapy to know current intensity, duration and frequency of headache of subject and for remedy, we applied meditative techniques and alternate therapies. For backup, we stored the data in Google Drive or Hard Disk to avoid any data loss.(Saini et al., 2019; Singhal et al., 2019)

FUNCTIONS OF EXPERIMENTAL APP

1. Our product measured the subject stress level in specified time and helped them to handle it as per their scores and stress intensity. 2. We are using dataset of SF-36 [Dataset for SF-36, n.d.] and we have clustered it into three clusters using k-means algorithm and after clustering we have modified and added the dataset with their respective clusters and used it as new dataset for training and testing of classification algorithms
2. We have used 70% data to train four classification algorithms Naïve Baye's, Logistic Regression, SVM and Decision tree and 30% for testing purpose.
3. Out of which Decision tree has most high accuracy in our case.
4. Now in Decision tree we have used various test cases given as the input to the trained model and by the help of outputs of these test cases we were able to find the range in which the new weight will be classified: low, medium or high.
5. We have used the same range limit in website for decided the stress level of the person depending upon the weights of the questions he has answered.

USER CHARACTERISTICS

Subject under considerations were users of all ages (18-65), genders, locality and is mainly focused on adolescents.

CONSTRAINTS

1. The system complied with all local regulatory policies and ethical committee.
2. The users had to answer all the questions honestly otherwise they may be classified into wrong stress level.
3. Our research work was based on EMG and GSR machines with are very costly and very hard to find and do analysis.
4. This product will be windows-based. So all the users must have windows operatingsystem running on their pc's.
5. Our product will use client server architecture and therefore be able to handle multiple participants at onetime.
6. Our product will use cookies to help identify the registered users attempting to use the product via the internet.
7. Our product will provide a backup capability to protect the data.

ASSUMPTIONS AND DEPENDENCIES

It is assumed that every user who will use our product will have windowsoperating system or Linux and all will satisfy the software and hardware requirements mentioned above.

APPORTIONING OF REQUIREMENTS

We may not be able to do thermal imaging. We only used questionnaires to measure the participant stress level. The different diagrams of Mental Health Analyzer(MHA) App are as below.

UML SPECIFICATIONS

Use Case Model

Use case model was used to exhibit the functions and activities of all users and participants of the study. It also demonstrates the functioning of the app shows the functions that can be done by a particular user according to their position.

In the figure 1,we can see that a particular participant can login, register on site, can take test, can get a result. An administrator can manage the whole database and login on website. The user will get the question set and the evaluation of stress level will be done which will be saved in the database. If the stress level is too high, then he will be advised to go to doctor or psychiatrist.

Figure 1. Use Case Model of MHA App

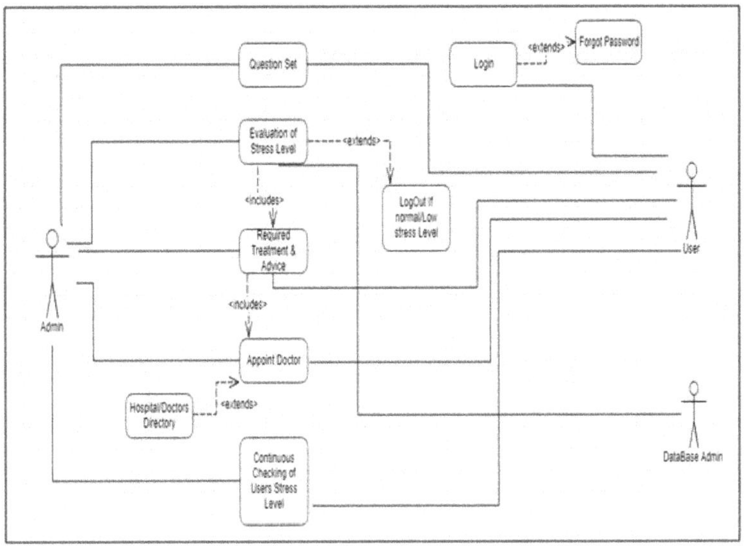

SYSTEM DESIGN AND METHODOLOGY

System Design & System Architecture

In figure 2, Flowchart shows the flow in which the whole work of site will go on. In this flowchart we can see that when the user will login into the site then they will counter a questionnaire. They will attempt that on basis of given answer their result will be calculated and remedies will be given to them, according to where they lie whether low, medium or high.

ACTIVITY DIAGRAM

Figure 3, the activity diagram shows all the activities performed in the project are shown.

DFD

In the figure 4, data flow diagram level 0 is shown.
   In the figure 5, data flow diagram level 1 is shown.
   In the figure 6, data flow diagram level 2 is shown.

ER DIAGRAM

In the figure 7, Entity relationship diagram is shown with entities, attributes and relationship that are used in the project.

Figure 2. Flowchart of MHA App

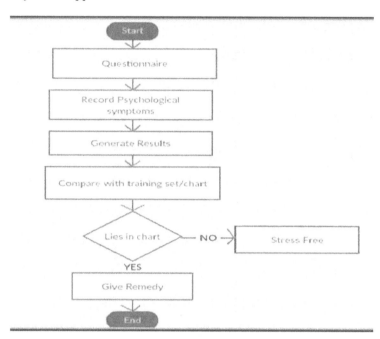

Figure 3. Activity Diagram of MHA App

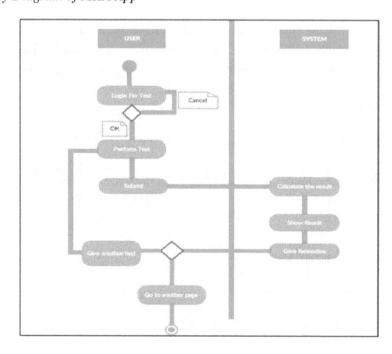

Figure 4. DFD level 0 of MHA app

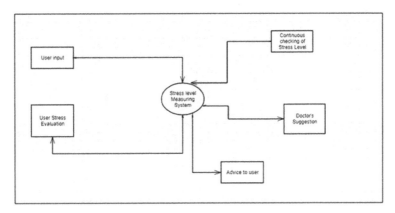

Figure 5. DFD level 1 of MHA app

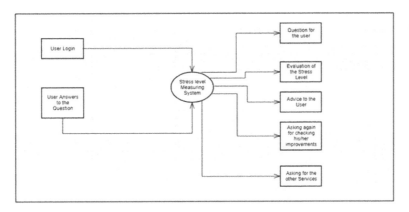

Figure 6. DFD level 2 of MHA app

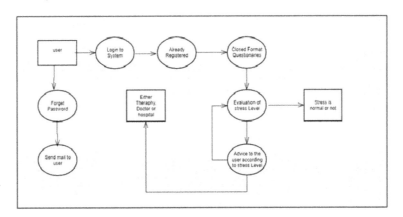

Figure 7. ER Diagram of MHA app

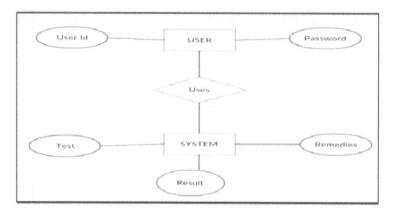

IMPLEMENTATION AND RESULTS

Software and Hardware Requirements

Software Requirements

1. Python 3.6
2. Angular 6
3. Node js 10.0.0
4. Express js
5. Mongo db 4.0
6. PyCharm
7. Angular CLI
8. Mongo shell
9. Visual Studio Code
10. Tablue (Data visualization)

Hardware Requirements

1. Operating System: Linux, Unix or Windows
2. Web Server: Node js and Express js provided by NPM package
3. Ram size: 8 GB
4. x86 - 64 processor
5. EMG (only used for research not for website)
6. GSR (only used for research not for website)

ASSUMPTIONS AND DEPENDENCIES

It is assumed that every user who will use our product will have windows operating system and will satisfy all the software and hardware requirements mentioned above.

IMPLEMENTATION DETAILS

Snapshots of Interfaces

In the figure 8, Home page which will be loaded on the screen of user

In the figure 9, Login screen will be shown after clicking on Know your mental health option the user will have to login or register if he is new to our website.

In the figure 10, Test page is shown in which the user will answer the questions and submit.

In the figure 11-14, dashboard is shown which will be opened after the user has given first time his test. This page will contain the result along with three other options to go with i.e. Retest, Remedy and Statics. He can again give retest or go to the remedy page.

In figure 15 remedies depending upon the stress level of the user is shown. It is expected from the user that they will follow the steps sincerely.

TEST CASES

1. If stress level lies in range of S >= 25 and S <=57.
2. If stress level lies in range of S >= 58 and S <=68.
3. If stress level lies in range of S >= 68 and S<=125.

Figure 8. Home Page of the MHA app

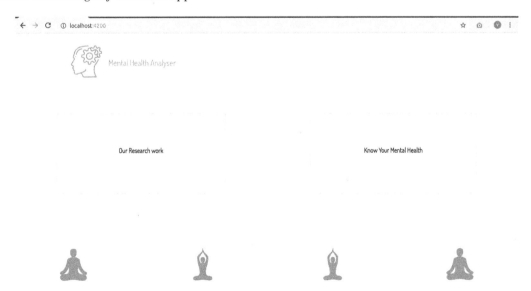

Figure 9. Login Page of MHA app

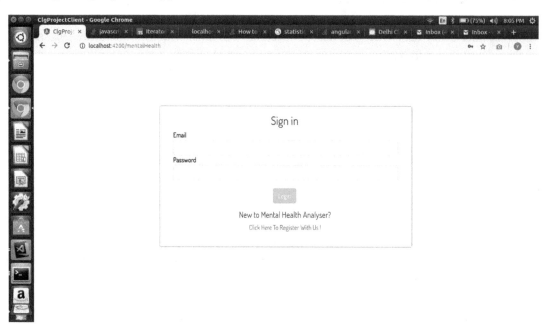

Figure 10. Test Page of MHA app

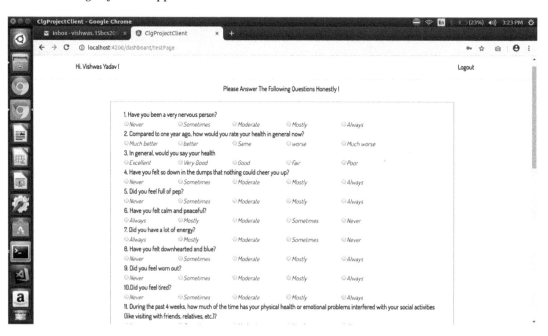

Figure 11. Dashboard of MHA app with Medium level of Stress

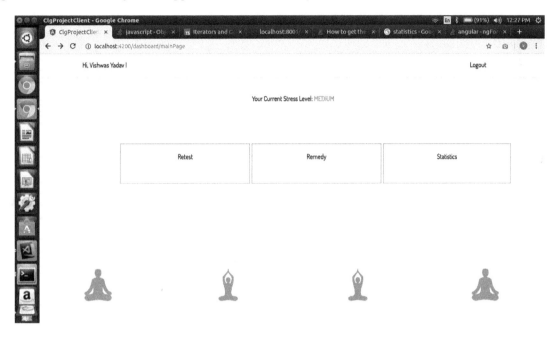

Figure 12. Dashboard of MHA app with Low level of Stress

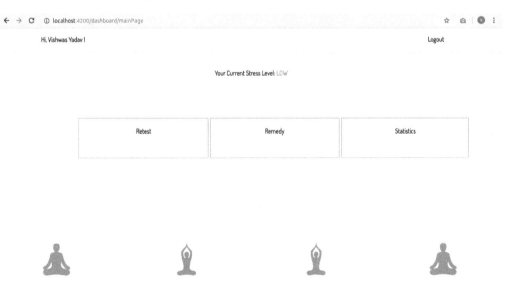

Figure 13. Dashboard of MHA app with High level of Stress

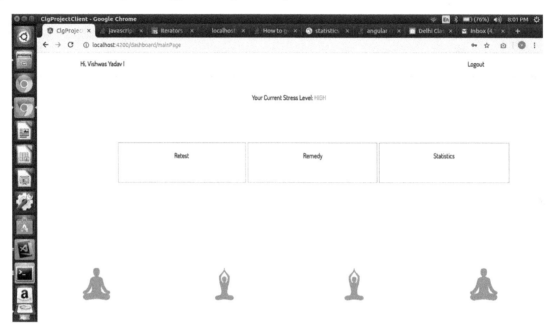

Figure 14. Log of Different responses by an user of MHA app

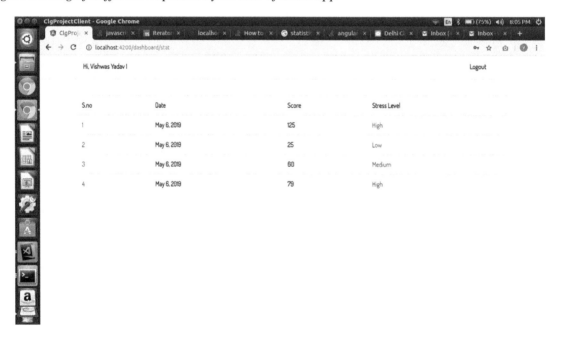

Figure 15. Remedies proposed of MHA app

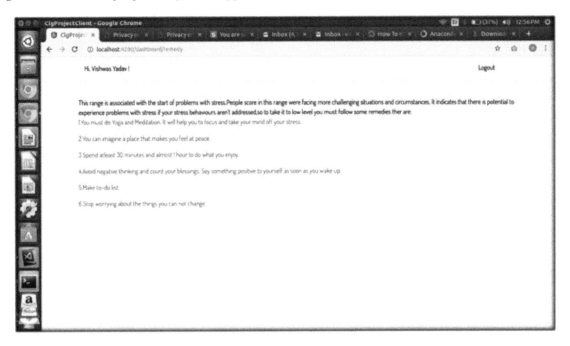

RESULTS

Result of our Research Work

We have find the result that EMG in Audio mode is best among all the other modesof EMG as well as it is also better than GSR in all modes i.e. Audio, Visual andAudio-visual. We have published this results in a book chapter. (Arora et al., 2019)

Results of Experiments

In the figure 16, mean calculated by the python code is shown. It is the mean of all the questions answered by 399 people as present in the dataset.

1. We have successfully clustered responses from dataset into three clusters i.e. low, medium & high stress level by the help of K-means algorithms and now we classify new user into one of these three classes.

The figure 17 shows the clusters that we have got using k-means algorithm on the dataset of 399 peoples response of SF-36 questionnaires (Dataset for SF-36, n.d.).

Cluster 1 represents Low Stress Level
Cluster 2 represents Medium Stress Level
Cluster 3 represents High Stress Level

Figure 16. Mean of all questions

q1	2.967419
q2	2.716792
q3	3.022556
q4	2.832080
q5	2.350877
q6	2.852130
q7	3.225564
q8	2.451128
q9	2.238095
q10	2.832080
q11	2.694236
q12	2.471178
q13	2.696742
q14	2.057644
q15	2.558897
q16	1.822055
q17	2.203008
q18	1.944862
q19	2.203008
q20	2.859649
q21	2.498747
q22	1.794486
q23	2.263158
q24	2.403509
q25	3.035088
Total	62.994987

Figure 17. Clusters of the Analyzed datasets

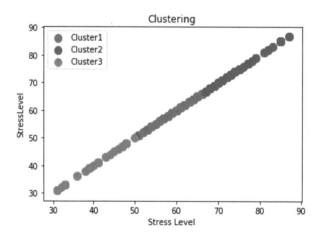

2. After making three clusters we have modified the dataset and added the respective clusters in each row and used the new dataset to train various classification algorithms that we have used: Logistic Regression, Naïve Bayes, SVM, Decision Tree algorithm.

3. For training the machines, we used 70% data and for testing and accuracy, 30% data was used for the purposes.

4. Out of all the algorithms Decision tree gives the best accuracy so we have find out the range of each class i.e. low, medium and high using various test cases onDecision tree algorithm and we have got range limits from it that we are using in ourwebsite for giving results.

The Figure 18 shows the accuracy of various classification algorithms that are used for classification.

CONCLUSION

Performance Evaluation

We have used 70% data for training and 30% for testing purposes.(Saini et al., 2019; Singh et al., 2019) Out of all the algorithms Decision tree gives the best accuracy as shown in table 1, so we have find out the range of each class i.e. low, medium and high using various test cases on Decision tree algorithm and we have got range limits from it that we are using in our website for giving results.

Figure 18. Accuracy of various algorithms applied

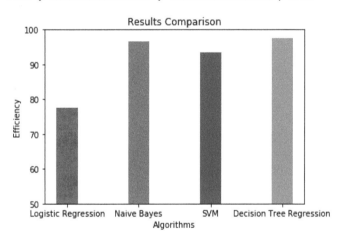

Table 1. Accuracy of various Algorithms applied

S.NO	Algorithm Name	Accuracy (%)
1.	Logistic Regression	77.5
2.	Naïve Bayes Classifier	96.667
3.	SVM	93.333
4.	Decision Tree Regression	97.5

EXPERIMENTAL RESEARCH BASED LEARNING

1. Different technologies like: Angular 6, Mongo db, Node js, Express js, Python, Tableu, k-mean clustering, logistic regression algorithm.
2. Practical implementation of tools like: Visual Studio, Tableu and Mongo Shell
3. Team Work.
4. Dividing and Managing the work.

FUTURE DIRECTIONS

1. Give suggestion of nearby hospitals or psychiatrists by tacking GPS location of the user's device.
2. Send the result with the remedies to the user through email.
3. Make a team for doing survey among people in our college and offices for getting larger dataset so that we may increase the accuracy.
4. Conducting awareness camps for telling people to use this type of application for getting better stress-free lifestyle.

ACKNOWLEDGMENT

Author is a research scholar on domain of scientific spirituality and thankful with gratitude for his guide and co-guides of various prestigious academic institutions to understand the concept well and for showing the path ahead. The Scientific spirituality is the emerging field of future and all spiritual organizations working for betterment of society and humanity in large are acknowledged for their great deeds. The acknowledgement to all those forces which choose us to make this world a better place to live in.

REFERENCES

Arora, N., Rastogi, R., Chaturvedi, D. K., Satya, S., Gupta, M., Yadav, V., Chauhan, S., & Sharma, P. (2019). Chronic TTH Analysis by EMG & GSR Biofeedback on Various Modes and Various Medical Symptoms Using IoT. In Big Data Analytics for Intelligent Healthcare Management. doi:10.1016/B978-0-12-818146-1.00005-2

Arora, N., Trivedi, P., Chauhan, S., Rastogi, R., & Chaturvedi, D. K. (2017). Framework for Use of Machine Intelligence on Clinical Psychology to study the effects of Spiritual tools on Human Behavior and Psychic Challenges. *Proceedings of NSC-2017(National System Conference)*.

Bansal, I., Rastogi, R., Chaturvedi, D. K., Satya, S., Arora, N., & Yadav, V. (2018). Intelligent Analysis for Detection of Complex Human Personality by Clinical Reliable Psychological Surveys on Various Indicators. *National Conference on 3rd MDNCPDR-2018 at DEI*.

Chaturvedi, D. K., Rastogi, R., Arora, N., Trivedi, P., & Mishra, V. (2017). Swarm Intelligent Optimized Method of Development of Noble Life in the perspective of Indian Scientific Philosophy and Psychology. *Proceedings of NSC-2017 (National System Conference).*

Chaturvedi, D.K., Rastogi, R., Satya, S., Arora, N., Saini, H., Verma, H., Mehlyan, K., & Varshney, Y. (2018). Statistical Analysis of EMG and GSR Therapy on Visual Mode and SF-36 Scores for Chronic TTH. *Proceedings of UPCON-2018.*

Chauhan, S., Rastogi, R., Chaturvedi, D. K., Satya, S., Arora, N., Yadav, V., & Sharma, P. (2018d). Analytical Comparison of Efficacy for Electromyography and Galvanic Skin Resistance Biofeedback on Audio-Visual Mode for Chronic TTH on Various Attributes. Proceedings of the ICCID.

Dataset for SF-36. (n.d.). https://www.kaggle.com/janiferroborts/sf-36-dataset,Janifer

Effects of Biofeedback on Stress. (n.d.). https://jillshultz.com/williamaltman/Courses/PSY_110/Sample%20Papers/Proposal-Effects-of-Biofeedback-on-Stress.pdf

Gulati, M., Rastogi, R., Chaturvedi, D. K., Sharma, P., Yadav, V., Chauhan, S., Gupta, M., & Singhal, P. (2019). Statistical Resultant Analysis of Psychosomatic Survey on Various Human Personality Indicators: Statistical Survey to Map Stress and Mental Health. In *Handbook of Research on Learning in the Age of Transhumanism*. Hershey, PA: IGI Global. doi:10.4018/978-1-5225-8431-5.ch022

Gupta, M., Rastogi, R., Chaturvedi, D. K., & Satya, S. (2019). Comparative Study of Trends Observed During Different Medications by Subjects under EMG & GSR Biofeedback. *IJITEE, 8*(6S), 748-756. https://www.ijitee.org/download/volume-8-issue-6S/

Khanna, A., Paul, M., & Sandhu, J. S. (2007). A study to compare the effectiveness of GSR biofeedback training and progressive muscle relaxation training in reducing blood pressure and respiratory rate among highly stressed individuals. *Indian J Physiol Pharmacol, 51*(3), 296-300.

Kikuchi, H., Yoshiuchi, K., Yamamoto, Y., Komaki, G., & Akabayashi, A. (2012). Diurnal variation of tension-type headache intensity and exacerbation: An investigation using computerized ecological momentary assessment. *Biopsychosoc Med., 6*(18). doi:10.1186/1751-0759-6-18

List of best 25 mobile apps used for mental and physical health. (n.d.). https://www.psycom.net/25-best-mental-health-apps

Ngo-Metzger, Sorkin, Mangione, Gandek, & Hays. (n.d.). *36-Item Short Form Survey (SF-36)*. https://www.rand.org/health-care/surveys_tools/mos/36-item-short-form.html

PyCharm. (n.d.). https://en.wikipedia.org/wiki/PyCharm

Rastogi, R., Chaturvedi, D. K., Satya, S., Arora, N., & Chauhan, S. (2018). An Optimized Biofeedback Therapy for Chronic TTH between Electromyography and Galvanic Skin Resistance Biofeedback on Audio, Visual and Audio Visual Modes on Various Medical Symptoms. *National Conference on 3rd MDNCPDR-2018 at DEI.*

Rastogi, R., Chaturvedi, D. K., Satya, S., Arora, N., Singhal, P., & Gulati, M. (2018). Statistical Resultant Analysis of Spiritual & Psychosomatic Stress Survey on Various Human Personality Indicators. *The International Conference proceedings of ICCI 2018*. DOI: 10.1007/978-981-13-8222-2_25

Rastogi, R., Chaturvedi, D. K., Satya, S., Arora, N., Sirohi, H., Singh, M., Verma, P., & Singh, V. (2018). *Which One is Best: Electromyography Biofeedback Efficacy Analysis on Audio, Visual and Audio-Visual Modes for Chronic TTH on Different Characteristics*. Proceedings of ICCIIoT- 2018. https://ssrn.com/abstract=3354375

Rastogi, R., Chaturvedi, D. K., Satya, S., Arora, N., Yadav, V., Chauhan, S., & Sharma, P. (2018). SF-36 Scores Analysis for EMG and GSR Therapy on Audio, Visual and Audio Visual Modes for Chronic TTH. Proceedings of the ICCIDA-2018.

Saini, H., Rastogi, R., Chaturvedi, D. K., Satya, S., Arora, N., Gupta, M., & Verma, H. (2019). An Optimized Biofeedback EMG and GSR Biofeedback Therapy for Chronic TTH on SF-36 Scores of Different MMBD Modes on Various Medical Symptoms. In Hybrid Machine Intelligence for Medical Image Analysis, Studies Comp. Intelligence, (Vol. 841). Springer Nature Singapore Pte Ltd. doi:10.1007/978-981-13-8930-6_8

Saini, H., Rastogi, R., Chaturvedi, D. K., Satya, S., Arora, N., Verma, H., & Mehlyan, K. (2018). *Comparative Efficacy Analysis of Electromyography and Galvanic Skin Resistance Biofeedback on Audio Mode for Chronic TTH on Various Indicators*. Proceedings of ICCIIoT- 2018. https://ssrn.com/abstract=3354371

Satya, S., Arora, N., Trivedi, P., Singh, A., Sharma, A., Singh, A., Rastogi, R., & Chaturvedi, D. K. (2019). *Intelligent Analysis for Personality Detection on Various Indicators by Clinical Reliable Psychological TTH and Stress Surveys*. Proceedings of CIPR 2019.

Satya, S., Rastogi, R., Chaturvedi, D. K., Arora, N., Singh, P., & Vyas, P. (2018). Statistical Analysis for Effect of Positive Thinking on Stress Management and Creative Problem Solving for Adolescents. *Proceedings of the 12th INDIA-Com*, 245-251.

Sharma, S., Rastogi, R., Chaturvedi, D. K., Bansal, A., & Agrawal, A. (2018). Audio Visual EMG & GSR Biofeedback Analysis for Effect of Spiritual Techniques on Human Behavior and Psychic Challenges. *Proceedings of the 12th INDIACom*, 252-258.

Singh, A., Rastogi, R., Chaturvedi, D. K., Satya, S., Arora, N., Sharma, A., & Singh, A. (2019). Intelligent Personality Analysis on Indicators in IoT-MMBD Enabled Environment. In *Multimedia Big Data Computing for IoT Applications: Concepts, Paradigms, and Solutions*. Springer. Advance online publication. doi:10.1007/978-981-13-8759-3_7

Singhal, P., Rastogi, R., Chaturvedi, D. K., Satya, S., Arora, N., Gupta, M., Singhal, P., & Gulati, M. (2019). Statistical Analysis of Exponential and Polynomial Models of EMG & GSR Biofeedback for Correlation between Subjects Medications Movement & Medication Scores. *IJITEE, 8*(6S), 625-635. https://www.ijitee.org/download/volume-8-issue-6S/

Vyas, P., Rastogi, R., Chaturvedi, D. K., Arora, N., Trivedi, P., & Singh, P. (2018). Study on Efficacy of Electromyography and Electroencephalography Biofeedback with Mindful Meditation on Mental health of Youths. *Proceedings of the 12th INDIA-Com*, 84-89.

What is biofeedback? (2008). Association for Applied Psychophysiology and Biofeedback.

Yadav, V., Rastogi, R., Chaturvedi, D. K., Satya, S., Arora, N., Yadav, V., Sharma, P., & Chauhan, S. (2018). Statistical Analysis of EMG & GSR Biofeedback Efficacy on Different Modes for Chronic TTH on Various Indicators. *Int. J. Advanced Intelligence Paradigms*, *13*(1), 251–275. doi:10.1504/IJAIP.2019.10021825

Chapter 21

Pre–Clustering Techniques for Healthcare System:
Evaluation Measures, Evaluation Metrics, Comparative Study of Existing vs. Proposed Approaches

Asadi Srinivasulu

Sree Vidyanikethan Engineering College, India

ABSTRACT

This chapter presents a comparative study of the proposed approaches (i.e., extended dark block extraction [EDBE], extended cluster count extraction [ECCE], and extended co-VAT approaches). This chapter evaluates pre-clustering and post-clustering algorithms on real-time data and synthetic datasets. Unlike traditional clustering algorithms, pre-clustering algorithms provide a prior clustering on different datasets. Simulation studies are carried out using datasets having both class-labeled and unlabeled information. Comparative studies are performed between results of existing pre-clustering and proposed pre-clustering approaches. A simulated RDI-based preprocessing method is also applied for data diversification. Extensive simulation on real and synthetic datasets shows that pre-clustering algorithms with simulated RDI-based pre-processing performs better compared to conventional post-clustering algorithms.

INTRODUCTION

This chapter presents a comparative study of the proposed approaches viz., Extended Dark Block Extraction (EDBE), Extended Cluster Count Extraction (ECCE), and Extended Co-VAT approaches. This chapter evaluates Pre-Clustering and Post-Clustering algorithms on real-time data and synthetic datasets. Unlike traditional clustering algorithms, Pre-Clustering algorithms provide a prior clustering on different datasets. Simulation studies are carried out using datasets having both class-labeled and unlabeled information. Comparative studies are performed between results of existing Pre-Clustering

DOI: 10.4018/978-1-7998-2742-9.ch021

and proposed Pre-Clustering approaches. A simulated RDI based preprocessing method is also applied for data diversification. Extensive simulation on real and synthetic datasets shows that Pre-Clustering algorithms with simulated RDI based pre-processing performs better compared to conventional Post-Clustering algorithms.

Comprehensive study has been conducted on cluster validation metrics for several Pre-Clustering approaches. For real time data, Pre-Clustering results are generated based on "dark blocks" concept with EDBE, ECCE and Extended Co-VAT approaches on *WINE* and *IRIS* data samples. It is important to compare various cluster validation metrics and select one that fits best with the "VAT" data distribution. Cluster validation is the process of assessing the quality and reliability of the cluster sets derived from various Pre-Clustering processes. A comparative study has been performed using four cluster validation metrics viz., clustering accuracy, clustering error, time complexity and cluster coefficient for assessing the quality of different pre-clustering approaches. The following Table 6.1 describes two datasets viz., *NUMERIC* and *IMAGE* dataset that consist of characteristics such as physical classes, attributes, size of the dataset and number of clusters. Pre-Clustering approaches are applied on different sizes of datasets in-order to detect the number of clusters.where N_1– N_4 stands for *NUMERIC* dataset, I_1- I_4 are *IMAGE* datasets.

The *NUMERIC* and *IMAGE* dataset characteristics i.e. size of datasets, physical classes, attributes, and number of clusters of EDBE, ECCE and Extended Co-VAT are summarized in Table 1.

Table 1. Datasets with Characteristics for the Proposed Approaches

Synthetic Dataset	Physical Classes	Attributes	Size (n)	Generated number of Clusters (C)		
				Extended Co-VAT	ECCE	EDBE
Numeric Dataset N_1	2	3	3*3	2	2	2
Numeric Dataset N_2	3	10	10*10	2	2	2
Numeric Dataset N_3	3	50	5000* 5000	3	3	3
Numeric Dataset N_4	5	100	100000* 100000	3	3	3
IMAGE Dataset I_1	2	3	3*3	2	2	2
IMAGE Dataset I_2	3	10	10*10	2	2	2
IMAGE Dataset I_3	3	50	5000* 5000	3	3	3
IMAGE Dataset I_4	5	100	100000* 100000	3	3	3

Evaluation Measures

One of the most important issues in cluster analysis is the evaluation of the clustering results. The evaluation of clustering results is the most difficult task within the whole clustering workflow.

The ways of evaluation are divided in two parts:

- Internal quality measures, and
- External quality measures.

In internal quality measures, the overall similarity measure is calculated based on the pair-wise similarity of documents and there is no external knowledge to be used. In external quality measures, some external knowledge for the data is required. In this thesis all internal quality measures viz., clustering accuracy, clustering error, time complexity and cluster coefficient are considered.

Evaluation Metrics

The performance of the proposed approaches is calculated using constraint partitioning K-Means algorithm and they are computed by means of four internal quality evaluation measures.

i)   Clustering Accuracy (C_a)
ii) Clustering Error (C_e)
iii) Time Complexity
iv) Clustering Co-efficient(C_c)

Clustering Accuracy

Clustering accuracy is a simple and transparent evaluation metric or measure. Accuracy is an external evaluation criterion for cluster quality. To compute accuracy, each cluster is assigned to the class which is most frequent in the cluster, and then the accuracy of this assignment is measured by counting the number of correctly assigned data points and dividing it by N_d. Clustering accuracy specifies quality of the clustering process, which is given as follows:

$$C_a\left(N, M\right) = \frac{1}{N_d} \sum_k \max_j \left| w_k \cap c_j \right|$$

where, N_d = Number of data points in the dataset.

$N = \{ w_1, w_2, \dots\dots w_k \}$ is the set of clusters.

$M = \{ c_1, c_2, \dots\dots\dots c_j \}$ is the set of classes. where w_k is interpreted as the set of data points in w_k and c_j as the set of data points in c_j in Equation 6.1. The following Figure 1 contains three clusters (i.e. red=x, green=o, blue=d). Majority class and number of members of the majority class for the three clusters are, (x,5) is for cluster 1, (o,4) is for cluster 2 and (d,3) is for cluster 3. Cluster Accuracy is (1/17)*(5+4+3) ≈ 0.71

Hopkins' statistic is used to assess the clustering tendency of a dataset by measuring the probability that a given dataset is generated by a uniform data distribution (or) it tests the spatial randomness of the data. In order to determine the cluster tendency of data using proposed approaches viz., EDBE, ECCE and Extended Co-VAT, grouping of data is calculated based on VAT algorithm. VAT image with RDI for the proposed approaches with integration of K-Means algorithm on two datasets viz., *IRIS* and *WINE* are as shown in Figure 1.

Figures 1(a) and 6.1(b) shows the formation of three clusters after running pre-clustering approaches viz., EDBE and ECCE respectively on *IRIS* and *WINE* datasets. The colors of the three clusters are indicated in green, red and blue.

Figure 1. (a) Cluster formation after running EDBE on IRIS dataset, (b) Cluster formation after running ECCE on WINE dataset

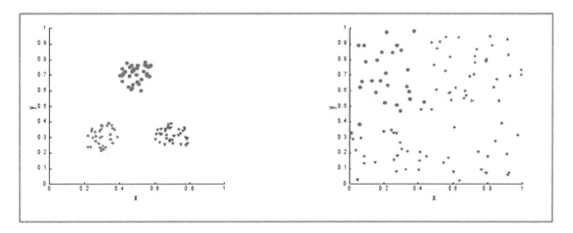

Clustering Error

Clustering error specifies the correlation between data points within cluster i.e. data element - by - data element within cluster. Consider statistical inference for regression when data are grouped into clusters, with regression model errors independent across clusters but correlated within clusters. Hence, data points in one cluster is 'R_x' i.e. within cluster correlation regression, 'R_e' is the within cluster error correlation and 'C_a' is the average cluster size. It is noticed about the importance of clustering error if there is an aggregate regression (i.e., $R_x = 1$).

Clustering error can be calculated by using below formula

$$C_e = R_x - R_e$$

where C_e = Clustering Error.

R_x = within-cluster correlation regression.

R_e = within-cluster error correlation regression.

Time Complexity

The code corresponding to EDBE, ECCE and Extended Co-VAT is run on the *IRIS, WINE* and *NUMERIC* datasets and it takes 1.130691 sec, 2.130691 sec and 3.130691 sec respectively to obtain the cluster count as the output.

Clustering Co-Efficient

A clustering coefficient 'C_c' for any cluster data point 'i' has at least two neighbors. A fundamental measure that has long received attention in both theoretical and empirical research is the clustering coefficient. Clustering coefficient is calculated based on the number of the nearest neighbors with data points connecting its nearest neighbor cluster group as follows

$$C_c = \frac{y}{(z(z-1)/2)}$$

where, 'z' is the number of nearest neighbors of clusters and 'y' is the number of data points of clusters i.e. the number of data points connected to its nearest neighbor cluster.

Comparative Study of Existing vs. Proposed Approaches

This section presents the comparative study of the proposed approaches with existing approaches. The results are compared with real-time datasets viz., *NUMERIC, IRIS,* and *WINE* with the evaluation metrics are Cluster accuracy, Cluster error, Time complexity and Cluster Co-efficient.

Results for *NUMERIC* dataset

Table 2 presents the Clustering accuracy of different pre-clustering approaches for the *NUMERIC* dataset by using the formula given section 6.2.1

Table 2. Pre-Clustering approaches vs. NUMERIC dataset Cluster Accuracy

Pre-Clustering Approaches	DBE	CCE	Co-VAT	EDBE	ECCE	Extended Co-VAT
Cluster accuracy	70.12%	50.95%	60.53%	90.23%	80.12%	80.50%

The above data is plotted through the bar chart as shown in Figure 6.2.

The above results indicate that EDBE is more accurate when compared with the pre-clustering approaches viz., DBE, CCE, Co-VAT, ECCE and Extended Co-VAT. Hence, it outperforms the other pre-clustering approaches.

Figure 2. Pre-Clustering Approaches vs. NUMERIC dataset Cluster Accuracy

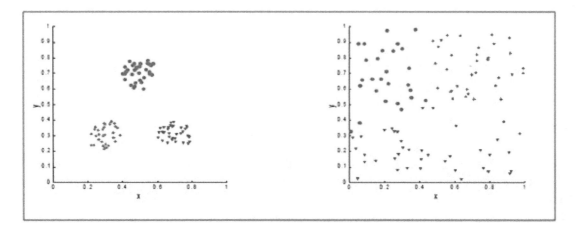

Table 3 presents the Cluster error of different pre-clustering approaches for *NUMERIC* dataset by using the formula given section 6.2.2

Table 3. Pre-Clustering Approaches vs. NUMERIC dataset Cluster Error

Pre-Clustering Approaches	DBE	CCE	Co-VAT	EDBE	ECCE	Extended Co-VAT
Cluster error	0.12	1.22	1.45	0.10	1.23	1.50

The above data is plotted through the bar chart as shown in Figure 3.

The above results indicate that EDBE has least cluster error when compared with the other pre-clustering approaches viz., CCE, Co-VAT, DBE, ECCE and Extended Co-VAT.

Figure 3. Pre-Clustering Approaches vs. NUMERIC dataset Cluster Error

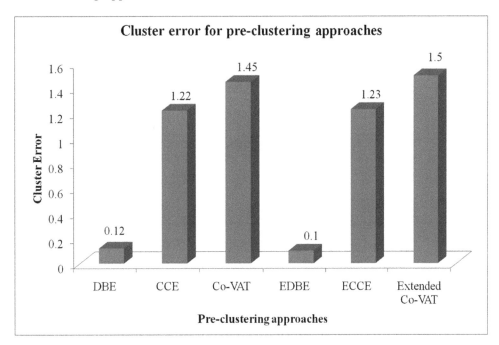

Table 4 presents the time complexity of different pre-clustering approaches for the *NUMERIC* dataset. The above data is plotted through the bar chart as shown in Figure 4.

Pre-Clustering Approaches vs. *NUMERIC* Dataset Time Complexity

The above results indicate that EDBE is less time complex when compared with the other pre-clustering approaches viz., DBE, CCE, Co-VAT, ECCE and Extended Co-VAT.

Table 4. Pre-Clustering Approaches vs. NUMERIC dataset Time Complexity

Pre-Clustering Approaches	DBE	CCE	Co-VAT	EDBE	ECCE	Extended Co-VAT
Time Complexity	2.1 Sec	3.1 Sec	4.1 Sec	1.1 Sec	2.2 Sec	3.12 Sec

Figure 4. Pre-clustering approaches vs. NUMERIC dataset Time Complexity

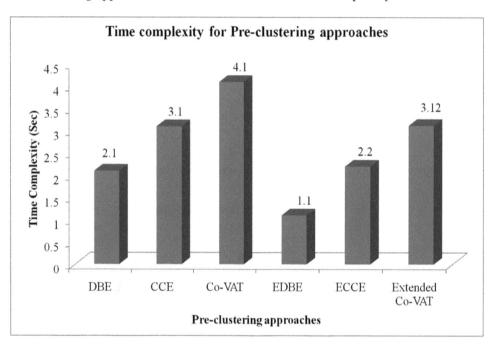

Results for *IRIS* dataset

Table 5 presents the Cluster accuracy of different pre-clustering approaches for the *IRIS* dataset by using the formula given section 6.2.1.

Table 5. Pre-Clustering Approaches vs. IRIS dataset with Cluster Accuracy (C_a)

Pre-Clustering Approaches	DBE	CCE	Co-VAT	EDBE	ECCE	Extended Co-VAT
Cluster Accuracy	71.0%	60.0%	65.0%	91.0%	80.0%	85.0%

The above data is plotted through the bar chart as shown in Figure 5.

The above results indicate that EDBE is more accurate when compared with the other pre-clustering approaches viz., DBE, CCE, Co-VAT, ECCE and Extended Co-VAT.

Figure 5. Pre-Clustering Approaches vs. IRIS dataset with Cluster Accuracy (C$_a$)

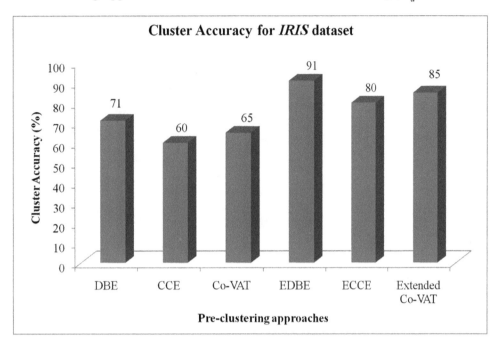

Table 6 presents the Cluster error of different pre-clustering approaches for the *IRIS* dataset by using the formula given section 6.2.2

Table 6. Pre-Clustering Approaches vs. IRIS dataset with Clustering Error (C$_e$)

Pre-Clustering Approaches	DBE	CCE	Co-VAT	EDBE	ECCE	Extended Co-VAT
Cluster Error	0.13	1.21	1.49	0.12	1.22	1.49

The above data is plotted through the bar chart as shown in Figure 6.

The above results indicate that EDBE has least Cluster error when compared with the other pre-clustering approaches viz., CCE, Co-VAT, DBE, Extended CCE and Extended Co-VAT.

Table 7 presents the time complexity of different pre-clustering approaches for the *IRIS* dataset.

Table 7. Pre-Clustering Approaches vs. IRIS dataset with Time Complexity

Pre-Clustering Approaches	DBE	CCE	Co-VAT	EDBE	ECCE	Extended Co-VAT
Time Complexity	2.1 Sec	3.1 Sec	4.1 Sec	1.1 Sec	2.2 Sec	3.1 Sec

Figure 6. Pre-Clustering Approaches vs. IRIS dataset with Clustering Error (C_e)

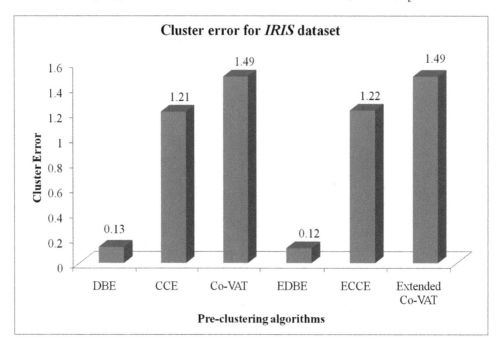

The above data is plotted through the bar chart as shown in Figure 7

The above results indicate that EDBE is less time complex when compared with the other pre-clustering approaches viz., DBE, CCE, Co-VAT, Extended CCE and Extended Co-VAT.

Figure 7. Pre-Clustering Approaches vs. IRIS dataset with Time Complexity

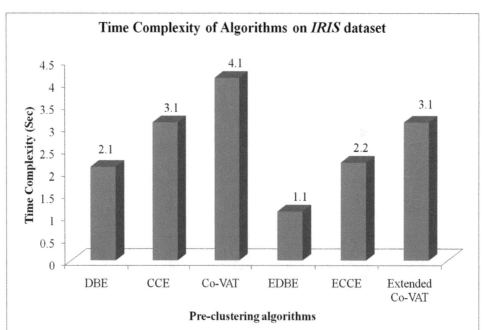

Results for *WINE* Dataset

Table 8 presents the Cluster accuracy of different pre-clustering approaches for the *WINE* dataset by using the formula given section 6.2.1

Table 8. Pre-Clustering Approaches vs. WINE dataset with Cluster Accuracy (C_a)

Pre-Clustering Approaches	DBE	CCE	Co-VAT	EDBE	ECCE	Extended Co-VAT
Cluster Accuracy	72.0%	62.0%	53.0%	93.0%	89.0%	81.0%

The above data is plotted through the bar chart as shown in Figure 8.

The above results indicate that EDBE is more accurate when compared with the other pre-clustering approaches viz., DBE, CCE, Co-VAT, EDBE, Extended CCE and Extended Co-VAT.

Figure 8. Pre-Clustering Approaches vs. WINE dataset with Cluster Accuracy (C_a)

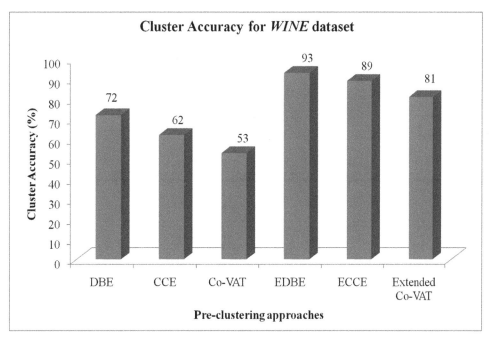

Table 9 presents the Cluster error of different pre-clustering approaches for the *WINE* dataset by using the formula given section 6.2.2

The above data is plotted through the bar chart as shown in Figure 9.

The above results indicate that EDBE has least Cluster error when compared with the other pre-clustering approaches viz., DBE, CCE, Co-VAT, Extended CCE and Extended Co-VAT.

Table 9. Pre-Clustering Approaches vs. WINE with Clustering Error (C_e)

Pre-Clustering Approaches	DBE	CCE	Co-VAT	EDBE	ECCE	Extended Co-VAT
Cluster Error	0.3	1.53	1.8	0.21	1.42	1.9

Figure 9. Pre-Clustering Approaches vs. WINE with Clustering Error (C_e)

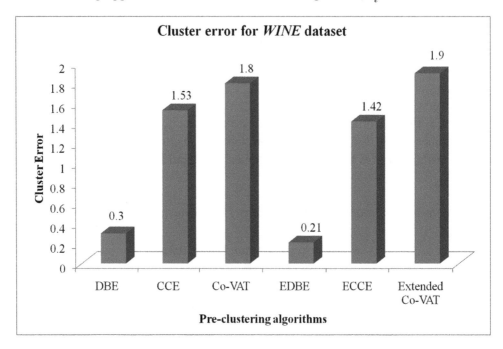

Table 10 presents the time complexity of different pre-clustering approaches for the *WINE* dataset.

Table 10. Pre-Clustering Approaches vs. WINE dataset with Time Complexity

Pre-Clustering Approaches	DBE	CCE	Co-VAT	EDBE	ECCE	Extended Co-VAT
Time Complexity	2.9 Sec	3.5 Sec	4.3 Sec	2.4 Sec	4.1 Sec	5.1 Sec

The above data is plotted through the bar chart as shown in Figure 10.

The above results indicate that EDBE is less time complex when compared with the other pre-clustering approaches viz., CCE, Co-VAT, DBE, Extended CCE and Extended Co-VAT.

Figure 10. Pre-Clustering Approaches vs. WINE dataset with Time Complexity

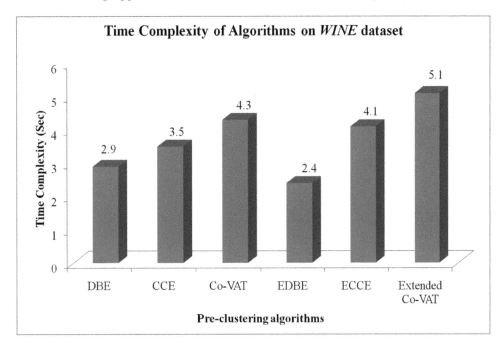

Table 11. Comparison of Real Datasets Characteristics and Results using Existing vs. Proposed Approaches

Pre-Clustering Approach	# Instances	# Attributes	# Clusters	Cluster Accuracy	Cluster Error(α)	Cluster Coefficient	Time Complexity (in Sec)
DBE	150	4	2	72.35	0.15	0.35	2.1306
CCE	150	4	2	60.10	1.25	0.45	3.1306
Co-VAT	150	4	2	65.00	1.50	0.55	4.1306
EDBE	500	8	3	92.35	0.15	0.33	1.1306
ECCE	500	8	3	80.10	1.25	0.55	2.1306
Extended Co-VAT	500	8	3	85.00	1.50	0.66	3.1306

The results obtained in sections 6.3.1, 6.3.2 and 6.3.3 are summarized in Table 6.11. The datasets viz., *NUMERIC*, *IRIS*, and *WINE* are from UCI Machine learning repository (https://archive.ics.uci.edu/ml/datasets.html). In each dataset, VAT image is calculated and the corresponding First-Order Derivative and Fast Fourier Transformations are also computed. The first order derivative signal is calculated by applying threshold value 0.03 to obtain Cluster Error (α). The above results indicates that EDBE is more accurate, less Time complex and results into minimal cluster error when compared with the other pre-clustering approaches viz., DBE, CCE, Co-VAT, Extended CCE and Extended Co-VAT.

SUMMARY

The performance of the proposed approaches i.e. EDBE, ECCE and Extended Co-VAT is evaluated by taking cluster accuracy, cluster error and computational time as metrics. The extended pre-clustering approaches are compared with existing approaches by considering the above said parameters. It is observed that these extended techniques significantly reduced the computational complexity of estimation of cluster count when compared with the existing DBE, CCE, Co-VAT algorithms. Hence, it is concluded that integration of pre and post-clustering approaches results in better computational cost and cluster count accuracy.

Chapter 22
Strategic Analysis in Prediction of Liver Disease Using Different Classification Algorithms

Binish Khan

https://orcid.org/0000-0003-2360-1741

University Institute of Technology, Rajiv Gandhi Proudyogiki Vishwavidyalaya, Bhopal, India

Piyush Kumar Shukla

University Institute of Technology, Rajiv Gandhi Proudyogiki Vishwavidyalaya, Bhopal, India

Manish Kumar Ahirwar

University Institute of Technology, Rajiv Gandhi Proudyogiki Vishwavidyalaya, Bhopal, India

Manish Mishra

University Institute of Technology, Rajiv Gandhi Proudyogiki Vishwavidyalaya, Bhopal, India

ABSTRACT

Liver diseases avert the normal activity of the liver. Discovering the presence of liver disorder at an early stage is a complex task for the doctors. Predictive analysis of liver disease using classification algorithms is an efficacious task that can help the doctors to diagnose the disease within a short duration of time. The main motive of this study is to analyze the parameters of various classification algorithms and compare their predictive accuracies so as to find the best classifier for determining the liver disease. This chapter focuses on the related works of various authors on liver disease such that algorithms were implemented using Weka tool that is a machine learning software written in Java. Also, orange tool is utilized to compare several classification algorithms in terms of accuracy. In this chapter, random forest, logistic regression, and support vector machine were estimated with an aim to identify the best classifier. Based on this study, random forest with the highest accuracy outperformed the other algorithms.

DOI: 10.4018/978-1-7998-2742-9.ch022

INTRODUCTION

Healthcare is regarded as a significant component in enhancing the health-related services for every individual. It makes a provision to improve the health by taking the certain essential measures into consideration and mainly deals with the enhancement of health through the diagnosis of diseases at the right time (Saritha et al., 2017). Thus, "The main aim behind the Healthcare System is to deliver the best quality of services and to predict the diseases at an early stage."

Liver is an imperative organ of our body. There is a great need for an early detection of liver disease so as to prevent complete liver failure, which can result in patient's death. For the proper diagnosis, it is necessary to evaluate some of the main attributes of liver patient's dataset (Vijayarani et al., 2015). Some of the main attributes of liver disease include, "Total_bilirubin, direct_bilirubin, alkaline_phosphotas, total_protein, albumin and globulin_ratio." Below, Figure 1 shows the various functions that are performed by the liver that makes it the second largest organ in our body.

Figure 1. Functions performed by the liver

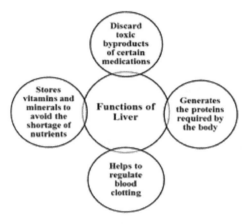

It is a rigorous task for doctors to detect the liver disease accurately. Various classifiers have been utilized to classify the data and to predict the disease through the liver patient's dataset (Ghosh et al., 2017). "Having access to classification algorithms with huge volume of data will help clinicians to come up with optimal decisions and ultimately improve the overall experience of the patient." This paper exhibits a survey about the techniques that can be utilized to reveal the disease and gives a roadmap for future work, such as which classification technique to be utilized further for diagnosis of the liver disease.

A. Tool Used

Weka Tool

Weka is an efficient machine learning software that is widely used to classify various parameters when different algorithmic approaches are applied based on the datasets. It is an accumulation of tools utilized for the purpose of visualization and algorithms for analyzing the data and predictive modelling.

Classification algorithms are implemented using Weka that are utilized for an early stage detection of disease (Pathan et al., 2018). The experimental results of classification algorithms provide ease to the doctors through the provision of accurate patient's pathological status. As shown in Figure 2, Weka can be utilized to perform several data mining tasks.

Figure 2. Data Mining Tasks performed by Weka

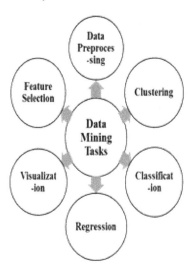

Orange Tool

Orange is a data mining tool that constitutes several components. It includes various widgets that are utilized for data analysis and visualization. In this tool, Python is used as a scripting language. It consists of several components for data preprocessing, modeling, ranking, test and scoring. It is compatible with Python, C and C++. Various features are utilized for data analytics. Also, it is an open source machine learning software build on Python. It has a better debugger than the other tools. Moreover, it can be efficiently utilized for comparison of several classification algorithms by analyzing various parameters such as accuracy and precision values. Further, this tool can be utilized to maintain the huge amount of data and to identify various patterns.

B. Classification Algorithms Used

Random Forest

Random forest is a machine learning algorithm that mainly deals with the construction of multiple decision trees. It follows a basic approach where a dataset is divided into a batch of random dataset such that a decision tree is created for each random dataset (Nahar et al., 2018). Thus, "The forest is an ensemble of decision trees that are trained and all of them come up with a decision such that a majority vote is considered which results in a final single decision." It can operate on large data set and maintains the accuracy for missing data.

Logistic Regression

Logistic Regression is utilized for predictive modelling and helps to calculate the possibility of a event taking place. It mainly deals with the group of independent variables to predict their binary outcomes and determine the discrete values. It performs the binary classification and predict the future outcomes based on training from the previous output (Arshad et al., 2018). It is an approach that is widely used for predictive analysis when the dependent variable is categorical.

Support Vector Machine

Support Vector Machine is a machine learning algorithm that can perform both linear and nonlinear classification as well as regression tasks. The main idea behind this algorithm is to separate two classes with a straight line. Also, it mainly deals with the identification of a hyperplane in an N-dimensional space that distinctly classifies the data points. Support Vectors are data points that are mainly responsible for the position of the hyperplane. They play a vital role in the formation of Support Vector Machine (Kefelegn et al., 2018).

C. Methodology

In this section, a flow diagram is demonstrated which consist of various classification algorithms that are evaluated and compared based on accuracy parameter. The algorithms are analyzed to find the best classifier, which can be further used to predict the liver disease (Jin et al., 2014). Based on accuracy, Random Forest algorithm with 100% accuracy outperformed other algorithms. Below, Figure 3 depicts the work flow diagram that is used to determine the best classification technique.

- **Dataset Collection**
  Firstly, dataset is collected from various sources such as UCI Machine learning Repository in order to initiate the process of data analysis.

- **Data Preprocessing**
  It involves data cleaning such that data is processed in such a way that there are no missing values. Various methods are utilized in order to deal with the missing data such as Drop the missing values, Replace the missing values or Leave the missing data.

- **Feature Extraction**
  It is an essential task that is utilized for the purpose of extracting a set of features from the dataset. Thus, data should be consistent and in proper format. Some essential features are selected that could be further utilized to improve the overall performance.

- **Comparison based on Accuracy**
  Random Forest, Separation Algorithm and Logical Regression were further compared on the basis of accuracy parameter in order to find the most accurate algorithm.

Figure 3. Flow Diagram

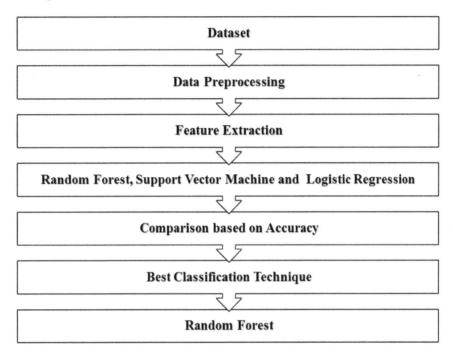

- **Best Classification Technique**

  On the basis of accuracy, Random Forest Algorithm outperformed the other algorithms such that this algorithm being the best classifier can be further utilized for the prediction of Liver Disease.

The remaining portion is arranged as follows, "Section 1 consists of Introduction that describes about the tool used and various classifiers that are required for an accurate prediction along with the methodology that contains a flowchart, Section 2 consists of Literature Survey that provides a description of the work performed by several authors and also include a table comparing the work of several authors, Section 3 consists of Proposed Methodology, Section 4 consists of a Conclusion that describes about the accomplishment of this study by providing the best classification technique that can be utilized for an accurate prediction of liver disease and followed by References."

LITERATURE SURVEY

B. Saritha et al. (Saritha et al., 2017), described an approach of Separation algorithm that could be further utilized in the diagnosis of liver disease. Separation of points by planes algorithm was used to distinguish healthy patients from the unhealthy patients and assisted in the diagnoses of liver disorder. Thus, "Separation algorithm could diagnose the liver disorder with the accuracy of 85.1% and the total time taken for completion of training is 1 second and testing is 1 second".

Dr. S. Vijayarani1 et al. (Vijayarani & Dhayanand, 2015), demonstrated the predictive analysis of liver disorder at an early stage. The proposed system was implemented using Matlab 2013 tool and evaluated the dataset that had been collected from UCI Repository. After the experimental results, it had been observed that Support Vector Machine outperformed Naïve Bayes Algorithm due to the highest classification accuracy and can be used further in the prediction of liver disease.

Ayesha Pathan et al. (Pathan et al., 2018), proposed the concept of diagnoses of liver disease. Various classification algorithms were used such as Naïve Bayes, Ada Boost, J48, Bagging and Random Forest. These algorithms were further compared based on the parameters such as Accuracy, Error rate and so on. Also, Pre-processing technique was utilized to divide the data into two groups- liver patients and non-liver patient that was accomplished using K means clustering algorithm. Further, the clustered dataset was applied to the various classification algorithms which were implemented through Weka. The overall comparison was done between Naïve Bayes, Ada Boost, J48, Bagging and Random Forest algorithms. After the comparison was performed, the comparative study showed that the Random Forest gave the better results as compared to the other algorithms.

Hoon Jin et al. (Jin et al., 2014), described the concept of various classification techniques that assist the doctors to determine the disease quickly and efficiently. These techniques were implemented using the Weka tool and dataset was collected from UCI Repository. The experimental results showed that in terms of precision, Naïve Bayes gave the better classification results whereas Logistic Regression and Random Forest gave better results in terms of recall and sensitivity.

Tapas Ranjan Baitharu et al. (Baitharu & Pani, 2016), presented an approach of diagnoses of liver disorder through an analysis of liver disorder datasets. The main focus of the research was to help the physicians with the medical decision making process. Several algorithms were compared on various parameters such as Naive Bayes, ANN, ZeroR, IBK, VFI, J48 and Multilayer Perceptron. The algorithms were implemented using the Weka tool and dataset was collected from UCI Repository. The experimental results showed that Multilayer Perceptron gave the better classification results as compared to other algorithms. Thus, Multilayer Perceptron can be further used to diagnose the liver disorder efficiently.

Rakhi Ray et al. (Ray, 2018), proposed the concept of healthcare management system using a data mining technique. Owing to the great advantages various organizations are using data mining technology. Healthcare is a vital part for everyone. Different new technologies are inventing to examine physical conditions and finding symptoms of the different disease. There is a huge amount of data involved with it including a patient's past medical records, examination history, and even the personal details. Since there are large amount of data related to the medical systems, an efficient method to find the appropriate data from the database is required. Thus, Data mining is one of the best solution for an appropriate prediction of diseases.

Below, Table 1 shows the comparison of various parameters that are utilized for an analysis of liver disease. Weka tool was utilized by the several authors in order to evaluate the results of various classification algorithms. On the basis of their performance, best algorithm was evaluated and analyzed for the prediction of liver disease.

Table 2 shows the comparison of various parameters utilized in different decision trees and classification algorithms by several authors. Weka tool was utilized in order to evaluate the results of various algorithms on the liver disease dataset. On the basis of performance, best algorithm was analyzed and evaluated for the detection of liver disorder.

Table 1. Comparison Table of parameters used in different Classification Algorithms for Liver Disease Prediction

Features	Hoon Jin et al. (2014)				Ayesha Pathan et al. (2018)				Tapas Ranjan Baitharu et al. (2016)			
Objective	To evaluate the results of classification algorithms for better prediction of liver disease.				To implement different classification algorithms using Weka in order to predict the liver disorder.				To forecast liver disease from Liver Function Test dataset using various classification algorithms.			
Dataset	UCI Repository (Liver Disease Dataset).				UCI Repository (Liver Disease Dataset).				UCI Repository (Liver Disease Dataset).			
Concerned Disease	Liver Disease				Liver Disease				Liver Disease			
Environment Used	Weka				Weka				Weka			
Attributes Used	11				11				7			
Algorithms Used	Naïve Bayes	Decision Tree	Multilayer Perceptron	k-NN	Naïve Bayes	Ada Boost	J48	Random Forest	J48	ZeroR	Naïve Bayes	Multilayer Perceptron
Specificity	0.952	0.352	0.303	0.467	-	-	-	-	-	-	-	-
Sensitivity	0.374	0.831	0.829	0.727	-	-	-	-	-	-	-	-
TP Rate	-	-	-	-	-	-	-	-	-	-	-	-
Precision	95.1	76.3	74.9	77.4	0.796%	0.508	0.872	1	-	-	-	-
F Measure	-	-	-	-	0.56	0.594	0.872	1	-	-	-	-
Accuracy	53.9	69.4	67.9	65.3	55.84%	71.31%	87.46%	100%	68.97	57.971	62.8986	60.2899
Error Rate	-	-	-	-	44.16%	28.69%	12.54%	0.00%	-	-	-	-
Recall	-	-	-	-	0.558	0.713	0.875	1	-	-	-	-
Kappa Statistics	-	-	-	-	-	-	-	-	0.3401	0	0.153	0.4023
Mean Absolute Error	-	-	-	-	-	-	-	-	0.3673	0.4874	0.4597	0.3543
Root Mean Squared Error	-	-	-	-	-	-	-	-	0.5025	0.4936	0.5083	0.4523
Relative Absolute Error	-	-	-	-	-	-	-	-	75.3511	100	102.9673	72.68
Best Algorithm	Naïve Bayes				Random Forest				Multilayer perceptron			
Result	In terms of precision, Naïve Bayes gave better classification results. Also, appropriate algorithms were evaluated and analyzed for prediction of the liver disease.				Random Forest Algorithm gave better performance results as compared to other algorithms.				Multilayer perceptron gave best accuracy results as compared to other classifiers.			

Table 2. Comparison Table of parameters used in different Classification Algorithms and Decision Trees for Liver Disease Prediction

Features	B.Saritha et al. (2017)	Han Ma et al. (2018)				Nazmun Nahar et al. (2018)		
Objective	Rapid Initial Diagnosis of the liver disease by classifying liver function data using the separation algorithm.	To predict the Non-alcoholic Fatty Liver Disease using various machine learning techniques.				To predict the liver disease using various decision tree techniques.		
Dataset	Medics Path Labs India private Limited, Hyderabad (**Liver Disease Dataset**).	College of Medicine, Zhejiang University, China (**Liver Disease Dataset**).				UCI Repository (**Liver Disease Dataset**).		
Concerned Disease	Liver Disease	Liver Disease				Liver Disease		
Environment Used	Weka	Weka and Keel				Weka		
Attributes Used	11	18				11		
Algorithms Used	Separation Algorithm	Logical Regression	Support Vector Machine	Naïve Bayes	Bayesian Network	Decision Stump	Hoeffding Tree	Logistic Model Tree
Accuracy	85.1%	83.41%	86.73%	81.31%	82.92%	70.67%	69.75%	69.47%
Specificity	-	0.934	0.946	0.913	0.878	-	-	-
Precision	-	0.713	0.725	0.644	0.636	0.499	0.634	0.632
Recall	-	0.518	0.452	0.496	0.675	0.707	0.700	0.695
F-measure	-	0.600	0.557	0.560	0.655	0.585	0.619	0.628
Tree Size	-	-	-	-	-	Single Level	1	1
Mean Absolute Error	-	-	-	-	-	0.4392	0.4091	0.4116
Kappa Statistics	-	-	-	-	-	0.379	0.0501	0.065
Runtime	-	-	-	-	-	0.01	0.12	0.88
Best Algorithm	Separation Algorithm	Bayesian Network				Decision Stump		
Result	The Separation algorithm could diagnose the liver disorder with the accuracy of 85.1% and the total time taken for completion of training is 1 second and testing is 1 second.	In this study, F-measure was considered as an evaluative measure due to which Bayesian Network with the highest F- measure demonstrated the best performance and could be used as a major classifier for the earlier diagnoses of liver disease.				Decision stump gave better accuracy results as compared to other algorithms.		

PROPOSED METHODOLOGY

Several Classification algorithms such as Random Forest, Logistic Regression and Support Vector Machine are compared and analyzed using an Orange Tool. It is a component based data mining tool based on Python that is mainly utilized for data analysis and data visualization.

Various steps involved in the process of determining the most accurate algorithm through Orange Tool are as follows:

Step1: Load the data in the File through the UCI Machine Learning Repository that consists of Indian Liver Patients Dataset. File shows all the attributes of the Indian Liver Patients Dataset (Figure 4).

Step2: Now establish the connection between the File and Data Table widget such that an output of File acts as an input to the Data Table. Data Table consists of all the values of the Indian Liver Patients Dataset (Figure 5).

Step 3: Data preprocessing is done in order to deal with the missing values. All the missing values are imputed and after preprocessing of data is done we get a new data table with the average or most frequent values in place of missing values (Figures 6, 7, and 8).

Step 4: Classification Algorithms such as Random Forest, Logistic Regression and Support Vector Machine were compared and through the Test and Score Widget the data was analyzed and it showed the accuracy, precision, recall, F1 and Area under Curve values (Figure 9).

Thus, Random Forest with 72% of accuracy outperformed the other algorithms as Logistic Regression has 70% and Support Vector Machine has 69% of accuracy.

Figure 4. Loading of Data

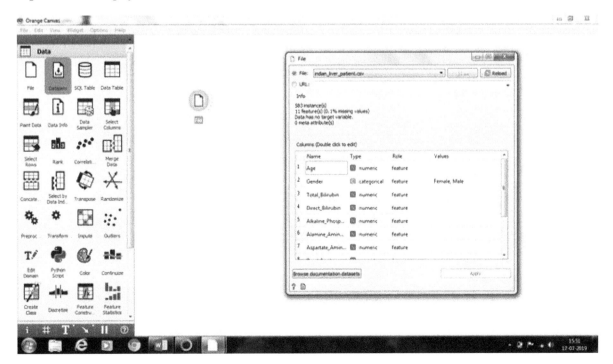

Figure 5. Establishment of Connection between File and Data Table widget

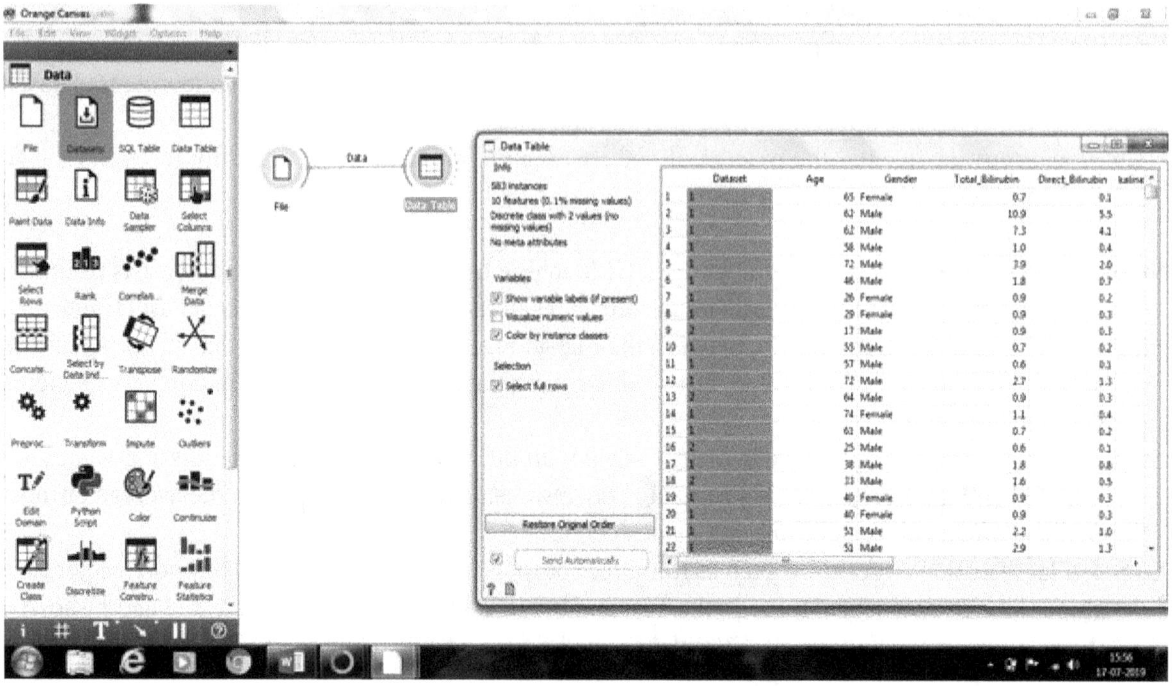

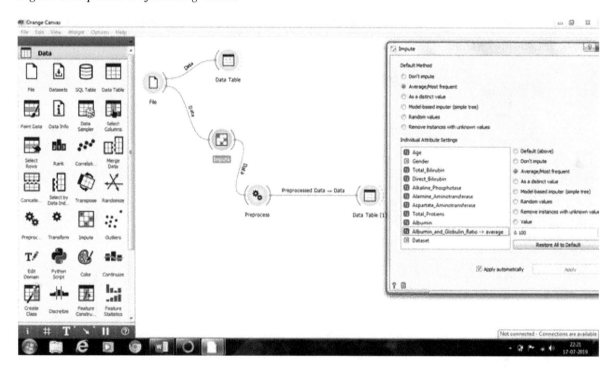

Figure 6. Imputation of Missing Values

Figure 7. Data Table with Missing Values

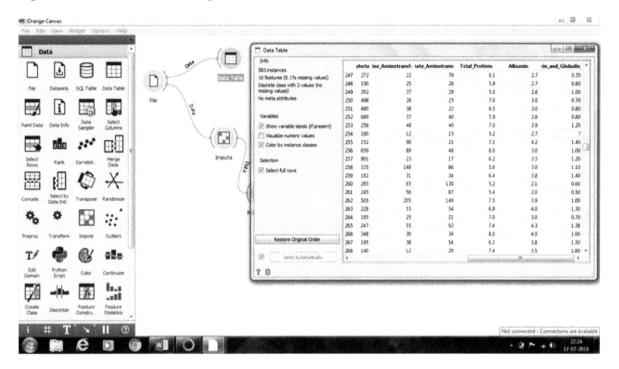

Figure 8. Data Table without Missing Values

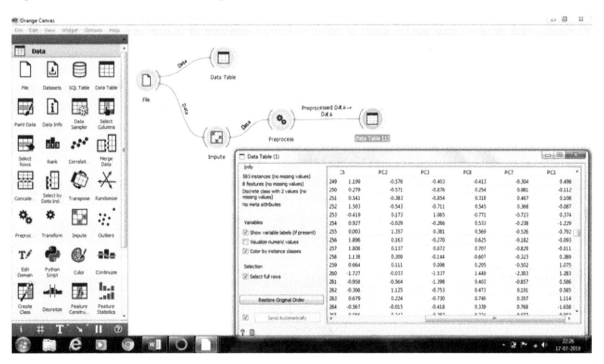

Figure 9. Evaluation Results

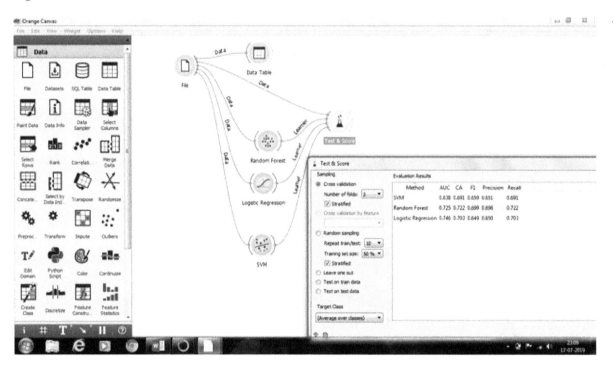

CONCLUSION

The main aim of this study was to provide an overview of different classification algorithms popular in the field of data driven prediction of liver disease. In this chapter, various classification algorithms were analyzed that can help doctors to predict the liver disease at an early stage. The purpose of this study was achieved by performing a comparative study of various papers. Thus, Random forest with 100% accuracy, Support Vector Machine with 86.73% accuracy and Logistic Regression with 83.4% accuracy were compared and analyzed as they have the better performance in terms of accuracy than other algorithms. Also, Orange Tool was utilized in order to compare and analyze the results of Random Forest, Logistic Regression and Support Vector Machine. Thus, after analysis Random forest scored 72% accuracy, Logistic Regression scored 70% accuracy and Support Vector Machine scored 69% accuracy. From this evaluation study, the authors conclude that Random Forest outperformed the other algorithms and should be further utilized for an accurate prediction of liver disease.

REFERENCES

Arshad, I., Dutta, C., Choudhury, T., & Thakra, A. (2018). Liver Disease detection due to excessive alcoholism using Data Mining Techniques. In *International Conference on Advances in Computing and Communication Engineering*, (pp. 163-168). 10.1109/ICACCE.2018.8441721

Baitharu, T. R., & Pani, S. K. (2016). Analysis of data mining techniques for healthcare decision support system using liver disorder dataset. *Procedia Computer Science*, *85*, 862–870. doi:10.1016/j.procs.2016.05.276

Ghosh, S. R., & Waheed, S. (2017). Analysis of classification algorithms for liver disease diagnosis. *Journal of Science, Technology & Environment Informatics*, 360-370.

Jin, H., Kim, S., & Kim, J. (2014). Decision Factors on Effective Liver Patient Data Prediction. *International Journal of Bio-Science and Bio-Technology*, 167-178.

Kefelegn, S., & Kamat, P. (2018). Prediction and Analysis of Liver Disorder Diseases by using Data Mining Technique: Survey. *International Journal of Pure and Applied Mathematics*, 765-769.

Nahar, N., & Ara, F. (2018). Liver Disease Prediction using different decision tree techniques. *International Journal of Data Mining & Knowledge Management Process*, 1-9.

Pathan, A., Mhaske, D., Jadhav, S., Bhondave, R., & Rajeswari, D. K. (2018). Comparative Study of Different Classification. *International Journal for Research in Applied Science and Engineering Technology*, *6*(2), 388–394. doi:10.22214/ijraset.2018.2056

Ray, R. (2018). Advances in Data Mining: Healthcare Applications. *International Research Journal of Engineering and Technology*.

Saritha, B., Ramana, S. V., Manaswini, N., Priyanka, R., Hiranmayi, D., & Eswaran, K. (2017). Classification of Liver data using a new algorithm. *4th International Conference on New Fronteirs of Engineering, Science, Management and Humanities*.

Vijayarani, D. S., & Dhayanand, D. S. (2015). Liver Disease Prediction using SVM and Naïve Bayes Algorithms. *International Journal of Science Engineering and Technology Research*, *4*(4), 816–820.

Chapter 23
Texture Segmentation and Features of Medical Images

Ashwani Kumar Yadav
iD https://orcid.org/0000-0001-5880-5491
Amity University Rajasthan, Jaipur, India

Vaishali
Manipal University, Jaipur, India

Raj Kumar
Shri Vishwakarma Skill University, Palwal, India

Archek Praveen Kumar
Malla Reddy College of Engineering for Women, Hyderabad, India

ABSTRACT

Texture analysis is one of the basic aspects of human visual system by which one can differentiate the objects and homogenous areas in an image. Manual diagnosis is not possible for huge database of images. Automatic diagnosis is required for greater accuracy in a shorter time. Texture analysis is required for effective diagnosis of medical images like functional MRI (magnetic resonance image) and diffusion tensor MRI, where only visualization is not sufficient to get the pathological information. This chapter explains the basic concepts of texture analysis and features available for analysis of medical images. Specifically, the intense review of texture segmentation and texture feature extraction and entropy measures of medical images have been done. The chapter also explores the available techniques for it. Common findings, comparative analysis, and gaps identified have also been mentioned on both issues.

DOI: 10.4018/978-1-7998-2742-9.ch023

INTRODUCTION

Texture Analysis is the most desirable technique to process images, mainly their classification. Texture Analysis has various application areas like computer vision, medical imaging, remote sensing, graphics and many more. In last few decades, various techniques have been proposed to achieve better classification, these techniques basically depend on statistics of the pixel values, modelling of images, image filtration using different kernels and multiple scale texture analysis. Most of work in this area has been motivated by human visual system. Medical imaging is a very important tool to obtain important information from normal and pathological processes related to health. Now a days without image processing we cannot think of living a healthy life. Various quantitative imaging techniques help to live a life in a healthy way by helping in diagnosis of various diseases, for example functional MRI and diffusion tensor MRI, where only visualization of the medical images are not sufficient to get the pathological information. Image processing is embedded in various important systems and applications, more extensively it is used in medicine from diagnosis of micro level disorder to therapy and surgery.

Evaluation of Texture Analysis

It is a very complex task to evaluate the performance and compare the different texture analysis techniques (Laws, 1980) and this has received huge attention from the researchers. Visual texture is an interesting area of research in the field of image processing in which the basic recognition and segmentation do not have much importance when the images are real. There are infinite types of textures (Richards & Polit, 1974) having different properties which creates confusion, due to this it is a complex task to evaluate the relative performance of a specific algorithm for different textures. In medical images it is also very difficult to identify the dissimilarities and uniform intensities but with the help of texture analysis (Haralick,1979) it can be done in effective way. Different feature sets have shown different performance rate for the same types of images. The performance can be measured for a specific application and for a particular set of images. A number of algorithms have been proposed by the researchers for a wide range of applications. In this chapter, theoretical concepts and literature of different texture analysis techniques has been discussed in the area of medical image processing.

Defining Texture

Texture has been defined by various researchers. According to David Marr, texture is defined as a symbolic representation of visual information that is designed in the interpretation process (Marr & Hildreth,1980).

A precise definition for texture is not possible to give, as it normally depends on the application. Few definitions with respect to various applications has been given by (Coggins, 1982). They are as given below:

- We may consider texture as a collection of macroscopic regions, its structure is attributed to the repetitive patterns (Tamura et al., 1978).
- Constant texture is a region of an image having constant set of local statistics (Sklansky, 1978).
- Image texture is nonfigurative in nature, a texture is considered as number of (tonal) primitives (Haralick,1979).

- Texture is a property of display, like coarseness, bumpiness, fineness etc. The set of all patterns without having enumerable components will include several textures (Richards & Polit, 1974).
- Texture mostly plays an important role in early processing to get visual information, specifically for practical classification. There is no such definition of texture which is globally accepted. It is a systems for representation at many different abstraction levels, these levels consists intensities, progress on edges and texture descriptors (Zucker & Kant, 1981).

The texture is related to the image's appearance, structure and arrangement of an object's partitions within the image. Image texture is the spatial variations present in the pixel intensities (gray values), it is useful for various applications and has been the latest topic of research. Image processing and pattern recognition is one of the application areas of texture analysis. Texture (Mallat, 1991) identifies the homogeneous regions present in an image. Generally, the extraction of features from image is done then classification of these features are done to differentiate the abnormal from the normal tissue. There are various features and it is very difficult to extract all the features from an image, so identification of the most informative features is also important issue.

The artificial textures present in any image can be due to the primitive rectangular regions in black or white. It is not difficult to segment single-color based regions and simple patterns recognition. The quality of an image can give enough information to understand it.

Feature Extraction

It is the initial step in the process of texture analysis of any medical image after pre-processing. Various feature of an image can be extracted with various techniques. The basic technique for feature extraction is GLCM (Gray level co-occurrence matrix) and GLCM. The features which can be extracted using these techniques are: Autocorrelation, Contrast, Correlation, Cluster Prominence, Cluster Shade, Dissimilarity, Energy, Entropy, Homogeneity, and Maximum Probability. In this chapter various texture analysis techniques has been discussed and also explored the texture segmentation, texture feature extraction and entropy measures for medical images.

LITERATURE REVIEW

Literature review done effectively will give us a complete background to conduct a noble research work. In this section a categorical review related to the texture segmentation and texture feature extraction and entropy measures has been discussed. Further including the common findings and gaps in the published research.

Review Outcome in the issue "Texture Segmentation"

Segmentation means to partition an image into different homogeneous regions.

[Wu Jianchao et al., 1989]

The segmentation techniques for B-scan images has been discussed in this work. Gray level sum and difference histogram were employed to extract texture features. Then K-mean clustering algorithm were used to segment the image into homogenous regions of texture. The performance of work is tested by the analysis of natural texture. At last the author applied it to the abdominal ultrasound images. In this paper, a method that enabled partitioning of ultrasound B-scan images is proposed, each of which can then be characterized by Module and Mode 2-D distribution (Jianchao et al., 1989).

[J. Peter et al., 1995]

In this work, the relaxation process is used for the segmentation decision, where each image pixel can be performed in parallel. This technique has shown higher performance in terms of the segmentation quality, time factor, and memory demand. Authors describe the structure of the neural network and basic operations involved in data compression. Signal statistics has been adjusted, also weight function and temporary assessment of the neighborhood influence in this work for segmentation process. The performance of the network in terms of efficiency discussed (J. Peter et al., 1995).

[Atkins & Mackiewich, 1998]

In this work an automatic segmentation algorithm has designed for brain MRI's, the main objective of this work is to segment the image under the influence of Radio Frequency (RF) in homogeneities. Anisotropic filters and contouring techniques has been used to achieve the objectives. This work has been done in three steps in first histogram analysis is done. In second step nonlinear anisotropic diffusion and automatic thresholding to create a mask, mask has been used to differentiating the regions of brain MRI's. In the third step an active contour model algorithm has been designed to detect the intracranial boundary. It is the multistage process, in which removal of the background noise, after that outline of the brain has been drawn, at last brain outline is converted into a final mask (Atkins & Mackiewich, 1998).

[Shareef et al., 1999]

In this paper, oscillator network known as locally excitatory globally inhibitory oscillator network (LEGION) is used for the segmentation. This is known as effective computational framework for identification of similar and dissimilar features in an image. An algorithm from LEGION dynamics is designed by the authors. Both the 2-D and 3-D computerized topography (CT) and magnetic resonance imaging (MRI) are used as input images. The experimental results obtained from the proposed algorithm has been compared with other and manual segmentation. Experimental results shows that it is very useful and efficient because of LEGION's computational and architectural properties (Shareef et al., 1999).

[Kontaxakis et al., 2003]

In this work authors proposed a discrete wavelet transform based method for feature extraction and image segmentation. Initially the pixel features were calculated with the help of directional filters, also these filters are used to divide the image into a set of sub images, where each image having an isolated angular section of the initial image spectrum. Pixel local energy is also stored and estimated. A novel feature extraction technique has been proposed and a multi component texture segmentation has been achieved in this work. Experiments has been done to do texture separation and their performance has been estimated. Results shows that the effectiveness of the discrete wavelet transform and its comparison with feature extraction techniques (Kontaxakis et al., 2003).

[Grande et al., 2004]

In this work multiscale texture analysis and segmentation was done for the polarimetric SAR images. Wavelet decomposition has been used for this purpose. At different level of decomposition local variance has been estimated. Two level decomposition has been done on the images derived by polarimetric power synthesis. After feature extraction, Feature reduction is done with the help of Multiple Discriminant Analysis (MDA) transform. Monte Carlo simulations is used for the experiment purpose, and identified the performance of proposed system w.r.t texture segmentation. Lastly the real SAR image acquired by the DLR E-SAR sensor has been used to prove the effective texture segmentation with proposed system (Grande et al., 2004).

[Vyas et al., 2006]

Authors proposed automated texture Analysis based on Gabor filter. Texture was depended on the features that were extracted from images. Texture features were extracted for each pixel position. Texture classified methods were Perturbed and Unperturbed. Unperturbed texture has been formed exact periodic repetitions of basic pattern. Perturbed texture was formed Texel arranged with arbitrary orientations and random overlaps. Gabor filter provided means for better spatial localization. Gabor transform signal could be represented in terms of sinusoids. Those were modulated by translated Gaussian windows. Gabor filter had been proved appropriate for texture segmentation in several senses. The filter was characterized with the help of orientation and spatial frequency. Gabor feature vectors were used as input for segmentation operator. Gabor filter minimized the effect of noise by implemented of texture segmentation algorithm. Gabor filter may not gave optimum result and not even detect the particular texture (Vyas et al., 2006).

[Ali et al., 2007]

In this paper a design of wavelet system by using genetic algorithm for texture discrimination. For best texture discrimination wavelet function had been used parameters (contrast, energy and PSNR) by genetic algorithm. Different texture feature vector had been calculated for better texture discrimination by new wavelet bases. Wavelet bases calculated these feature vectors in multi-resolution environment. Multi- resolution decomposition had provided framework for texture discrimination at different-different resolution. After applied wavelet, original image had represented as sub-images. These sub images were in multi-scale representation of original image. Feature extraction was an important stage of texture analysis for texture discrimination. By wavelet bases analyzed different regions by using sample of satellite images which was based on textural properties. The different samples were followed as: land sample, low mountain terrain sample, desert area sample, high mountain sample and plateau sample. PSNR values were calculated of these samples which were showed as 0.001db, 0.008db, 0.005db, 0.043db, 0.024db. Performance had been also checked by calculate accuracy of each sample. Accuracy was showed: land sample= 85%, low mountain terrain sample=81%, desert area sample=72%, high mountain sample=69% and plateau sample =72%. For shorter length filter had been given better result for texture discrimination (Ali et al., 2007).

[Basile et al., 2010]

A diagnosis system has been developed for the light microscope images of human oocytes. The proposed system having three main blocks, segmentation, feature extraction and clustering. Region of interest is extracted from the images with the help of morphological and Hough transform for segmentation. Then features are extracted from that region. Fuzzy clustering has been used. Comparison of proposed work with other related methods for feature extraction and clustering (Basile et al., 2010).

[Gao et al., 2011]

In this paper Image segmentation and registration has been done. Quantitative analysis of medical CT images are a complex task. Chest CT images are used for experimental results, in this work region growing method is used for the segmentation of CT image, their applications are also discussed. Results achieved authenticate the performance of the developed system and comparison of result has been discussed. This work will help in the diagnosis (Gao et al., 2011).

[Chang et al., 2011]

In the proposed work, authors developed an automatic algorithm for CT images segmentation. Variability in shape of the prostate is identified manually. The fitness of each individual is identifies with the help texture of enclosed regions. Gold standard segmentations results has been compared with the results of proposed automatic segmentation, and results shows promising results and clinical application (Chang et al., 2011).

[Korchiyne et al., 2012]

In this paper authors proposed an algorithm for texture segmentation of medical images by using Multifractal analysis. The problem of classical methods had been eliminated by this segmentation algorithm. The proposed algorithm was used to segment the image into regions with similar properties like: gray level, color, texture, brightness, and contrast. Algorithm had been showed the relationship between multifractel analysis and medical characteristics for understand the medical images. Segmentation had been identifying region of interest, study of anatomical structure, measure the volume of tissue and help in treatment planning by Multifractal analysis. The texture segmentation and classification of image in digital image processing had been analyzed by Multifractal method. Multifractal had been calculated the fractal dimensions and spectrum of each point with the help of Hausdorff dimension. Hausdorff dimension was complex method but it had given important information to understand the fractal dimensions. The Multifractal segmented the images by performed different stages which were: Load MR Image, Divide the image into sub-images, calculate sum for each pixel, Divide sub-images into different intensity period, Calculate FD and Segmentation. For measuring sum of image of brain and chest, author was applied segmentation algorithm by using Multifractal. By this algorithm images were found as correct segmentation and visualization. It had obtained more accuracy as ~93% (Korchiyne et al., 2012).

[Mohammad et al., 2013]

Authors has been proposed segmentation of optic nerve in retinal images by Hough transform and Snake method. Hough transform had solved three main problems in optic nerve segmentation. The problems were (1) Ingoing and outgoing blood vessels unclear part of the optic nerve boundary, (2) Contrast around the optic nerve and (3) Clarification of the retina image is not uniform. Comparison of Hough transform and Snake had been tested by using edge detector. Hough transform and Snake methods had been used two texture measurements for optic nerve texture segmentation. Hough transform had been balanced between high quality description and low computational requirements for good texture descriptor. The texture descriptor was based on BRIEF. It had combined the pixel classification and template matching for segmentation of optic nerve. The BRIEF measurement had chosen for clarification of issues in retinal images. For texture measurement, Hough transform and Snake had tested 196 images. After testing it was classified as 10 healthy retina images and 86 glaucomatous images. The obtained average ratio between true optic nerve region and segmented region was 0.81 and 0.82. The obtained accuracy for Hough transform was 88% and for Snake was 85% (Mohammad et al., 2013).

[Materka et al., 2013]

Authors proposed a system for MRI non-uniformity based on application of texture analysis. MRI non-uniformity was recommended by ROI normalization. Nonuniformity was considered large images and volume of uniform texture by MRI. Texture descriptor was depended on ROI properties. Intensity of images was computed by ROI. T.A application for MRI of brain, bone, breast, liver, myocardium and prostate. Spatial pattern of the image intensity that originate in the structure of tissues were computed by MRI texture descriptors. Information of large organs and detain of internal organs were contained by the MR scanner.MRI had two main symptoms of osteoporosis like reduce bone mass and changes in bone micro-architecture. Texture liver images were corrected by additive and Multiplicative model. Texture analysis main issue was calculation of numerical descriptors presented in 2D, 3D, and 4D images. A good separation of texture classes were actually caused by image intensity inhomogeneity fields (Materka et al., 2013).

[Jui et al., 2014]

In this work a segmentation algorithm has been developed for medical images. First of all MR images are de-noised with the help of wavelet transform and then segmentation is done with the help of Fuzzy C-Means (FCM). In this filter is designed to reduce the noise and that filter is incorporated with FCM algorithm. With the help of FCM not only spatial information is explored also useful in reducing clustering errors occurs due to noise present in medical images. Results obtained with the experimental setup shows the importance of FCM in the area of de-noising and segmentation of MR images, Results are verified in terms of visual quality (Jui et al., 2014).

[Hamedi et al., 2015]

Authors proposed an algorithm based on fuzzy support vector machine to segmentation of the basil ganglia of brain. Support vector machine could be calculate the shape of surface, texture and classify the basil ganglia in brain MRI image processing. The classification performance of SVM had improved by combining fuzzification method. Fuzzy SVM would be classified the error rate for various educational sample in image segmentation. By clustering algorithm (k-means, fuzzy C-means), SVM had evaluated contrast which was leading to optimal solution. SVM had followed two steps: 1) feature extraction, 2) classification of image pixels. In first step, features of image were selected and extracted each pixel for next statistical processing. In second step, classification had done in two stages learning and recognition, where learning create data model for class attribute. Recognition had applied classification by using data model which was created by learner. 40 images of brain MRI image were collected where 75% for training and 25% for test. By applied Fuzzy SVM for segmentation of each image, the accuracy had been measured of this method. For check the performance of this method, measured accuracy, specificity and sensitivity. The proportion of sample were categorized correctly that checked by measuring accuracy. Sensitivity had been defined that the positive data were classified correctly and specificity for negative data. The measured accuracy was 76.34% for brain MRI image by fuzzy support vector machine. By compared to other methods Fuzzy SVM was better in all medical diagnostic images (Hamedi et al., 2015).

[Dhage et al., 2015]

In this paper a technique for tumor cases of clinical MRI's has been developed. The Watershed segmentation has been implemented on MRI data. The MRI Image were used as an input in the experimentation and proposed algorithm is very much efficient to identify the location and size of the tumor. Various parameters like perimeter, eccentricity, entropy and centroid were estimated for the identification of the tumor shape and position precisely (Dhage et al., 2015).

[Goswami et al., 2016]

Authors proposed an algorithm for segmentation of X-ray images by edge detection method. X-ray was an oldest device which had captured the human bones and analyzed abnormality. Image could be segmented into meaningful regions with its characteristics such as intensity, contrast, color and texture. Segmentation, pattern recognition and object detection in image analysis had been performed by edge detection methods. The image intensity function computed of each image point (edge) which was defined by edge detection. Edges of image had changed its brightness continuously because of discontinuously changes in surface orientation; object occludes each other and appeared a shadow line. Identification of region of interest, measurement of tissue volume, treatment planning and differentiate anatomic structure had been performed by edge detection. For experiment, four distinct X-ray images had been used by author. The clarification of each image with its boundary detection had been shown by applying edge detection method. Edge detection method had been computed standard deviation and mean of resultant images. The obtained mean of images were 0.0198, 0.0217, 0.0149 and 0.0166; standard deviation was 0.1392, 0.1457, 0.1211 and 0.1278 (Goswami et al., 2016).

[Anitha et al., 2016]

In this work a system has been proposed which uses the adaptive pillar K-means algorithm for successful segmentation. In this features are extracted with the help of different decomposition level of discrete wavelet transform. After feature extraction the classification is done with the help of two-tier classification system. The validation of the proposed system has been checked with the help of real data sets and results proved that the performance is quite good with other techniques (Anitha et al., 2016).

2.1.1 Comparative Analysis of Solution Approaches for "Texture Segmentation".

Texture Segmentation is one of the issues, in which Researchers use these approaches for this issue. They are DWT, Wavelet Transform, Gabor filter, PTPSA (piecewise-Triangular-prism Surface area), Edge Detection, Chest Radiograph, Bayesian Classifier and SVM, k-Gabor, MRI non-uniformity and Integrated Method.

2.1.2 Common Finding From the Issue of "Texture Segmentation"

- Image texture could be analyzed by MAZDA software, which is an efficient and reliable tool.
- Fuzzy C-Means (FCM) is identified as a good technique for de-noising and segmentation.
- Region growing method shown good results to identify the homogenous regions, it is better technique for image segmentation and registration.
- K-mean clustering and Mean Shift algorithm provides a robust feature space analysis approach which can be applied to discontinuity preserving, smoothing and image segmentation problems.
- The N-cut method was applied directly to the image pixels, which were typically of very large size. It was applied to perform globally optimized clustering and could get the final segmentation result.
- Thresholding techniques are used for the segmentation, it is the oldest, fastest technique.
- In global thresholding, single threshold value is selected from the entire image.
- The problem of texture classification and texture segmentation had been solved in many ways by Gabor filters.
- Discrete wavelet transformation having better capabilities to deal with medical images in terms of texture analysis.

2.1.3 Gaps Found in the Review of Texture Segmentation

- Further Study required to understand anatomical structure of medical images more accurately.
- Perfect Identification of Region of Interest is required i.e. locate tumor, lesion and other abnormalities
- Advanced algorithms are required to deal with the presence of artifacts.
- Results are not promising where closeness in gray level of different soft tissue are present.
- The filters may not have almost perfect structure, so, the separation of images was not accurate.
- The contrast between regions of images may be not sufficient for an edge detector to identify the edges along the boundary.
- New methods for segmentation are need to be developed for better results for complex images.

Table 1. Comparative analysis of review on texture segmentation

Authors	Input			Segmentation method	Result		Description
	Type (image)	Area	Format		Segmentation Performance	Quality Measurement	
Jianchao et al., 1989	Ultrasound images	Abdominal	Gray	K-mean clustering	Gray level sum and difference histogram	Natural texture	Characterized by Module and Mode 2-D distribution
[Peter et al., 1995]	MRI	Brain	Gray	Constraint satisfaction neural network	Local spatial neighbourhood	Segmentation quality, time factor, and memory demand	Signal statistics has been adjusted
[Atkins et al., 1998]	MRI	Brain	Gray	active contour model	Radio Frequency (RF)in homogeneities	Intracranial boundary	Anisotropic filters and contouring techniques has been used.
[Shareef et al., 1999]	computerized topography (CT) & MRI	Brain	Gray	locally excitatory globally inhibitory oscillator network (LEGION)	Useful and efficient because of LEGION's computational and architectural properties.	Similar and dissimilar features in an image	Better because its architectural properties
[Kontaxakis et al., 2003]	Digital Image	Texture	Binary	Discrete wavelet transform	Pixel local energy is also stored and estimated	Pixel features	Texture separation and their performance has been estimated
[Grande et al., 2004]	SAR image	Forest	Color	Wavelet decomposition	MonteCarlo simulations	Non-redundant representation	Multiscale texture analysis and segmentation is done.
[Vyas, et al., 2006]	Microscopic photography	Forest	Color	Gabor filter	Detect the particular texture	Discontinuities at texture boundaries	Gabor filter was transform texture differences into detectable filter output
[Ali et al., 2007]	Satellite images	Land, desert area	Color	Wavelet transform	Calculate accuracy of each sample is above 81%	PSNR values	For shorter length filter had been given better result
[Gao, 2011]	CT images	Chest	Gray	Region growing method	Detection of various homogenious regions	Homogenous texture	Image segmentation and registration has been done
[Korchiyne et al., 2012]	MR Images	Brain and Chest	Gray	Hausdorff dimension	It had obtained more accuracy as ~93%	Divide sub-images into different intensity period	Algorithm images were found as correct segmentation and visualization
[Mohammad et al., 2013]	Retinal images	Optic nerve	Gray	Hough transform	The obtained accuracy for Hough transform was 88%	Binary Robust Independent Elementary Features (BRIEF) and a rotation invariant BRIEF	Hough transform had tested 196 images
[Jui et al., 2014]	MR Images	Brain	Gray	Fuzzy C-Means (FCM).	Reducing clustering errors	Results are verified in terms of visual quality	Importance of FCM in the area of de-noising and segmentation of MR images is shown
[Hamedi et al., 2015]	MR Images	Brain	Gray	Fuzzy support vector machine	The measured accuracy was 76.34% for brain MRI image	Accuracy, specificity and sensitivity	40 images has been used to authenticate the results
[Goswami et al., 2016]	X-ray images	Human bones	Gray	Edge detection methods	The obtained mean of images were 0.0198, 0.0217, 0.0149 and 0.0166	Standard deviation and mean of resultant images	Identification of region of interest, measurement of tissue volume has been done.

- PSNR value and accuracy was low which had been giving by CAD model.

Review on the Issue of "Texture Feature Extraction and Entropy Measures"

[Haralick et al., 1973]

In this paper textural features were described based on gray tone spatial dependencies which can be described easily and also the application of these features were also discussed. Three types of images were used like photomicrographs, earth resources technology satellite (ERTS) and aerial photographs. Two different decision rules were used: convex pollyhedra and rectangular parallelpipeds. Images were divided into two parts training and testing data images, different accuracy has been achieved with different images 89%, 82%, and 83% for photomicrographs, aerial photographic imagery and satellite images respectively. This paper opens the scope in the image classification and the features acceptability for wide application areas (Haralick et al., 1973).

[Jernigan & Astoush, 1984]

In this work a system has been developed for the measurement of entropy in the spatial frequency domain. Texture discrimination is addressed in this work with entropy measure. Entropy features are calculated from the images and their performance with other features like gray level co-occurrence contrast features to check the effectiveness of entropy features. For this comparison purpose frequency scaling is also done. Entropy is an important feature for the analysis of medical images is the main outcome of this work (Jernigan & Astoush, 1984).

[Desoky & Hall, 2002]

A texture analysis technique has proposed in which various transform methods are used to calculate the entropy. Various images of different types were used for the testing of proposed system. Entropy calculation has been done from various images with the help of various transform methods like, fast-Fourier transform (FFT), transform components using the discrete-cosine transform (DCT), and the transform coefficients of the fast-Hadamard transform (FHT). Basically entropy is depend on gray-level components and frequency components, so four entropy computation methods were implemented. In this entropy is calculated from the gray-levels histogram, FFT, DCT and FHT. Experimental results shows that FHT is the fastest (Desoky & Hall, 2002).

[Shareha et al., 2008]

In this paper author introduces a thresholding method based on textured Renyi Entropy for images, which was depend on a novel combination method. The Renyi Entropy is advanced version of its priori, where overall functionality is preserved. In this work optional priori is introduced to improve the accuracy. Due to the priori modification addition of texture information can be achieved in effective way. Also it helps in accurate thresholding. Moreover, the proposed system allow to add other features after some normalization. Modified priors has been proved as good method to add multiple features simultaneously (Shareha et al., 2008).

[Pharwaha & Singh, 2009]

In this work texture feature extraction has been addressed for digital mammogram. Gray level histogrammoments statistical texture analysis method has been implemented has shown excellent results. The main focus of work is on entropy that is considered as an important texture feature, Classification of the mammograms has been done as abnormal and normal with the help of entropies of the different regions of mammograms. Where Non-Shannon entropies are better than Shannon entropy in terms of dynamic range, at different scattering conditions. The database of mammogram images are created with the help of mini-MIAS database (Mammogram Image Analysis Society database (UK)). Detection of breast cancer is effectively done with this computer aided decision (CAD) system from mammogram images (Pharwaha & Singh, 2009).

[Zhang & Gao, 2010]

In this work authors has been developed an algorithm with the help of canny operator and the non-sub-sampled contour let transform. This novel algorithm is designed for the feature extraction from medical image. Canny operator is normally used to detect edges and the non-subsampled contour let transform effective for multi-scale. In this work edges were detected and then decomposed with non-subsampled contour let transform. Geometry moments of the non-subsampled contour let coefficient at different scales and with different directions are considered as the different features of image. Also Similarity measurement is done effectively with the help of Euclidean distance between the features of query image and images in database. Experimental results has been compared with the retrieval based wavelet transform and proved that proposed system is efficient (Zhang & Gao, 2010).

[Khehra and Pharwaha, 2011]

The main focus of this work is on non-Shannon measures (Havrda & Charvat, Renyi and Kapur) of entropy and comparison with Shannon entropy. This work proves that non-Shannon entropy is more advantageous. Images used for the testing of proposed algorithm was taken from mini-MIAS database. Validation of the results has been done with the help of different types of test images (fatty, fatty-glandular and dense-glandular) taken from mini-MIAS database. In this work the effect of the various parameters in thresholding has been identified. Experimental results shows that non-Shannon measures of entropy is more effective for all types of mammograms. The main advantage of this proposed system is to identify the early breast cancer (Khehra & Pharwaha, 2011).

[Lundervold, 2011]

In this paper authors proposed a system for the texture analysis of 2D and 3D images. In this spatial distribution of signal intensity variations within local regions in images has been identified. Some outcomes has been concluded in this work like, enabling to detect signal signatures and biology-related information etc. Also statistical and mathematical measures can be achieved with the help of texture analysis. In this paper six basic textural properties are considered for texture analysis like, coarseness, regularity, contrast, line-likeness, directionality, and roughness has been discussed in detail and their effectiveness in texture analysis. Also different patient groups are discriminated with the help of texture analysis (Lundervold, 2011).

[Zare et al., 2011]

The main aim of this paper is to design a content-based image retrieval (CBIR) system. Low level features like, shape and texture are calculated for the classification of medical X-ray image. The main features extracted in this work are based on Gray level Co-occurrence Matrix, Local Binary Pattern, Canny Edge Operator and pixel level information of the images. These features are used to train the classifier, Support Vector Machine (SVM) is used for classification purpose. Experimental results shows the performance of classifier and features combination. The implementation of proposed work was done to identify the116 different classes of 11,000 X-ray images. Overall classification accuracy achieved by the system was 90.7% that is quite high (Zare et al., 2011).

[Barabas et al., 2012]

In this work authors conducted a systematic study for the medical image analysis. The main focus was on all the main steps involved in analysis like, pre-processing, segmentation, edge detection and Hough man transform. Various literature has been discussed in this field. The images which has been discussed in detail are CT and MR Images. Also a detailed study of software was conducted to explain how the viewing of individual slices, slice reconstruction in various projections of these medical image modalities. Detailed analysis of slices are done in this work with 3D reconstruction of desired objects (Barabas et al., 2012).

[Natarajan et al., 2012]

In this paper a morphological processing technique has been used for the extraction and filtering purpose. The proposed technique is used to detect and segment brain tumor from MR images. Testing images having different size and shape of the tumor. The morphological operators are used to change the structure of the image according to application. Operators like open, spur, dilate and close has been proved as good in extracting the brain tumor from the MR Images. Before applying morphological operation, Pre-processing was done with the help of gray scaling, histogram equalization and filtration. For the better results threshold segmentation has been also done to identify the region of interest (Natarajan et al., 2012).

[Sharma et al., 2012]

In this work authors proposed a threshold selection technique for the segmentation of color images, which approximately preserves the colors in different segments. The simulation results performed in MATLAB on the MRI images. In this work the threshold value is dependent on the type of the entropy chosen, also this entropy effects the segmentation results. In the proposed approach, threshold selection in each of the three component (RGB) images is done on the basis of different entropy measures. It was further observed that the segmentation results calculated by Havrda-Charvat entropy measures are considered as better results w.r.t other entropy measures. Preservation of colors in different segments are taken as quality parameters (Sharma et al., 2012).

[Gautam et al., 2013]

In this paper a system has been proposed for threshold selection in the area of image segmentation. Grayscalebrain MRI scans are used as the input images. Entropy value has been used for effective segmentation. The segmentation results obtained with different entropies are compared, which shows Havrda-Charvat entropy measures are better than other entropy measures. The entropy function versus individual RGB component level plot for both entropies. The experimental results shows that, only 8% error was shown by the system. A metastasis level tumor or a cancer of level 2 or above can be detected by the system effectively (Gautam et al., 2013).

[Mathur & Gupta, 2014]

In this paper authors has used the Shannon and non-Shannon entropy measures like Renyi, Vajda etc. are used to getanspecific threshold value to do image segmentation effectively. In this work color image segmentation has been done, with colors in different segments preservation. The segmentation of the color images has been done with the help of different entropies measured. Experiment results of image segmentation has been shown with different entropy performance (Mathur & Gupta, 2014).

[Urooj & Singh, 2016]

In this work an automatic object detection from a large-scale database has been developed. The main concept of the proposed work is pattern recognition. Image retrieval has been performed for the images which are deformed by some geometric deformation. Moments and their invariants are calculated as the features. Due to their invariance properties like rotation, scale, and translation they are considered as very useful for invariant feature extraction. In this work, authors utilize Hu's moments for geometric transformation issues. The experiments are done with different properties like, scale invariant, rotation invariant, and combined rotation and scale invariance (Urooj & Singh, 2016).

[Naik & Reddy, 2016]

In this work a simplified method for filtering electrocardiogram (ECG) signal has been proposed. Gaussian Mean Variant is used for the filtration purpose and for feature extraction Integrated Peak Analyzer has been used. Initially the signals are filtered and smoothen with the help of conventional filters like low pass filter, Butterworth filter, Finite impulse (FIR) filter, least mean squares (LMS) filter and the proposed filter. In the second stage feature extraction has been done using peak estimations of QRS complexes and their pulse transit time (PTT) estimations. For feature extraction, a novel model, Integrated Peak Analyzer is used. Comparison of the proposed work has been done with adaptive filters (Naik & Reddy, 2016).

Table 2. Comparative analysis of review on different features (entropy)

Author	Solution Approach	Data used	Performance Measures(Threshold Value)						Results
[Mathur et al., 2014]	Shannon and non-Shannon Entropy	jpg image	Entropy	Kaju.jpg		Algae.jpg		America.jpg	Havrda-Charvat entropy is better to segment the gray scale images compared to other entropy measures.
			Shannon	10		83		197	
			Kapur	26		140		211	
			Vajda	5		141		209	
			Renyi	122		140		211	
			Havrda	83		113		161	
[Gautam et al., 2013]	Shannon and Non-shannon Entropy	Color Image	Entropy	Component					RGB component are plotted individually for Shannon and non-Shannon entropy measures.
				R			G	B	
			Havrda-Charvat Entropy	124			42	55	
			Shannon Entropy	17			39	106	
			Renyi Entropy	234			15	39	
[Shareha et al., 2008]	Renyi's entropy	Synthetic Images	Image No.	Threshold using the original Entropy	Threshold using Textured Renyi				The experimental results show that the proposed method enhances the thresholding result and reduce the error rate.
			1	T=187	T=177				
			2	T=155	T=86				
			3	T=55	T=55				
			4	T=154	T=74				
			5	T=153	T=149				
			6	T=133	T= 133				
			7	T=178	T= 172				
			8	T=157	T= 154				
[Desoky & Hall,2002]	Entropy calculation from transform components	Gray Image of size 512* 480	Measure Entropy percentage change	Time(Sec.)	Histogram		FHT	FFT	FHT is much faster than Histogram and FFT.
				34.14	6.08		1.30	1.31	
				35.58	-1.50		-7.92	-8.04	
				41.11	-8.62		-75.33	-74.85	
[Sharma et al., 2012]	Shannon and Non-Shannon Entropy	Ball Image	Entropy	Component					Havrda-Charvat entropy is better for segmentation.
				R		G		B	
			Kapur	20		23		71	
			Havrda-Charvat	117		138		141	
			Shannon	64		80		198	
			Renyi	216		215		73	
			Vajda	10		21		72	

continues on following page

Table 2. Continued

Author	Solution Approach	Data used	Performance Measures(Threshold Value)				Results
[Jernigan & Astoush, 1984]	Havrda-Charvat Entropy	Brodatz images(pressed cork, erringbone weave, and Wood grain etc.	Sub Image Size			$d^2_{(x,\,mc)}$	Entropy measure within spatial frequency is used for texture discrimination.
			16 * 16			309.64	
			32 * 32			19.57	
			64 * 64			3.97	
			128 *128			7.68	
			Texture			$d^2_{(x,\,mc)}$	
			Random			130.97	
			Herringbone			431.95	
			Wood			1380.80	
[Singh et al., 2009]	Shannon and Non-Shannon Entropy Measures	Mammogram Image Analysis Society Database	Images Sample	S	R α=0.5	HC α=0.7	K α=0.5β=0.7	Results have demonstrated that Havrda&Charvat entropy based feature for classifying normal and abnormal mammogram images.
			Mam1	4.76	6.92	8.79	7.99
			Mam2	5.17	6.90	9.05	7.79
			Mam3	5.24	7.01	9.34	7.88
			Mam4	5.16	6.71	8.63	7.57
			Mam5	4.84	6.78	8.51	7.81
			Mam6	5.10	6.79	8.71	7.72
[Khehra et al.,2011]	Shannon and non-shannon Entropy	mini-MIAS database (Mammogram Image Analysis Society database	Test Image	t^S	t^R	t^{HC}	t^k	The result show that it is useful for radiologists to find suspicious regionin mammogram.
			mdb218	180	191	194	193
			mdb236	186	200	201	201
			mdb238	171	179	178	177
			mdb219	185	194	198	198
			mdb222	186	193	194	194
			mdb227	184	193	194	194
			mdb240	198	210	210	210
			mdb245	177	198	200	199
			mdb248	177	192	193	194
			mdb253	191	203	205	205

2.2.1 Comparative Analysis of Review on Feature Extraction and Entropy Measure Issue

Comparative analysis of review on feature extraction techniques and various entropy measure methods are shown in the table 2.4.

2.2.2 Common Finding From the Review of Features Extraction and Entropy Issue

- Almost technique had used for feature extraction and classification of medical images like MRI, CT, X-Ray and PET etc. After feature extraction, these techniques got additional information or sensitive information which had been helped for classification to better accuracy.

- The watershed transformation algorithm could extract shape and form related information from images precisely.
- The Vajda entropy measures is very much faster than the Kapur's entropy measure.
- Havrda-Charvat entropy is the best for image segmentation for gray scale images as compared to other entropy measures.
- Gabor Wavelet method was highly significant in the process of texture feature extraction. It had higher recognition rate
- GLCM (gray level co-occurrence Matrix) method applied for CT image (feature extraction) analysis. It computed the variance, Co-relation and sum average.
- Edge detection algorithms for object detection were used in several areas like, medical image processing, biometrics etc.
- Pre-processing and segmentation is quite important for better feature extraction.

2.2.3 Gaps in the Area of Feature Extraction and Entropy Measures

There are certain gaps observed in this issue are:

- Very few works has been done in order to extract important features with maximum information.
- More features need to be identified for advanced processing of MR images.
- GLCM is good to extract but need to be used with better pre-processing technique and classification techniques.
- The wavelet based features are not used at very large scale.
- Specific feature performance was not identified by any researchers feature extraction techniques are compared.
- Different wavelets performance are not addressed by any researchers.
- Importance of decomposition levels and feature extraction with each level is required.

REFERENCES

Ali, C. M. (2007). Design of appropriate wavelet bases for texture discrimination. *Kuwait Journal of Science & Engineering, 34*(2).

Anitha, V., & Murugavalli, S. (2016). Brain tumour classification using two-tier classifier with adaptive segmentation technique. *IET Computer Vision, 10*(1), 9–17. doi:10.1049/iet-cvi.2014.0193

Atkins, M. S., & Mackiewich, B. T. (1998). Fully automatic segmentation of the brain in MRI. *IEEE Transactions on Medical Imaging, 17*(1), 98–107. doi:10.1109/42.668699 PMID:9617911

Barabas, J., Babusiak, B., Gala, M., Radil, R., & Capka, M. (2012). Analysis, 3D Reconstruction and Anatomical Feature Extraction from Medical Images. *International Conference on Biomedical Engineering and Biotechnology*, 731-735. 10.1109/iCBEB.2012.72

Basile, T. M., Caponetti, L., Castellano, G., & Sforza, G. (2010). A Texture-Based Image Processing Approach for the Description of Human Oocyte Cytoplasm. *IEEE Transactions on Instrumentation and Measurement*, *59*(10), 2591–2601. doi:10.1109/TIM.2010.2057552

Chang, Q., Zhang, B., & Liu, R. (2011). Texture analysis method for shape-based segmentation in medical image. *International Congress on Image and Signal Processing*, 1146-1149. 10.1109/CISP.2011.6100395

Coggins, J. M. (1982). *A framework for texture analysis based on spatial filtering* (Ph.D Thesis). Michigan State University.

Desoky, A. H., & Hall, S. A. (1990). Entropy measures for texture analysis based on Hadamard transform. *IEEE Proceedings on Southeastcon*, *2*, 467-470.

Dhage, P., Phegade, M. R., & Shah, S. K. (2015). Watershed segmentation brain tumor detection. *Pervasive Computing (ICPC), International Conference*, *1*, 5.

Gao, H., Dou, L., Chen, W., & Xie, G. (2011). The applications of image segmentation techniques in medical CT images. *Proceedings of the 30th Chinese Control Conference*, 3296-3299.

Gautam, V., & Lakhwani, K. (2013). Implementation of Non Shannon Entropy measures for Color Image Segmentation and Comparison with Shannon Entropy Measures. *International Journal of Scientific Research (Ahmedabad, India)*, *2*(5), 391–394.

Goswami, B., & Mishra, S. K. (2016). Analysis of various Edge detection methods for X-ray images. *International Conference on Electrical, Electronics, and Optimization Techniques (ICEEOT)*. 10.1109/ICEEOT.2016.7755185

Grande, G. D., Hoekman, D., Lee, J. S., Schuler, D., & Ainsworth, T. (2004). A wavelet multiresolution technique for polarimetric texture analysis and segmentation of SAR images. *IGARSS, IEEE International Geoscience and Remote Sensing Symposium*, 713-719.

Hamedi, S. M., Vahidi, J., & Hamedi, S. M. (2015). Automatic MRI image threshold using fuzzy support vector machines. *International Conference on Knowledge-Based Engineering and Innovation (KBEI)*, 207-210. 10.1109/KBEI.2015.7436047

Haralick, R. (1979). Statistical and Structural approaches to texture. *Proceedings of the IEEE*, *67*(5), 786–804. doi:10.1109/PROC.1979.11328

Haralick, R. M., Shanmugam, K., & Kinstein, I. (1973). Texture features for image classification. *IEEE Transactions on Systems, Man, and Cybernetics*, *8*(6), 610–621. doi:10.1109/TSMC.1973.4309314

Jernigan, M. E., & Astoush, F. D. (1984). Entropy-Based Texture Analysis in the Spatial Frequency Domain. *IEEE Transactions on Pattern Analysis and Machine Intelligence*, *PAMI-6*(2), 237–243. doi:10.1109/TPAMI.1984.4767507 PMID:21869187

Jianchao, W., Mengyang, L., & Sixian, W. (1989). Texture segmentation of ultrasound B-scan image by sum and difference histograms. *Images of the Twenty-First Century. Proceedings of the Annual International Engineering in Medicine and Biology Society*, *2*, 417-418.

Jui, S. L. (2014). Fuzzy C-Means with Wavelet Filtration for MR Image Segmentation. *IEEE, Sixth World Congress on Nature and Biologically Inspired Computing (NaBIC)*, 12-16. 10.1109/NaBIC.2014.6921884

Khehra, B. S., & Pharwaha, A. P. S. (2011). Digital Mammogram Segmentation using Non-Shannon Measures of Entropy" *Proceedings of the World Congress on Engineering, WCE*, 2.

Kontaxakis, I., Sangriotis, E., & Martakos, D. (2003). Directional analysis of image textures for feature extraction and segmentation. *3rd International Symposium on Image and Signal Processing and Analysis, ISPA, 1*, 78-83. 10.1109/ISPA.2003.1296872

Korchiyne, R., Sbihi, A., Farssi, S. M., Touahni, R., & Alaoui, M. T. (2012). Medical image texture segmentation using Multifractal analysis. *International Conference on Multimedia Computing and Systems*, 422-425. 10.1109/ICMCS.2012.6320316

Laws, K. I. (1980). *Texture image segmentation* (Ph.D thesis). University of Southern California.

Lundervold, A. (2011). Lecture: Analysis of texture: Practice. *19th Annual Meeting of the International Society for Magnetic Resonance in Medicine(ISMRM)*.

Mallat, S. G. (1991). Zero-crossing of a wavelet transform. *IEEE Transactions on Information Theory, 37*(4), 1019–1033. doi:10.1109/18.86995

Marr, D., & Hildreth, E. (1980). Theory of edge detection. *Proceedings of the Royal Society of London. Series B, Biological Sciences, 207*(1167), 187–217. doi:10.1098/rspb.1980.0020 PMID:6102765

Materka, A., & Strzelecki, M. (2013). *On the importance of MRI non-uniformity correction for texture analysis. In Signal Processing: Algorithms, Architectures, Arrangements, and Applications*. SPA.

Mathur, S., & Gupta, M. (2014). An Analysis on Color Preservation Using Non-Shannon Entropy Measures for Gray and Color Images. *Fourth International Conference on Advances in Computing and Communications*, 109-112. 10.1109/ICACC.2014.32

Mohammad, S., Morris, D. T., & Thacker, N. (2013). Texture Analysis for the Segmentation of Optic Disc in Retinal Images. *IEEE International Conference on Systems, Man, and Cybernetics*, 4265-4270. 10.1109/SMC.2013.727

Naik, G. R., & Reddy, K. A. (2016). A new model for ECG signal filtering and feature extraction. *IEEE International Conference on Computer and Communications (ICCC)*, 765-768. 10.1109/Comp-Comm.2016.7924806

Natarajan, P., Krishnan, N., Kenkre, N. S., Nancy, S., & Singh, B. P. (2012). Tumor detection using threshold operation in MRI brain images. *IEEE International Conference on Computational Intelligence and Computing Research*, 1-4. 10.1109/ICCIC.2012.6510299

Peter, J., Muller, T., & Freyer, R. (1995). Optimized constraint satisfaction neural network for medical image segmentation. *Neural Networks, Proceedings, IEEE International Conference on, 5*, 2592-2595.

Pharwaha, A. P. S., & Singh, B. (2009). Shannon and Non-Shannon Measures of Entropy for Statistical Texture Feature Extraction in Digitized Mammograms. *Proceedings of the World Congress on Engineering and Computer Science, WCECS*, 2.

Richards, W., & Polit, A. (1974). Texture Matching. *Kybernetic, 16*(3), 155–162. doi:10.1007/BF00271719 PMID:4437126

Shareef, N., Wang, D. L., & Yagel, R. (1999). Segmentation of medical images using LEGION. *IEEE Transactions on Medical Imaging, 18*(1), 74–91. doi:10.1109/42.750259 PMID:10193699

Shareha, A. A. A., Rajeswari, M., & Ramachandram, D. (2008). Textured Renyi Entropy for Image Thresholding. *Fifth International Conference on Computer Graphics, Imaging and Visualisation*, 185-192. 10.1109/CGIV.2008.48

Sharma, K. K., Sharma, N., & Sharma, S. (2012). Comparison of Shannon and Non Shannon Entropy Measures for Threshold Selection in Color Image Segmentation Problems. *International Conference on Electronics Computer Technology,* 533.

Sklansky, J. (1978). Image Segmentation and Feature Extraction. *IEEE Transactions on Systems, Man, and Cybernetics, 8*(4), 237–247. doi:10.1109/TSMC.1978.4309944

Tamura, H., Mori, S., & Yamawaki, Y. (1978). Textural features corresponding to visual perception. *IEEE Transactions on Systems, Man, and Cybernetics, 8*(6), 460–473. doi:10.1109/TSMC.1978.4309999

Urooj, S., & Singh, S. P. (2016). Geometric invariant feature extraction of medical images using Hu's invariants. *3rd International Conference on Computing for Sustainable Global Development (INDIA-Com)*, 1560-1562.

Vyas, V. S., & Rege, P. (2006). Automated texture analysis with Gabor filter. *GVIP Journal, 6*(1), 35–41.

Zare, M. R., Mueen, A., Seng, W. C., & Awedh, M. H. (2011). Combined Feature Extraction on Medical X-ray Images. *Third International Conference on Computational Intelligence, Communication Systems and Networks*, 264-268. 10.1109/CICSyN.2011.63

Zhang, Q., & Gao, L. (2010). A Novel Medical Image Feature Extraction Algorithm. *Third International Conference on Intelligent Networks and Intelligent Systems*, 56-59. 10.1109/ICINIS.2010.172

Zucker, S., & Kant, K. (1981). Multiple- level representations for texture discrimination. *Proceedings of the IEEE Conference on pattern Recognition and Image Processing*, 609-614.

Chapter 24

Towards Integrating Data Mining With Knowledge-Based System for Diagnosis of Human Eye Diseases:
The Case of an African Hospital

Nilamadhab Mishra

(iD) https://orcid.org/0000-0002-1330-4869

School of Computing Science and Engineering, VIT Bhopal University, India

Johny Melese Samuel

Debre Berhan University, Ethiopia

ABSTRACT

The eye is the most important sensory organ of vision function. But some eye diseases can lead to vision loss, so it is important to identify and treat eye disease as early as possible. Eye care professionals can help protect their patients from vision loss or blindness by recognizing common eye diseases and recommending for an eye exam. Eye diseases with early detection, treatment, and appropriate follow-up care, vision loss, and blindness from eye disease can be prevented or delayed. In this study, rule-based eye disease identification and advising the knowledge-based system are projected. The projected system is targeting using hidden knowledge extracted by employing the extraction algorithm of data mining. To identify the best prediction model for the diagnosis of eye disease, four experiments for four classification algorithms were performed. Finally, the researchers decided to use the rules of the J48 pruned classification algorithm for further use in the development of a knowledge base of KBS because it exhibited better performance with a 98.5% evaluation result.

DOI: 10.4018/978-1-7998-2742-9.ch024

INTRODUCTION

Eye problems have been recognized worldwide as one of the major public health problems, particularly in developing countries where 90% of the blind live and international actions to prevent avoidable blindness has been gaining momentum over the last decade. According to the world health organization (WHO), about 37 million people are blind and 124 million people have low vision worldwide [**HeMavatHi et al, 2014; World Health Organization, 2006; Aemero et al, 2015; Abdulkerim, 2013**]. A large proportion of low vision (91.2%) and blindness (87.4%) are due to avoidable (either preventable or treatable) causes. Females and rural residents carry greater risk for eye problems. The burden of eye disease is believed to pose huge economic and social impacts on individuals, society, and the nation at large [**Fayyad et al, 1996, August; Prentzas et al, 2007; Oprea, 2006**]. A computer-based system (expert system), over-dependence on human experts, can be minimized. Knowledgebase (KBS) benefits the individual by providing a high-quality decision within a given time frame and facilitating job security and personal development [**Shiferaw et al, 2015; Berhane et al, 2007; Akerkar et al, 2010**]. Also, artificial expertise (AE) has some features that make it more beneficial over human expertise such as permanent, easy to transfer, easy to document, consistent, and affordable [**Schreiber et al, 1993; Datta et al, 2011**].

Classification is the process of classifying a data instance into one of several predefined categorical classes based on the training set containing known observations. A regression task begins with data instances in which the target values are known. The relationships between predictors and the target are summarized in a regression model that can be applied to different data instances in which the target values are unknown [**Covington et al, 1996; Fayisa et al, 2018; 15. Brose et al, 2009**]. Classification is the derivation of a function or model which determines the class of an object based on its attributes. A set of objects is given as the training set in which every object is represented by a vector of attributes along with its class. A classification function or model is constructed by analysing the relationship between the attributes and the classes of the objects in the training set. Such a classification function or model can be used to classify future objects and develop a better understanding of the classes of the objects in the database [**Han et al, 2011; Morgan, 2006**]. As mentioned in [**Jackson, 2002; Phyu, 2009, March; Serapião et al, 2013**] and [**Quinlan, 2014; Tayel et al, 2013**], classification is also called supervised learning. It is called supervised learning because it works on labeled attributes in which there is a specially chosen attribute and the aim is to use the data given to predict the values of that attribute for instances that have not yet been seen. The chosen attributes in classification are categorical such as 'high', 'low' or medium', [**Esseynew, 2011; Sasikumar et al, 2007; Mishra et al, 2019; Achour et al, 1999**]. Classification is a two-step process [**Prasad et al, 2012; DeKock, 2005**] consisting of model construction and model usage. In the first step, a classifier is built describing a predetermined or labeled set of data classes or concepts. This is the learning step (or training phase), where a classification algorithm builds the classifier by analysing or learning from a training set made up of database instances and their associated class labels. This step is called model construction. Generally, classification is a process of construction model that defines data class and used to predict the class of objects whose class label is unknown. It finds out the relationship between predictor value and the target value. The model is based on the analysis of a set of training data. The data; historical, for classification is typically divided into two datasets: one for building the model; the other for testing the model. [Dokas, 2005, September; Schmoldt et al,2012]Thus the various classification approaches can be employed on medical data for obtaining specific information and disease diagnosis. Decision tree, Byes classifier, neural network, support vector machine, and rule-based learning are some of the classification data mining techniques. The general objective of this study is to construct a knowledge base system prototype that can update its knowledge base using the hidden knowledge extracted from Eye disease dataset by using data mining classification techniques. The following are the research specific objectives that help to achieve the general objective of the study. To understand methods, approaches, techniques, and tools from works of literature, to apply different data mining (DM) algorithms and select suitable data mining classification algorithms for constructing predictive models, to acquire knowledge from the predictive model, for knowledge base construction, to build an integrator aiming at automatically building a knowledge base from the predictive model, to update knowledge base based on the new knowledge obtained from data mining, and to evaluate the performance and user acceptance levels of the knowledge-based system[Al-Saiyd et al, 2011; Efraim, 2011; Levesque, 1986; Mishra et al, 2014, December; Mishra, 2018]. The knowledge acquisition for the knowledge-based system is effected automatically by employing data mining techniques rather than undertaking an interview with experts. Data mining results are integrated into the knowledge base by using the integrator application. The integrator directly creates knowledge after mining rules from the dataset. It has a graphic user interface for selecting evaluated rules which are developed by using SWI-Prolog, Net beans IDE programming tools. The advice after detecting and identifying an Eye disease is targeted mainly for beginner Eye care professionals and primary health care workers. However, the prototype does not give detail treatment advising services by using medications. To treat Eye patients with medication it requires selection of the appropriate medicine, dosage, duration, frequency of the medication, etc. It needs a detailed study on those medications. Due to the short time available for the research, the study does not address all the treatment planning.

Also, the time and resources constraints are limited to cover the entire KBS of all diseases in this study. Hence, this study does not include the diagnosis of all diseases of Eye. The disease covered includes the following eye disease; Bacterial conjunctivitis, Cataract, Viral Conjunctivitis, Trachoma, Glaucoma, Chalazion, Corneal ulcer, Blepharitis, Nearsightedness (Myopia), and Farsightedness (Hyperopia). Thus, the proposed system covers the diagnosis of common diseases which can be identified by the domain experts with differential diagnosis of clinical patient complain, Eye condition, and symptoms. Knowledge Discovery in Database (KDD) model is followed for the data mining task. Knowledge Discovery Databases is the process of extracting and refining useful knowledge from large databases [**Žarko et al, 2014, June; Gubbi et al, 2013**]. KDD has been used by different researchers to discover knowledge from a large collection of records. KDD has been used by different researchers to discover knowledge from a large collection of records. It has seven steps such as Data cleaning, Data integration, Data selection, Data transformation, Data mining, Pattern evaluation, and Knowledge presentation [**Anantharam et al, 2013, June; Mishra et al, 2015; Dagnino et al, 2014, July**]. The knowledge that the researcher acquired from Data mining classification techniques is in the form of rules. Rules are constructed in the form of an if-then format. These if-then rules statements are used to formulate the conditional statements that constitute the knowledge base. Rule-based representation is highly expressive, is easy to interpret and easy to generate. To mine the hidden knowledge from the pre-processed dataset and compare the performance of classifiers, the researchers used WEKA 3.9.0 data mining tool. Also, to develop an application that maps the knowledge acquired from the data mining classifiers with knowledge-based system Java NetBeans IDE 8.2 with JDK 1.8.0 is employed. NetBeans offers easy and efficient project management, has the best support for the latest Java technologies, and can be installed on all operating systems supporting Java. To represent rules in the knowledge base and constructing the Rule-based Eye diagnosis and advising Knowledge-based system PROLOG is used. PROLOG is used because the researcher is more familiar than other AI programming languages used to develop a knowledge-based system. SWI-PROLOG editor is used to represent rules. The Prolog program consists of a set of facts accompanied by a set of conditions that the solution must satisfy; the computer can figure out for itself how to infer the solution from the given facts that are called logic programming [**Chang et al, 2015**]. Prolog is based on formal logic and solves problems by applying techniques originally developed to prove theorems in logic. It is a versatile language. Also, it classifies new instances rapidly. Hence, rules are used to represent knowledge for the knowledge-based system. The set of discovered rules has to be verified for accuracy, consistency, or no redundant or contradictory rules and usefulness (rules showing the decision-making process) for the knowledge base being developed. The accuracy of the models developed using data mining techniques is evaluated based on finding the accuracy of classifiers, Precision, Recall, F-measure, and True Positive rate. The researcher also evaluated the KBS using system performance testing by preparing test cases and users' acceptance testing questionnaire which helps the researcher to make sure that whether the potential users would like to use the proposed system frequently and whether the proposed systems meets user requirements. The main benefits of using a knowledge-based system are increased output and productivity, improved quality, reduced downtime, capturing scarce expertise, flexibility, and reliability, integrated knowledge, educational benefits/ease of training, enhance the problem-solving capability, and knowledge documentation and ease of knowledge transfer. With the proper utilization of knowledge, the KBS increases productivity and enhances problem-solving capabilities most flexibly. Such systems also have document knowledge for future use and training. This leads to increased quality in the problem-solving process. In this work, the integration is done between the J48 pruned classifier and PROLOG and converted from rule representation to PROLOG understandable format. Thus, SWI-Prolog 7.6.4 has used to implement the prototype of eye disease advising KBS and Java Net Beans IDE 8.2 with JDK 1.8.0 to integrate the model.

The rest of this paper is organized as follows. Section 2 discusses the integrated framework outline of a data mining model with the knowledge-based system. Our implementation and analysis are deliberated in section 3. Section 4 highlights the discussion of the classifier models. Finally, section 5 concludes this paper along with future work.

INTEGRATED FRAMEWORK OUTLINE

The purpose of this research is to integrate data mining results for the development of a knowledge-based system. The knowledge base is the core of a certain knowledge-based system. For that knowledge, the acquisition is done using the J48 pruned rule extraction algorithm, which achieves the best for Eye disease dataset. The challenge here is how is it possible to integrate data mining and knowledgebase system? The following sections discuss the combination of this issue. **Figure 1** suggests the general system design and structure of integrating data mining extracted hidden knowledge about Eye disease and their types based on Eye disease dataset with the knowledge-based system. The Structure shows that the data mining tasks used for generating knowledge from a collection of Eye disease datasets. Then following the validation of rules, the generated ruleset is encoded to the knowledge base.

In the context of the Data pre-processing, raw data cannot be used directly for processing with the machine learning algorithms. They first need to be pre-processed into the machine-understandable format. Raw data can be stored in several formats, including text, Excel, or other database types of files. Sometimes the raw data is not in any format. Having data already in a format understandable by algorithms can result in better time efficiency concerning the processing of the data [**Žarko et al, 2014, June**].

Figure 1. The proposed integrated knowledge-based system framework

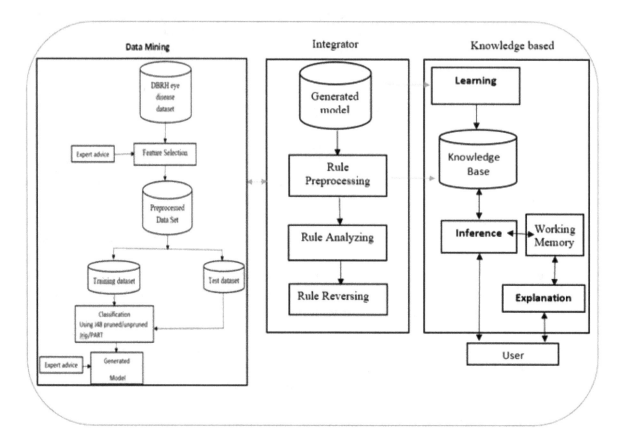

After the collected 1120 instances of the KDD dataset for this study, 53 of them are found redundant from Bacterial conjunctivitis, Nearsightedness, Farsightedness, and Blepharitis disease type. Therefore, before the actual mining task is performed, these instances are removed at the data pre-processing stage. Designed for building a predictive model that classifies instances into labeled classes rule extraction algorithms is used. In this study, algorithms such as J48 pruned, J48 unpruned, PART, and JRIP which are capable of generating rules are selected and employed for the mining task. Extraction algorithms produce knowledge in the form of rules from the dataset. These rules should be validated to make sure that they are a reproduction of the dataset. Attributes or combinations of attributes together form the rules. These rules should be evaluated to make sure that the attributes and values of the attributes represent or reveal the conclusion. For this study, several rules are generated by the algorithm to identify an instance of the KDD dataset as Bacterial conjunctivitis, Cataract, Viral Conjunctivitis, Trachoma, Glaucoma, Chalazion, Corneal ulcer…. For that, most rules used a combination of attributes and a small number of them used a single attribute with the respective values for attributes. Therefore, before using the generated rules as part of the knowledge base, the rules are evaluated in consultation with domain experts. Knowledge Base is a container of rules about Eye disease which are generated by the J48 pruned rule extraction algorithm after planned by the integrator to PROLOG logical format. User Interface is the interaction point between the user and the system. The user interface can be a graphical user interface (GUI). In the sequence of integration of data mining with a knowledge-based system, Graphical User

Interface for the integrator for the knowledge-based system. In this study, an attempt is made to design an automatic integration of the result of the data mining model with the knowledge base. To achieve this Java NetBeans IDE 8.2 with JDK 1.8.0 and PROLOG has been used. This is done by understanding the standard format followed by J48 pruned rule construction and PROLOG formalism [**Mishra et al, 2015**].

Next, the mining is accomplished, the result is written as a text file. The rule Pre-processor element is responsible for removing some special characters, removing unwanted tokens, replacing some logical operator by another logical operator, and replacing comparison operator with another comparison operator. The replacement and removal of special characters, logical operators, and comparison operators are based on the tokenization process illustrated in **table 1**. Hence, all the rules are pre-processed in the same fashion. Then fact And Rule Generator module continues its task of reversing the right-hand side to the left-hand side from the tokenized rules.

Table 1. Rules before and after tokenization

Before rule preprocessing	After rule preprocessing
IF A2 =YES AND A14=YES AND A20=NO THEN Bacterial conjunctivitis	A2 =YES, A14=YES,A20=NO: - bacterial conjunctivitis
IF A1=YES AND A2=YES AND A10=YES AND A13=YES THEN **Viral Conjunctivitis**	A1=YES, A2=YES, A10=YES, A13=YES:- **Viral Conjunctivitis**
IF A 20=YES THEN **Corneal ulcer**	20=YES:- **Corneal ulcer**
IF A1=YES AND A8=YES AND A15=YES A17=YES AND A20=YES THEN **Corneal ulcer**	A1=YES, A8=YES, AND A15=YES, A17=YES, A20 =YES:- **Corneal ulcer**
IF A18=YES THEN **Nearsightedness(Myopia)**	A18=YES:- **Nearsightedness(Myopia)**

After rules are cleaned by using the rule Pre-processor section, the next step is integrating rules and facts following the syntax of PROLOG for creating the knowledge base needed to enhance the reasoning process. This requires reversing the order of the rules from IF…THEN construct to THEN…IF construct for backward chaining. Hence this section exchanges the position of the left-hand side and right-hand side of J48 pruned rules. Prolog rules have both head and body but facts have only heads. Hence, the component first builds the heads of the rules having the format: 'predicate (conclusion):-'. After that ':-' is concatenated which means IF in PROLOG. To make it a complete rule, the body part (antecedents) must be concatenated with the heads.

IMPLEMENTATION AND ANALYSIS

A total of four experiments targeting building predictive models are undertaken. In this study, 1055 instances are ready for experimentation after data pre-processing. The dataset contains 22 attributes and all of them are involved in all experiments. Also after undertaking several experiments, the default value of parameters is taken into consideration for each classifier algorithm since it allows achieving better accuracy compared to modifying the default parameters 'values.

The first experiment shows that the model built using a J48 pruned classifier involving its default value of parameters and 10-fold cross-validation is selected as a test option. Hence, the model developed using J48 pruned classifier has a tree of size 39 and the number of leaves 20. The algorithm has correctly classified 1039 instances and only 16 instances are classified incorrectly taking 0.05 seconds to build the model. An overview is given in **Table 2**.

Table 2. Confusion matrix for the J48 pruned classification algorithm

	Classified as										
Actual Class	a	b	C	d	e	f	g	h	i	j	
	138	0	0	0	0	0	0	0	0	0	a = Bacterial conjunctivitis
	0	133	0	0	0	0	0	0	0	0	b = Cataract
	0	0	144	0	0	0	0	0	0	0	c = Viral Conjunctivitis
	0	0	0	119	0	0	0	0	0	0	d = Trachoma
	0	0	0	0	106	0	0	0	7	0	**e =** Glaucoma
	0	0	0	0	0	76	0	0	0	0	f= Chalazion
	0	0	0	2	0	1	85	0	5	0	g = Corneal ulcer
	0	0	0	0	0	0	0	80	1	0	h = Blepharities
	0	0	0	0	0	0	0	0	80	0	i=Nearsightedness (Myopia)
	0	0	0	0	0	0	0	0	0	78	j=Farsightedness (Hyperopia)

The second experiment indicates that the model built using the J48 Unpruned decision tree algorithm. This experiment has involved the unpruned "True" parameters with respective values and 10-fold cross-validation test mode. Then, the algorithm registered prediction accuracy of 98.2938% in which J48 unpruned has correctly classified 1037 instances out of 1055, which means it has incorrectly classified 18 instances taking 0.04 seconds to build the model. An overview of performance analysis classifiers is given in **Table 3**.

Table 3. Model Performance analysis by class for J48 unpruned classification algorithm

Classifier	TP Rate	Precision	Recall	F-measure	Class
J48 unpruned	1.000	1.000	1.000	1.000	Bacterial conjunctivitis
	1.000	1.000	1.000	1.000	Cataract
	1.000	0.986	1.000	0.993	Viral Conjunctivitis
	1.000	0.983	1.000	0.992	Trachoma
	0.920	1.000	0.920	0.959	Glaucoma
	1.000	0.987	1.000	0.993	Chalazion
	0.914	1.000	0.914	0.955	Corneal ulcer
	0.988	1.000	0.988	0.994	Blepharities
	1.000	0.860	1.000	0.925	Nearsightedness(Myopia)
	1.000	1.000	1.000	1.00	Farsightedness (Hyperopia)

In this experiment, the PART rule induction algorithm is employed. It generated 16 rules by involving all the attributes of the dataset and a 10-fold cross-validation test option. The algorithm registered prediction accuracy of 98.2938% in which 1037 instances out of 1055 are correctly classified. The algorithm has incorrectly classified only 18 instances by taking 0.06 seconds to build the model (**Table 4**).

Table 4. Model Performance analysis by class for the PART classification algorithm

Classifier	TP Rate	Precision	Recall	F-measure	Class
	1.000	1.000	1.000	1.000	Bacterial conjunctivitis
	1.000	1.000	1.000	1.000	Cataract
	1.000	0.986	1.000	0.993	Viral Conjunctivitis
	1.000	0.983	1.000	0.992	Trachoma
PART	0.920	1.000	0.920	0.959	Glaucoma
	1.000	0.987	1.000	0.993	Chalazion
	0.914	1.00	0.914	0.955	Corneal ulcer
	0.988	1.00	0.988	0.994	Blepharities
	1.000	0.860	1.000	0.925	Nearsightedness (Myopia)
	1.000	1.000	1.000	1.000	Farsightedness (Hyperopia)

The other rule induction algorithm selected for this study is JRip. Therefore, to generate IF-THEN rules from the experimental Eye disease dataset JRip algorithm with its default values of the parameter and 10-fold cross-validation test mode is employed. JRip correctly classified 1036 instances from 1055. The number of incorrectly classified instances is 24. The algorithm has generated 19 rules. The algorithm takes 0.08 seconds to develop the model (**Table 5**).

Table 5. Model Performance analysis by class for JRip classification algorithm

Classifier	TP Rate	Precision	Recall	F-measure	Class
	1.00	1.00	1.00	1.000	Bacterial conjunctivitis
	0.985	1.00	0.985	0.992	Cataract
	1.00	0.986	1.00	0.993	Viral Conjunctivitis
	1.00	0.983	1.00	0.992	Trachoma
JRip	0.938	1.00	0.938	0.968	Glaucoma
	1.000	0.974	1.000	0.987	Chalazion
	0.903	1.00	0.903	0.949	Corneal ulcer
	0.988	1.00	0.988	0.994	Blepharities
	1.000	0.860	1.000	0.925	Nearsightedness (Myopia)
	1.000	1.000	1.000	1.000	Farsightedness (Hyperopia)

Table 6. Summarised Performance of Classifiers

Classifier	Correctly classified instances		Incorrectly classified instances		Time take to build the model(in second)
	No.	percentage	No.	percentage	
J48 pruned	**1039**	**98.4834%**	**16**	**1.5166%**	**0.05**
J48 unpruned	1037	98.2938%	18	1.7062%	0.01
JRip	1036	98.1991%	19	1.8009%	0.08
PART	1037	98.2938%	18	1.7062%	0.06

As described in **figure 2**, there is a minor difference among the classifiers in terms of classifying the dataset correctly. Even if their minor difference, J48 pruned has registered the best prediction accuracy by classifying 1039 instances out of 1055 correctly. Results of J48 unpruned and PART show that an equal number of incorrectly classified instances. The highest incorrect classification is registered by the JRip algorithm. The Prediction accuracy shows us the general classification accuracy of the algorithms. Apart from prediction accuracy, classifiers are also evaluated to measure how they correctly classified each class to their correct class or incorrectly classified to another class. As stated earlier, pruned and unpruned decision trees and two decision rule induction algorithms are used for the experiments. All the selected algorithms allow generating rules from the dataset. The results of the algorithms are evaluated based on prediction accuracy in classifying the instances of the dataset into Bacterial conjunctivitis, Viral Conjunctivitis, Trachoma, Glaucoma, Corneal ulcer, Cataract, Blepharitis, Chalazion, Nearsightedness (Myopia), and Farsightedness (Hyperopia). The Prediction accuracy shows us the general classification accuracy of the algorithms. Apart from prediction accuracy, classifiers are also evaluated to measure how they correctly classified each class to their correct class or incorrectly classified to another class. Hence, to evaluate the performance of the classifiers employed in this study True Positive rate, Precision, Recall, and F-measure are used as discussed in **figure 3**.

Figure 2. Accuracy of J48pruned, J48Unpruned, JRip and PART Algorithms

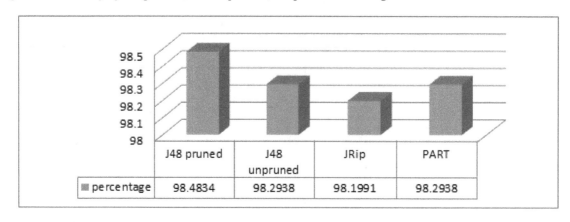

Figure 3. Performance Comparison of the Classifier Models

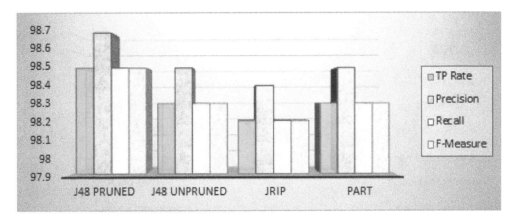

. J48 pruned has registered the best result in terms of precision, recall, and F-measure values as compared to another classification algorithm. Moreover, the True Positive rate of classifiers is also compared. Table 3-11 also shows from the result the highest TP Rate of 98.5% was scored by J48 pruned model followed by the J48 unpruned model and PART that achieved 98.3%. The least TP Rate of 97.2% was scored by JRip.

From the precision values, the highest scores of 98.7% were registered by J48 pruned followed by the J48 unpruned model and PART that achieved 98.5%. The least scores of 98.4% were registered by JRip. When we come to the Recall and F-Measure results, J48 pruned model with all attributes achieved the highest scores of 98.5% and 98.5%respectively, whereas the least Recall rate of 98.2% and F-Measure of 98.2% were presented by the JRip.

The rule acquired from the classifier algorithms is used for constructing the knowledge base.

To develop an effective knowledge base system, acquiring relevant rules is dominant. Hence from the four algorithms, the researcher selected the classifier which best performed on classifying the dataset. J48 pruned has the best performance among the four classifiers. Its prediction accuracy and TP rate for all types of diseases are above 98.48% which is a great performance in predicting identifying and diagnosis each disease correctly. The FP rate is almost minor for most diagnosis class. This shows the model developed using J48 pruned is acceptable for constructing the rule base of the knowledge base system. Speed refers to the execution time it takes a classifier to be trained. To build this model, JRip, PART, J48 pruned and J48 unpruned classifier took much time respectively.

J48 pruned classifiers have generated 20 rules but among them, 17 rules are selected for implementation which is correctly identifying disease which has proved by the domain expert. The rules involved 14 features/attributes among the 22 features/attributes from the sample dataset. The algorithm generated 1 rule for each Eye disease namely, viral conjunctivitis, Nearsightedness (Myopia), Farsightedness (Hyperopia), and Chalazion and two rules for each Bacterial conjunctivitis, Corneal ulcer, Glaucoma, Trachoma and Blepharitis Eye disease and the remaining three generated rules for cataract eye disease identification.

This page consists of components such as the combo box and command buttons. The command buttons of the GUI are used to fire a Prolog query. Combo boxes allow users to select alternatives given by the inference engine. The Diagnose command button links with other dialog boxes to display the results of the detected diagnosis and recommendation to users (**figure 4**).

Figure 4. Prototype of an Integrated Knowledge Base System

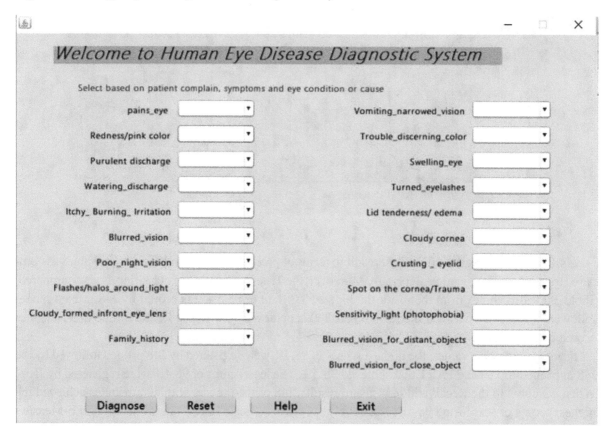

The disease of eye diagnosis is started when the user can select "Yes" or "No" option from a combo box based on patient complain, symptom and eye condition or case which is listed in the label Then, the user clicking "Diagnose" command button and if match with encoded rule the system immediately gives the result of the detected disease followed by its recommendation to assist the practitioner to take action. **Figure 5** shows the results of detected bacterial conjunctivitis eye disease and its advice or rec-

Figure 5. diagnosis and recommendation of bacterial conjunctivitis after "Diagnose"

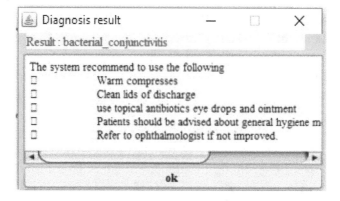

ommendation. To assure that Eye disease diagnostic system-KBS meets the requirement it is developed for, it has to be tested. Test cases are one of the predominant evaluation mechanisms for evaluating the performance of the proposed system which helps the researcher to compare and contrast the domain experts' judgment. The system performance testing focuses on testing the behavior of the knowledge-based system to check that it is satisfactory in the eyes of the user. But accurate in performance measures is the system, how complete the knowledge-based system is, it will be difficult if the system doesn't meet user requirements. It does not take into consideration the internal mechanics of the system and tends to be subjective. To make the model into industrial applicability, the Eye disease diagnostic system (EDDS-KBS) has met the desired performance with the least errors.

DISCUSSIONS

As discussed in the evaluation section, the proposed system achieves favorable results with a 90.1% system performance testing result and an 86% user acceptance testing result. The overall performance of the prototype system is 88.1%. This indicates that using integrated knowledge acquisition techniques is better than using manual knowledge acquisition techniques separately.

In the beginning, this study has four research questions to answer, and let's discuss how these questions have been answered with this study. The first research question of this study was "Is it possible to use rules resulted from production rules in data mining to construct the rule-based knowledge-based system and provide advice for the user?" To answer this question, four experiments for rule classification algorithms namely J48 pruned, J48 unpruned, PART, and JRip under ten-fold Cross-Validation test option/mode was conducted and the experiments showed that J48 pruned classification algorithm is the best rules classifications resulted to develop the prediction model that can predict the type of eye disease. It records better performance with 98.4 and the researcher decided to use the results for further use in the development of the knowledge base of KBS then collect the advice for each detected disease from the domain expert to encode with a prototype. The second question was "How it is possible to describe the knowledge-based system from knowledge extracted using data mining techniques?" To answer this question, the first eye disease dataset was collected from DBRH's future selection and pre-processing was undertaken. Secondly, to extract hidden knowledge rule classification algorithms were conducted. Finally, the best rule classification results were pre-processed, converted into Prolog understandable able to format to integrate with a knowledge base, and describe it.

The third question was "How Data Mining results could be integrated with Knowledge-Based System for Diagnosis and advice of Human Eye disease?" To answer this question, a prototype Knowledge

Based were developed using the knowledge that is acquired from discovered knowledge and which enabled us to integrate the WEKA result automatically with the knowledge base. Then to call the knowledge base that is constructed with Prolog from Java, the researcher has added a JPL file in Java library.

The fourth question was "How to evaluate the performance and user acceptance of the prototype?" To answer this question, system performance was undertaken by preparing test cases that help to compare domains' judgment with the proposed system's responses. In this case, the test case included 21 samples of eye disease instances and 22 attributes with a respected value which was unlabelled. Finally, 19 eye disease instances were correctly labeled out of 21 which shows 90.1% system performance is correct.

CONCLUSIONS AND FUTURE WORK

In this study, the possibility of integrating data mining models with the knowledge-based system is comprehended and discovered. The integration process begins by taking samples of the DBRH eye disease dataset which is found in the Amara region Debre Birhan Hospital, Ethiopia, Africa. The dataset is preprocessed and made suitable for mining steps. Then the researcher extracted knowledge in the form of rules using the WEKA data mining tool. Data mining has demonstrated to extract hidden knowledge from a large collection of the dataset. Hence, four experiments for four classification algorithms namely J48 pruned, J48 unpruned, PART, and JRip under ten-fold Cross-Validation test option/mode were conducted. Finally, the data mining classifier, J48 pruned is employed for the knowledge acquisition step since it has performed best among the selected classifiers with an accuracy of 98.4834%. The implementation of the prototype system is accomplished by using the SWI-Prolog tool which supports GUI integration for the user interface. The user interface is designed by using the Net Beans IDE Java program and connected to the Prolog knowledge base system via the Prolog inference engine. The study reveals further research investigation to fully implement the integrating of data mining with Knowledge-Based Systems in eye health care and disease diagnosis in the domain area. Based on the results of the study, the following recommendations are suggested for further investigation on the applicability of integration of data mining with a Knowledge-Based System in eye health care. We conducted the research on a selected sample of diseases of the eye which could be differentiated by common typical symptoms by applying differential diagnosis techniques. To fully implement, further investigation should be made to incorporate all eye health problems by incorporating emerging computing technologies.

CONFLICT OF INTERESTS

The author declares that there is no conflict of interest regarding the publication of this paper.

ACKNOWLEDGMENT

The authors would like to express thanks to the School of Computing Sciences and Engineering, VIT Bhopal University, India, and College of Computing, Debre Berhan University, Ethiopia, Africa for supporting this research.

REFERENCES

Abdulkerim, M. (2013). *Towards integrating data mining with knowledge based system: the case of network intrusion detection* (Doctoral dissertation). Addis Ababa University.

Achour, S. L., Dojat, M., Rieux, C., Bierling, P., & Lepage, E. (1999). Knowledge acquisition environment for the design of a decision support system: application in blood transfusion. In *Proceedings of the AMIA Symposium* (p. 187). American Medical Informatics Association.

Aemero, A., Berhan, S., & Yeshigeta, G. (2015). Role of health extension workers in eye health promotion and blindness prevention in Ethiopia. *JOECSA, 18*(2).

Akerkar, R., & Sajja, P. (2010). *Knowledge-based systems*. Jones & Bartlett Publishers.

Al-Saiyd, N. A., Mohammad, A. H., Al-Sayed, I. A., & Al-Sammarai, M. F. (2011). Distributed knowledge acquisition system for software design problems. *European Journal of Scientific Research, 62*(3), 311–320.

Anantharam, P., Barnaghi, P., & Sheth, A. (2013, June). Data Processing and Semantics for Advanced Internet of Things (IoT) Applications: modeling, annotation, integration, and perception. In *Proceedings of the 3rd International Conference on Web Intelligence, Mining and Semantics* (pp. 1-5). 10.1145/2479787.2479821

Berhane, Y., Worku, A., Bejiga, A., Adamu, L., Alemayehu, W., Bedri, A., ... Kebede, T. D. (2007). National survey on blindness, low vision and trachoma in Ethiopia: Methods and study clusters profile. *The Ethiopian Journal of Health Development, 21*(3), 185–203.

Brose, L. S., & Bradley, C. (2009). Psychometric development of the retinopathy treatment satisfaction questionnaire (RetTSQ). *Psychology Health and Medicine, 14*(6), 740–754. doi:10.1080/13548500903431485 PMID:20183546

Chang, H. T., Mishra, N., & Lin, C. C. (2015). IoT big-data centred knowledge granule analytic and cluster framework for BI applications: A case base analysis. *PLoS One, 10*(11), e0141980. doi:10.1371/journal.pone.0141980 PMID:26600156

Covington, M. A., Nute, D., & Vellino, A. (1996). *Prolog programming in depth*. Prentice-Hall, Inc.

Dagnino, A., & Cox, D. (2014, July). Industrial Analytics to Discover Knowledge from Instrumented Networked Machines. In SEKE (pp. 86-89). Academic Press.

Datta, R. P., & Saha, S. (2011). *An Empirical comparison of rule based classification techniques in medical databases* (No. 1107). Academic Press.

De Kock, E. (2005). *Decentralising the codification of rules in a decision support expert knowledge base* (Doctoral dissertation). University of Pretoria.

Dokas, I. M. (2005, September). Developing Web Sites For Web Based Expert Systems: A Web Engineering Approach. In ITEE (pp. 202-217). Academic Press.

Efraim, T. (2011). *Decision support and business intelligence systems*. Pearson Education India.

Esseynew, S. (2011). *Prototype Knowledge Based System for Anxiety Mental Disorder Diagnosis* (Doctoral dissertation). Addis Ababa University.

Fayisa, D. (2018). *Integrated Predictive Model and Knowledge Based System for Wheat Disease Detection: Case of Arsi Zone* (Doctoral dissertation). ASTU.

Fayyad, U. M., Piatetsky-Shapiro, G., & Smyth, P. (1996, August). Knowledge Discovery and Data Mining: Towards a Unifying Framework. In KDD (Vol. 96, pp. 82-88). Academic Press.

Gubbi, J., Buyya, R., Marusic, S., & Palaniswami, M. (2013). Internet of Things (IoT): A vision, architectural elements, and future directions. *Future Generation Computer Systems*, *29*(7), 1645–1660. doi:10.1016/j.future.2013.01.010

Han, J., Pei, J., & Kamber, M. (2011). *Data mining: concepts and techniques*. Elsevier.

HeMavatHi, P. S., & SHenoy, P. (2014). Profile of microbial isolates in ophthalmic infections and antibiotic susceptibility of the bacterial isolates: A study in an eye care hospital, Bangalore. *Journal of Clinical and Diagnostic Research: JCDR*, *8*(1), 23. PMID:24596715

Jackson, J. (2002). Data mining; a conceptual overview. *Communications of the Association for Information Systems*, *8*(1), 19.

Levesque, H. J. (1986). Knowledge representation and reasoning. *Annual Review of Computer Science*, *1*(1), 255–287. doi:10.1146/annurev.cs.01.060186.001351

Mining, W. I. D. (2006). Data mining: Concepts and techniques. *Morgan Kaufinann*, *10*, 559–569.

Mishra, N. (2018). Internet of Everything Advancement Study in Data Science and Knowledge Analytic Streams. *International Journal of Scientific Research in computer science and Engineering*, *6*(1), 30-36.

Mishra, N., Chang, H. T., & Lin, C. C. (2015). An Iot knowledge reengineering framework for semantic knowledge analytics for BI-services. *Mathematical Problems in Engineering*, *2015*, 2015. doi:10.1155/2015/759428

Mishra, N., Lin, C. C., & Chang, H. T. (2014, December). A cognitive oriented framework for IoT big-data management prospective. In *2014 IEEE International Conference on Communiction Problem-solving* (pp. 124-127). IEEE. 10.1109/ICCPS.2014.7062233

Mishra, N., Thangavel, G., & Samuel, J. M. (2019). A Case Assessment Of Knowledge-Based Fit In Frame For Diagnosis Of Human Eye Diseases. *Journal of Critical Reviews*, *7*(6), 2020.

Oprea, M. (2006). On the Use of Data-Mining Techniques in Knowledge-Based Systems. *Ecological Informatics*, *6*, 21–24.

Phyu, T. N. (2009, March). Survey of classification techniques in data mining. In *Proceedings of the International MultiConference of Engineers and Computer Scientists* (*Vol. 1*, pp. 18-20). Academic Press.

Prasad, T. V. (2012). *Hybrid systems for knowledge representation in artificial intelligence*. arXiv preprint arXiv:1211.2736

Prentzas, J., & Hatzilygeroudis, I. (2007). Categorizing approaches combining rule-based and case-based reasoning. *Expert Systems: International Journal of Knowledge Engineering and Neural Networks*, *24*(2), 97–122. doi:10.1111/j.1468-0394.2007.00423.x

Quinlan, J. R. (2014). *C4. 5: programs for machine learning*. Elsevier.

Sasikumar, M., Ramani, S., Raman, S. M., Anjaneyulu, K. S. R., & Chandrasekar, R. (2007). *A practical introduction to rule based expert systems*. Narosa Publishing House.

Schmoldt, D. L., & Rauscher, H. M. (2012). *Building knowledge-based systems for natural resource management*. Springer Science & Business Media.

Schreiber, G., Wielinga, B., & Breuker, J. (Eds.). (1993). *KADS: A principled approach to knowledge-based system development* (Vol. 11). Academic Press.

Serapião, A., & Bannwart, A. C. (2013). Knowledge discovery for classification of three-phase vertical flow patterns of heavy oil from pressure drop and flow rate data. *Journal of Petroleum Engineering*.

Shiferaw, B., Gelaw, B., Assefa, A., Assefa, Y., & Addis, Z. (2015). Bacterial isolates and their anti-microbial susceptibility pattern among patients with external ocular infections at Borumeda hospital, Northeast Ethiopia. *BMC Ophthalmology*, *15*(1), 103. doi:10.118612886-015-0078-z PMID:26268424

Tayel, S., Reif, M., & Dengel, A. (2013). Rule-based Complaint Detection using RapidMiner. In *Conference: RCOMM* (pp. 141-149). Academic Press.

World Health Organization. (2006). *Sight test and glasses could dramatically improve the lives of 150 million people with poor vision*. WHO.

Žarko, I. P., Pripužić, K., Serrano, M., & Hauswirth, M. (2014, June). Iot data management methods and optimisation algorithms for mobile publish/subscribe services in cloud environments. In *2014 European conference on networks and communications (EuCNC)* (pp. 1-5). IEEE.

Chapter 25
Use of IoT and Different Biofeedback to Measure TTH:
An Approach for Healthcare 4.0

Rohit Rastogi
https://orcid.org/0000-0002-6402-7638
ABES Engineering College, India

Devendra Kumar Chaturvedi
https://orcid.org/0000-0002-4837-2570
Dayalbagh Educational Institute, Agra, India

Mayank Gupta
Tata Consultancy Services, India

ABSTRACT

This chapter applied the random sampling in selection of the subjects suffering with headache, and care was taken that they ensure to fulfill the International Headache Society criteria. Subjects under consideration were assigned the two groups of GSR-integrated audio-visual feedback, GSR (audio-visual)- and EMG (audio-visual)-integrated feedback groups. In 10 sessions, the subjects experienced the GSR and EMG BF therapy for 15 minutes. Twenty subjects were subjected to EEG therapy. The variables for stress (pain) and SF-36 (quality of life) scores were recorded at starting point, 30 days, and 90 days after the starting of GSR and EMG-BF therapy. To reduce the anxiety and depression in day-to-day routine, the present research work is shown as evidence in favor of the mindful meditation. The physical, mental, and total scores increased over the time duration of SF-36 scores after 30- and 90-days recordings (p<0.05). Intergroup analysis has demonstrated the improvement. EMG-audio visual biofeedback group also showed highest improvement in SF-36 scores at first and third month follow up. EEG measures the Alpha waves for the subjects after meditation. GSR, EMG, and EEG-integrated auditory-visual biofeedback are efficient in solution of stress due to TTH with most advantage seen.

DOI: 10.4018/978-1-7998-2742-9.ch025

1. INTRODUCTION

1.1 IOT

It is a technology that has made the non-connectivity appliance a connectivity appliance. The appliances that contain technology that helps us to communicate us with human and technology. Let us take some example the GPS is a latest technology that are inbuilt in car help the driver to make it easy to travel within the road, i.e. it is that technology in which we require internet base technique.(Rubin, 1999)

1.1.1 History Of IoT

IoT has evolved when the major language that are not famous on that days such as machine language, commodity analysis etc. Now a days Automation, control system, wireless sensor networks that are connect to internet and helps us to make us easier to do work.

Kevin Ashton in 1999 was first who coined the term IoT i.e. "Internet of Things". But in earlier the concept of IoT was purposed in Carnegie Mellon University in 1982 that work on the concept of Network smart devices.

Now a days the technology is increasing day by day is increasing day by day like CISCO is introducing a new technology and in future the technology will replace every human work with this technology. (Rubin, 1999)

1.1.2 Applications

The application of IoT is usually bifurcated among infrastructure, industry, commercial and consumer spaces. Many technologies have being evolved in this field some are describing as-

a-Smart Home: It is a future upcoming home in this world. These technologies include the theory of Automation. This include smart lighting, smart lock system, smart kitchen, even we has wireless technology to which we can speak like GOOGLE assistance, amazon echo, SIRI in apple IOS and, many other. This technology helps to make our work easier and make interactive home design that help and attract the other. This technology is basically helps to upgrade our system. Many companies are now being evolving now days like APPLE, SAMSUNG and LENOVO etc.(Rubin, 1999)

b- IoT as Medical Health Care: IoT helps in medical field to make our future bright such as, major technology has being evolved in this field such as pacemaker.

With the help of IoT we can create digitalized health care facilities; we can connect to medical resources easily and can get medical facilities easier.

Devices enabled with IoT services are applicable for remote health monitoring and especially in emergency notification facilities. They may help us in from blood pressure and heart rate monitors and latest gadgets like pacemakers to monitor specialized implants.

Now a days "smart beds" can be seen in the medical facilities that is a another a feature of IoT. Doctor can interrogate their patient with the help of video call from far away from the place, even the nurses can be appointed through internet facilities. A 2015 Goldman Sachs reported that by increasing revenue and decreasing cost, gadgets being used for health care devices in USA are helping to save nearly $300 billion in annual expenditures in health sector.

Moreover a special monitoring sensor is being setup in the parks, shop, medical shops, hospitals etc... To ensure the medical health care of the people. These sensor are being connected to a data base system that are been collected server and information is being gather out. This ways scientists are researching their on the human being that how they are developing day by day.

Machines are being built on the bases of application on IoT that help doctor to study properly to their patients and collect and store data in the form of big data that is sub class of IoT. Many researches are being done by collecting the data from the sensor. Chronic Disease control and prevention of them is being wisely cared by IoT in health sector plays a fundamentally. Mighty wireless connections have proved remote monitoring a reality; this fast connectivity has made easy the application of recording of subject data and analysis of complex algorithms on it (Rubin, 1999).

1.1.3 Future Perspective of IoT

With the base of IoT wireless design has been made which can enhance our technology and made our work easier. Much wireless technology has been developed and these technology has been categorized in three ways i.e. short, medium and long range wireless.

- **Short Range Wireless-** With short frequency and applied for home purpose.
- **Bluetooth Mesh Networking–** Applied with large no. of nodes and using BLE, it is used in application layer.
- **Light-Fidelity (Li-Fi)–** Same as wi-fi, uses visible light communication for high bandwidth.
- **Near-Field Communication (NFC)–** Protocols making capable communication of 2 devices in four centimetre range..
- **Radio-Frequency Identification (RFID)–** Tags are embedded in items, applies EM fields to retrieve data.
- **Wi-Fi –** Devices communicate through a shared access point or directly between individual devices.LAN based method on IEEE 802.11 standard.
- **Medium Range Wireless-** For company purpose.
- **LTE-Advanced–** High-speed communication specification for mobile networks. Enhancements to the LTE standard. Extended coverage, higher throughput, and lower latency.
- **Long Range Wireless-** Establish connect within a country, state etc.(Rastogi, Chaturvedi, Satya, Arora, & Chauhan, 2018)

1.1.4 Concluding Remarks for IoT

IoT is a very useful technology in every field because it play crucial role in every filed. In the field of medical it is very important and by this we can help the people and save them even they are suffering from TTH, stress, or any other disease.

1. **Low-Power Wide-Area Networking (LPWAN)** – Wireless networks, allows Low data rate communication in long-rang, decreases power and cost for transmission. Available LPWAN technologies and protocols: LoRaWan, Sigfox, NB-IoT, Weightless.
2. **Very Small Aperture Terminal (VSAT)–** Uses small dish antennas for narrowband and broadband data with Satellite communication technology,

1.2 Big Data

The large collection of data is referred as big data which are very much big and highly complex to process for commonly used data processing software. It consists of data sets which are too large to be stored, organized, integrated, managed and processed within a certain elapsed time by common software. (Fumal & Scohnen, 2008)

1.2.1 Characteristics

There are major four characteristics of Big data, namely volume, variety, velocity and veracity. Volume is the quantity of the data which is to be stored and which determines whether a data set is large enough to be considered big data or not. The nature and type of generated data is known as variety whereas the processing speed of data and its generation to handle a specific need is called velocity. Veracity characterizes the quality and value of the available data. (Fumal & Scohnen, 2008)

1.2.2 Applications of Big Data

Healthcare

Big data finds a major application in the healthcare industry. Nowadays, in major hospitals and large healthcare centers, there is a huge influx of patients suffering from a wide variety of ailments. Thus, the doctors rely more on the patient's clinical health record which means gathering huge amount of data and that too for different patients. This is not possible with the help of traditional data processing and storing software. Hence, big data comes into the picture.

Predictive analysis is an important result of big data which ensures the patient's quality care and safety. It helps the doctors to give the right prescriptions to their patients keeping their medical histories in mind. Analytics can also be used by the medical researchers to observe the recovery rates of various cancer patients which may help them to find the treatments that have the highest rates of success. As the number of patients' increases, the volume of medical records also increases which stems the need of adopting a new approach called Electronic Health Records (EHRs), that organizes this data and makes it easier to have access to such data. Various real time monitoring systems and tools are offered by many healthcare centers to their patients like new wearable sensors which keep track of the patient's health trends right at their home, which will reduce the patient's visits to the clinics.(Chaturvedi et al., 2018)

Media and Entertainment

The media and entertainment sector is rapidly developing day by day. Development brings about creation of new content and an improvement in marketing and distribution. Many actionable points of action are provided by big data about thousands of individuals which are collected through various different data mining activities. Big data helps this sector by:

- Considering the needs and requirements of the audience
- Being open to optimization
- Consumer targeting for advertisement and marketing purposes
- New content development and content monetization (Boureau et al., 2001)

Government

In government processes, the same sets of data are used again and again across multiple platforms. Big data allows this and also offers cost innovation and productivity, thus allowing different departments to work together in association. As the government works in almost all the important sectors, the role of big data increases. Some major areas include:

- **Crime Prevention and Prediction**: Real time analytic systems can be used by the police and intelligence departments to observe and track crime patterns and criminal behavior.
- **Weather Forecasting:** Large amount of data at every instance of each day by using high end sensors and then use this information to predict the forecast for coming instances of time as used by NOAA.
- **Tax Fraud Identification**: Tax organizations can use big data to identify suspicious behavior and multiple or duplicate identities.
- **Drug Evaluation:** Big data can be used to access large amounts of data and help in the evaluation of treatment and drugs and thus save millions of dollars for the pharmaceutical companies.
- **Traffic Optimization:**The real time traffic data collected from sensors, GPS navigators, CCTV cameras, etc. can be used to solve the traffic problems in dense or congested areas by adjusting transportation routes accordingly.(Boureau et al., 2001; Chaturvedi et al., 2018)

Internet of Things (IoT)

Relation between IoT and Big Data

The quantity of gadgets inetrjoined to the internet is growing day by day at a rapid rate. These devices will obviously generate a huge amount of data which will increase in quantity with the number of devices. This data will need to be stored, organized and processed and hence, big data comes into the picture.

Role of Big Data in IoT

In big data system, heavy quantity of unorganized data is generated by IoT devices and stored. Then this data can be processed or organized accordingly. Analysis of this data can be done using tools like Spark or Hadoop, Map-Reduce. This data needs light fastening speed of analysis as it is collected through the internet.

Interdependence Between Big Data and IoT

Big Data and IoT are not only mutually dependent but also hugely impact each other. As the number of IoT devices will increase, the demand for Big Data services will also increase gradually. This is because as the quantity of the generated data increases, traditional storage technology will be pushed to its limits and the demand for Big Data, which is a more advanced and developed data storage technology, will increase drastically. Therefore, more and more organizations will update, develop and work on their Big Data storage systems.(Arora et al., 2017)

1.2.3 Big Data Tools

For storage and analysis of the Big data, the main tools are:

a- Apache Hadoop: Java based free software framework to store a heavy amount of data effectively in the form of a cluster, Runs in parallel on a cluster to enable the user to process data across all the nodes.

b- Microsoft HD Insight: Big Data solution by Microsoft, using Azure Blob storage as the default file system, provides high availability with low cost.

c- Big Data in Excel: MS Excel can be used to access Big Data. MS Excel 2013 has a feature which allows the user to access the stored data in a Hadoop platform.

d- Presto: Open source Query engine, developed by Facebook, used to handle large amounts of data, not works on Map-Reduce data and can quickly retrieve data.

e- Poly Base: Works on SQL Server 2012 Parallel Data Warehouse (PDW), accesses the data stored in PDW, an appliance for data warehousing to process any related data and provide connectivity with Hadoop as well.(Haynes et al., 2005)

1.2.4 Big Data Security

It is a term used for all measures and techniques to secure the data and all the data analysis processes. The threats to data can include information thefts which can endanger critical and confidential information stored online. There are several ways to implement data security. One simple way is encryption. Encrypted data is useless to any third party as long as it does not have the key to access it. Data stays protected during both input and output processes. Another way of securing the data is by building a strong firewall, which act as strong data filters and avoid any external sources or third parties.(Rastogi, Chaturvedi, Satya, Arora, Yadav et al, 2018)

1.3 TTH (TENSION TYPE HEADACHE)

TTH stand for tension type headache. It is a condition of body in which one experiences ache/ pain like a physical weight or a tight band around your head. It can generally last for some days or can even continue long. TTH is different from migraine as it can be affected due to everyday activities, which is not in the case of TTH.

Tension type headache arises due to

- Constant stress
- Incomplete sleep
- Anxiety
- Depression
- Emotional Disturbance

More than half of the world experiences TTH in one form or the other. It has been called by different names over the years for example: tension headache, muscle contraction etc.(Cassel, 1997)

It is not accompanied by nausea or vomiting and is also not affected by physical factors. Thus one will continue to do his daily task without even knowing if he is suffering from such headache or not. It also does not have any visual disturbances. The pain in TTH spreads all over the head unlike migraine which pains only on a particular side of your head.

Symptoms of TTH include:

- Feeling of pressure across the forehead
- Aching head all over the area
- Tenderness of head and neck muscles etc.(Cassel, 1997)

TTH can be divided into two main types: Chronic and Episodic

Episodic Tension Headaches:

They can last from 30 minutes to about a week. It can also vary from 15 days in a month to about 3 months. It can also become chronic. One can have migraines if episodic headaches occur frequently.

Chronic Tension Headaches:

If the headache last for 15-20 days out of a month continuing for about 3 months it becomes chronic. It occurs early in the morning and its symptoms include: poor appetite, restlessness, lack of concentration and depression.

TTH varies in intensity, duration and location. Use of alcohol, stress, caffeine, cold, dental problem, eye strain, excessive smoking, tiredness etc. are the triggers of tension headaches. However one must remember they are not a brain disease.

An individual may suffer with this TTH in any age group however they are normal in adult age and older teens. It generally runs in families and is common in women.

Earlier reports which show the occurrence of tension type headaches is given below:

Figure 1. Stats of Occurrence of TTH as per different Countries (Episodic vs. Chronic)(Boureau et al., 2001)

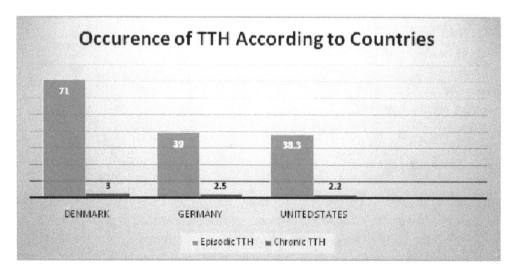

This graph shows various countries in which Episodic TTH and Chronic TTH is experienced by the people whether it is man or women. Around 71% and 3% people in Denmark are suffering, 39% & 2.5% in Germany and around 38.3% & 2.2% all are suffering by this disease.

1.3.1 Treatment

Massaging scalp, temples or bottom of your neck can help to relieve pain in a headache.

Over the countries pain killers such as ibuprofen, aspirin, paracetamol and naproxen are mostly used by patients suffering from TTH. These painkillers are used when the condition of headache becomes uncontrollable and interferes with your physical activities. However the treatment of TTH can vary according to the symptoms and triggers causing it.

Taking painkillers more than thrice a weak can be harmful and thus avoided by the patient. An individual is suggested to be in relaxation stage and tension free to avoid TTH. It is also suggested by experts to have a full sleep of 7-8 hours a day in order to be away from headaches. Other way is the use of tricyclic antidepressants. If your headache is caused due to psychological factors it may be hard to tackle. It is then advised to see a counselor or psychotherapist. If home remedies do not work then medical assistance may be needed by the doctor. Consumption of high quantity of acetaminophen can damage the liver. The heavy dose of analgesic like ibuprofen or aspirin can disturb one's stomach or damage the kidneys too.

When To Seek Medical Emergency?

One must seek medical emergency if

- Loss of balance, vision, speech, etc. occurs
- Headache starts suddenly and becomes uncontrollable
- Headache accompanied with high fever
- Headache pattern changes
- Medicines fail
- One has side effects from medicines such as pale skin, rashes, depression, nausea, vomiting, cramps, dry mouth etc.
- One is pregnant

One needs to learn to keep balance among alternative therapy with no-drug consumption, using right and necessary medications only and nurturing healthy habits. It is not necessary that one is having TTH only whenever headache happens. There may be sufficient chances of brain tumor or rupture of a weakened blood vessel also known as aneurysm in heavy TTH cases. One might also face headaches after a severe head injury. Protecting your head from such injuries is very important. Tension headaches are very common and it mars the QoL and efficiency and productivity in job along with life satisfaction. Such kind of aches checks an individual from active participation in different activities. One may need to take a break from job and be at home or even if one goes to work it may make your work impaired. (Satya et al., 2019; Wenk-Sormaz, 2005)

1.3.2 Preventions

Biofeedback Training: It is used to check some predefined body responses in constrained environment to decrease the pain. Some important body indications are used as parameters like muscle tension, heart rate and blood pressure.

Cognitive Behavioral Therapy: The method supports individual to learn how to handle stress and helps to shorten the frequency and severity of one's headaches.

Other Relaxation Techniques: Includes effective alternate therapies like deep breathing, yoga, meditation and progressive muscle relaxation etc.

As per different studies and reports, it has been found and established that TTH is directly correlated with demographical conditions, social culture across region as per age, gender of individual and stats analysis of data assessment. Large range of risk factors, new researches in genetic and neurobiological research have given a clear insight and in depth know how for TTH.

A majority of people with TTH do not seek medical attention thus it has been proven to be difficult to completely diagnose the exact effects, causes and preventions of TTH. Even adults with new bodily changes are likely to go through TTH. This report thus proves that further research is very necessary on this particular topic and must be done by the medical associations. (Carlson, 2013)

1.4 Biofeedback Therapy

Biofeedback Therapy is the process of collecting knowledge about the different psychological functions using some specific instruments. The major objective is to control and manipulate these functions. Some of these controllable functions or processes are important body functions like skin conductance, brainwaves, heart rate, pain perception and muscle tone. It may also be used to rectify psychological changes related to altering emotions, thoughts and human behaviour. This therapy is useful for treating migraines and headaches.(Chauhan et al., 2018)

1.4.1 History

The concept of homeostasis, i.e. the tendency of the body to stay hold in inner environment, was introduced by Claude Bernard in the year 1865. It was shown by J.R. Tarchanoff in the year 1885 that the voluntary control of the heart rate could be precisely direct without changing the breathing rate. The voluntary control of the retrahensaurem muscle which wriggles the ear was studied by J.H. Blair in the ear 1901. He discovered that this skill was learnt by the subjects by inhibiting interfering muscles and by the demonstration of the self regulation of the skeletal muscles. Conscious efforts were made by Alexander Graham Bell used 2 devices, the phonautograph invented by Edouard-Leon Scott's and a manometric flame, where he tried best to enable a deaf to speak. A theory was developed by mathematician Norbert Wiener proposing that control of systems is possible by monitoring their results. The popular word 'biofeedback' was given by feedback of Wiener in the conference in Santa Monica in 1969. As a result, the Bio-Feedback Research Society was founded that allowed isolated researchers to collaborate with each other and it popularised the term 'biofeedback' as well. (Chauhan et al., 2018)

1.4.2 Biofeedback And TTH

It is a non-pharmacologic, majorly used to treat the stress and headache and tension type headache. The key factors of efficiency, specificity and treatment moderators are measured by the meta-analysis of biofeedback for TTH.

It is suggest that biofeedback is good exercise for overcoming headache mainly tension type headache. Many studies has been carried out for Biofeedback for treatment of TTH and migraine. It was revealed that out off last three months at least four patients were been arm by this technique to cure headache.

Now a days the rate of headache and migraine disease is been increased upto 6 to 12. Mean patient age, where reported, ranged from 10.3 to 66.7 years (overall mean 35.9 years). The proportion of female patients varied from 43 per cent to 100 per cent (overall 71 per cent). Duration of TTH varied from 1.2 to 42.4 years (overall mean 13.9 years) (Chaturvedi et al., 2017).

Many techniques were used to survey this problem one of the technique is electromyography feedback (EMG-FB). Many factors are been observed for making the survey like Temperature feedback, galvanic skin response feedback and electroencephalography feedback. Many teenagers in this world are facing this problem a lot and they all are unaware of this technique. Biofeedback techniques is simply cure of TTH and other headache problem.

1.4.3 Biofeedback Application in Headache

Biofeedback is a technique where our body is been carried out by electrical sensor to monitors. It monitors oursthat function activities that is not able to recognize by our physical body.

Biofeedback take many measurement, like the important human body parameters heart rate, blood pressure, brain waves, skin temperature, anxiety, breathing rate etc. This helps us recognized that what inner problem our body is facing and we are not able to cure that in time.

By this treatment we are able to cure our headache and other problem like anxiety, high blood pressure etc. But in today world TTH i.e. tension type headache is a main problem that every single person in present generation is facing day by day. So it is a simple technique to cure headache. By doing many physical activities instead of eating medicines that can affect our body biofeedback technique in which person is not being effected by other problem.

1.4.4 Social Impact of TTH

TTH though is not very harmful as it is present in majority of the population. But to be true there are various social impacts of TTH. They can be described as below:

- It can result in lack of concentration at work.
- One may not be able to go to work due to this and constantly stay unhappy.
- It can also lead to anger and disturbed state of mind leading to unhealthy relationships with others.
- One may not be able to spend quality time with friends and family.
- Person suffering TTH may stay in depression and anxiousness for prolonged period of time.
- Person will find it difficult to stay socially active.

1.5 Social Records of TTH According to Gender And Age

Figure 2. Represents the Impact of TTH on Age Between Male and Female(Haynes et al., 2005)

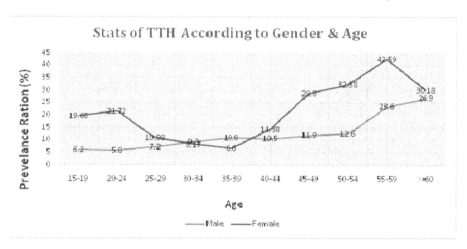

According to Type of TTH

Figure 3. Prevalence of Different Types of TTH [J. of Neurology & Neuroscience]

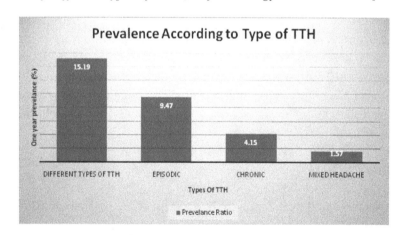

2 MENTAL HEALTH

2.1 Importance of Mental Health, Stress And Emotional Needs and Significance of Study

From ages, human has always been in search of peace. From 5000 B.C. to till date in first quarter of 21st century, from long time, man has developed many methods for recreation, entertainment and synergy.

As much as the life style went on hectic, population was increasing, limited resources of earth were not enough for all. To grab more and more resources, the natural life style vanished and the human race was collectively gripped into materialistic culture and accumulating tendency with consumerist life style.

It generated mass of stress and consequently clashes, disharmony, anxiety, depression and in extreme situation, the suicidal tendency. To meet these issues, the psychiatrist, psychologist, social analysts did in depth studies in their own ways and they found many alternative methods and treatments for same. In recent studies of this century, it has been well established that most of the human body diseases and abnormality is psycho somatically generated. In this research, the scholar have tried best the recent method(s) of alternative therapy like biofeedback which are getting popular due to their ease of applicability and no side effects on human brain and body.(Satya et al., 2018)

The Biofeedback therapies have been popular for long for the treatment of various mental challenges, stress and chronic headache like TTH type headache. Stress due to TTH headache is a very frequent occurrence in all our lives. A TTH symptom experienced for long by an individual with no relief or with increased frequency, it is termed as "distress". Weakened cognitive and physiological control is due to TTH originated stress and results in performance reduction. It can lead to symptoms like headache, gastrointestinal disturbances, elevated blood pressure, chest-pain, insomnia, peptic ulcers, sexual dysfunction, skin ailments, etc.(Satya et al., 2018)

The Life may be divided in four major stages of kid-life, childhood, adolescence and adulthood where the third one is having a transition and transformation. The misbalance of increasing Harmon, physical, mental and all kind of growths, body changes disturb the individual's mental piece in lack of right guidance and care.

In this crucial time, mostly the teenagers lose their mental balance, get violent and are unable to handle the pressure from peer, friends, parents and society. In opposition to this, those parents who rightly care their youngsters and treat them friendly behave sympathetically, less suffer with these issues in their families.

Major emotions of an individual are fear, anger, love, jealousy, guilt and worries. Wise people handle them carefully and stops the cycle within them instead of spreading them. They enjoy their family relations, office work and social relations and treat them as their duty. So in this research work, the author team tried to find the impact of positive ideas on mood states of personality for mental health (Anxiety, Stress, Depression, Aggression, Fatigue, Guilt, Extraversion and Arousal on the students and technocrats of our institutes. [DSVV and ABES Engineering College Ghaziabad].(Rastogi, Chaturvedi, Satya, Arora, Singhal et al, 2018; Scott & Lundeen, 2004)

2.2 Mental Health Introduction

Mental Health has been always the prime concern of intellectuals, behavioral scientists and social study makers. Now a days, its of a prime concern and happiness index has been considered as an integral part of progress of any country. Less wok has been experimented in South Ashian region regarding mental health correlated with social parameters of age, gender

Defined by Kornhauser (1965)"connotates those behaviours, perceptions and feelings that determines a person's overall level of personal effectiveness, success, happiness and excellence of functioning as a person."(Sharma et al., 2018)

It depends on the development and retention of goals that are neither too high nor too low to permit realistic successful maintenance of belief in one's self as a worthy, effective human being (Lakshminarayan & Prabhakaran, 1993). So a mentally healthy person is firm in his intentions and is least distributed by strains and stresses of day to day life.(Haddock et al., 1997)

As per the Medilexicon's medical dictionary, "A state of emotional and psychological wellbeing in which an individual is able to use his or her cognitive and emotional capabilities, function in society, and meet the ordinary demands of everyday life."

WHO has also accepted the fact and reframe its definition of complete health as individual mental, physical, social and spiritual well being is termed as complete health.

Therefore has found a balance in his or her social, emotional and psychological areas of life. – [John M. Grohol, Psy.D]

In 2007, WHO has stated, Mental health is about: the feeling for ourselves, others and our demands from life. It has also stated the difference between mental ill health and illness. It states that mental unfitness vanishes the chance of potentials and causes serious problems.

In case of mental issues, the recovery/management may be ensured in the form of counseling or psychotherapy, drug treatment and lifestyle changes. Stats says that approximately 25% of the people in UK have a mental health problems during their lives whereas the USA is said to have the highest incidence of people diagnosed with mental health .(Arora et al., 2019; Vyas et al., 2018)

2.3 Factors Affecting Mental Health

According to Joel L. Young M.D, there are 9 main symptoms or components that challenge to individual's mental health- Daily exercise and social activity Level, Smoking, Diet pattern, Physical activity in form of bodily work, Abuse or misbehave, Social and Community Activities in residence, Relationships with peer and office mates, practice of meditation and other relaxation techniques, use of alternate therapies and priority to healthy sleep.(McCrory et al., 2001; Rastogi, Chaturvedi, Satya, Arora, Sirohi et al, 2018)

2.4 Problems and Needs of Adolescents

On the basis of age group adolescence is categorized into (20-26)years of age or according to early principles (13-18)years that mainly depends on physical growth and development.

Physical, Emotional, Social and Intellectual Development are 4 major types.

Following needs and life goals appear to be a source of many emotional problems of adolescents.

Need for social status, acceptance and security, independence, adventure, self-support, belongingness. Adjustment to personal appearance, physical and psychological changes, Use of alcohol and drugs, Need of heterosexual relations and a theory of life.(Saini et al., 2018; Turk et al., 2008)

3. BIOFEEDBACK

3.1 Biofeedback With EEG Instrument (Earlier Experiments)

Biofeedback is a method of neuro therapy, a forward moving regression and self controlled relaxation technique to handle the stress and TTH (Wenk-Sormaz, 2005). It helps subject to know the current stress level and to handle them.

The Biofeedback is an alternative popular therapy used for QoL and strengthen the adjustment skills. (Baum, Herberman, & Cohen, 1995). Mcdowell (2015) found that silent meditation, yoga and Indian spiritual exercises have very deep effect on the subconscious of patient and refines their ill personality factors. Chambers et al.,(2008) in their research, recruited 20 mediation practitioners for 10 days meditative therapy process and established the high reported concentration, confidence and peace of mind. They also reported the decrement in the negative emotions and ill effects as compared to non experimental control group. They also witnessed less demotivating components and reduced rumination. (Fig.7)

3.2 Sensor Modalities

Popularly 3 standard organizations responsible for controlling and marking the biofeedback process, therapy, symptoms and effects are AAPB, BCIA and ISNR,they unanimously reached the common definition of biofeedback in 2008: "Biofeedback is a process to make capable an individual to learn to alter physiological activity to strengthen the purposes rectifying the health and performance. There are very high accurate instruments to record physiological activity through body functions like brainwaves, heart function, breathing, muscle activity, and skin temperature. These instruments rapidly and accurately 'feedback' information to the user. As time passes, these alterations can sustain without rapid use of an instrument (Rastogi, Chaturvedi, Satya, Arora, Singhal et al, 2018)".

Types of Biofeedback

Electroencephalography (EEG): It is an electrophysiological monitoring technique which is used to track the brain's electrical activity. EEG is generally non-invasive, electrodes are placed along the scalp, although sometimes invasive electrodes may be used too. Brain neurons have ionic current which is measured by voltage fluctuations. It is generally used to diagnose epilepsy. It can also be used to diagnose coma, brain death, sleep disorders, encephalopathy, depth of anaesthesia, stroke, tumours and other brain disorders.(Rastogi, Chaturvedi, Satya, Arora, Singhal et al, 2018)

Electrocardiography (ECG): The process of generating an electrocardiogram, electrodes are placed on the skin, is called electrocardiography (ECG). Small electrical changes produced as a result of the cardiac muscle polarisation and depolarisation during each heartbeat are detected by these electrodes. Inadequate artery blood flow, electrolyte disturbances and numerous cardiac abnormalities can result in changes in the normal ECG pattern.(Scott & Lundeen, 2004)

Electromyography (EMG): The electro diagnostic technique used to track and evaluate the electrical activity of the skeletal muscles is known as electromyography (EMG). It is carried out by using an instrument known as electromyograph, which generates a record called electromyogram. The electric potential produced by the electrically or neurologically activated muscle cells is detected by the electromyograph. Upon evaluation and analysis, to analyse the biomechanics of human and animal movement, these signals can be used to detect recruitment order, medical abnormalities or activation level.(Sharma et al., 2018)

Galvanic Skin Response (GSR): The features and characteristic of our body where rapid variations on electrical characteristic of skin are measured I very important biofeedback indicator. The gadget to record this feature is called Galvanic Skin Response (GSR). The resistance of the skin changes as per nature of the sweat glands in the individual's skin. Skin conductance indicates physiological or psychological arousal. If the sympathetic nervous system gets aroused, then sweat gland activity increases, which results in the increase of skin conductance. Skin conductance measures the sympathetic and emotional responses. Recent studies show that there is much more about GSR than meets the eye, and further research and study is going on this field. It is also known as Electro dermal activity (EDA), Electro dermal response (EDR), skin conductance, psychogalvanic reflex (PGR), etc.(Haddock et al., 1997)

Electrical characteristic of the skin of human body are measured under electro dermal activity (EDA) (Fig.8) EDA has also been known as Skin Conductance, Galvanic Skin Response (GSR), Electro Dermal Response (EDR), Psycho Galvanic Reflex (PGR), Skin Conductance Response (SCR), Sympathetic Skin Response (SSR) and Skin Conductance Level (SCL).(Rastogi, Chaturvedi, Satya, Arora, Sirohi et al, 2018)

At Subconscious state, the cognitive and emotional level of human behaviour are modulated by autonomous way for sympathetic activity of skin conductance. So it helps to get right evaluation of autonomous emotional regulation. Fingers, palms, and soles of feet and other human extremities exhibit various bio-electrical phenomena.(McCrory et al., 2001)

Figure 4. Experiment of Biofeedback Machines   *Figure 5. Recording of Biofeedback Data*

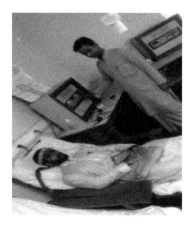
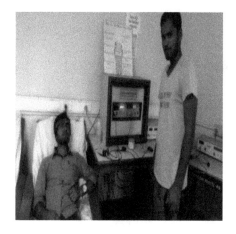

Figure 6. Eight Factors of Mood State(Arora et al., 2019)

DEPENDENT VARIABLE:-

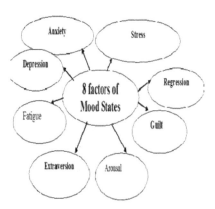

Figure 7. Process of Mind(Arora et al., 2019)

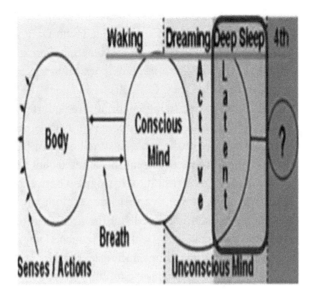

Table 1. Primary and secondary Variables of EMG-GSR Biofeedback Process (Haynes et al., 2005)

Variables	EMG	GSR	Control
Average frequency of headache per week	56	55.9	25.8
Average intensity of headache per week	58.2	56.3	46.5
Average duration of headache per week	75.7	63.6	49
SF-36 physical score	25	26	21
SF-36 mental score	25.1	19.5	21.7
SF-36 total score	28.5	30.5	21.7

4. LITERATURE REVIEW

There are various researches are carried out on stress and illness. Design of EMG model for biofeedback is efficient and it decides some protocol that would be for TTH. The main mode to treat people who are affected from TTH is Pharmacotherapy, it is very effective in decreasing the extent and duration of TTH. But it also have drawback as it is all over used as antidepressant medicine and those have risk of having adverse effect. Other than that it has potential risk for analgesic medication because of the overuse. In 2008 there was an article which state the efficiency of biofeedback in treating TTH. Galvanic skin resistance(GSR) therapies are used to treat these headaches and are found very effective. At times,it can be very severe that it becomes difficult to differentiate among tension type headache and migraine attack. The most commonly used preventive measures include medications such as allopathic treatments and non-medication treatments such as biofeedback therapies. The term "tension type headache" (TTH) has been declared through the International Classification Headache Diagnosis I (ICHD I). The terms "tension" and "type" represents its different meanings and reflect that there are sort of mental or physical tension could cause an impact. However, studies at large extent at this topic shows that there somehow a doubt about its neurobiological nature(McCrory, D., 2001).

TTH is the most basic form of headache occurring in about three quarters of the world. Tension type headache can usually last from 31 minutes to 8 days. The pain is generally mild and moderate in most of the times and sometimes it is worst. There are no diagnosis tests to conform Tension type headache(TTH). Galvanic skin resistance(GSR) therapies are used to treat these headaches and are found very effective. At times, it can be very severe that it becomes difficult to distinguish between tension type headache and migraine attack. The most commonly used preventive measures include medications such as allopathic treatments and non-medication treatments such as biofeedback therapies. The term "tension type headache" (TTH) has been declared by the International Classification Headache Diagnosis I (ICHD I). The terms "tension" and "type" represents its different meanings and reflect that some sort of mental or muscular tension could cause a impact. However, studies at large extent at this topic shows that there somehow a doubt about its neurobiological nature(Rubin, A., 1999). It is one of the common form for headache and in normal cases people took it lightly and they don't consult to the doctor and they treat themselves with various drugs in most cases people got cured but sometime the drugs have chronic impact on the health which could be severe(Kropotov, 2009; Millea & Brodie, 2002).To our knowledge no study has been done so far to find out the effectiveness of auditory, visual or integrated (audio- visual) EMG feedback in TTH patients.(Bansal et al., 2018; Kropotov, 2009; Millea & Brodie, 2002)

In a study, auditory EMG BF was used in TTH patients and it was found that the subjects were not only able to maintain low frontalis EMG levels but also managed to remain headache free during follow-up11. Similar studies utilizing only auditory BF have been performed in both TTH and migraine patients (Arora et al., 2017; Carlson, 2013; Chaturvedi et al., 2017; Chauhan et al., 2018). Visual EMG BF has been used less compared to auditory feedback15. In another study, TTH patients received both visual and audio EMG feedback and found significant decrease in headache (Crystal & Robbins, 2010; Mullaly et al., 2009).

Though there is evidence pointing out the efficacy of BF in tension headache patients, it is not advocated very frequently in India which could due to the cost of the equipment involved and hence the added cost to the patient as well. Most BF equipment provide both visual and audio feedback, hence if the equipment could be designed to provide only the form of feedback which is the most effective, it could automatically reduce the equipment cost as well as the cost to the patient making it more economical for both practitioner as well as patient.

No controlled trials have been done so far to compare the efficacy of visual EMG feedback or auditory EMG BF separately in tension type headache. This study therefore was conducted to find out relative efficacy of visual and auditory BF in isolation or combination in TTH subjects.(Lee & Yoon, 2017; Zanella et al., 2004)

5. STUDY PLOT

5.1 Independent Variable

5.1.1 Emotional Fulfillment

Basic human needs for emotional fulfillment are universal and include:

Love, Acceptance, Affection, Feeling valued, Appreciated, Secure, Companionship, Admiration, Trust, Respect, Understanding, Conversation, Communication.

In the theory of Self Actualization, Maslowin 1954 has given a hierarchy of human needs which are Psychological, safety, belonging, love, esteem needs and need of self-actualization.

Murrayin his studies proposed 12 physical needs and 28 psychological needs. Among them 20 important needs are as follows:Dominance, Sentience, Deference, Exhibition, Autonomy, Play, Aggression, Affiliation, Abasement, Rejection, Achievement, Succorance, Sex, Nurturance, avoidance, Ham avoidance, Dependence, Order, Counteraction, Understanding.

5.2 10 Steps to Emotional Fulfillment in Psychology Today (2012)

We all want to feel happy, and each one of us has different ways of getting there .Here are ten steps that help us to bring more happiness in our life.1-Be with others who make you smile.2-Hold on to your values. 3-Accept the good. 4-Imagine the best. 5-Do things you love. 6-Find purpose. 7-Listen to your heart. 8-Push yourself and not others. 9-Be open to change.10-Bask in the simple pleasure.(Binder & Blettner, 2015)

5.3 Stress

5.3.1-Models of Stress (Headache):3 Models in practice

1-General Adaptation Syndrome (Fig.9 and Fig.10) Stages:-Alarm, Resistance, Exhaustion2-Selye Eustress and Distress (Fig.11) 3-Lazarus: Cognitive appraisal Model

5.4-Types of Stress

Stress management can be very much worrying and disturbing, with three types of stress Acute stress containing Emotional Problem, Muscular Pressure, episodic acute stress and chronic stress each with its own characteristics, symptoms, duration and treatment approaches.(Fig.12 and Fig.13)

Figure 8. Stress and Syndromes(Arora et al., 2019)

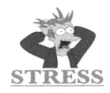

Figure 9. Phases of Stress(Arora et al., 2019)

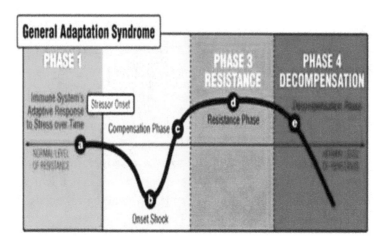

Figure 10. Graphical updates for Stress(Arora et al., 2019)

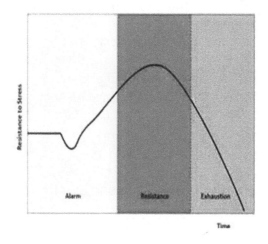

Figure 11. Different Body / Mood States(Arora et al., 2019)

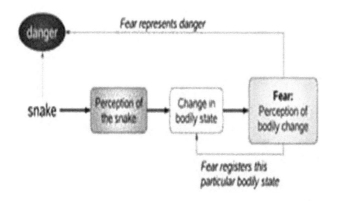

Figure 12. Stress Vs. Distress(Arora et al., 2019)

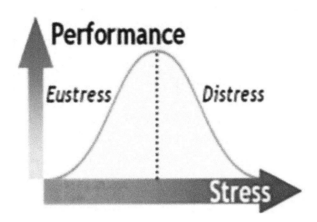

Figure 13. Levels of Stress(Arora et al., 2019)

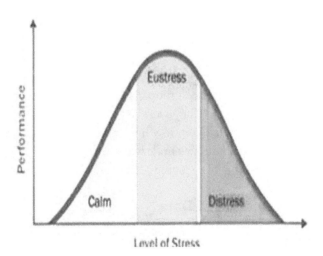

5.4.1-Causes of stress

In 1965, Korchin differentiated categories panic situations as below
1-Uncertainty and under stimulation, 2-Informative overload, 3-Danger, 4-Ego control failure, 5-Ego-mastery failure, 6-Self-esteem danger, 7-Other esteem danger .

5.4.1-Symptoms of Stress: Stress Warning indicators and Symptoms are as below

Cognitive symptoms consists of memory problem, inability to concentrate, poor judgment, seeing only the negative, anxious or reaching thoughts, constant worrying, the emotional symptoms deals with moodiness, Irritability or short temper, agitation, inability to relax, feeling overwhelmed, sense of loneliness and isolation, depression or general unhappiness and physical symptoms covers aches and pains, diarrheal or constipation, nausea, dizziness, chest pain, rapid heartbeat, low of sex drive, frequent colds, there is last variety of behavioural symptoms which deals with procrastinating or neglecting responsibilities, isolating oneself from others, sleeping too much or too little, eating more or less, nervous habits (e.g. nail biting, pacing), using alcohol, cigarettes, or drugs to relax.(Costa, 2014; Yadav et al., 2018)

5.5 Background and Purpose of Study With Experimental Setup

All the experiments are done in randomized, single blinded and protected environment so that the results wouldn't deviate much. Topics are taken from various neurology clinics and subjects referred by neurologists to the OPD of Hardwar Physiotherapy University.

5.5.1 Study Duration and Approval from Candidates

The candidates were taken from Middle of January '17 tillMay'18 and uptoJuly 2018. Candidates were taken in the experiment only after when we got a consent approval signed from them. Another information-Consent Form was signed by the ethical committee was got completed by the subjects and clinical verification for the experiment was recorded and clearance was given by the ethical committee formed by the University.

5.5.2 Intervention

When all the candidates are divided into three groups, all the candidates are informed about the treatment that is going to be tested upon them. They were given biofeedback training in a separated room of, Hardwar research laboratory, which had very low lighting and negligible external noise, so that they could remain in relaxation state. All candidates underwent respective (EMG/GSR) BF training for 20 minutes per session for 07 sessions(Turk, D. C. et al., 2008 and(Kropotov, J. D., 2009).

5.6 Methodology and Collection of Data

a- **Study Design:** This study will be a randomized, single blinded, prospective controlled trial.(Costa, 2014; Yadav et al., 2018)
b- **Source of Data:** Data will be obtained from the subjects recruited from various neurology clinics and subjects referred by neurologists to the outpatient department of Department of psychology, DevSanskritiVishwavidyalaya, Hardwar, Uttarakhand and ABESEC, Ghaziabad for biofeedback therapy.
c- **Study Duration:** Subjects will be recruited from June-2019 up to June-2020 and followed up till October-2020.
d- **Informed Consent:** Subjects will be recruited in the trial only after obtaining informed consent from them. (Informed Consent Form approved by the ethical committee attached).
e- **Sampling design:** Simple random sampling will be used with lottery method for allocation of subjects to seven groups. Subjects with stress and TTH(Tension Type Headache) will be enrolled in the study. Subjects who will not give consent and who will not meet the eligibility criteria will be excluded from the study. The rest of the subjects will be randomized using the lottery method for allocation. They will also be scrutinized after 30 days, 60 days.

f- **Allocation Procedure:** Chits numbered one to seven will be placed in a bowl and the subjects will be asked to pick the chits. Subjects with the following chit numbers will be allocated to the corresponding groups:

1: EMG auditory biofeedback (EMGa) group
2: EMG visual biofeedback (EMGv) group
3: EMG auditory +visual (EMGav) group
4: GSR auditory (GSRa) group
5: GSR visual (GSRv) group
6: GSR auditory +visual (GSRav) group
7: Control group

g- **Sample Size:** Sample size will be calculated using the following formula:

Probability of Type I error will be set at 0.05 Power of the study is expected to set at 80% (0.8).

Let p1= 1.0 and p2=0.75 are the mean differences of pre and post (baseline to one year) average frequency of headache per month in the EMG biofeedback training group and pain management group respectively from a study by (Mullay et al., 2009).

Let p=0.875 was calculated as (p1+p2)/2 and q=0.125 was calculated as 1-p. The sample size thus calculated was 26.6 per group. To accommodate for drop outs the sample size was chosen as 30 per group.(Binder & Blettner, 2015; Gupta et al., 2019; Singhal et al., 2019)

h- **Universe and Sample:** This study will be a randomized single blinded controlled prospective study. We will select a no. of recruited subjects n, h (f and m males) will be randomly assigned to seven groups receiving electromyography feedback auditory (EMGa) (let n =27), visual (EMGv) (let n=28), combined audio-visual (EMGav) (let n=27), galvanic skin resistance biofeedback auditory (GSRa) (let n =26), visual (GSRv) (let n=29) and combined audio-visual (GSRav) (let n=28) and a control group (let n = 27). Each subject (except the control group) will receive 10 sessions of respective biofeedback for 15 minutes each in an isolated room. The control group will receive only medication prescribed by their treating doctor. Each patient will be kept blinded to the type of biofeedback (EMG or GSR) being given. Pain variables (average frequency, duration and intensity of headache per week), SF-36 quality of life scores will also be measured from survey to all n subjects.

All the psycho challenged cases living in Uttarakhand and NCR region (Delhi, Meerut, Ghaziabad, Faridabad, Gurugram, Modinagar and Muradnagar) will be the universe of study. The college going students and Technocrats of different giant MNCs will be under study.

A control group of around 100 to 150 persons will be chosen and for carrying out this work the methodology employed shall be as follows:

(a). Literature survey.
(b). Identification of the location (Cluster near the region of NCR-national capital region Zone) and perform the study of different given parameters of the psychosomatic disorders due to life deregulation which disturb one's complete health.

(c). Development of a model of Biofeedback based experiments which will be performed at Research Labs and Scientific Spirituality Centers of DevSanskritiVishwaVidyalaya, Hardwar and Patanjali Research Foundations, Uttarakhand.

(d). Experimental investigation of Mental and spiritual health will be on various medical parameters.

(e). We will Apply some spiritual techniques as per the symptoms observed, suitable to the patient as per his/ her age, diet, culture and habits.

(f). Data Analysis of the Comparative study of both EMG and GSR machines with various spiritual techniques (Guided meditations) will be applied over the patients and their performance.

(g). Analysis of the results obtained and verification of the efficiency of the technique and suggesting appropriate one will be done in repeated process in case the method doesn't work.

(h). Impact of the result obtained on the society, the employee, company/ college and environment.

(i). 25% area (approximately 25 wards) out of 103 wards will be selected as sample purposively.

In the present study, samples of 95 adolescents are selected from ABESEC, Ghaziabad and DSVV Hardwar of graduation. Among these sample 55 are from urban area i.e. Lalquan and 50 are from rural area i.e. near to Pilkhua township in Ghaziabad.(Gulati et al., 2019; Saini et al., 2019; Singh et al., 2019)

6. RESULT AND DISCUSSIONS

6.1 Experiments and Results

Hypothesis:-There is a significant effect of Bio Feedback based self Guided meditation on Mental Health, stress management (Headache). There is a significant increase in the level of Stress Management (TTH) and emotional Needs by meditation practices.

-There is no significance difference in the mental health of adolescents due to meditation and therapy by EEG, GSR and EMG integrated audio-visual BioFeedback.

-There is no significant relation between mental health and stress relief practices.

Variables in the Study: Independent Variable- EEG inputs, Audio-visual EMG and GSR Biofeedback therapy, Mindful Meditation, Spiritual Attitude.

Dependent Variable- Stress Management, Tension Type Headache, Mental Health of Adolescents.

6.2 Experiments With EMG and GSR

Experiment with Audio-Visual EMG & GSR

Graphs were plotted in Anaconda Framework with the help of python programming.

Analysis (Fig. 14)-SF-36 test was applied on different subjects who experienced the audio-visual EMG therapy and graph shows the SF-36 Scores of 27 patients over the period of starting point, 30 days, 90 days, 180 days and 365 days, from the bar graph it is observed that the relative scores of all the patients have been increased.

Figure 14. Graph shows the SF-36 Scores of 27 patients over the period of starting point, 30 days, 90 days, 180 days and 365 days with EMGav therapy

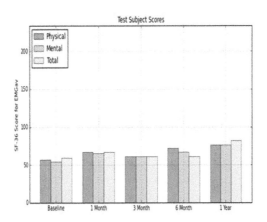

Analysis (Fig. 15)-The above graph shows the SF-36 Scores of 28 patients which were give audio-visual GSR therapy for 10 sessions each of 15 mins. And records were taken over the period of starting point, 30 days, 90 days, 180 days and 365 days, from the graph we may conclude that the relative scores of all the patients have been increased, so it validates the utility of therapy.

Figure 15. Graph shows the SF-36 Scores of 28 patients which were given audio-visual GSR therapy for 10 sessions each of 15 mins

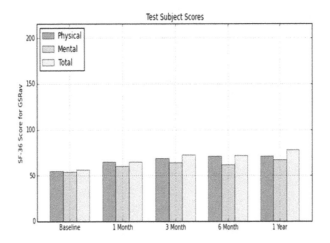

Analysis (Fig. 16)- 27 other subjects chosen for non experiment group and their SF-36 scores were recorded but it has been observed that over the period of Baseline, 1 Month, 3 Month, 6 Month, 1 Year. From the graph it is observed that the above scores increased.

From all of the 3 bar graphs, simultaneous observations may be made that relatively EMG and GSR group has experienced more growth than control group in their physical, mental and total scores than control group. BFB therapy application has shown significant reduction in stress (TTH).

Figure 16. SF-36 scores of 27 subjects chosen for non experiment (Control) group were recorded over a period of baseline

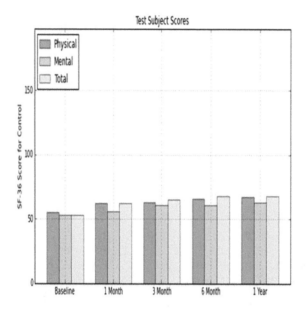

In EMG, Physical scores were constant around for 6 months and gradually increased in next half. In GSR, Physical scores kept on varying to increment continuously. In EMG, Mental scores were continuously increasing. In GSR, Physical scores kept on increasing continuously. Total scores in both were under fluctuation and varying but increasing timely.

Analysis(Fig. 17)-The above line graph shows the relation between Physical scores of audio-visual EMG, GSR, Control categories over the period of starting point, 30 days, 90 days, 180 days and 365 days,. From the graphs it is clear that the physical scores of EMG and GSR were better than have increased over the period of time. Initially the GSR superseded the EMG therapy up to around 6 months but in next half, EMG therapy showed significant increment over GSR and control groups.

Figure 17. Line graph shows the relation between Physical scores of audio-visual EMG, GSR, Control categories over the period of starting point, 30 days, 90 days, 180 days and 365 days

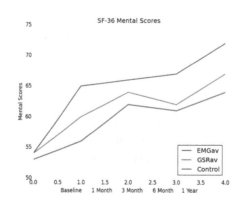

Analysis (Fig. 18)- The line graph showing the relation between Mental scores of audio-visual EMG, GSR, Control categories over the time period of Baseline, 1 Month, 3 Month, 6 Month, 1 Year. From very starting point, the EMG therapy showed the drastic increment continuously over GSR and control groups in overall experiment period.

Figure 18. Graph showing the relation between Mental scores of audio-visual EMG, GSR, Control categories over the time period of Baseline, 1 Month, 3 Month, 6 Month, 1 Year

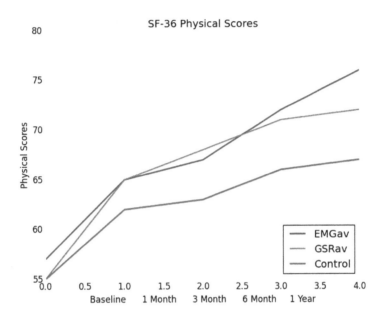

Analysis (Fig. 19): In overall score of EMG, GSR and control categories, we found that initially GSR and EMG were competing but in later half, EMG showed a clear win over GSR technique in dealing with the stress issue of subjects.

Analysis (Fig. 20): The above line graph shows the relation between Average frequency of headache for audio-visual EMG category over the period of starting point, 30 days, 90 days, 180 days and 365 days,. From the graphs it is clear that the frequency of EMG and GSR were decreased over the period of time.

Analysis (Fig. 21): The above line graph shows the relation between Average frequency of headache for audio-visual GSR category over the period of starting point, 30 days, 90 days, 180 days and 365 days,. From the graphs it is clear that the frequency of EMG and GSR were decreased over the period of time.

Analysis (Fig. 22): The above line graph shows the relation between Average frequency of headache for control category over the period of starting point, 30 days, 90 days, 180 days and 365 days,. From the graphs it is clear that the frequency of EMG and GSR were decreased over the period of time. On the other hand their control groups do show such results.

Analysis (Fig. 23): The following graph shows the score of REMG & VAS of 51 patients. X axis shows the score of VAG and REMG score is shown on Y axis. The X axis is also shows the serial number of patients. Graph shows the Fluctuating records of different patients with respect to their relative EMG scores and Visual analogue Score of Headache intensity in scale of 10.

Figure 19. Shows the overall score of EMG, GSR and Control categories

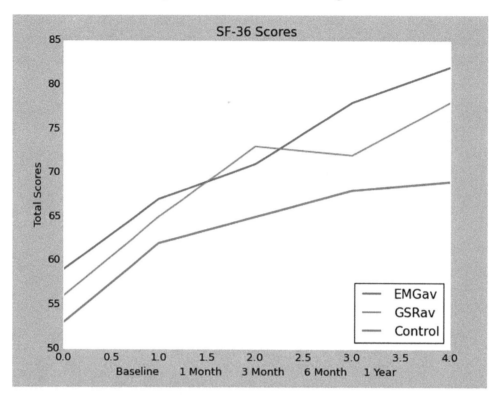

Figure 20. Above line graph shows the relation between Average frequency of headache for audio-visual EMG category over the period of starting point, 30 days, 90 days, 180 days and 365 days

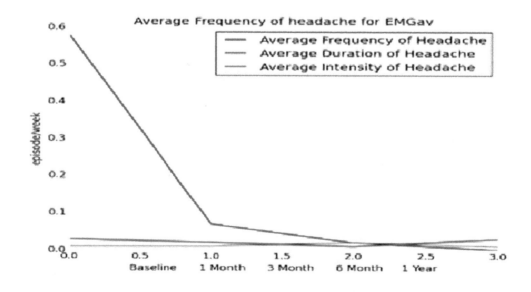

Figure 21. Line graph shows the relation between Average frequency of headache for audio-visual GSR category over the period of starting point, 30 days, 90 days, 180 days and 365 days

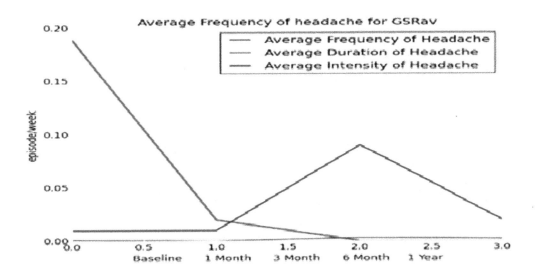

Figure 22. Line graph shows the relation between Average frequency of headache for control category over the period of starting point, 30 days, 90 days, 180 days and 365 days

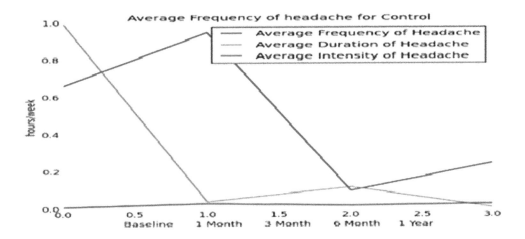

Analysis (Fig. 25): The waves are categorised majorly into four type's i.e. alpha, beta, gamma and theta. Alpha waves are considered to be the best while theta to be the worst. The coolest form of waves is the alpha waves which are considered to be released during meditation process.

Our experiment focussed on to measure the alpha waves before and after meditation and also considering the use of EEG for the same. The EEG machine we have done experiment is 32 channels and the 64 channels could not be used because it was costly. Observations were recorded with and without EEG machine and for pre and post meditation.

Figure 23. graph shows the score of REMG & VAS of 51 patients

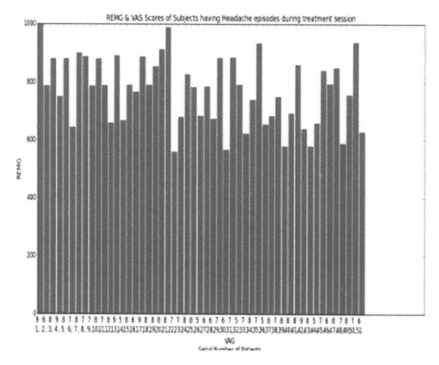

Table 2. EEG Recording in first Experiment

M1	3.84
M2	6.94
r	0.18
SDx	0.53
Sdy	1.06
SED	0.25
t-value	12.6

Table 3. EEG Recording in first Experiment

Name		Reading						Reading			
	Pre	Post	Alpha Waves/sec. .X	x=X-M1	x2	Pre	Post	Alpha Waves/sec. .Y	y-Y-M2	y2	X+Y
Raj	10	34	3.4	-0.44	0.189225	10	59	5.9	-1.04	1.0816	0.452
Radha	10	46	4.6	0.765	0.585225	10	56	5.6	-1.34	1.7956	-1.03
Monika	10	29	2.9	-0.94	0.874225	10	67	6.7	-0.24	0.0576	0.224
Harish	10	43	4.3	0.465	0.216225	10	89	8.9	1.96	3.8416	0.911
Ganga	10	32	3.2	-0.64	0.403225	10	49	4.9	-2.04	4.1616	1.295
Mradul	10	44	4.4	0.565	0.319225	10	66	6.6	-0.34	0.1156	-0.19
Mukesh	10	32	3.2	-0.64	0.403225	10	69	6.9	-0.04	0.0016	0.025

Table 4. EEG Recording in first Experiment

Savitri	10	29	2.9	-0.94	0.874225	10	79	7.9	0.96	0.9216	-0.9
Jaya	10	39	3.9	0.065	0.004225	10	74	7.4	0.46	0.2116	0.03
Rekha	10	44	4.4	0.565	0.319225	10	84	8.4	1.46	2.1316	0.825
Poornima	10	39	3.9	0.065	0.004225	10	62	6.2	-0.74	0.5476	-0.05
Manoj	10	37	3.7	-0.14	0.018225	10	87	8.7	1.76	3.0976	-0.24
Mukul	10	44	4.4	0.565	0.319225	10	72	7.2	0.26	0.0676	0.147
Suresh	10	33	3.3	-0.54	0.286225	10	72	7.2	0.26	0.0676	-0.14
Savita	10	46	4.6	0.765	0.585225	10	69	6.9	-0.04	0.0016	-0.03
Anmol	10	38	3.8	-0.04	0.001225	10	72	7.2	0.26	0.0676	-0.01
Mradul	10	36	3.6	-0.24	0.055225	10	49	4.9	-2.04	4.1616	0.479
Veerendra	10	39	3.9	0.065	0.004225	10	67	6.7	-0.24	0.0576	-0.02
Akhilesh	10	42	4.2	0.365	0.133225	10	72	7.2	0.26	0.0676	0.095
Nupur	10	41	4.1	0.265	0.070225	10	74	7.4	0.46	0.2116	0.122
		Sum	76.7	Ex	5.6655			138.8	Ey	22.668	Exy 2.012
		M1	3.835		0.283275		M2	6.94		1.1334	
				SD1	0.532236				SD2	1.0646	

Figure 24. Graph shows the alpha waves for some subjects recorded within a particular interval of time

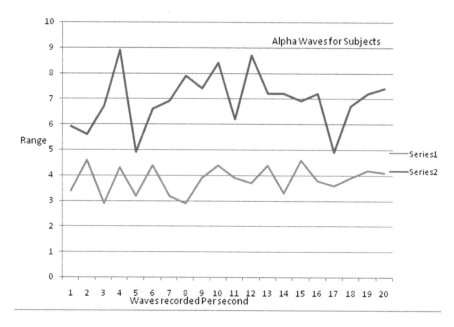

Figure 25. Graph shows the alpha waves of subjects recorded after meditation

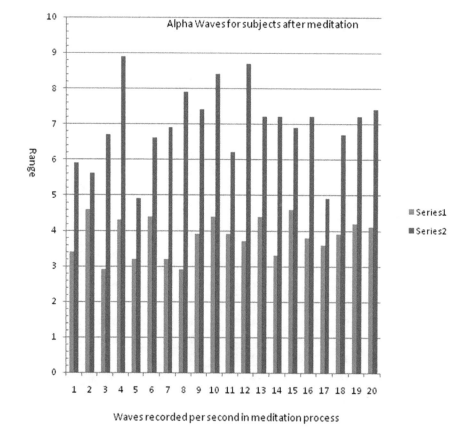

Table 5. Second Experiment Readings on EEG

Name	Age	Sex	Pre	Post	Alpha Waves/sec..X	x=X-M1	x^2	Pre	Post	Alpha Waves/sec..Y	y=Y-M2	y2		X*Y
				Alpha EEG for combined Before experiment						Alpha EEG for combined After Experiment Reading				
Rakhi	23	F	10	51.7	5.17	0.04	1.600E-03	10	92.7	9.27	2.25	5.0625		0.09
Anamika	24	F	10	41.3	4.13	-1	1.000E+00	10	72.3	7.23	0.21	0.0441		-0.21
Sanjeev	23	M	10	60	6	0.87	7.569E-01	10	100.3	10.03	3.01	9.0601		2.6187
Sudha	25	F	10	73.7	7.37	2.24	5.018E+00	10	97	9.7	2.68	7.1824		6.0032
Ankita	26	F	10	46.7	4.67	-0.46	2.116E-01	10	63	6.3	-0.72	0.5184		0.3312
Satyendra	24	M	10	63	6.3	1.17	1.369E+00	10	78	7.8	0.78	0.6084		0.9126
Sumit	21	M	10	29.7	2.97	-2.16	4.666E+00	10	64	6.4	-0.62	0.3844		1.3392
Jitendra	22	M	10	56	5.6	0.47	2.209E-01	10	68.7	6.87	-0.15	0.0225		-0.0705
Chhaya	22	F	10	44.7	4.47	-0.66	4.356E-01	10	102.3	10.23	3.21	10.3041		-2.1186
Aneeta	24	F	10	41.3	4.13	-1	1.000E+00	10	70.7	7.07	0.05	0.0025		-0.05
Shobheet	32	M	10	44	4.4	-0.73	5.329E-01	10	63.3	6.33	-0.69	0.4761		0.5037

Table 6. Second Experiment Readings on EEG

Name	Age	Sex	Pre	Post	X	x=X-M1	x^2	Pre	Post	Y	y=Y-M2	y2		X*Y
Ajeet	25	M	10	47.3	4.73	-0.4	1.600E-01	10	60.7	6.07	-0.95	0.9025		0.38
Swati	24	F	10	43	4.3	-0.83	6.889E-01	10	67.7	6.77	-0.25	0.0625		0.2075
Naveen	24	M	10	53.3	5.33	0.2	4.000E-02	10	59	5.9	-1.12	1.2544		-0.224
Meenakshi	23	F	10	47.7	4.77	-0.36	1.296E-01	10	43.3	4.33	-2.69	7.2361		0.9684
Anshu	21	M	10	67.7	6.77	1.64	2.690E+00	10	52	5.2	-1.82	3.3124		-2.9848
Surakhsha	21	M	10	40.7	4.07	-1.06	1.124E+00	10	64.3	6.43	-0.59	0.3481		0.6254
Sheela	24	M	10	52.3	5.23	0.1	1.000E-02	10	52	5.2	-1.82	3.3124		-0.182
Asif	24	M	10	60.3	6.03	0.9	8.100E-01	10	52.7	5.27	-1.75	3.0625		-1.575
Sameer	26	M	10	64.3	6.43	1.3	1.690E+00	10	63.5	6.35	-0.67	0.4489		-0.871
				Sum	102.87	Ex					138.75	Ey	Exy	5.694
				M1	5.134				M2	7.02				0.2847
						SD1	1.02				SD2	1.62		

Table 7. Second Experiment Readings on EEG

Alpha EEG-Combine			Alpha EEG-For Male			Alpha EEG-For Female	
M1	5.134		M1	4.98		M1	5.28
M2	7.02		M2	5.94		M2	4.73
N	20		N	10		N	10
r	0.52		r	0.24		r	0.71
SDx	1.02		SDx	0.87		SDx	1.26
SDy	1.62		SDy	0.79		SDy	1.55
SEMx	0.24		SEMx	0.29		SEMx	0.42
SEMy	0.37		SEMy	0.26		SEMy	0.52
SED	0.108		SED	0.115		SED	0.14
t-value	0.01		t-value	8.42		t-value	20.16
Sig	0.01		Sig	0.01		Sig	0.01

The initial experiment was for a group of 13 subjects of different genders. The readings for alpha waves without using EEG were 3.4,4.6,2.9,4.3 and so on while for after using EEG were 5.9,5.6 and so on respectively. We then calculated the standard derivative and the rank relation coefficient for the two values and concluded that they are very very less correlated (0.18). The values of SD1 and SD2 were 0.53 and 1.06 respectively. Also the test conducted result in a t-value of 12.6.

Experiment 2

Figure 26. Graph shows the alpha EEG for subjects recorded after stress relief exercises

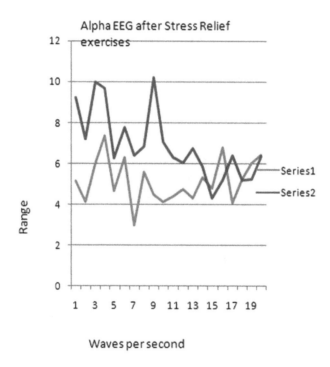

Analysis (Fig. 26, 27)

The same experiment was repeated for another 18 subjects for pre and post stress relief exercises. The observations were recorded as they were previously done. The alpha waves measured for before experiment were recorded to be 5.17, 4.13, 6, 7.37 and so on. The observations were however this time divided based on gender and also a combined observation was recorded. The readings were different for some subjects while same for some subjects and differed for each subject. The value of SD1 and SD2 for combined data was recorded to be 1.02 and 1.62 respectively. The rank correlation coefficient was 0.52. However a very low value of T was recorded i.e. 0.01. The study could be better experimented using 64 channel EEG but due to some limitations we were unable to do so. The 64 channel EEG machine is costly and can be used for a large sample of data.

Figure 27. Bar graph showing alpha EEG after for subjects after stress relief exercises

Alpha EEG after Stress Relief exercises

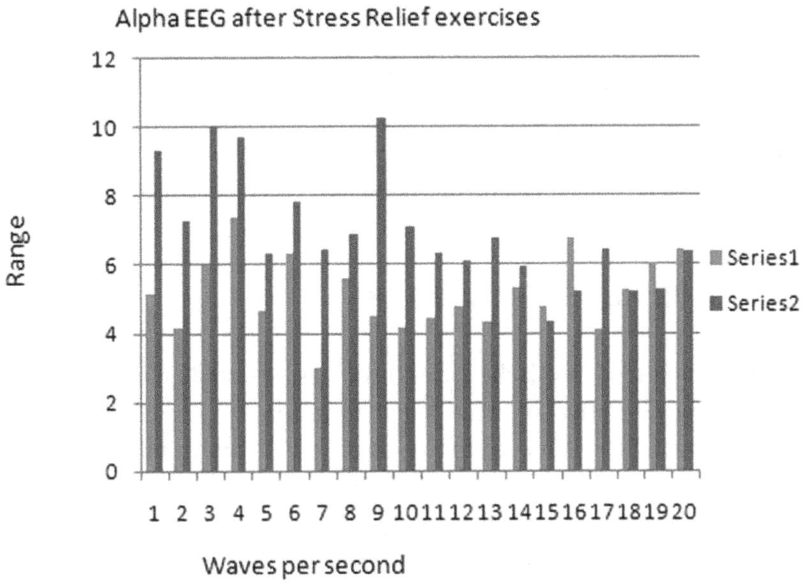

6.4 The Discussion on Quality of Life

Since in the duration of 1 year, only 22 subjects participated fully so we are considering only them. Likewise BF too is a learning process which therefore can be assumed to be facilitated by providing audio and visual cues to the patients. In our study there was significant improvement of stress variables and SF-36 sum and sub-scores in audio-visual EMG group indicating that integrated feedback is effective than that of GSR.

Increasing stress levels in people nowadays is creating higher tension levels ultimately results in chronic headaches. One of the most prominent headache is Tension Type Headache (TTH) creating unendurable mental disorders. Main life events such as divorce, surgery and loss of close relatives, family members inculcate major negative effects. Such events in the previous year have been considerably related to the persistence of headache.

The main aim of our research is to study the effects of tension type headache using biofeedback therapies on various modes such as audio modes, visual modes and audio- visual modes. The experiment was conducted on 90 people out of which 78 people remains till the end of medical treatment. In 78 people, 46 were females and 32 were males and it was recorded that females had higher levels of headaches in younger ages. The groups were randomly allocated for Galvanic Skin Resistance (GSR) therapies and the other one was control group (the group which was not under any type of allopathic or other medications).Except control group, other groups were treated in a session for 20 minutes in isolated chambers. The results were recorded over a specific period of time say 1 month, 6 months or 12 months.

In this study, authors have also tried their best to check the effect of TTH over Age and Gender. TTH is one of harmful headache, TTH is produced by Stress, it may start at any stage of life. Subjects usually suffer from two type of TTH i.e. for short time and for long time. When subjects suffer from long time, then it affects both mind and body. So, one may check at which age it started and how the gender is affected by this problem.

Another study similar to ours in terms of methodology, in which EMG and GSR BF were used for relaxation training. In this study the subjects were randomly assigned to four groups:1) group receiving EMG-GSR audio BF with eyes closed, 2) group receiving EMG-GSR audio BF with eyes open, 3) group receiving EMG-GSR visual BF and4)control group which received no feedback. It was reported that group which received EMG audio BF with eyes closed showed better decrease in frontalis muscle activity as compared to other groups. However, integrated feedback was not used in this study.

7 NOVELTIES IN THIS RESEARCH WORK

Till date the field of tension type Headache (stress) was less covered area, the time, a systematic study has been conducted to show the effect of other than medication therapies like BFB therapy and comparing the results of EMG and GSR techniques for the effect of positive thinking to manage daily life stress and increase the capacity of problem solving. The study also shows the betterment of Bio Feedback mechanism in a long duration of 1 year, subsequently recorded the SF-36 scores in 4 quarters and ignites the path of alternative medication techniques to overcome stress, anxiety and depression like psycho challenges. That means we can use this term commonly but stress is not so easy to explain. Stress as a word means "to draw tight" and has been used to describe hardship, affliction, force, pressures, strain or strong effort. There are two higher mental processes. Problem solving has been conceived by psychologists as discovery of correct response to a problem or situation that is new and difficult to the individual. But decision-making refers to selection of a correct response, out of several correct responses already brought out and had been found that as people are getting older and older their problem solving ability is reducing. The paper has shown a clear path to find the relation of stress(headache), problem solving, decision making and physical and mental well being of individual.

Nowadays, stress is associated with everyone's life and every person of any society at some levels is affected by stress problems and thus suffer TTH. The work in this research is unique as it aims at reducing the headache level and to control the analgesic and prophylactic medications. Based on results it was seen the transfer of people from one group to other. As the number of sufferings are increasing in the society and the world, these type of researches provide a means to treat various disorders according to(Millea, J.P., Brodie, J.J., 2002) and (Mullaly, J.W., 2009).

8 FUTURE SCOPE, LIMITATIONS AND POSSIBLE APPLICATIONS

In our research work, the experiment was conducted on a limited and fixed number of patients. And depending on the needs, it may be experimented on various patients based on different type of factors like age, gender, climate, etc. Biofeedback therapies provide a way to treat mental disorders with minimal use of medications and these therapies conducted on different age groups, genders of various countries. Biofeedback therapies help individuals to improve their physical and mental health by gaining control on their bodies and minds. These therapies increase awareness of these functions,so patients can control stress and physical ailments. Although it is bit costly for common people and efforts have been made to make this therapy accessible to every group of society. These therapies are also useful in treating:

1. Alcohol use disorder
2. Drug addiction
3. Insomnia
4. Anxiety
5. Chronic pains
6. Migraines
7. Nausea

Various scientists believe that these therapies will bring a revolution in the treatment of TTH.The patients will be able to control their own pains and can record their real time reactionsas per(Crystal SC, Robbins MS, 2010) and (Zanella A. et al., 2004).

Our study based on TTH and the IOT will be very useful for studying on this topic in the future coming projects. It will be very useful and will aim to find effective solution to TTH in a tech effective manner. The development on this topic will prove very useful as each and every one around this world is suffering from TTH in one way or the other. Hence future scope regarding this topic is not just limited to studying it but will result in effective applications in coming future.

Limitation:

There have been several studies regarding TTH and use of IOT in such field but the studies have been limited merely to writings. The solution to TTH and its perfect cure is not yet found. With such high prevalence rate it becomes a necessity for researchers to have discussion over this topic and come to a final conclusion rather than relating to its symptoms and their cures. Thus important information must be deprived to plan the optimal treatment for TTH patients.

Significance:

This study covers all possible aspects of TTH, IOT and big data and their applications to field of medical study. It is done in a very short period of time but covers. As large area of population suffer from TTH thus it becomes a necessity to have a worthy and fruitful discussion and research on this topic. Topics like the causes, effects, cures, biofeedback therapies, future scope etc. have all been covered by the researchers but its effective application is yet to come. These studies will prove to be useful at the time of its application. This study needs to be done on a large scale in order to prove useful and bring out a solution.

9 CONCLUSION

From above experimentation, we may conclude that EEG, audio-visual EMG-BF and GSR-BF are effective in the treatment of stress (TTH), with facts of EMG-BF being more effective than GSR-BF. In this study, the experimental group showed significant reduction in the level of stress. Hence it can be proved by EMG and GSR biofeedback therapy concluded that continuous positive thinking has the capacity to reduce stress among students and increase their working performance.

In EMG and GSR, a prophylactic is a treatment used to prevent diseases from occurring. "Prevention is better than cure"; these treatments works on this principle. They are used to prevent something from happening, for example, a prophylactic hepatitis vaccine prevents the patient from getting hepatitis. These are also called anti-depressants as they help to reduce headaches. Results show that there is significant effect of the GSR therapy on the prophylactic treatment.

The license for practicing varies based on different health care provider and different countries. Though the practice of alternative medicine is illegal, yet it is promoted by various practitioner in cancer treatment. Alternative medicine is criticized for taking advantage of the weakest members of society. PM- Prophylactic Medication, other Anti-Depressants and AM- Alternative Medicines. Prophylactic id basically a Greek word which means "an advanced guard". A prophylactic medication of a treatment or a medication which is designed to prevent a disease which a subject is suffering from. EEG is also proved to be effective therapy.

ACKNOWLEDGMENT

Our Sincere thanks to all direct and indirect supporters and well wishers. Esteem gratitude to Management of Dev Sanskriti Vishwavidyalaya Hardwar and Shantikunj where the Bio Feedback experiments and study were conducted. Also the control group were designed at ABESEC so for the infrastructure, staff support and students of ABESEC, Ghaziabad. We Are specially thanked for their time contribution to be part of this study. We also convey gratitude to officers of DayalBagh Educational Institute for their mentorship and timely valuable suggestions.

REFERENCES

Arora, N., Rastogi, R., Chaturvedi, D. K., Satya, S., Gupta, M., Yadav, V., Chauhan, S., & Sharma, P. (2019). Chronic TTH Analysis by EMG & GSR Biofeedback on Various Modes and Various Medical Symptoms Using IoT. In Big Data Analytics for Intelligent Healthcare Management. doi:10.1016/B978-0-12-818146-1.00005-2

Arora, N., Trivedi, P., Chauhan, S., Rastogi, R., & Chaturvedi, D. K. (2017). Framework for Use of Machine Intelligence on Clinical Psychology to study the effects of Spiritual tools on Human Behavior and Psychic Challenges. *Proceedings of NSC-2017 (National System Conference).*

Bansal, I., Rastogi, R., Chaturvedi, D. K., Satya, S., Arora, N., & Yadav, V. (2018). *Intelligent Analysis for Detection of Complex Human Personality by Clinical Reliable Psychological Surveys on Various Indicators.* National Conference on 3rd MDNCPDR-2018 at DEI, Agra.

Binder, H., & Blettner, M. (2015). Big Data in Medical Science—a Biostatistical View. *DeutschesÄrzteblatt International, 112*(9), 137.

Boureau, F., Luu, M., & Doubrere, J. F. (2001). Study of experimental pain measures and nociceptive reflex in Chronic pain patients and normal subjects. *Pain, 44*(3), 131–138. PMID:2052379

Carlson, N. (2013). *Physiology of Behavior.* Pearson Education, Inc.

Cassel, R. N. (1997). Biofeedback for developing self-control of tension and stress in one's hierarchy of psychological states. *Psychology: A Journal of Human Behavior, 22*(2), 50-57.

Chaturvedi, D. K., Rastogi, R., Arora, N., Trivedi, P., & Mishra, V. (2017). Swarm Intelligent Optimized Method of Development of Noble Life in the perspective of Indian Scientific Philosophy and Psychology. *Proceedings of NSC-2017 (National System Conference).*

Chaturvedi, D.K., Rastogi, R., Satya, S., Arora, N., Saini, H., Verma, H., Mehlyan, K., & Varshney, Y. (2018). Statistical Analysis of EMG and GSR Therapy on Visual Mode and SF-36 Scores for Chronic TTH. *Proceedings of UPCON-2018.*

Chauhan, S., Rastogi, R., Chaturvedi, D. K., Satya, S., Arora, N., Yadav, V., & Sharma, P. (2018). Analytical Comparison of Efficacy for Electromyography and Galvanic Skin Resistance Biofeedback on Audio-Visual Mode for Chronic TTH on Various Attributes. Proceedings of the ICCIDA-2018.

Costa, F. F. (2014). Big Data in Biomedicine. *Drug Discovery Today, 19*(4), 433–440. doi:10.1016/j.drudis.2013.10.012 PMID:24183925

Crystal, S. C., & Robbins, M. S. (2010). Epidemiology of tension-type headache. *Current Pain and Headache Reports, 14*(6), 449–45. doi:10.100711916-010-0146-2 PMID:20865353

Fumal, A., & Scohnen, J. (2008). Tension-type headache: Current research and clinical management. *Lancet Neurology, 7*(2), 70–83. doi:10.1016/S1474-4422(07)70325-3 PMID:18093564

Gulati, M., Rastogi, R., Chaturvedi, D. K., Sharma, P., Yadav, V., Chauhan, S., Gupta, M., & Singhal, P. (2019). Statistical Resultant Analysis of Psychosomatic Survey on Various Human Personality Indicators: Statistical Survey to Map Stress and Mental Health. In *Handbook of Research on Learning in the Age of Transhumanism.* Hershey, PA: IGI Global. doi:10.4018/978-1-5225-8431-5.ch022

Gupta, M., Rastogi, R., Chaturvedi, D. K., & Satya, S. (2019). Comparative Study of Trends Observed During Different Medications by Subjects under EMG & GSR Biofeedback. *IJITEE, 8*(6S), 748-756. https://www.ijitee.org/download/volume-8-issue-6S/

Haddock, C. K., Rowan, A. B., Andrasik, F., Wilson, P. G., Talcott, G. W., & Stein, R. J. (1997). Home-based behavioral Treatments for chronic benign headache: A meta-analysis of controlled trials. *Cephalalgia, 17*(1), 113–118. doi:10.1046/j.1468-2982.1997.1702113.x PMID:9137849

Haynes, S. N., Griffin, P., Mooney, D., & Parise, M. (2005). Electromyographic BF and Relaxation Instructions in the Treatment of Muscle Contraction Headaches. *Behavior Therapy, 6*(1), 672–678.

Kropotov, J. D. (2009). *Quantitative EMG, event-related potentials and neurotherapy.* Academic Press.

Lee, C. H., & Yoon, H. J. (2017). Medical big data: Promise and challenges. *Kidney Research and Clinical Practice, 36*(1), 461–475. doi:10.23876/j.krcp.2017.36.1.3

McCrory, D., Penzien, D. B., Hasselblad, V., & Gray, R. (2001). *Behavioral and physical treatments for tension Type and cervocogenic headaches.* Foundation for Chiropractic Education and Research.

Millea, J.P., & Brodie, J.J. (2002). Tension type headache. *American Family Physician, 66*(5), 797-803.

Mullaly, J. W., Hall, K., & Goldstein, R. (2009, November/December). Efficacy of BF in the Treatment of Migraine and Tension Type Headaches. *Pain Physician, 12*(1), 1005–1011. PMID:19935987

Rastogi, R., Chaturvedi, D. K., Satya, S., Arora, N., & Chauhan, S. (2018). *An Optimized Biofeedback Therapy for Chronic TTH between Electromyography and Galvanic Skin Resistance Biofeedback on Audio, Visual and Audio Visual Modes on Various Medical Symptoms.* National Conference on 3rd MDNCPDR-2018 at DEI, Agra.

Rastogi, R., Chaturvedi, D. K., Satya, S., Arora, N., Singhal, P., & Gulati, M. (2018). Statistical Resultant Analysis of Spiritual & Psychosomatic Stress Survey on Various Human Personality Indicators. *The International Conference Proceedings of ICCI 2018.* DOI: 10.1007/978-981-13-8222-2_25

Rastogi, R., Chaturvedi, D. K., Satya, S., Arora, N., Sirohi, H., Singh, M., Verma, P., & Singh, V. (2018). Which One is Best: Electromyography Biofeedback Efficacy Analysis on Audio, Visual and Audio-Visual Modes for Chronic TTH on Different Characteristics. *Proceedings of ICCIIoT-2018.* https://ssrn.com/abstract=3354375

Rastogi, R., Chaturvedi, D. K., Satya, S., Arora, N., Yadav, V., Chauhan, S., & Sharma, P. (2018). SF-36 Scores Analysis for EMG and GSR Therapy on Audio, Visual and Audio Visual Modes for Chronic TTH. Proceedings of the ICCIDA-2018.

Rubin, A. (1999). Biofeedback and binocular vision. *Journal of Behavioral Optometry, 3*(4), 95–98.

Saini, H., Rastogi, R., Chaturvedi, D. K., Satya, S., Arora, N., Gupta, M., & Verma, H. (2019). An Optimized Biofeedback EMG and GSR Biofeedback Therapy for Chronic TTH on SF-36 Scores of Different MMBD Modes on Various Medical Symptoms. In Hybrid Machine Intelligence for Medical Image Analysis. Springer Nature Singapore Pte Ltd. doi:10.1007/978-981-13-8930-6_8

Saini, H., Rastogi, R., Chaturvedi, D. K., Satya, S., Arora, N., Verma, H., & Mehlyan, K. (2018). Comparative Efficacy Analysis of Electromyography and Galvanic Skin Resistance Biofeedback on Audio Mode for Chronic TTH on Various Indicators. *Proceedings of ICCIIoT-2018.* https://ssrn.com/abstract=3354371

Satya, S., Arora, N., Trivedi, P., Singh, A., Sharma, A., Singh, A., Rastogi, R., & Chaturvedi, D.K. (2019). Intelligent Analysis for Personality Detection on Various Indicators by Clinical Reliable Psychological TTH and Stress Surveys. *Proceedings of CIPR 2019.*

Satya, S., Rastogi, R., Chaturvedi, D. K., Arora, N., Singh, P., & Vyas, P. (2018). Statistical Analysis for Effect of Positive Thinking on Stress Management and Creative Problem Solving for Adolescents. *Proceedings of the 12th INDIA-Com*, 245-251.

Scott, D. S., & Lundeen, T. F. (2004). Myofascial pain involving the masticatory muscles: An experimental model. *Pain, 8*(2), 207–215. doi:10.1016/0304-3959(88)90008-5 PMID:7402684

Sharma, S., Rastogi, R., Chaturvedi, D. K., Bansal, A., & Agrawal, A. (2018). Audio Visual EMG & GSR Biofeedback Analysis for Effect of Spiritual Techniques on Human Behavior and Psychic Challenges. *Proceedings of the 12th INDIACom*, 252-258.

Singh, A., Rastogi, R., Chaturvedi, D. K., Satya, S., Arora, N., Sharma, A., & Singh, A. (2019). Intelligent Personality Analysis on Indicators in IoT-MMBD Enabled Environment. In *Multimedia Big Data Computing for IoT Applications: Concepts, Paradigms, and Solutions*. Springer. Advance online publication. doi:10.1007/978-981-13-8759-3_7

Singhal, P., Rastogi, R., Chaturvedi, D. K., Satya, S., Arora, N., Gupta, M., Singhal, P., & Gulati, M. (2019). *Statistical Analysis of Exponential and Polynomial Models of EMG & GSR Biofeedback for Correlation between Subjects Medications Movement & Medication Scores*. IJITEE, 8(6S), 625-635. https://www.ijitee.org/download/volume-8-issue-6S/

Turk, D. C., Swanson, K. S., & Tunks, E. R. (2008). Psychological approaches in the treatment of chronic pain patients- -When pills, scalpels, and needles are not enough. *Canadian Journal of Psychiatry*, 53(4), 213–223. doi:10.1177/070674370805300402 PMID:18478824

Vyas, P., Rastogi, R., Chaturvedi, D. K., Arora, N., Trivedi, P., & Singh, P. (2018). Study on Efficacy of Electromyography and Electroencephalography Biofeedback with Mindful Meditation on Mental health of Youths. *Proceedings of the 12th INDIA-Com*, 84-89.

Wenk-Sormaz, H. (2005). Meditation can reduce habitual responding. *Advances in Mind-Body*, 3(4), 34–39.

Yadav, V., Rastogi, R., Chaturvedi, D. K., Satya, S., Arora, N., Yadav, V., Sharma, P., & Chauhan, S. (2018). Statistical Analysis of EMG & GSR Biofeedback Efficacy on Different Modes for Chronic TTH on Various Indicators. *Int. J. Advanced Intelligence Paradigms*, 13(1), 251–275. doi:10.1504/IJAIP.2019.10021825

Zanella, A., Bui, N., Castellani, A., Vangelista, L., & Zorzi, M. (2004). Internet of things for smart cities. *IEEE Internet Things J.*, 1(1), 22–32. doi:10.1109/JIOT.2014.2306328

Chapter 26
ACO_NB–Based Hybrid Prediction Model for Medical Disease Diagnosis

Amit Kumar
Sanaka Educational Trust's Group of Institutions, India

Manish Kumar
Vellore Institute of Technology, Chennai, India

Nidhya R.
Madanapalle Institute of Technology & Science, India

ABSTRACT

In recent years, a huge increase in the demand of medically related data is reported. Due to this, research in medical disease diagnosis has emerged as one of the most demanding research domains. The research reported in this chapter is based on developing an ACO (ant colony optimization)-based Bayesian hybrid prediction model for medical disease diagnosis. The proposed model is presented in two phases. In the first phase, the authors deal with feature selection by using the application of a nature-inspired algorithm known as ACO. In the second phase, they use the obtained feature subset as input for the naïve Bayes (NB) classifier for enhancing the classification performances over medical domain data sets. They have considered 12 datasets from different organizations for experimental purpose. The experimental analysis advocates the superiority of the presented model in dealing with medical data for disease prediction and diagnosis.

INTRODUCTION

In recent years, the world has encountered huge challenges with respect to early detection and prediction of diseases (Ilayaraja & Meyyappan, 2013). A useful matching pattern, related information or information extraction is not at all a simple task. Due to unavailability of related tools and technique, the world

DOI: 10.4018/978-1-7998-2742-9.ch026

is facing problem in medical field. As the medical data belong to natural domain, therefore there is a possibility for the dataset for being imbalance, impure and may have vagueness. Due to above mentioned points and due to less information available in the literature, it is quite difficult to develop a disease prediction model for predicting the diseases (Matsumoto et.al. 2002).

In the recent past, due to the development of new technologies and related research, extracting medical data and availability of the same is easier than earlier. With availability of data, authors can now help in the discovery of disease diagnosis which can directly contribute in the knowledge discovery related to medical diseases and practitioners. As said earlier, the availability of medical data will help to improve the disease diagnosis and will help in the treatment methodology for numbers of diseases. Now days, several new technologies such as Cloud computing, IoT and Big data has emerged as a boom for information retrieval and mining of medical data. Many authors have proposed a centralized medical database for the recording and analysis of medical data at one place. These centralized databases are considered with the application of new technologies such as Cloud Computing and IoT (Aswin & Deepak, 2012). If authors can able to develop any such kind of medical centralized database for keeping the health records of the patients and related diseases details, then it will be easier for the doctors and medical practitioners to cure the disease (Seera & Lim, 2014). Industries and organizations have to come forward in order to build such kind of centralized system for medical data. Similarly, authors need to have some decision support tools for stepping forward in the direction of medical disease diagnosis. Furthermore, this can also be achieved if authors implement or use the Artificial Intelligence techniques. In the literature, a number of decision support tools have been proposed. Seera and Lim (Seera & Lim, 2014). have proposed a fuzzy min-max neural network which came out to be an efficient hybrid classification system for medical data. Another proposal given by Kahramanli and Allahverdi (Kahramanli & Allahverdi 2008) which is based on the application of artificial and fuzzy neural network. This classification system is developed for the diagnosis of diabetes and heart diseases. Similarly, in 2011 Lee and Wang (Lee & Wang 2011) designed a fuzzy based expert system to diagnosis diabetes. In 2014, another such kind of diseases prediction system was purposed by Kalaiselvi and Nasira (Kalaiselvi & Nasira, 2014). The presented method in (Kalaiselvi & Nasira, 2014) gives a model which is useful for diabetes diagnosis as well as cancer disease prediction. The model was based on Adaptive Neuro Fuzzy Inference System (ANFIS). Many review and comparisons were also presented by various authors round the globe for Medical Disease Diagnosis. In (Garg et.al 2005) Garg et al. presented an extensive review which shows the importance of computerized clinical decision support systems on patient outcomes and practitioner performances. Similarly, Kawamoto et al.(Kawamoto et.al. 2005) presented a systematic review for identifying the important feature and parameters in order to improve and enhance the clinical practices using decision support system. Another approach was presented by Narasinga rao et al. (Narasinga rao et al. 2009), who designed a decision support system for diabetes with the application of multilayer neural networks. Moving further, authors in (Srimani & Koti, 2014) used a rough set method for producing optimal rule sets for medical related data. Ye et al. (Ye et al 2002) made research and development for finding the degree of malignancy in brain glioma by using fuzzy sets. As said in the previous paragraphs, Syeda-Mahmood (Syeda Mahmood 2015) has given a plenary talk on the role and application of machine learning algorithms in modern clinical decision support systems. Wagholikar et al. (Wagholikar et al. 2012)has made a survey report on modeling paradigms for medical diagnostic decision systems. Recently, an investigation for developing an intelligent system were purposed with the help of computer vision and image procession (Martis et.al 2015). Similar to the above concept presented in (Martis et.al 2015), Rajinikanth et al. (Rajinikanth et al. 2017) also presented an approach for segmentation of the brain tumor from MR Images using TLBO approach. Recently, in 2018, Kumar and Sarkar (Kumar,& Sarkar 2018) proposed a hybrid predictive model integrating C4.5 and Decision Table classifiers for medical data sets. Kumar and Sarkar (Kumar,& Sarkar 2017) also proposed a performance analysis of GA-based iterative and non-iterative learning approaches for medical domain data sets. In 2018, Kumar and Sarkar (Kumar,& Sarkar 2018) also proposed a hybrid classifier by combining GA with DTNB for medical data diagnosis.

In the proposal of Soliz et al (Soliz et.al 2008), authors presented an approach for extracting image-based features for classifying Age Related Macula Degeneration (AMD) in digital retinal image. In this approach, hundreds of images were classified into thousand different categories based on the visual characteristics of the disease. In (Soliz et.al 2008), the concept of Independent Components Analysis (ICA) is being used for feature selection and for giving input to classifiers. By referring to various literature studies, authors can assume that ICA technique is very much capable for robustly detect and characterized features in funds images, and also to extract mathematical features from each image in order to define the phenotype.

Authors (Deka & Sarma, 2012) used the application of ANN technique, Principle Component Analysis (PCA) and singular value decomposition (SVD) for diabetes detecting. The results so obtained is very much reliable in terms of cost and accuracy. The feature extraction methods presented in (Deka & Sarma, 2012) can be utilized for some related diseases such as ophthalmologists.

Considering the above paragraphs and literature studies mentioned in this article, authors can clearly say that there is a tremendous awareness observed in the field of medical disease diagnosis. The presented study says that how the world of medical science is moving towards the use of automated system and new techniques such as Artificial intelligence and fuzzy sets. Using these techniques, clearly projects toward the risk forecasting and prediction for numerous diseases. In spite of the several developments mentioned above, there is still need for the development of standard feature selection tools and techniques. Referring to various literature studies, it can be said that an efficient subset selection criteria is needed in order to improve the results of the classifiers.

For this study, authors have consider a bio-inspired algorithm (ACO) which will act over real dataset to select the real set of feature and then a well-known naïve Bayes classifier is applied to train over the medical domain data sets. Finally, the knowledge gained by classifier is used for evaluating the test case and comparison of test result.

The coming sections are arranged as follows: Next section will highlight the related terms that may be useful for the reader for having an insight view of the presented article. Thereafter, the proposed approach is presented i.e hybrid model for disease diagnosis. Moving further, result, analysis and conclusion is presented in the sections that follows.

BACKGROUND

Feature Selection

Feature selection is a method of filtering the valid elements or attributes by discarding the redundant or irrelevant data. These irrelevant data may increases unnecessary search space, and overhead which may led to a problematic situation at the time of processing the data. Feature selection is the selection of best feature among all available features. In (Ladha et al 2011) and authors in their study of feature selection presented and compared different feature selection algorithm.

ACO

ACO is a new bio-inspired meta-heuristic optimization technique which work on the principle of real activities and functions of ants. The concept of ACO was presented way back in 1990 by M. Dorigo and colleagues. This concept of ACO was developed based on the movement and activities followed by the ant and their colonies. In this technique, ethnologists made one experimental approach to find the optimal path followed by a swarm of ants in search of food. It was also observed that, while ant moves towards food they communicate with other ant by releasing a chemical substance known as pheromones also known as pheromones trail. In case, suppose an ant gets isolated from the group, then it uses the pheromones to decide which path to follow in search of group of ants or food. Such a repeating process is categorized by a positive feedback loop.

(i) Specifying the number of ants followed the previously constructed path or modify a path.
(ii) Updating the pheromone trail.

The construction or modification of a solution path is performed in a probabilistic way. The pheromone trails are modified keeping in mind the quality of current solution and evaporation rate.

Naive Bayes

Naïve Bayes is one of the most studied Bayesian classifier since 1950s. This classifier is used to calculate the probabilities of different classes given some observed evidence in the purpose of classification. This classifier is called naïve due to its feature in which it assumes that all attributes are independent of each other and are not related at all. This kind of methods are well suited for high dimensional input data. Naive Bayes models work on the principle of applying the method to maximum likelihood for estimation of parameters. Although, it is well known fact that authors don't have any complicated iterative parameter estimation technique for naïve Bayes learners. Generally, it has been observed that Naïve Bayes performs well indifferent verities of complex and real world problems. In the current scenario of research and development, the classifier techniques and methods are well accepted for classifying natural and artificial related domains.

Proposed Hybrid Model

In this section, a detailed description of ACO based hybrid classification model is presented. Here, the presented model of ACO and naïve Bayes classifier tries to justify a separate classification model. The exact hybrid model presented here consists of two phases in sequence. In order to have a better understanding of the proposed model, authors have drawn a sketch for the same shown in Figure-1.

The presented model is made to receives a medical data as input with a given *features*. In the beginning phase, the process is started with generating a number of ants, m, that can be placed on the graph randomly, i.e. each ant starts with a random feature. From this phase, ants traverse edges probabilistically until and unless a stopping condition for traversal is met. The resulting subsets that are received from the

Figure 1. Proposed Hybrid Model

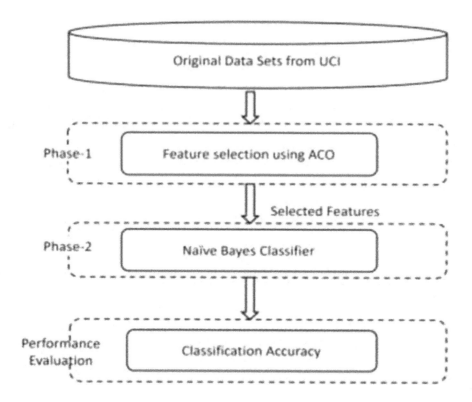

previous phase are combined and then evaluated. If an optimal subset in terms of results is achieved or there is small difference after a certain number of iteration, then it is assumed that the obtained result is the best optimal result that authors can have. If both the above criteria fails to give a satisfactory result, then one`s again a new set of ant is created, pheromones are updated and the process goes for iteration one`s again. At last, authors have a reduced feature set of medical data. The process of ACO feature selection shown in Figure-2.

In the next phase, the 5-fold cross validation technique is used to calculate the overall classification performance of the proposed model.

EXPERIMENTAL DESIGN AND ANALYSIS

This section detailed the experimental design and their result analysis.

Experiments

In order to judge the performance of the presented model, experiments were conducted which are denoted by E_1 and E_2. In E_1 authors are performing the selection of relevant features by using ACO whereas in E_2 the selected feature is operated using naïve Bayes. Weka package 3.7.2 is used for experimental analysis and implementation of Bayesian classifier NB. Furthermore, an ACO-based feature selection

Figure 2. Feature selection using ACO

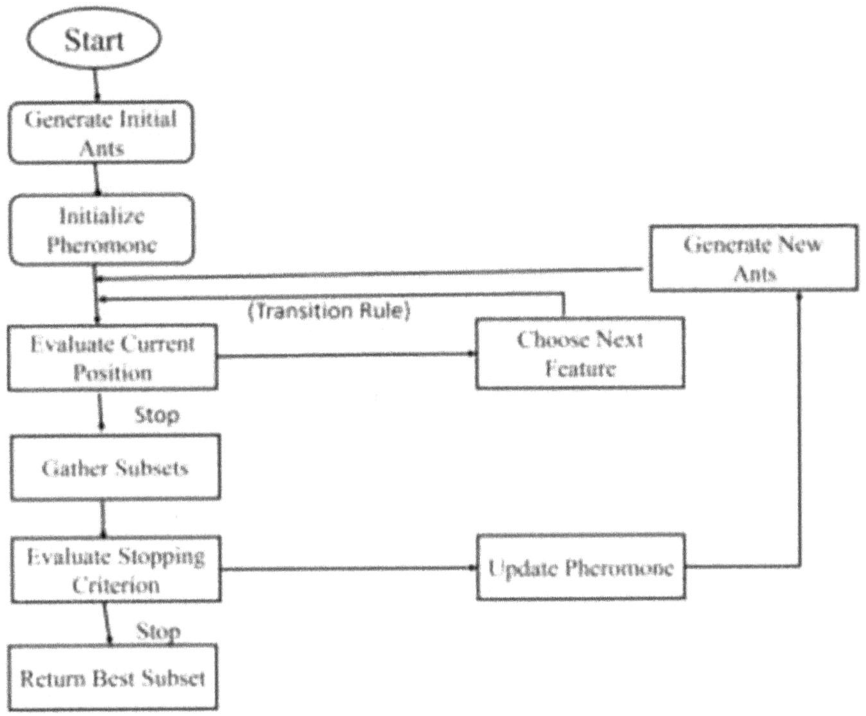

method is also implemented and executed by using Weka package 3.7.2. The presented model now is experimentally analyzed over 12 standard medical data sets taken from UCI repository and evaluated over correctly classified instances which are measured in terms of accuracy.

Results and Discussions

For the experimental purpose, authors have adopted 5-fold cross validation technique to measure the performance of the classifier (in terms of mean percentage accuracy) for diseases prediction. In addition to above, the in-built implementation technique of Weka package has also been considered. In each fold, the classifier is trained which is used to test the other fold for calculation of average trained accuracy. Here, authors have taken a sum of 100 outcomes of the classifier to calculate the average accuracy over each fold. Furthermore, authors have also evaluated the proposed classifier over F-measure, error rate, recall and precision. All these factors helped to achieve a comparative result when compared to other classifier available in the same field. For a better understanding, a small description of the parameter used for evaluation are mentioned hereunder:

Accuracy: This may be seen as correct tuples or test cases classified by a classifier in terms of percentage.

Error rate: It is the misclassification rate.
Precision: This factor is related to the true features.

Recall or **Sensitivity:** It is known as the measure of completeness or the positive rate.
F-Measure: It is used to show the robustness and preciseness of the classifier.

This may please be noted that, the sensitivity factor which is discussed above is directly correlates to the prediction accuracy w.r.t a particular class (assume positive class), whereas accuracy is the prediction accuracy over all the available classes. Here, authors can say that recall and precision are related to an individual and are known as relevance measures.

Parameter Settings

The experiments demonstrated in this article are performed using an open software implementation tool for data mining known as Weka 3.7.2 package. The combination factor of both ACO and CFS base subset has been used to generate best feature subset. The parameter setting for ACO is as follows: population size = 1000, maximum generation = 100, $\alpha = 1.0$ and $\beta = 2.0$. Rest settings are assumed as default.

Table 1. Experimental results of ACO_NB based hybrid classifier

Problem name	Number of original features	Number of selected features	Accuracy (%)	Mean Error	Precision	Recall	F-Measure
Breast Cancer (Wisconsin)	15	4	55.78	0.487	0.778	0.846	0.647
Dermatology	38	19	89.89	0.018	0.995	0.849	0.648
Ecoli	9	8	78.45	0.049	0.765	0.748	0.751
Heart (Cleveland)	15	5	87.14	0.077	0.764	0.641	0.878
Heart (Hungarian)	18	2	81.48	0.117	0.648	0.849	0.699
Heart (Swiss)	15	5	52.79	0.278	0.402	0.317	0.247
Hepatitis	22	12	84.19	0.157	0.948	0.647	0.791
Lung Cancer	60	8	72.48	0.348	0.789	0.618	0.781
Lymphography	14	18	84.21	0.124	0.765	0.613	0.615
New-thyroid	6	10	98.74	0.029	0.815	0.819	0.832
Pima-Indians	9	7	87.14	0.279	0.874	0.647	0.798
Primary Tumor	19	21	43.87	0.058	0.548	0.579	0.579

The result depicted in table 2, shows the improvement of Baysian classifier over other nature –inspired algorithms [19][20]. Its also advocates the superiority of the presented approach when compared to other standard methods from the same field. The presented approach also speeded up the computational time for modeling the classifier. This says that the relevant feature selection through ACO contributes an effective role to design a good model. The experimental analysis presented in this study are performed on ACERASPIRE notebook computer with P6200 @ 2.13 GHZ CPU running Microsoft Windows 10 and 4 GB RAM.

Table 2. Comparative results of ACO_NB, GA_NB and PSO_NB hybrid classifiers

Problem Name	GA_NB	PSO_NB	ACO_NB
Breast Cancer (Wisconsin)	74.87	74.82	**78.25**
Dermatology	98.08	98.36	**98.79**
Ecoli	85.41	**86.01**	74.48
Heart (Cleveland)	84.15	82.50	**89.47**
Heart (Hungarian)	**83.67**	80.95	82.14
Heart (Swiss)	39.02	38.21	**49.27**
Hepatitis	86.45	83.87	**98.65**
Lung Cancer	**75.01**	59.37	67.79
Lymphography	80.40	**83.10**	67.25
New-thyroid	97.20	97.20	**98.74**
Pima-Indians	77.47	74.80	**79.87**
Primary Tumor	47.78	44.24	**51.78**

Figure 3. Comparative mean accuracy percentage chart for proposed model

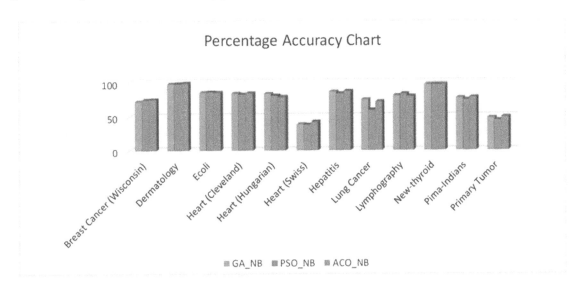

In order to have a better visualization of the presented result in Table 2, the same has been presented in the form of graph in Figure 3.

CONCLUSION AND FUTURE SCOPE

A large number of classification methods for medical disease diagnosis were proposed in recent past. But, all have certain drawback with respect to vagueness of patient's data and disease specificity. This study present a comparative analysis of most of the standard data set related to medical disease diagnosis. On the basis of the claimed results, it can be concluded that the model presented in this article outperformed most of the standard models (i.e. GA_NB and PSO_NB) in treatment and diagnosis of distinct diseases. It improves the reliability over medical domain data sets. However, the presented model proved to be insufficient when tested over lymphography ecoli, lung cancer and heart (Hungarian) related data set. The main reason behind the failure of the proposed model for some datasets is their complex structure.

REFERENCES

Aswin, V., & Deepak, S. (2012). Medical Diagnostics Using Cloud Computing with Fuzzy Logic and Uncertainty Factors. *International Symposium on Cloud and Services Computing*, 107-112. 10.1109/ISCOS.2012.29

Deka, A., & Sarma, K. (2012). SVD and PCA Feature for ANN Based Detection of Diabetes Using Retinopathy. *Proceedings of the CUBE International Information Technology Conference*, 38-44. 10.1145/2381716.2381725

Garg, A. X., Adhikari, N. K., McDonald, H., Rosas-Arellano, M. P., Devereaux, P. J., Beyene, J., Sam, J., & Haynes, R. B. (2005). Effects of computerized clinical decision support systems on practitioner performance and patient outcomes: A systematic review. *Journal of the American Medical Association*, *293*(10), 1223–1238. doi:10.1001/jama.293.10.1223 PMID:15755945

Ilayaraja, M., & Meyyappan, T. (2013). Mining medical data to identify frequent diseases using Apriori algorithm. *International Conference on Pattern Recognition, Informatics and Mobile Engineering*. 10.1109/ICPRIME.2013.6496471

Kahramanli, H., & Allahverdi, N. (2008). Design of a hybrid system for the diabetes and heart diseases. *Expert Systems with Applications*, *35*(1), 82–89. doi:10.1016/j.eswa.2007.06.004

Kalaiselvi, C., & Nasira, G. M. (2014). A new approach for diagnosis of diabetes and prediction of cancer using ANFIS. *Computing and Communication Technologies (WCCCT), World Congress, IEEE*, 188-190.

Kawamoto, K., Houlihan, C. A., Balas, E. A., & Lobach, D. F. (2005). Improving clinical practice using clinical decision support systems: A systematic review of trials to identify features critical to success. *BMJ (Clinical Research Ed.)*, *330*(7494), 765. doi:10.1136/bmj.38398.500764.8F PMID:15767266

Kumar, A., & Sarkar, B.K .(2017). Performance analysis of GA-based Iterative and Non-iterative Learning Approaches for Medical Domain Data Sets. *International Journal on Intelligent Decision Technologies, 11*(3), 321-334.

Kumar A., & Sarkar, B.K. (2018). A Hybrid Predictive Model Integrating C4.5 and Decision Table Classifiers for Medical Data Sets. *Journal of Information Technology Research, 11*(2), 150-167.

Kumar, A., & Sarkar, B. K. (2018). GA_DTNB: A Hybrid Classifier for Medical Data Diagnosis. *6th International Conference on Frontiers in Intelligent Computing Theory and Applications (FICTA-2018)*, *2*, 139-148. 10.1007/978-981-10-7566-7_15

Kumar, A., & Sarkar, B. K. (2018). Performance analysis of nature inspired algorithms based Bayesian prediction models for medical data sets. *Soft Computing Based Non-linear Control Systems Design, 7,* 134–155.

Ladla, L., & Deepa, T. (2011). Feature Selection Methods And Algorithms. *International Journal on Computer Science and Engineering, 3*(5), 1787–1797.

Lee, C. S., & Wang, M. H. (2011). A fuzzy expert system for diabetes decision support application. *IEEE Transactions on Systems, Man, and Cybernetics. Part B, Cybernetics, 41*(1), 139–153. doi:10.1109/TSMCB.2010.2048899 PMID:20501347

Martis, R.J., Lin, H., Gurupur, V.P., & Fernandes, S. L. (2017). *Frontiers in development of intelligent applications for medical imaging processing and computer vision.* Academic Press.

Matsumoto, T., Ueda, Y., & Kawaji, S. (2002). A software system for giving clues of medical diagnosis to clinician. *Proceedings of 15th IEEE Symposium on Computer-Based Medical Systems (CBMS 2002),* 65-70. 10.1109/CBMS.2002.1011356

Narasingarao, M.R., Manda, R., Sridhar, G.R., Madhu, K., & Rao, A.A. (2009). *A clinical decision support system using multilayer perceptron neural network to assess well being in diabetes.* Academic Press.

Rajinikanth, V., Satapathy, S. C., Fernandes, S. L., & Nachiappan, S. (2017). Entropy based Segmentation of Tumor from Brain MR Images–A study with Teaching Learning Based Optimization. *Pattern Recognition Letters, 94,* 87–95. doi:10.1016/j.patrec.2017.05.028

Seera, M., & Lim, C. P. (2014). A hybrid intelligent system for medical data classification. *Expert Systems with Applications, 41*(5), 2239–2249. doi:10.1016/j.eswa.2013.09.022

Soliz, P., Russell, S. R., Abramoff, M. D., Murillo, S., Pattichis, M., & Davis, H. (2008). Independent component analysis for vision-inspired classification of retinal images with age-related macular degeneration. *South authors Symposium on Image Analysis and Interpretation,* 65-68.

Srimani, P.K., & Koti, M.S. (2014). *Rough set (RS) approach for optimal rule generation in medical datawork.* Academic Press.

Syeda-Mahmood, T. F. (2015). *Role of machine learning in clinical decision support (Presentation Recording). In SPIE Medical Imaging.* International Society for Optics and Photonics.

Wagholikar, K. B., Sundararajan, V., & Deshpande, A. W. (2012). Modeling paradigms for medical diagnostic decision support: A survey and future directions. *Journal of Medical Systems, 36*(5), 3029–3049. doi:10.100710916-011-9780-4 PMID:21964969

Ye, C. Z., Yang, J., Geng, D. Y., Zhou, Y., & Chen, N. Y. (2002). Fuzzy rules to predict degree of malignancy in brain glioma. *Medical & Biological Engineering & Computing, 40*(2), 145–152. doi:10.1007/BF02348118 PMID:12043794

KEY TERMS AND DEFINITIONS

Ant Colony Optimization (ACO): It is a probabilistic technique for solving computational problems which can be reduced to finding good paths through graphs by the ants.

Classifiers: A classifier is a machine-based learning methodology that can be used to discriminate different objects based on certain useful features.

Data Mining: It is a technique used to turn raw data into some useful information. By using software to look for patterns in large batches of data, companies can learn more about their customers to develop more effective marketing strategies, in order to increase sales and decrease costs.

Feature Selection: It is a method of filtering the valid attributes or elements by discarding the irrelevant or redundant data.

Medical Disease Diagnosis: It is a method of determining the disease by analyzing the symptoms from which a person is suffering.

Medical Technology: It is a broad field where innovation plays a crucial role in sustaining health. Areas like biotechnology, pharmaceuticals, AI, ML, Cloud Computing, IoT, information technology, the development of medical devices and equipment, and more have made significant contributions to improving the health of people across the globe.

Naïve Bayes: A Naive Bayes classifier is a probabilistic machine learning model that is used for classification tasks.

Compilation of References

Abdulkerim, M. (2013). *Towards integrating data mining with knowledge based system: the case of network intrusion detection* (Doctoral dissertation). Addis Ababa University.

Abecasis, G. R., Auton, A., Brooks, L. D., DePristo, M. A., Durbin, R. M., Handsaker, R. E., ... McVean, G. A. (2012). An integrated map of genetic variation from 1,092 human genomes. *Nature*, *491*(7422), 56–65. doi:10.1038/nature11632 PMID:23128226

Acharya, R., Kumar, A., Bhat, P. S., Lim, C. M., Iyengar, S. S., Kannathal, N., & Krishnan, S. M. (2004). Classification of cardiac abnormalities using heart rate signals. *Medical & Biological Engineering & Computing*, *42*(3), 288–293. doi:10.1007/BF02344702 PMID:15191072

Achour, S. L., Dojat, M., Rieux, C., Bierling, P., & Lepage, E. (1999). Knowledge acquisition environment for the design of a decision support system: application in blood transfusion. In *Proceedings of the AMIA Symposium* (p. 187). American Medical Informatics Association.

Activation functions in Neural Networks. (n.d.). https://www.geeksforgeeks.org/activation-functions-neural-networks/

Aemero, A., Berhan, S., & Yeshigeta, G. (2015). Role of health extension workers in eye health promotion and blindness prevention in Ethiopia. *JOECSA, 18*(2).

Agrawal, R., & Srikant, R. (1994). Fast Algorithms for Mining Association Rules. *Proc. of 20th International Conference on Very Large Data Bases,* 487–499. Retrieved from citeseer.ist.psu.edu/agrawal94fast.html

Agrawal, R., Somani, A., & Xu, Y. (2001). Storage and querying of e-commerce data. *VLDB, 1,* 149–158.

Ahmetov, I. I., & Fedotovskaya, O. N. (2015). Current Progress in Sports Genomics. *Advances in Clinical Chemistry*, *70*, 247–314. doi:10.1016/bs.acc.2015.03.003 PMID:26231489

Aich, S., Kim, H. C., Hui, K. L., Al-Absi, A. A., & Sain, M. (2019, February). A Supervised Machine Learning Approach using Different Feature Selection Techniques on Voice Datasets for Prediction of Parkinson's Disease. In *2019 21st International Conference on Advanced Communication Technology (ICACT)* (pp. 1116-1121). IEEE. 10.23919/ICACT.2019.8701961

Akdeniz, F., & Kayikcioglu, T. (2018). Detection of ECG arrhythmia using Zhao-Atlas Mark time-frequency distribution. *26th Signal Processing and Communications Applications Conference (SIU)*, Izmir, Turkey. 10.1109/SIU.2018.8404585

Akerkar, R., & Sajja, P. (2010). *Knowledge-based systems*. Jones & Bartlett Publishers.

Aksakal, B. (2014). Solving vehicle routing problem with time windows and spesific demands of a company by using genetic algorithm (Msc). Istanbul Technical University, İstanbul.

Alberto, J. V. (2011). Insights into the area under the receiver operating characteristic curve (AUC) as a discrimination measure in species distribution modelling. *Journal of Microbiology (Seoul, Korea)*.

Ali, L., Hussain, A., Li, J., Zakir, U., & Yan, X. (2014). Intelligent image processing techniques for cancer progression detection, recognition and prediction in the human liver. Proceedings on Computational Intelligence in Healthcare and e-health. doi:10.1109/CICARE.2014.7007830

Ali, C. M. (2007). Design of appropriate wavelet bases for texture discrimination. *Kuwait Journal of Science & Engineering, 34*(2).

Alqahtani, E. J., Alshamrani, F. H., Syed, H. F., & Olatunji, S. O. (2018, April). Classification of Parkinson's Disease Using NNge Classification Algorithm. In *2018 21st Saudi Computer Society National Computer Conference (NCC)* (pp. 1-7). IEEE. 10.1109/NCG.2018.8592989

Al-Saiyd, N. A., Mohammad, A. H., Al-Sayed, I. A., & Al-Sammarai, M. F. (2011). Distributed knowledge acquisition system for software design problems. *European Journal of Scientific Research, 62*(3), 311–320.

Altman, D. G., & Bland, J. M. (1994). Diagnostic tests. 1: Sensitivity and specificity. *BMJ*.

Ameta, M. A., & Jain, M. K. (2017, Feb.). Data Mining Techniques for the Prediction of Kidney Diseases and Treatment: A Review. *International Journal of Engineering and Computer Science*.

Amin, D., & Raja Azlina, R.M. (2013). Feature Selection Based on Genetic Algorithm and Support Vector Machine for Intrusion Detection System. *SDIWC*.

Amir, A., & Lipika, D. (2007). *A k-mean clustering algorithm for mixed numeric and categorical data*. Elsevier.

Amir, G., & Murtaza, H. (2015). *Beyond the hype: Big data concepts, methods, and analytics*. Elsevier.

Anand, A., & Shakti, D. (2015, September). Prediction of diabetes based on personal lifestyle indicators. In *2015 1st International Conference on Next Generation Computing Technologies (NGCT)* (pp. 673-676). IEEE. 10.1109/NGCT.2015.7375206

Anantharam, P., Barnaghi, P., & Sheth, A. (2013, June). Data Processing and Semantics for Advanced Internet of Things (IoT) Applications: modeling, annotation, integration, and perception. In *Proceedings of the 3rd International Conference on Web Intelligence, Mining and Semantics* (pp. 1-5). 10.1145/2479787.2479821

Anderson, R. M., & May, R. M. (1991). *Infectious Diseases of Humans: Dynamics and Control*. Oxford University Press.

Andreao, R., Dorizzi, B., & Boudy, J. (2006). ECG signal analysis through hidden Markov models. *IEEE Transactions on Biomedical Engineering, 53*(8), 1541–1549. doi:10.1109/TBME.2006.877103 PMID:16916088

Anitha, V., & Murugavalli, S. (2016). Brain tumour classification using two-tier classifier with adaptive segmentation technique. *IET Computer Vision, 10*(1), 9–17. doi:10.1049/iet-cvi.2014.0193

Ansari, S., Duda, M., Horan, K., Andersson, H. B., Goldberger, Z. D., Nallamothu, B. K., & Najarian, K. (2015). A Review of Automated Methods for Detection of Myocardial Ischemia and Infarction using Electrocardiogram and Electronic Health Records. *IEEE Reviews in Biomedical Engineering*.

Antonini, M., Barlaud, M., Mathieu, P., & Daubechies, I. (1992). Image coding using wavelet transform. *IEEE Transactions on Image Processing, 1*(2), 205–220. doi:10.1109/83.136597 PMID:18296155

Anuradha, B., & Reddy, V. (2008). ANN classification of cardiac arrhythmias. *Journal of Engineering and Applied Sciences (Asian Research Publishing Network), 3*(3), 1–6.

Arasu, S. D., & Thirumalaiselvi, R. (2017, February). A novel imputation method for effective prediction of coronary Kidney disease. In *2017 2nd International Conference on Computing and Communications Technologies (ICCCT)* (pp. 127-136). IEEE. 10.1109/ICCCT2.2017.7972256

Arı, A., & Berberler, M. E. (2017). Interface Design for Prediction and Classification Problems with Artificial Neural Networks. *Acta INFOLOGICA, 1*(2), 55–73.

Armon, C. (2003). An evidence-based medicine approach to the evaluation of the role of exogenous risk factors in sporadic amyotrophic lateral sclerosis. *Neuroepidemiology, 22*(4), 217–228. doi:10.1159/000070562 PMID:12792141

Aron, J. L., & May, R. M. (1982). *The Population Dynamics of Infectious Disease: Theory and Applications*. Chapman and Hall.

Astorino, A., Fuduli, A., Gaudioso, M., & Vocaturo, E. (2019, June). Multiple Instance Learning Algorithm for Medical Image Classification. SEBD.

Astorino, A., Fuduli, A., Veltri, P., & Vocaturo, E. (2020). Melanoma detection by means of Multiple Instance Learning. *Interdisciplinary Sciences, Computational Life Sciences, 12*(1), 24–31. doi:10.100712539-019-00341-y PMID:31292853

Astrid, S., & Gerhard, H. (2010). Linear Regression Analysis. *Deutsches Ärzteblatt International*. PMID:21116397

Aswin, V., & Deepak, S. (2012). Medical Diagnostics Using Cloud Computing with Fuzzy Logic and Uncertainty Factors. *International Symposium on Cloud and Services Computing*, 107-112. 10.1109/ISCOS.2012.29

Atkins, M. S., & Mackiewich, B. T. (1998). Fully automatic segmentation of the brain in MRI. *IEEE Transactions on Medical Imaging, 17*(1), 98–107. doi:10.1109/42.668699 PMID:9617911

Auton, A., Brooks, L. D., Durbin, R. M., Garrison, E. P., Kang, H. M., Korbel, J. O., ... Abecasis, G. R. (2015). A global reference for human genetic variation. *Nature, 526*(7571), 68–74. doi:10.1038/nature15393 PMID:26432245

Awad, H. A. (2006). *A novel particle swarm-based fuzzy control scheme*. Paper presented at the 2006 IEEE International Conference on Fuzzy Systems. 10.1109/FUZZY.2006.1681969

Ayday, E., Raisaro, J. L., McLaren, P. J., Fellay, J., & Hubaux, J. P. (2013). Privacy-preserving Computation of Disease Risk by Using Genomic, Clinical, and Environmental Data. *USENIX Workshop on Health Information Technologies*.

Ayub, S., & Saini, J. P. (2011). ECG classification and abnormality detection using cascade forward neural network. *International Journal of Engineering Science and Technology, 3*(3), 41–46. doi:10.4314/ijest.v3i3.68420

Bailey, N. T. J. (1975). *The Mathematical Theory of Infectious Diseases*. Griffin.

Bakare, E. A., Nwagwo, A., & Danso-Addo, E. (2014). Optimal Control Analysis of an SIR Epidemic Model with Constant Recruitment. *International Journal of Applied Mathematical Research, 3*(3), 273–285. doi:10.14419/ijamr.v3i3.2872

Baker, D. B., Kaye, J., & Terry, S. F. (2016). Governance through privacy, fairness, and respect for individuals. *EGEMS (Washington, DC), 4*(2), 1207. doi:10.13063/2327-9214.1207 PMID:27141520

Bala, S., & Kumar, K. (2014). A literature review on kidney disease prediction using data mining classification technique. *International Journal of Computer Science and Mobile Computing, 3*(7), 960–967.

Baldi, P., Baronio, R., & Cristofaro, E. D. (2011). Countering GATTACA: efficient and secure testing of fully-sequenced human genomes, *Proceedings of the 18th ACM Conference on Computer and Communications Security*. 691-702. 10.1145/2046707.2046785

Barabas, J., Babusiak, B., Gala, M., Radil, R., & Capka, M. (2012). Analysis, 3D Reconstruction and Anatomical Feature Extraction from Medical Images. *International Conference on Biomedical Engineering and Biotechnology*, 731-735. 10.1109/iCBEB.2012.72

Barman, T., Ghongade, & Ratnaparkhi, A. (2016). Rough set based segmentation and classification model for ECG. *IEEE Conference on Advances in Signal Processing (CASP)*, 18-23. 10.1109/CASP.2016.7746130

Basheer, I. A., & Hajmeer, M. (2000). Artificial neural networks: Fundamentals, computing, design, and application. *Journal of Microbiological Methods*, *43*(1), 3–31. doi:10.1016/S0167-7012(00)00201-3 PMID:11084225

Basile, T. M., Caponetti, L., Castellano, G., & Sforza, G. (2010). A Texture-Based Image Processing Approach for the Description of Human Oocyte Cytoplasm. *IEEE Transactions on Instrumentation and Measurement*, *59*(10), 2591–2601. doi:10.1109/TIM.2010.2057552

Batra, A., & Jawa, V. (2016). Classification of Arrhythmia using Conjunction of Machine Learning Algorithms and ECG Diagnostic Criteria. *International Journal of Biology and Biomedicine*, *1*, 1–7.

Batra, S. S. S., & Sachdeva, S. (2016). Organizing standardized electronic healthcare records data for mining. *Health Policy and Technology*, *5*(3), 226–242. doi:10.1016/j.hlpt.2016.03.006

Bayindir, R., & Sesveren, Ö. (2008). Design of a visual interface for ANN based systems. *Pamukkale University Journal of Engineering Sciences*, *14*(1), 101–109.

Beale T. (2008). The openEHR archetype model-archetype object model. *The openEHR Release, 1*(2).

Beale T., Heard S., Kalra D., & Lloyd D. (2006). *OpenEHR architecture overview*. The OpenEHR Foundation.

Beale, T., Heard, S., Kalra, D., & Lloyd, D. (2007). *The OpenEHR Reference Model*. EHR Information Model.

Bedi, C. S., & Goyal, H. (2010). Qualitative and Quantitative Evaluation of Image Denoising Techniques. *International Journal of Computers and Applications*, *8*(14), 31–34. doi:10.5120/1313-1775

Behadada, O., & Chikh, M. A. (2013). An interpretable classifier for detection of cardiac arrhythmias by using the fuzzy decision tree. *Artificial Intelligence Research*, *2*(3), 45–58. doi:10.5430/air.v2n3p45

Behjat, A. R., Mustapha, A., Nezamabadi-pour, H., Sulaiman, M. N., & Mustapha, N. (2013). A PSO-Based Feature Subset Selection for Application of Spam /Non-spam Detection. *Communications in Computer and Information Science, 378 CCIS*, 183–193. doi:10.1007/978-3-642-40567-9_16

Bellotti, T., Nouretdinov, I., Yang, M., & Gammerman, A. (2014). *Conformal Prediction for Reliable Machine Learning. Theory, Adaptations and Applications*. Morgan Kaufmann.

Bengio, Y. (2009). *Learning deep architectures for AI*. Now Publishers Inc. doi:10.1561/9781601982957

Bensujin, Vijila, C.K., & Hubert, C. (2014). Detection of ST Segment Elevation Myocardial Infarction (STEMI) Using Bacterial Foraging Optimization Technique. *International Journal of Engineering and Technology, 6*(2), 1212-1224.

Bentley, P. (1999). An introduction to evolutionary design by computers. *Evolutionary Design by Computers*, 1-73.

Berhane, Y., Worku, A., Bejiga, A., Adamu, L., Alemayehu, W., Bedri, A., ... Kebede, T. D. (2007). National survey on blindness, low vision and trachoma in Ethiopia: Methods and study clusters profile. *The Ethiopian Journal of Health Development*, *21*(3), 185–203.

Bhoi, A. K., Sherpa, K. S., & Khandelwal, B. (2015). Classification probabil-ity analysis for arrhythmia and ischemia using frequency domain fea-tures of QRS complex. *International Journal Bioautomation*, *19*(4).

Bishop, C. M. (2006). *Pattern recognition and machine learning*. Springer.

Biswas, M. H. A. (2014). Optimal Control of Nipah Virus (NiV) Infections: A Bangladesh Scenario. *Journal of Pure and Applied Mathematics: Advances and Applications*, *12*(1), 77–104.

Boregowda, S., Handy, R., Sleeth, D., & Merryweather, A. (2016). Measuring Entropy Change in a Human Physiological System. *Journal of Thermodynamics*, *2016*, 1–8. doi:10.1155/2016/4932710

Borislava, M., Andrew, B., Anthony, O., & Simon, G. T. (2011). Review of statistical methods for analysing healthcare resources and costs. *Health Economics*, *20*(8), 897–916. doi:10.1002/hec.1653 PMID:20799344

Borkar, V. R., Carey, M. J., & Chen, L. (2012). Big data platforms: What's next? *ACM Crossroads*, *19*(1), 44–49. doi:10.1145/2331042.2331057

Bräysy, O. (2001). *Local search and variable neighborhood search algorithms for the vehicle routing problem with time windows*. Vaasan yliopisto.

Breiman, L. (2001). Random forests. *Machine Learning*, *45*(1), 5–32. doi:10.1023/A:1010933404324

Breiman, L., Friedman, J., Stone, C. J., & Olshen, R. A. (1984). *Classification and regression trees*. CRC Press.

Breslow, L. A., & Aha, D. W. (1997). Simplifying decision trees: A survey. *The Knowledge Engineering Review*, *12*(1), 1–40. doi:10.1017/S0269888997000015

Broder, C. C., Xu, K., Nikolov, D. B., Zhu, Z., Dimitrov, D. S., Middleton, D., & Wang, L. F. (2013). A treatment for and vaccine against the deadly Hendra and NipahViruses. *Antiviral Research*, *100*(1), 8–13. doi:10.1016/j.antiviral.2013.06.012 PMID:23838047

Brose, L. S., & Bradley, C. (2009). Psychometric development of the retinopathy treatment satisfaction questionnaire (RetTSQ). *Psychology Health and Medicine*, *14*(6), 740–754. doi:10.1080/13548500903431485 PMID:20183546

Bruha, I. (2000). From machine learning to knowledge discovery: Survey of preprocessing and postprocessing. *Intelligent Data Analysis*, *4*(3-4), 363–374. doi:10.3233/IDA-2000-43-413

Bur, A., Holcomb, A., Goodwin, S., Woodroof, J., Karadaghy, O., Shnayder, Y., Kakarala, K., Brant, J., & Shew, M., (2019, March). Machine learning to predict occult nodal metastasis in early oral squamous T cell carcinoma. In *2019 Elsevier* (pp. 20-25). Elsevier.

Burges, C. J. (1998). A tutorial on support vector machines for pattern recognition. *Data Mining and Knowledge Discovery*, *2*(2), 121–167. doi:10.1023/A:1009715923555

Burges, C. J., Smola, A. J., & Scholkopf, B. (1999). *Advances in Kernel Methods-Support Vector Learning*. MIT Press.

Butte, A. J., & Kohane, I. S. (2006). Creation and implications of a phenome-genome network. *Nature Biotechnology*, *24*(1), 55–62. doi:10.1038/nbt1150 PMID:16404398

Camilla, L. W., Jayna, M. H., David, L. S., & Sharon, E. S. (2010). Does This Patient Have Delirium? Value of Bedside Instruments. *Journal of the American Medical Association*. PMID:20716741

Cantú-Paz, E. (2003). *Pruning neural networks with distribution estimation algorithms*. Paper presented at the Genetic and Evolutionary Computation Conference. 10.1007/3-540-45105-6_93

Carbonneau, R., Kevin, L., & Rustam, V. (2008). *Application of machine learning techniques for supply chain demand forecasting*. Elsevier.

Carneiro, G., Zheng, Y., Xing, F. & Yang, L. (2017). Review of Deep Learning Methods in Mammography, Cardiovascular, and Microscopy Image Analysis. *Springer Advances in Computer Vision and Pattern Recognition*, 11-32. doi:10.1007/978-3-319-42999-1_2

Caroprese, L., Veltri, P., Vocaturo, E., & Zumpano, E. (2018, July). Deep learning techniques for electronic health record analysis. In *2018 9th International Conference on Information, Intelligence, Systems and Applications (IISA)* (pp. 1-4). IEEE. 10.1109/IISA.2018.8633647

Çavuşlu, M. A., Karakuzu, C., & Şahin, S. (2010). Hardware Implementation of Artificial Neural Network Training Using Particle Swarm Optimization on FPGA. *Journal of Polytechnic, 13*(2), 83–92.

Celin, S., & Vasanth, K. (2017). Survey on the Methods for Detecting Arrhythmias Using Heart Rate Signals. *Journal of Pharmaceutical Sciences and Research., 9*(2), 183–189.

Çetin, E. (2007). *Artificial Intelligence Applications*. Seçkin Publishing.

Çevik, K. K., & Dandıl, E. (2012). Development of Visual Educational Software for Artificial Neural Networks on. Net Platform. *Journal of Information Technology, 5*(1), 19–28.

Çevik, K. K., & Koçer, H. E. (2013). A Soft Computing Application Based On Artificial Neural Networks Training by Particle Swarm Optimization. *Suleyman Demirel University Journal of Natural and Applied Science, 17*(2), 39–45.

Ceylan, R., Ozbay, Y., & Karlik, B. (2009). A novel approach for classification of ECG arrhythmias: Type-2 fuzzy clustering neural network. *Expert Systems with Applications, 36*(3), 6721–6726. doi:10.1016/j.eswa.2008.08.028

Chadha, M. S., Comer, J. A., Lowe, L., Rota, P. A., Rollin, P. E., Bellini, W. J., & Mishra, A. (2006). Nipah virus-associated encephalitis outbreak, Siliguri, India. *Emerging Infectious Diseases, 12*(2), 235–240. doi:10.3201/eid1202.051247 PMID:16494748

Chang, H. T., Mishra, N., & Lin, C. C. (2015). IoT big-data centred knowledge granule analytic and cluster framework for BI applications: A case base analysis. *PLoS One, 10*(11), e0141980. doi:10.1371/journal.pone.0141980 PMID:26600156

Chang, Q., Zhang, B., & Liu, R. (2011). Texture analysis method for shape-based segmentation in medical image. *International Congress on Image and Signal Processing*, 1146-1149. 10.1109/CISP.2011.6100395

Chen, C., Tiong, L. K., & Chen, I.-M. (2019). Using a genetic algorithm to schedule the space-constrained AGV-based prefabricated bathroom units manufacturing system. *International Journal of Production Research, 57*(10), 3003–3019.

Cheng, H. D., Shan, J., Ju, W., Guo, Y., & Zhang, L. (2010). Automated breast cancer detection and classification using ultrasound images: A survey. *Journal of Pattern Recognition, 43*(1), 299–317. doi:10.1016/j.patcog.2009.05.012

Chen, L. H., & Wilson, M. E. (2006). Dengue and chikungunya infections in travelers. *Current Opinion in Infectious Diseases, 5*, 438–444. PMID:20581669

Chen, Y., Wang, T., Wang, B., & Li, Z. (2009). A survey of fuzzy decision tree classifier. *Fuzzy Information and Engineering, 1*(2), 149–159. doi:10.100712543-009-0012-2

Chen, Z., Lee, L., Chen, J., Collins, R., Wu, F., Guo, Y., Linksted, P., & Peto, R. (2005). Cohort profile: The Kadoorie Study of Chronic Disease in China (KSCDC). *International Journal of Epidemiology, 34*(6), 1243–1249. doi:10.1093/ije/dyi174 PMID:16131516

Ching, P. K. G., de los Reyes, V. C., Sucaldito, M. N., Tayag, E., Columna-Vingno, A. B., Malbas, F. F. Jr, Bolo, G. C. Jr, Sejvar, J. J., Eagles, D., Playford, G., Dueger, E., Kaku, Y., Morikawa, S., Kuroda, M., Marsh, G. A., McCullough, S., & Foxwell, A. R. (2015). Outbreak of henipavirus infection, Philippines, 2014. *Emerging Infectious Diseases*, *21*(2), 328–331. doi:10.3201/eid2102.141433 PMID:25626011

Chow, D. S., Qi, J., Guo, X., Miloushev, V. Z., Iwamoto, F. M., Bruce, J. N., Lassman, A. B., Schwartz, L. H., Lignelli, A., Zhao, B., & Filippi, C. G. (2014). Semiautomated volumetric measurement on postcontrast MR imaging for analysis of recurrent and residual disease in glioblastoma multiforme. *AJNR. American Journal of Neuroradiology*, *35*(3), 498–503. doi:10.3174/ajnr.A3724 PMID:23988756

Chuan, Z. (2018). *PPDP: An efficient and privacy-preserving disease prediction scheme in cloud-based e-Healthcare system*. Elsevier.

Clenshaw, C. W., & Hayes, J. G. (1965). Curve and Surface Fitting. *IMA Journal of Applied Mathematics*, *1*(2), 164–183. doi:10.1093/imamat/1.2.164

Clifford, M. H., & Chih-ling, T. (1989). Regression and time series model selection in small samples. *Biometrika*.

Codd, E. F. (1970). A relational model of data for large shared data banks. *Communications of the ACM*, *13*(6), 377–387. doi:10.1145/362384.362685

Coggins, J. M. (1982). *A framework for texture analysis based on spatial filtering* (Ph.D Thesis). Michigan State University.

Collins, F. S., & Varmus, H. (2015). A new initiative on precision medicine. *The New England Journal of Medicine*, *372*(9), 793–795. doi:10.1056/NEJMp1500523 PMID:25635347

Comparison of non-linear activation functions for deep neural networks on MNIST classification task. (n.d.). https://arxiv.org/pdf/1804.02763.pdf

Correa, R., Arini, P. D., Correa, L. S., Valentinuzzi, M., & Laciar, E. (2014). Novel technique for ST-T interval characterization in patients with acute myocardial ischemia. *Computers in Biology and Medicine*, *50*, 49–55. doi:10.1016/j.compbiomed.2014.04.009 PMID:24832353

Correa, R., Arini, P. D., Correa, L. S., Valentinuzzi, M., Laciar, E., & ... (2016). Identification of patients with myocardial infarction. *Methods of Information in Medicine*, *55*(3), 242–249. doi:10.3414/ME15-01-0101 PMID:27063981

Corwin, J., Silberschatz, A., Miller, P. L., & Marenco, L. (2007). Dynamic tables: An architecture for managing evolving, heterogeneous biomedical data in relational database management systems. *Journal of the American Medical Informatics Association*, *14*(1), 86–93. doi:10.1197/jamia.M2189 PMID:17068350

Cotta, C., Alba, E., Sagarna, R., & Larrañaga, P. (2002). Adjusting weights in artificial neural networks using evolutionary algorithms. In *Estimation of distribution algorithms* (pp. 361–377). Springer. doi:10.1007/978-1-4615-1539-5_18

Covington, M. A., Nute, D., & Vellino, A. (1996). *Prolog programming in depth*. Prentice-Hall, Inc.

Cristianini, N., & Shawe-Taylor, J. (2000). *An introduction to support vector machines and other kernel-based learning methods*. Cambridge University Press. doi:10.1017/CBO9780511801389

Curry, B., & Morgan, P. (1997). Neural networks: A need for caution. *Omega*, *25*(1), 123–133. doi:10.1016/S0305-0483(96)00052-7

Cynthia, D. (2006). Differential privacy. *International Colloquium on Automata, Languages and Programming*, *4052*, 1–12.

Daamouche, A., Hamami, L., Alajlan, N., & Melgani, F. (2012). A wavelet optimization approach for ECG signal classification. *Biomedical Signal Processing and Control*, *7*(4), 342–349. doi:10.1016/j.bspc.2011.07.001

Dagnino, A., & Cox, D. (2014, July). Industrial Analytics to Discover Knowledge from Instrumented Networked Machines. In SEKE (pp. 86-89). Academic Press.

Dalal, S., & Birok, R. (2016). Analysis of ECG Signals using Hybrid Classifier. *International Advanced Research Journal in Science. Engineering and Technology, 3*(7), 89–95.

Dallali, A., Kachouri, A., & Samet, M. (2011). Classification of Cardiac Arrhythmia Using WT, HRV, and Fuzzy C-Means Clustering. *Signal Processing: An Int. J., 5*(3), 101-109.

Dallali, A., Kachouri, A., & Samet, M. (2011). Fuzzy c-means clustering, Neural Network, wt, and Hrv for classification of cardiac arrhythmia. *ARPN J. of Eng. and Appl. Sci., 6*(10), 112–118.

Damian. (2017). Predicting Diabetic Readmission Rates: Moving Beyond Hba1c. *Current Trends in Biomedical Engineering & Bioscience, 7*(3).

Dandıl, E., & Gürgen, E. (2019). Prediction of Photovoltaic Panel Power Outputs using Artificial Neural Networks and Comparison with Heuristic Algorithms. *European Journal of Science and Technology,* (16), 146-158.

Daniel, B. K. (Ed.). (2016). *Big data and learning analytics in higher education: Current theory and practice.* Springer.

Das, M. K., & Ari, S. (2014). ECG Beats Classification Using Mixture of Features. *International Scholarly Research Notices, 2014,* 1–12. doi:10.1155/2014/178436 PMID:27350985

Data Augmentation | How to use Deep Learning when you have Limited Data — Part 2. (n.d.). https://medium.com/nanonets/how-to-use-deep-learning-when-you-have-limited-data-part-2-data-augmentation-c26971dc8ced

Datta, R. P., & Saha, S. (2011). *An Empirical comparison of rule based classification techniques in medical databases* (No. 1107). Academic Press.

De Gaetano, A., Panunzi, S., Rinaldi, F., Risi, A., & Sciandrone, M. (2009). A patient adaptable ECG beat classifier based on neural networks. *Applied Mathematics and Computation, 213*(1), 243–249. doi:10.1016/j.amc.2009.03.013

De Kock, E. (2005). *Decentralising the codification of rules in a decision support expert knowledge base* (Doctoral dissertation). University of Pretoria.

De Pierrefeu, A., Löfstedt, T., Laidi, C., Hadj-Selem, F., Leboyer, M., Ciuciu, P., ... Duchesnay, E. (2018, June). Interpretable and stable prediction of schizophrenia on a large multisite dataset using machine learning with structured sparsity. In *2018 International Workshop on Pattern Recognition in Neuroimaging (PRNI)* (pp. 1-4). IEEE. 10.1109/PRNI.2018.8423946

de Wit, E., & Munster, V. J. (2015). Animal models of disease shed light on Nipah virus pathogenesis and transmission. *The Journal of pathology, 235*(2), 196–205. doi:10.1002/path.4444de

Dean, A., & Will, D. (2014). *Data mining and predictive analytics.* Abbottanalytics-blog.

Deary, I. J., Johnson, W., & Houlihan, L. M. (2009). Genetic foundations of human intelligence. *Human Genetics, 126*(1), 215–232. doi:10.100700439-009-0655-4 PMID:19294424

Deja, A. W., & Paszek, P. (2003). Applying rough set theory to Multi stage medical diagnosing. *Fundamenta Informaticae, 54*(4), 387–408.

Deka, A., & Sarma, K. (2012). SVD and PCA Feature for ANN Based Detection of Diabetes Using Retinopathy. *Proceedings of the CUBE International Information Technology Conference,* 38-44. 10.1145/2381716.2381725

Derek, G. (2014). The 2014 Ebola virus disease outbreak in West Africa. *Journal of General Virology.*

Desoky, A. H., & Hall, S. A. (1990). Entropy measures for texture analysis based on Hadamard transform. *IEEE Proceedings on Southeastcon, 2*, 467-470.

Devi, J. C. (2014). Binary Decision Tree Classification based on C4. 5 and KNN Algorithm for Banking Application. *International Journal of Computational Intelligence and Informatics, 4*(2), 125–131.

Dhage, P., Phegade, M. R., & Shah, S. K. (2015). Watershed segmentation brain tumor detection. *Pervasive Computing (ICPC), International Conference, 1*, 5.

Dheva Rajan, S., IyemPerumal, A., Kalpana, D., & Rajagopalan, S.P. (2013a). SPR_SODE Model for dengue fever. *International Journal of Applied Mathematical and Statistical Sciences, 2*(3), 41-46.

Dheva Rajan, S., Iyemperumal, A., Kalpana, D., & Rajagopalan, S.P. (2013d). A support investigation for SPR_SODE Model for dengue. *American Journal of Sustainable City and Society, 1*(2), 204-212.

Dheva Rajan, S., IyemPerumal, A., Kalpana, D., & Rajagopalan, S.P. (2014a). Existence of the solution and disease-free equilibrium of SPR_SODE Model. *International Journal of Pure and Applied Mathematical Sciences, 7*(1), 1-7.

Dheva Rajan, S., Iyemperumal, A., Kalpana, D., & Rajagopalan, S.P. (2014b). A Critical analysis on bifurcation of SPR_SODE Model for the spread of dengue. *International Journal of Advanced Natural Sciences, 3*(1), 33-40.

Dheva Rajan, S., IyemPerumal, A., Kalpana, D., & Rajagopalan, S.P. (2013b). Improved SPR_SODE Model for dengue fever. *International Journal of Advanced Scientific and Technical Research, 5*(3), 418–425.

Dheva Rajan, S., IyemPerumal, A., Kalpana, D., & Rajagopalan, S.P. (2013c). Asymptotic Stability Of SPR_SODE Model for Dengue. *International Journal of Research in Applied.Natural and Social Sciences, 1*(6), 59–64.

Dheva Rajan, S., IyemPerumal, A., Kalpana, D., & Rajagopalan, S.P. (2014c). Bifurcation Analysis of SPR_SODE Model for the spread of dengue. *International Journal Applied Engineering Research, 9*(6), 643–651.

Dheva Rajan, S., IyemPerumal, A., Kalpana, D., & Rajagopalan, S.P. (2014d). Sensitivity Analysis of SPR_SODE Model for the spread of dengue. *International Journal Applied Environmental Sciences, 9*(4), 1237–1250.

Diekmann, O., & Heesterbeek, J. A. P. (2000). *Mathematical Epidemiology of Infectious Diseases: Model Building, Analysis and Interpretation*. John Wiley.

Diekman, O., Heesterbeek, J. A. P., & Metz, J. A. J. (1990). On the definition and the computation of the basic reproduction ratio R_0 in models for infectious diseases in heterogeneous populations. *Journal of Mathematical Biology, 28*, 365–382. PMID:2117040

Dietterich, T. G. (2000, June). Ensemble methods in machine learning. In *International workshop on multiple classifier systems* (pp. 1-15). Springer.

Dietz, K., Molineaux, L., & Thomas, A. (1990). A dengue model tested in the African Savannah. *Bulletin of the World Health Organization, 50*, 347–357. PMID:4613512

Dimitrov, D. V. (2016). Medical internet of things and big data in healthcare. *Healthcare Informatics Research, 22*(3), 156–163. doi:10.4258/hir.2016.22.3.156 PMID:27525156

Dinesh, K. G., Arumugaraj, K., Santhosh, K. D., & Mareeswari, V. (2018, March). Prediction of Cardiovascular Disease Using Machine Learning Algorithms. In *2018 International Conference on Current Trends towards Converging Technologies (ICCTCT)* (pp. 1-7). IEEE. 10.1109/ICCTCT.2018.8550857

Dinu, V., & Nadkarni, P. (2007). Guidelines for the effective use of entity–attribute–value modeling for biomedical databases. *International Journal of Medical Informatics*, *76*(11-12), 769–779. doi:10.1016/j.ijmedinf.2006.09.023 PMID:17098467

Dinu, V., Nadkarni, P., & Brandt, C. (2006). Pivoting approaches for bulk extraction of Entity–Attribute–Value data. *Computer Methods and Programs in Biomedicine*, *82*(1), 38–43. doi:10.1016/j.cmpb.2006.02.001 PMID:16556470

DiviyaPrabha & Ratthipriya. (2018). Prediction of Hyperglycemia using Binary Gravitational Logistic Regression (BGLR). *International Journal of Pure and Applied Mathematics*, *118*(16).

Dokas, I. M. (2005, September). Developing Web Sites For Web Based Expert Systems: A Web Engineering Approach. In ITEE (pp. 202-217). Academic Press.

Donald, W. D. (1999). The bombe a remarkable logic machine. *J Cryptologia*.

Donoho, D. L. (1995). Denoising by soft-thresholding. *IEEE Transactions on Information Theory*, *41*(3), 613–627. doi:10.1109/18.382009

Donoho, D. L., & Johnstone, I. M. (1994). Ideal spatial adaptation *via* wavelet shrinkage. *Biomefrika*, *81*(3), 425–455. doi:10.1093/biomet/81.3.425

Dorigo, M. (1992). *Optimization, learning and natural algorithms* (PhD Thesis). Politecnico di Milano.

Dorigo, M., & Di Caro, G. (1999). *Ant colony optimization: a new meta-heuristic.* Paper presented at the Proceedings of the 1999 congress on evolutionary computation-CEC99 (Cat. No. 99TH8406). 10.1109/CEC.1999.782657

Dropout in (Deep) Machine learning. (n.d.). https://medium.com/@amarbudhiraja/https-medium-com-amarbudhiraja-learning-less-to-learn-better-dropout-in-deep-machine-learning-74334da4bfc5

Dropout Regularization in Deep Learning Models With Keras. (n.d.). https://machinelearningmastery.com/dropout-regularization-deep-learning-models-keras/

Dua, D., & Taniskidou, E. K. (n.d.). *UCI Machine Learning Repository*. Retrieved March 2018, from http://archive.ics. uci. edu/ml

Dubey, A. (2015). A classification of ckd cases using multivariate k-means clustering. *International Journal of Scientific and Research Publications*, *5*(8), 1–5.

Duskalov, I., Dotsinsky, I. A., & Christov, I. I. (1998). Developments in ECG acquisition, preprocessing, parameter measurement, and recording. *IEEE Engineering in Medicine and Biology Magazine*, *17*(2), 50–58. doi:10.1109/51.664031 PMID:9548081

Du, W., & Zhan, Z. (2002). Building decision tree classifier on private data. In *International conference on Privacy, security and data mining* (pp. 1-8). IEEE.

ECG signals (1000 fragments). (n.d.). https://data.mendeley.com/datasets/7dybx7wyfn/3

Efraim, T. (2011). *Decision support and business intelligence systems.* Pearson Education India.

Efthymioua, S., Manolea, A., & Houlden, H. (2016). Next-generation sequencing in neuromuscular diseases. *Current Opinion in Neurology*, *29*(5), 527–536. doi:10.1097/WCO.0000000000000374 PMID:27588584

Ehud, R., & Robert, D. (1997). Building applied natural language generation systems. *Natural Language Engineering*, *3*(1), 57–87. doi:10.1017/S1351324997001502

El-Dahshan, E. (2010). Genetic algorithm and wavelet hybrid scheme for ECG signal denoising. *Telecommunication Systems*, *46*(3), 209–215. doi:10.100711235-010-9286-2

Elisseeff, A., & Guyon, I. (2003). An Introduction to Variable and Feature Selection. *Journal of Machine Learning Research*, 1157–1182. http://www.jmlr.org/papers/v3/guyon03a.html

Elomaa, T., & Rousu, J. (1999). General and efficient multisplitting of numerical attributes. *Machine Learning*, *36*(3), 201–244. doi:10.1023/A:1007674919412

ELU-Networks. (n.d.). *Fast and Accurate CNN Learning on ImageNet*. http://image-net.org/challenges/posters/JKU_EN_RGB_Schwarz_poster.pdf

Emel, G. G., & Taşkın, Ç. (2002). Genetic Algorithms and Applications. *Uludağ University Journal of Faculty of Economics and Administrative Sciences*, *21*(1), 129–152.

Enriko, I. K., Suryanegara, M., & Gunawan, D. (2018). Heart Disease Diagnosis System with k-Nearest Neighbors Method Using Real Clinical Medical Records. In *International Conference on Frontiers of Educational Technologies*, (pp. 127-131). 10.1145/3233347.3233386

Esfahani, H. A., & Ghazanfari, M. (2017, December). Cardiovascular disease detection using a new ensemble classifier. In *2017 IEEE 4th International Conference on Knowledge-Based Engineering and Innovation (KBEI)* (pp. 1011-1014). IEEE. 10.1109/KBEI.2017.8324946

Espinoza, J., Good, S., Russell, E., & Lee, W. (2013). Does the use of automated fetal biometry improve clinical work flow efficiency. *Journal of Ultrasound in Medicine*, *32*(5), 847–850. doi:10.7863/jum.2013.32.5.847 PMID:23620327

Esseynew, S. (2011). *Prototype Knowledge Based System for Anxiety Mental Disorder Diagnosis* (Doctoral dissertation). Addis Ababa University.

Estivill-Castro, V. (2002). Why so many clustering algorithms: A position paper. *SIGKDD Explorations*, *4*(1), 65–75. doi:10.1145/568574.568575

Euan, A. A. (2015). The Precision Medicine Initiative-A New National Effort. *Journal of the American Medical Association*. PMID:25928209

Exarchos, T. P., Papaloukas, C., Fotiadis, D. I., & Michalis, L. K. (2006). An association rule mining-based methodology for automated detection of ischemic ECG beats. *IEEE Transactions on Biomedical Engineering*, *53*(8), 1531–1540. doi:10.1109/TBME.2006.873753 PMID:16916087

Exploring the different types of nosql databases part ii. (n.d.). Retrieved June 22, 2017, from https://www.3pillarglobal.com/insights/exploring-the-different-types-of-nosql-databases

Eykhoff, P. (1974). *System Identification: Parameter and State Estimation*. Wiley & Sons.

Faisal, M. I., Bashir, S., Khan, Z. S., & Khan, F. H. (2018, December). An Evaluation of Machine Learning Classifiers and Ensembles for Early Stage Prediction of Lung Cancer. In *2018 3rd International Conference on Emerging Trends in Engineering, Sciences and Technology (ICEEST)* (pp. 1-4). IEEE. 10.1109/ICEEST.2018.8643311

Farooq, A., Anwar, S., Awais, M., & Rehman, S. (2017, October). A deep CNN based multi-class classification of Alzheimer's disease using MRI. In *2017 IEEE International Conference on Imaging systems and techniques (IST)* (pp. 1-6). IEEE. 10.1109/IST.2017.8261460

Faruque, M. F., & Sarker, I. H. (2019, February). Performance Analysis of Machine Learning Techniques to Predict Diabetes Mellitus. In *2019 International Conference on Electrical, Computer and Communication Engineering (ECCE)* (pp. 1-4). IEEE. 10.1109/ECACE.2019.8679365

Fayisa, D. (2018). *Integrated Predictive Model and Knowledge Based System for Wheat Disease Detection: Case of Arsi Zone* (Doctoral dissertation). ASTU.

Fayyad, U. M., Piatetsky-Shapiro, G., & Smyth, P. (1996, August). Knowledge Discovery and Data Mining: Towards a Unifying Framework. In KDD (Vol. 96, pp. 82-88). Academic Press.

Fei, T., Ying, C., LiDa, X., Lin, Z., & Li, B.H. (2015). CCIoT-CMfg: Cloud Computing and Internet of Things-Based Cloud Manufacturing Service System. IEEE.

Field, H., Young, P., Yob, J. M., Mills, J., Hall, L., & Mackenzie, J. (2001). The natural history of Hendra and Nipah viruses. *Microbes and Infection*, *3*(4), 307–314. doi:10.1016/S1286-4579(01)01384-3 PMID:11334748

Fığlalı, A. E. O. (2002). Reproduction operator optimization of Genetic Algorithms in flowshop scheduling problems *ITU. Engineering Journal (New York)*, *1*(1), 1–6.

Finlay, D., Bond, R., Kennedy, A., Guldenring, D., Moran, K., & McLaughlin, J. (2015). The effects of electrode placement on an automated algorithm for detecting ST segment changes on the 12-lead ECG. *Computers in Cardiology*, *42*, 1161–1164. doi:10.1109/CIC.2015.7411122

Fogel, D. B. (1998). *Artificial intelligence through simulated evolution*. Wiley-IEEE Press.

Foster, K. R., Jenkins, M. E., & Toogood, A. C. (1998). The Philadelphia Yellow Fever Epidemic of 1793. *Scientific American*, *279*(2), 88–93. doi:10.1038cientificamerican0898-88 PMID:9674172

Foster, P., & Tom, F. (2013). Data science and its relationship to big data and data-driven decision making. *Big Data*.

Friedman, N., Geiger, D., & Goldszmidt, M. (1997). Bayesian network classifiers. *Machine Learning*, *29*(2-3), 131–163. doi:10.1023/A:1007465528199

Fuduli, A., Veltri, P., Vocaturo, E., & Zumpano, E. (2019). Melanoma detection using color and texture features in computer vision systems. Advances in Science. *Technology and Engineering Systems Journal*, *4*(5), 16–22. doi:10.25046/aj040502

Fujimoto, A., Kimura, R., Ohashi, J., Omi, K., Yuliwulandari, R., Batubara, L., Mustofa, M. S., Samakkarn, U., Settheetham-Ishida, W., Ishida, T., Morishita, Y., Furusawa, T., Nakazawa, M., Ohtsuka, R., & Tokunaga, K. (2008). A scan for genetic determinants of human hair morphology: EDAR is associated with Asian hair thickness. *Human Molecular Genetics*, *17*(6), 835–843. doi:10.1093/hmg/ddm355 PMID:18065779

FunctionsA. (n.d.). https://ml-cheatsheet.readthedocs.io/en/latest/activation_functions.html

Fung, R. Y., Tang, J., & Wang, D. (2002). Extension of a hybrid genetic algorithm for nonlinear programming problems with equality and inequality constraints. *Computers & Operations Research*, *29*(3), 261–274. doi:10.1016/S0305-0548(00)00068-X

Galit, S., & Otto, R. K. (2011). Predictive Analytics in Information Systems Research. *MIS*, *3*, 553–572.

Gao, D., Madden, M., Schukat, M., Chambers, D., & Lyons, G. (2004). Arrhythmia Identification from ECG Signals with a Neural Network Classifier Based on a Bayesian Framework. *Twenty-fourth SGAI International Conference on Innovative Techniques and Applications of Artificial Intelligence*, *3*(3), 390-409.

Gao, H., Dou, L., Chen, W., & Xie, G. (2011). The applications of image segmentation techniques in medical CT images. *Proceedings of the 30th Chinese Control Conference*, 3296-3299.

Garcia, J., Astrom, M., Mendive, J., Laguna, P., & Sornmo, L. (2003). ECG-based detection of body position changes in ischemia monitoring. *IEEE Transactions on Biomedical Engineering*, *50*(6), 677–685. doi:10.1109/TBME.2003.812208 PMID:12814234

Garcia, J., Sornmo, L., Olmos, S., & Laguna, P. (2000). Automatic detection of ST-T complex changes on the ECG using filtered RMS difference series: Application to ambulatory ischemia monitoring. *IEEE Transactions on Biomedical Engineering*, *47*(9), 1195–1201. doi:10.1109/10.867943 PMID:11008420

Garg, A. K., Chouhan, P., & Sharma, B. (2019). Fundamental Tenets of Nipah Virus Infection in Ayurveda and its Management: A Multidisciplinary Investigation. *International Journal of Ayurveda and Pharmaceutical Chemistry*, *10*(2), 48–64.

Garg, A. X., Adhikari, N. K., McDonald, H., Rosas-Arellano, M. P., Devereaux, P. J., Beyene, J., Sam, J., & Haynes, R. B. (2005). Effects of computerized clinical decision support systems on practitioner performance and patient outcomes: A systematic review. *Journal of the American Medical Association*, *293*(10), 1223–1238. doi:10.1001/jama.293.10.1223 PMID:15755945

Gary, K., & Langche, Z. (2001). Logistic Regression in Rare Events Data. *J Oxford*.

Gaudioso, M., Giallombardo, G., Miglionico, G., & Vocaturo, E. (2019). Classification in the multiple instance learning framework via spherical separation. *Soft Computing*, 1–7.

Gautam, V., & Lakhwani, K. (2013). Implementation of Non Shannon Entropy measures for Color Image Segmentation and Comparison with Shannon Entropy Measures. *International Journal of Scientific Research (Ahmedabad, India)*, *2*(5), 391–394.

Gehrke, J., Ramakrishnan, R., & Ganti, V. (2000). RainForest-a framework for fast decision tree construction of large datasets. *Data Mining and Knowledge Discovery*, *4*(2-3), 127–162. doi:10.1023/A:1009839829793

Genton, M. G. (2001). Classes of kernels for machine learning: A statistics perspective. *Journal of Machine Learning Research*, *2*(Dec), 299–312.

Gharibdousti, M. S., Azimi, K., Hathikal, S., & Won, D. H. (2017). Prediction of chronic kidney disease using data mining techniques. In *IIE Annual Conference. Proceedings* (pp. 2135-2140). Institute of Industrial and Systems Engineers (IISE).

Ghoshal, S. P. (2004). Optimizations of PID gains by particle swarm optimizations in fuzzy based automatic generation control. *Electric Power Systems Research*, *72*(3), 203–212. doi:10.1016/j.epsr.2004.04.004

Ghosh, B., Indurkar, M., & Jain, M. K. (2013). ECG: A Simple Noninvasive Tool to Localize Culprit Vessel Occlusion Site in Acute STEMI. *Indian Journal of Clinical Practice*, *23*(10), 590–595.

Gillespie, D.T. (1976). A general method for numerically simulating the stochastic time evolution of coupled chemical reactions. *Journal of Computational Physics, 22*, 403–434. doi:10.1016/0021-9991(76)90041-3

Gillespie, D. T. (1977). Exact stochastic simulation of coupled chemical reactions. *Journal of Physical Chemistry*, *81*(25), 2340–2361. doi:10.1021/j100540a008

Glover, F. (1977). Heuristics for integer programming using surrogate constraints. *Decision Sciences*, *8*(1), 156–166. doi:10.1111/j.1540-5915.1977.tb01074.x

Go, A., Mozaffarian, D., Roger, V. L., Benjamin, E. J., Berry, J. D., Blaha, M. J., Dai, S., Ford, E. S., Fox, C. S., Franco, S., Fullerton, H. J., Gillespie, C., Hailpern, S. M., Heit, J. A., Howard, V. J., Huffman, M. D., Judd, S. E., Kissela, B. M., Kittner, S. J., ... Turner, M. B. (2014). Executive summary: heart disease and stroke statistics—2014 update: a report from the American Heart Association. *Circulation*, *129*(3), 399–410. doi:10.1161/01.cir.0000442015.53336.12 PMID:24446411

Goel, S., Tomar, P., & Kaur, G. (2016). A Fuzzy Based Approach for Denoising of ECG Signal using Wavelet Transform. *International Journal of Bio-Science and Bio-Technology*, *8*(2), 143–156. doi:10.14257/ijbsbt.2016.8.2.13

Goh, K. J., Tan, C. T., Chew, N. K., Tan, P. S. K., Kamarulzaman, A., Sarji, S. A., Wong, K. T., Abdullah, B. J. J., Chua, K. B., & Lam, S. K. (2000). Clinical features of Nipah virus encephalitis among pig farmers in Malaysia. *The New England Journal of Medicine*, *342*(17), 1229–1235. doi:10.1056/NEJM200004273421701 PMID:10781618

Goldberg, D. E., & Holland, J. H. (1988). Genetic algorithms and machine learning. *Machine Learning*, *3*(2), 95–99. doi:10.1023/A:1022602019183

Goldberger, J., & Hinton, G. E. (2005). Neighbourhood components analysis. *Advances in Neural Information Processing Systems*, ●●●, 513–520.

Goletsis, Y., Papaloukas, C., Fotiadis, D. I., Likas, A., & Michalis, L. K. (2004). Automated ischemic beat classification using genetic algorithms and multicriteria decision analysis. *IEEE Transactions on Biomedical Engineering*, *51*(10), 1717–1725. doi:10.1109/TBME.2004.828033 PMID:15490819

Gonzalez, B., Valdez, F., Melin, P., & Arechiga, G. P. (2015). Fuzzy logic in the gravitational search algorithm for the optimization of modular neural networks in pattern recognition. *Expert Systems with Applications*, *42*(14), 5839–5847. doi:10.1016/j.eswa.2015.03.034

Gopinathan, K. M., Biafore, L. S., Ferguson, W. M., Lazarus, M. A., Pathria, A. K., & Jost, A. (1998). *Fraud detection using predictive modeling*. US Patent. 5,819,226. https://hackernoon.com/ http://predictiveanalyticstoday.com/

Goswami, B., & Mishra, S. K. (2016). Analysis of various Edge detection methods for X-ray images. *International Conference on Electrical, Electronics, and Optimization Techniques (ICEEOT)*. 10.1109/ICEEOT.2016.7755185

Grabe, H. J., Assel, H., Bahls, T., Dorr, M., Endlich, K., Endlich, N., ... Fiene, B. (2014). Cohort profile: Greifswald approach to individualized medicine (GANI_MED). *Journal of Translational Medicine*, *12*(1), 144. doi:10.1186/1479-5876-12-144 PMID:24886498

Grande, G. D., Hoekman, D., Lee, J. S., Schuler, D., & Ainsworth, T. (2004). A wavelet multiresolution technique for polarimetric texture analysis and segmentation of SAR images. *IGARSS, IEEE International Geoscience and Remote Sensing Symposium*, 713-719.

Grant, C., Lo Iacono, G., Dzingirai, V., Bett, B., Winnebah, T. R., & Atkinson, P. M. (2016). Moving interdisciplinary science forward: Integrating participatory modelling with mathematical modelling of zoonotic disease in Africa. *Infectious Diseases of Poverty*, *5*(1), 17. doi:10.118640249-016-0110-4 PMID:26916067

Grover, S., Bhartia, S., Yadav, A., & Seeja, K. R. (2018). Predicting Severity of Parkinson's Disease Using Deep Learning. *Procedia Computer Science*, *132*, 1788–1794. doi:10.1016/j.procs.2018.05.154

Gubbi, J., Buyya, R., Marusic, S., & Palaniswami, M. (2013). Internet of Things (IoT): A vision, architectural elements, and future directions. *Future Generation Computer Systems*, *29*(7), 1645–1660. doi:10.1016/j.future.2013.01.010

Gulcher, J. R., Jonsson, P., Kong, A., Kristjansson, K., Frigge, M. L., Karason, A., ... Sigurthoardottir, S. (1997). Mapping of a familial essential tremor gene, FET1, to chromosome 3q13. *Nature Genetics*, *17*(1), 84–87. doi:10.1038/ng0997-84 PMID:9288103

Güleç, D. (2014). *Optimization of user accessibility in architectural design using genetic algorithm- aDA:Case study on health campuses* (PhD). Istanbul Technical University. Retrieved from http://archive.ics.uci.edu/ml/datasets/Breast+Cancer

Guler, I., & Ubeyli, E. D. (2007). Multiclass support vector machines for EEG signals classification. *IEEE Transactions on Information Technology in Biomedicine*, *11*(2), 117–126. doi:10.1109/TITB.2006.879600 PMID:17390982

Gupta, S., Chauhan, R. C., & Saxena, S. C. (2005). Locally adaptive wavelet domain Bayesian Processor for denoising medical ultrasound images using speckle modeling based on Rayleigh distribution. Proceeding on Vision, Image and Signal Processing, 152(1), 129-135.

Gupta, S., Kaur, L., Chauhan, R.C. & Saxena, S.C. (2003). A wavelet based statistical approach for speckle reduction in medical ultrasound images. *Proceedings on Convergent Technologies for Asia-Pacific Region*, 534-537. doi:10.1109/TENCON.2003.1273218

Gupta, J. N., & Sexton, R. S. (1999). Comparing backpropagation with a genetic algorithm for neural network training. *Omega, 27*(6), 679–684. doi:10.1016/S0305-0483(99)00027-4

Gupta, K. O., & Chatur, P. N. (2012). ECG Signal Analysis and Classification using Data Mining and Artificial Neural Networks. *International Journal of Emerging Technology and Advanced Engineering, 2*(1), 56–60.

Gupta, S., Chauhan, R. C., & Saxena, S. C. (2004). A wavelet based statistical approach for speckle reduction in medical ultrasound images. *Medical & Biological Engineering & Computing, 42*(2), 189–192. doi:10.1007/BF02344630 PMID:15125148

Gupta, S., Kaur, L., Chauhan, R. C., & Saxena, S. C. (2007). A versatile technique for visual enhancement of medical ultrasound images. *Digital Signal Processing, 17*(3), 542–560. doi:10.1016/j.dsp.2006.12.001

Gustavo, C., Georgescu, B. & Good, S. (2008). Knowledge-based automated fetal biometrics using syngo Auto OB measurements. *Siemens Medical Solutions*, 67.

Hadjem, M., Nait-Abdesselam, F., & Khokhar, A. (2016). ST-segment and T-wave anomalies prediction in an ECG data using RUSBoost. *IEEE 18th International Conference on e-Health Networking, Applications and Services (Healthcom)*, 1–6.

Hamedi, S. M., Vahidi, J., & Hamedi, S. M. (2015). Automatic MRI image threshold using fuzzy support vector machines. *International Conference on Knowledge-Based Engineering and Innovation (KBEI)*, 207-210. 10.1109/KBEI.2015.7436047

Hammoud, D. A., Lentz, M. R., Lara, A., Bohannon, J. K., Feuerstein, I., Huzella, L., Jahrling, P. B., Lackemeyer, M., Laux, J., Rojas, O., Sayre, P., Solomon, J., Cong, Y., Munster, V., & Holbrook, M. R. (2018). Aerosol exposure to intermediate size Nipah virus particles induces neurological disease in African green monkeys. *PLoS Neglected Tropical Diseases, 12*(11), e0006978. doi:10.1371/journal.pntd.0006978 PMID:30462637

Han, J., Pei, J., & Kamber, M. (2011). *Data mining: concepts and techniques*. Elsevier.

Haralick, R. (1979). Statistical and Structural approaches to texture. *Proceedings of the IEEE, 67*(5), 786–804. doi:10.1109/PROC.1979.11328

Haralick, R. M., Shanmugam, K., & Kinstein, I. (1973). Texture features for image classification. *IEEE Transactions on Systems, Man, and Cybernetics, 8*(6), 610–621. doi:10.1109/TSMC.1973.4309314

Harrington, P. (2012). *Machine learning in action*. Manning Publications Co.

Hastie, T., Tibshirani, R., Friedman, J., & Franklin, J. (2005). The elements of statistical learning: Data mining, inference and prediction. *The Mathematical Intelligencer, 27*(2), 83–85. doi:10.1007/BF02985802

Haykin, S. S. (2009). *Neural networks and learning machines*. Academic Press.

Health Level Seven International - Homepage. (n.d.). Retrieved June 22, 2017, from http://www.hl7.org/

Hearn-Stebbins, B. (1995). Normal fetal growth assessment: A review of literature and current practice. *Journal of Diagnostic Medical Sonography: JDMS, 11*(4), 176–187. doi:10.1177/875647939501100403

Heartbeat Categorization DatasetE. C. G. (n.d.). https://www.kaggle.com/shayanfazeli/heartbeat

Heesterbeek, H., Anderson, R. M., Andreasen, V., Bansal, S., De Angelis, D., Dye, C., Eames, K. T. D., Edmunds, W. J., Frost, S. D. W., Funk, S., Hollingsworth, T. D., House, T., Isham, V., Klepac, P., Lessler, J., Lloyd-Smith, J. O., Metcalf, C. J. E., Mollison, D., Pellis, L., ... Viboud, C. (2015). Isaac Newton Institute IDD Collaboration (2015). *Modeling infectious disease dynamics in the complex landscape of global health. Science, 347*(6227), aaa4339. Advance online publication. doi:10.1126cience.aaa4339 PMID:25766240

HeMavatHi, P. S., & SHenoy, P. (2014). Profile of microbial isolates in ophthalmic infections and antibiotic susceptibility of the bacterial isolates: A study in an eye care hospital, Bangalore. *Journal of Clinical and Diagnostic Research: JCDR, 8*(1), 23. PMID:24596715

Hethcote, H. (2000). The Mathematics of Infectious Diseases. *SIAM Review, 42*(4), 599–653. doi:10.1137/S0036144500371907

Hiremath, P. S., & Tegnoor, J. R. (2014). Fuzzy inference system for follicle detection in ultrasound images of ovaries. *Soft Computing, 18*(7), 1353–1362. doi:10.100700500-013-1148-x

Hoekstra, C., Zhao, Z. Z., Lambalk, C. B., Willemsen, G., Martin, N. G., Boomsma, D. I., & Montgomery, G. W. (2008). Dizygotic twinning. *Human Reproduction Update, 14*(1), 37–47. doi:10.1093/humupd/dmm036 PMID:18024802

Hoffmann, T. J., Kvale, M. N., Hesselson, S. E., Zhan, Y., Aquino, C., Cao, Y., Cawley, S., Chung, E., Connell, S., Eshragh, J., Ewing, M., Gollub, J., Henderson, M., Hubbell, E., Iribarren, C., Kaufman, J., Lao, R. Z., Lu, Y., Ludwig, D., ... Risch, N. (2011). Next generation genome-wide association tool: Design and coverage of a high-throughput European-optimized SNP array. *Genomics, 98*(2), 79–89. doi:10.1016/j.ygeno.2011.04.005 PMID:21565264

Hofmeyr, S. A., & Forrest, S. (2000). Architecture for an artificial immune system. *Evolutionary Computation, 8*(4), 443–473. doi:10.1162/106365600568257 PMID:11130924

Holland, J. H. (1992). *Adaptation in natural and artificial systems: an introductory analysis with applications to biology, control, and artificial intelligence.* MIT Press. doi:10.7551/mitpress/1090.001.0001

Hornoch, T. P. (2013). A survey of informatics approaches to whole-exome and whole-genome clinical reporting in the electronic health record. *Genetics in Medicine, 15*(10), 824–832. doi:10.1038/gim.2013.120 PMID:24071794

Host and Vector. (2019). *Infectious Diseases: In Context.* Retrieved August 27, 2019 from Encyclopedia.com: https://www.encyclopedia.com/media/educational-magazines/host-and-vector

How to Accelerate Learning of Deep Neural Networks With Batch Normalization. (n.d.). https://machinelearningmastery.com/how-to-accelerate-learning-of-deep-neural-networks-with-batch-normalization/

Hsu, V. P., Hossain, M. J., Parashar, U. D., Ali, M. M., Ksiazek, T. G., Kuzmin, I., Breiman, R. F., & ... . (2004). Nipah virus encephalitis reemergence, Bangladesh. *Emerging Infectious Diseases, 10*(12), 2082–2087. doi:10.3201/eid1012.040701 PMID:15663842

Huang, X. M., & Zhang, Y. H. (2003). A new application of rough set to ECG recognition. *Int. Conference on Machine Learning and Cybernetics, 3*, 1729-1734.

Hu, C., Ju, R., Shen, Y., Zhou, P., & Li, Q. (2016, May). Clinical decision support for Alzheimer's disease based on deep learning and brain network. In *2016 IEEE International Conference on Communications (ICC)* (pp. 1-6). IEEE. 10.1109/ICC.2016.7510831

Huyvaert, K. P., Russell, R. E., Patyk, K. A., Craft, M. E., Cross, P. C., Garner, M. G., & Walsh, D. P. (2018). Challenges and Opportunities Developing Mathematical Models of Shared Pathogens of Domestic and Wild Animals. *Veterinary Sciences*, *5*(4), 92. doi:10.3390/vetsci5040092 PMID:30380736

HYP. (n.d.). www.mathworks.com/access/helpdesk/help/toolbox/images

Ilayaraja, M., & Meyyappan, T. (2013). Mining medical data to identify frequent diseases using Apriori algorithm. *International Conference on Pattern Recognition, Informatics and Mobile Engineering.* 10.1109/ICPRIME.2013.6496471

Iram, S. (2014). *Early Detection of Neurodegenerative Diseases from Bio-Signals: A Machine Learning Approach* (Doctoral dissertation). Liverpool John Moores University.

Ismaeel, S., Miri, A., & Chourishi, D. (2015, May). Using the extreme learning machine (ELM) technique for heart disease diagnosis. In *2015 IEEE Canada International Humanitarian Technology Conference (IHTC2015)* (pp. 1-3). IEEE. 10.1109/IHTC.2015.7238043

ISO 13606-1. 2008. Health informatics -- Electronic health record communication -- Part 1: Reference Model. Retrieved June 22, 2017, from https://www.iso.org/standard/40784.html

ISO/DIS 13606-2 - Health informatics -- Electronic health record communication -- Part 2: Archetype interchange specification. Retrieved June 22, 2017, from https://www.iso.org/standard/62305.html

Jackson, J. (2002). Data mining; a conceptual overview. *Communications of the Association for Information Systems*, *8*(1), 19.

Jadhav, S., Nalbalwar, S. L., & Ghatol, A. (2012). Artificial Neural Network Models based Cardiac Arrhythmia Disease Diagnosis from ECG Signal Data. *International Journal of Computers and Applications*, *44*(15), 8–13. doi:10.5120/6338-8532

Jager, F., Mark, R., Moody, G., & Divjak, S. (1992). *Analysis of transient ST segment changes during ambulatory monitoring using the Karhunen-Loeave transform. In Computers in Cardiology 1992, Proceedings of, IEEE. IEEE Comput. Soc. Press.*

Jager, F., Moody, G. B., & Mark, R. G. (1998). Detection of transient ST segment episodes during ambulatory ECG monitoring. *Computers and Biomedical Research, an International Journal*, *31*(5), 305–322. doi:10.1006/cbmr.1998.1483 PMID:9790738

Jahangir, M., Afzal, H., Ahmed, M., Khurshid, K., & Nawaz, R. (2017, September). An expert system for diabetes prediction using auto tuned multi-layer perceptron. In *2017 Intelligent Systems Conference (IntelliSys)* (pp. 722-728). IEEE. 10.1109/IntelliSys.2017.8324209

Jalalian, A., Mashohor, S. B., Mahmud, H. R., Saripan, M. I., Ramli, A. R., & Karasfi, B. (2013). Computer-aided detection/diagnosis of breast cancer in mammography and ultrasound: A review. *Clinical Imaging*, *37*(3), 420–426. doi:10.1016/j.clinimag.2012.09.024 PMID:23153689

Jaleel, A., Tafreshi, R., & Tafreshi, L. (2016). An expert system for differential diagnosis of myocardial infarction. *Journal of Dynamic Systems, Measurement, and Control*, *138*(11), 111012. doi:10.1115/1.4033838

Jambukia, S. H., Dabhi, V. K., & Prajapati, H. B. (2015). Classification of ECG signals using Machine Learning Techniques: A Survey. *International Conference on Advances in Computer Engineering and Applications.*

James, H., Colin, M., Sidney, M. B., John, H., Barney, P., Charlton, C., ... Richard, A. N. (2018). Nextstrain: Real-time tracking of pathogen evolution. *Bioinformatics (Oxford, England).* PMID:29790939

Janghel, R. R., Mehra, A., Shukla, A., & Tiwari, R. (2011). Intelligent Diagnostic System for the diagnosis and prognosis of Breast Cancer using ANN. *Journal of Computing, 3*(3), 93–98.

Jayanthi, N., Vijaya Babu, B., & Sambasiva Rao, N. (2017). Survey on Clinical Prediction Models for Diabetes prediction. *Journal of Big Data, 4*(1), 26. doi:10.118640537-017-0082-7

Jeffry, F. (2000). Review of Metamathematics of fuzzy logics. *The Bulletin of Symbolic Logic, 6*(3), 342–346.

Jena, L., & Kamila, N. K. (2015). Distributed data mining classification algorithms for prediction of chronic-kidney-disease. *Int. J. Emerg. Res. Manag. &Technology, 9359*(11), 110–118.

Jernigan, M. E., & Astoush, F. D. (1984). Entropy-Based Texture Analysis in the Spatial Frequency Domain. *IEEE Transactions on Pattern Analysis and Machine Intelligence, PAMI-6*(2), 237–243. doi:10.1109/TPAMI.1984.4767507 PMID:21869187

Jeyalakshmi, M. S., & Robin, C. (2016). Fuzzy based Expert system for sleep apnea diagnosis. *International Journal of Engineering Trends and Technology, 35*(12), 555–558. doi:10.14445/22315381/IJETT-V35P312

Jianchao, W., Mengyang, L., & Sixian, W. (1989). Texture segmentation of ultrasound B-scan image by sum and difference histograms. *Images of the Twenty-First Century. Proceedings of the Annual International Engineering in Medicine and Biology Society, 2*, 417-418.

John, P. H., & Fredrik, R. (2001). MRBAYES: Bayesian inference of phylogenetic tree. *Bioinformatics (Oxford, England).*

Johnson, K. A., Fox, N. C., Sperling, R. A., & Klunk, W. E. (2012). Brain imaging in Alzheimer disease. *Cold Spring Harbor Perspectives in Medicine, 2*(4), a006213. doi:10.1101/cshperspect.a006213 PMID:22474610

Johnson, S. B. (1996). Generic data modeling for clinical repositories. *Journal of the American Medical Informatics Association, 3*(5), 328–339. doi:10.1136/jamia.1996.97035024 PMID:8880680

Johnston, S. C., Briese, T., Bell, T. M., Pratt, W. D., Shamblin, J. D., Esham, H. L., & Honko, A. N. (2015). Detailed analysis of the African green monkey model of Nipah virus disease. *PLoS One, 10*(2), e0117817. doi:10.1371/journal.pone.0117817 PMID:25706617

Jo, J. H., & Gero, J. S. (1998). Space layout planning using an evolutionary approach. *Artificial Intelligence in Engineering, 12*(3), 149–162. doi:10.1016/S0954-1810(97)00037-X

Jordan, M. I., & Mitchell, T. M. (2015). Machine learning: Trends, perspectives, and prospects. *Science, 349*(6245), 255–260. doi:10.1126cience.aaa8415 PMID:26185243

Joshi, D., & Ghongade, R. (2013). Performance analysis of feature extraction schemes for ECG signal classification. *Int. J. of Elect. Electron. And Data Commun., 1*, 45–51.

Joshi, N. P., & Topannavar, P. S. (2014). Support vector machine based heartbeat classification. *Proc. of 4th IRF Int. Conf.*, 140-144.

Juang, C.-F., & Lu, C.-F. (2006). Load-frequency control by hybrid evolutionary fuzzy PI controller. *IEE Proceedings. Generation, Transmission and Distribution, 153*(2), 196–204. doi:10.1049/ip-gtd:20050176

Jui, S. L. (2014). Fuzzy C-Means with Wavelet Filtration for MR Image Segmentation. *IEEE, Sixth World Congress on Nature and Biologically Inspired Computing (NaBIC)*, 12-16. 10.1109/NaBIC.2014.6921884

Junifer, J., & Suharjito, P. (2014). Diagnosis of Diabetes Mellitus Using Extreme Learning Machine. In *International Conference on Information Technology Systems and Innovation (ICITS)* (pp. 1-6). Academic Press.

Kaabi, J., & Harrath, Y. (2019). Permutation rules and genetic algorithm to solve the traveling salesman problem. *Arab Journal of Basic and Applied Sciences*, 26(1), 283–291. doi:10.1080/25765299.2019.1615172

Kahramanli, H., & Allahverdi, N. (2008). Design of a hybrid system for the diabetes and heart diseases. *Expert Systems with Applications*, 35(1-2), 82–89. doi:10.1016/j.eswa.2007.06.004

Kalaiselvi, C., & Nasira, G. M. (2014). A new approach for diagnosis of diabetes and prediction of cancer using ANFIS. *Computing and Communication Technologies (WCCCT), World Congress, IEEE*, 188-190.

Kalyan, K., Jakhia, B., Lele, R.D., Joshi, M. & Chowdhary, A. (2014). Artificial Neural Network Application in the Diagnosis of Disease Conditions with Liver Ultrasound Images. *Advances in Bioinformatics*, 1-14, doi: /708279 doi:10.1155/2014

Kalyan, K., Jain, S., Lele, R. D., Joshi, M., & Chowdhary, A. (2013). Application of artificial neural networks towards the determination of presence of disease conditions in ultrasound images of kidney. *International Journal of Computer Engineering & Technology*, 4(5), 232–243.

Kamiński, B., Jakubczyk, M., & Szufel, P. (2018). A framework for sensitivity analysis of decision trees. *Central European Journal of Operations Research*, 26(1), 135–159. doi:10.100710100-017-0479-6 PMID:29375266

Kampouraki, A., Manis, G., & Nikou, C. (2009). Heartbeat Time Series Classification with Support Vector Machines. *IEEE Transactions on Information Technology in Biomedicine*, 1(4), 512–518. doi:10.1109/TITB.2008.2003323 PMID:19273030

Kanan, H. R., Faez, K., & Taheri, S. M. (2007). Feature selection using Ant Colony Optimization (ACO): A new method and comparative study in the application of face recognition system. Lecture Notes in Computer Science, 4597, 63–76. doi:10.1007/978-3-540-73435-2_6

Kanani, P., & Padole, M. (2018). Recognizing Real Time ECG Anomalies Using Arduino, AD8232 and Java. In M. Singh, P. Gupta, V. Tyagi, J. Flusser, & T. Ören (Eds.), *Advances in Computing and Data Sciences. ICACDS 2018. Communications in Computer and Information Science* (Vol. 905). Springer. doi:10.1007/978-981-13-1810-8_6

Kannathal, N., Acharya, U. R., Lim, C. M., Sadasivan, P. K., & Krishnan, S. M. (2003). Classification of cardiac patient states using artificial neural networks. *Experimental and Clinical Cardiology*, 8(4), 206–211. PMID:19649222

Karaboga, D. (2005). An idea based on Honey Bee Swarm for Numerical Optimization. *Technical Report TR06, Erciyes University*, (TR06), 10.

Karaboga, D., & Basturk, B. (2007). A powerful and efficient algorithm for numerical function optimization: Artificial bee colony (ABC) algorithm. *Journal of Global Optimization*, 39(3), 459–471. doi:10.100710898-007-9149-x

Karaylan, T., & Kılıç, Ö. (2017, October). Prediction of heart disease using neural network. In *2017 International Conference on Computer Science and Engineering (UBMK)* (pp. 719-723). IEEE. 10.1109/UBMK.2017.8093512

Karen, Y. (2017). Big Data analytics for genomic medicine. *International Journal of Molecular Sciences*, 18(2), 412. doi:10.3390/ijms18020412 PMID:28212287

Karthik, Tyagi, Raut, Saxena, & Kumar. (n.d.). *Implementation of Neural Network and feature extraction to classify ECG signals*. https://arxiv.org/ftp/arxiv/papers/1802/1802.06288.pdf

Kaur, P., Singh, G. & Kaur, P. (2019). An Intelligent Validation system for diagnosis and prognosis of Ultrasound Fetal Growth Analysis using Neuro-Fuzzy based on Genetic Algorithm. *Egyptian Informatics Journal*, 20(1), 55-87. doi:10.1016/j.eij.2018.10.002

Kaur, P., Singh, G., & Kaur, P. (2016), Image Enhancement of Ultrasound Images using Multifarious Denoising Filters and GA. *IEEE International Conference on Advances in Computing, Communications and Informatics (ICACCI)*, 2375-2384.

Kaur, G., & Sharma, A. (2017, November). Predict chronic kidney disease using data mining algorithms in hadoop. In *2017 International Conference on Inventive Computing and Informatics (ICICI)* (pp. 973-979). IEEE. 10.1109/ICICI.2017.8365283

Kaur, L., Gupta, S., & Chauhan, R. C. (2002). Image denoising using wavelet thresholding. *Proceedings of Indian conference on computer vision, graphics and image processing*, 1-4.

Kaur, L., Gupta, S., Chauhan, R. C., & Saxena, S. C. (2007). Medical ultrasound image compression using joint optimization of thresholding quantization and best-basis selection of wavelet packets. *Digital Signal Processing*, *17*(1), 189–198. doi:10.1016/j.dsp.2006.05.008

Kawamoto, K., Houlihan, C. A., Balas, E. A., & Lobach, D. F. (2005). Improving clinical practice using clinical decision support systems: A systematic review of trials to identify features critical to success. *BMJ (Clinical Research Ed.)*, *330*(7494), 765. doi:10.1136/bmj.38398.500764.8F PMID:15767266

Kennedy, J. E. R. (1995). Particle swarm optimization. *Proceedings of IEEE International Conference on Neural Networks IV*. 10.1109/ICNN.1995.488968

Keras: The Python Deep Learning library. (n.d.). https://keras.io/

Kermack, W., & McKendrick, A. (1991a). Contributions to the mathematical theory of epidemics—I. *Bulletin of Mathematical Biology*, *53*(1–2), 33–55. doi:10.1007/BF02464423 PMID:2059741

Kermack, W., & McKendrick, A. (1991b). Contributions to the mathematical theory of epidemics—II. The problem of endemicity. *Bulletin of Mathematical Biology*, *53*(1–2), 57–87. doi:10.1007/BF02464424 PMID:2059742

Kermack, W., & McKendrick, A. (1991c). Contributions to the mathematical theory of epidemics—III. Further studies of the problem of endemicity. *Bulletin of Mathematical Biology*, *53*(1–2), 89–118. doi:10.1007/BF02464425 PMID:2059743

Khalaf, W., Astorino, A., d'Alessandro, P., & Gaudioso, M. (2017). A DC optimization-based clustering technique for edge detection. *Optimization Letters*, *11*(3), 627–640. doi:10.100711590-016-1031-7

Kharya, S. (2012). *Using data mining techniques for diagnosis and prognosis of cancer disease.* arXiv preprint arXiv:1205.1923

Khazaee, A. (2013). Heart Beat Classification Using Particle Swarm Optimization. *Int. J. of Intelligent Syst. and Applicat.*, *5*(6), 25–33. doi:10.5815/ijisa.2013.06.03

Khehra, B. S., & Pharwaha, A. P. S. (2011). Digital Mammogram Segmentation using Non-Shannon Measures of Entropy" *Proceedings of the World Congress on Engineering, WCE*, 2.

Khorrami, H., & Moavenian, M. (2010). A comparative study of DWT, CWT and DCT transformations in ECG arrhythmias classification. *Expert Systems with Applications*, *37*(8), 5751–5757. doi:10.1016/j.eswa.2010.02.033

Kirkpatrick, S., Gelatt, C. D., & Vecchi, M. P. (1983). Optimization by simulated annealing. *Science, 220*(4598), 671-680.

Koella, J. C., & Boete, C. (2003). A model for the co-evolution of immunity and immune evasion in vector-borne disease with implications for the epidemiology of malaria. *American Naturalist*, *161*(5), 698–707. doi:10.1086/374202 PMID:12858279

Kontaxakis, I., Sangriotis, E., & Martakos, D. (2003). Directional analysis of image textures for feature extraction and segmentation. *3rd International Symposium on Image and Signal Processing and Analysis, ISPA, 1*, 78-83. 10.1109/ISPA.2003.1296872

Kora, P., & Kalva, S. R. (2015). Improved Bat algorithm for the detection of myocardial infarction. *SpringerPlus*, *4*(1), 666. doi:10.118640064-015-1379-7 PMID:26558169

Korchiyne, R., Sbihi, A., Farssi, S. M., Touahni, R., & Alaoui, M. T. (2012). Medical image texture segmentation using Multifractal analysis. *International Conference on Multimedia Computing and Systems*, 422-425. 10.1109/IC-MCS.2012.6320316

Korurek, M., & Dogan, B. (2010). ECG beat classification using particle swarm optimization and radial basis function neural network. *Expert Systems with Applications*, *37*(12), 7563–7569. doi:10.1016/j.eswa.2010.04.087

Köse, U. (2010). *Developing Education Software For Fuzzy Logic And Artificial Neural Networks* (Msc). Afyon Kocatepe University, Afyon.

Kotsiantis, S. B., Zaharakis, I., & Pintelas, P. (2007). Supervised machine learning: A review of classification techniques. *Emerging Artificial Intelligence Applications in Computer Engineering*, *160*(1), 3-24.

Kovács, P. (2012). ECG signal generator based on geometrical features. *Annales Universitatis Scientiarum Budapestinensis de Rolando Eötvös Nominatae. Sectio Computatorica. 37*.

Kropf, M., Heyn, D., & Schreeler, G. (2017). ECG Classification Based on Time and Frequency Domain Features Using Random Forests. *Computers in Cardiology*, *44*, 1–4. doi:10.22489/CinC.2017.168-168

Kumar A., & Sarkar, B.K. (2018). A Hybrid Predictive Model Integrating C4.5 and Decision Table Classifiers for Medical Data Sets. *Journal of Information Technology Research, 11*(2), 150-167.

Kumar Tyagi, & Shamila. (2019). *Spy in the Crowd: How User's Privacy is getting affected with the Integration of Internet of Thing's Devices.* Elsevier.

Kumar, A., & Sarkar, B.K .(2017). Performance analysis of GA-based Iterative and Non-iterative Learning Approaches for Medical Domain Data Sets. *International Journal on Intelligent Decision Technologies, 11*(3), 321-334.

Kumar, P. S., & Pranavi, S. (2017, December). Performance analysis of machine learning algorithms on diabetes dataset using big data analytics. In *2017 International Conference on Infocom Technologies and Unmanned Systems (Trends and Future Directions) (ICTUS)* (pp. 508-513). IEEE. 10.1109/ICTUS.2017.8286062

Kumar, A., & Sarkar, B. K. (2018). GA_DTNB: A Hybrid Classifier for Medical Data Diagnosis. *6th International Conference on Frontiers in Intelligent Computing Theory and Applications (FICTA-2018), 2*, 139-148. 10.1007/978-981-10-7566-7_15

Kumar, A., & Sarkar, B. K. (2018). Performance analysis of nature inspired algorithms based Bayesian prediction models for medical data sets. *Soft Computing Based Non-linear Control Systems Design*, *7*, 134–155.

Kumar, B. P., Prathap, C., & Dharshith, C. N. (2013). An Automatic Approach for Segmentation of Ultrasound Liver Images. *International Journal of Emerging Technology and Advanced Engineering*, *3*(1), 337–340.

Kumari, V. S. R., & Kumar, P. R. (2013). Cardiac Arrhythmia Prediction using improved Multilayer Perceptron Neural Network. *Research for Development*, *3*(4), 73–80.

Kumar, K., & Abhishek, B. (2012). *Artificial neural networks for diagnosis of kidney stones disease.* GRIN Verlag. doi:10.5815/ijitcs.2012.07.03

Kumar, V., Chhabra, J. K., & Kumar, D. (2014). Performance evaluation of distance metrics in the clustering algorithms. *INFOCOMP Journal of Computer Science*, *13*(1), 38–52.

Kunwar, V., Chandel, K., Sabitha, A. S., & Bansal, A. (2016, January). Chronic Kidney Disease analysis using data mining classification techniques. In 2016 6th International Conference-Cloud System and Big Data Engineering (Confluence) (pp. 300-305). IEEE. doi:10.1109/CONFLUENCE.2016.7508132

Kusiak, A., Dixon, B., & Shah, S. (2005). Predicting survival time for kidney dialysis patients: A data mining approach. *Computers in Biology and Medicine, 35*(4), 311–327. doi:10.1016/j.compbiomed.2004.02.004 PMID:15749092

Laciar, E., Jane, R., & Brooks, D. H. (2003). Improved alignment method for noisy high-resolution ECG and Holter records using multiscale cross-correlation. *IEEE Transactions on Biomedical Engineering, 50*(3), 344–353. doi:10.1109/TBME.2003.808821 PMID:12669991

Lacson, R. C., Baker, B., Suresh, H., Andriole, K., Szolovits, P., & Lacson, E. Jr. (2019). Use of machine-learning algorithms to determine features of systolic blood pressure variability that predict poor outcomes in hypertensive patients. *Clinical Kidney Journal, 12*(2), 206–212. doi:10.1093/ckjfy049 PMID:30976397

Ladla, L., & Deepa, T. (2011). Feature Selection Methods And Algorithms. *International Journal on Computer Science and Engineering, 3*(5), 1787–1797.

Lahiri, T., Kumar, U., Mishra, H., Sarkar, S., & Roy, A. D. (2009). Analysis of ECG signal by chaos principle to help automatic diagnosis of myocardial infarction. *Journal of Scientific and Industrial Research, 68*(10), 866–870.

Lampinen, J., Laaksonen, J., & Oja, E. (1997). *Neural network systems, techniques and applications in pattern recognition*. Helsinki University of Technology.

Laws, K. I. (1980). *Texture image segmentation* (Ph.D thesis). University of Southern California.

Lee, C. S., & Wang, M. H. (2011). A fuzzy expert system for diabetes decision support application. *IEEE Transactions on Systems, Man, and Cybernetics. Part B, Cybernetics, 41*(1), 139–153. doi:10.1109/TSMCB.2010.2048899 PMID:20501347

Lei, W. K., Li, B. N., Dong, M. C., & Vai, M. I. (2007). AFC-ECG: An Intelligent Fuzzy ECG Classifier. In book. *Soft Computing in Industrial Applications, 39*, 189–199. doi:10.1007/978-3-540-70706-6_18

Levesque, H. J. (1986). Knowledge representation and reasoning. *Annual Review of Computer Science, 1*(1), 255–287. doi:10.1146/annurev.cs.01.060186.001351

Li, W., Han, J., & Pei, J. (2001). CMAR: Accurate and efficient classification based on multiple class-association rules. *Proceedings - IEEE International Conference on Data Mining, ICDM,* 369–376. 10.1109/icdm.2001.989541

Liaw, A., & Wiener, M. (2002). Classification and regression by random Forest. *R News,* ●●●, 18–22.

Li, L. (2014, November). Diagnosis of diabetes using a weight-adjusted voting approach. In *2014 IEEE International Conference on Bioinformatics and Bioengineering* (pp. 320-324). IEEE. 10.1109/BIBE.2014.27

Li-Ping, Z., Huan-Jun, Y., & Shang-Xu, H. (2005). Optimal choice of parameters for particle swarm optimization. *Journal of Zhejiang University. Science A, 6*(6), 528–534. doi:10.1631/jzus.2005.A0528

Li, Q., & Nishikawa, R. M. (Eds.). (2015). *Computer-aided detection and diagnosis in medical imaging*. Taylor & Francis. doi:10.1201/b18191

Liu, B., Hsu, W., Ma, Y., & Ma, B. (1998). Integrating Classification and Association Rule Mining. *Data Mining and Knowledge Discovery,* 80–86.

Liu, Y. (2015). Image denoising method based on threshold, wavelet trans-form and genetic algorithm. International Journal of Signal Processing. *Image Processing and Pattern Recognition, 8*(2), 29–40. doi:10.14257/ijsip.2015.8.2.04

Lo Presti, A., Cella, E., Giovanetti, M., Lai, A., Angeletti, S., Zehender, G., & Ciccozzi, M. (2015). Origin and evolution of Nipah virus. *Journal of Medical Virology, 88*(3), 380–388. doi:10.1002/jmv.24345 PMID:26252523

Long, N. C., Meesad, P., & Unger, H. (2015). A highly accurate firefly based algorithm for heart disease prediction. *Expert Systems with Applications, 42*(21), 8221–8231. doi:10.1016/j.eswa.2015.06.024

Loughna, P., Chitty, L., Evans, T., & Chudleigh, T. (2009). Fetal size and dating: Charts recommended for clinical obstetric practice. *Ultrasound, 17*(3), 160–166. doi:10.1179/174313409X448543

Luby, S. P., Gurley, E. S., & Hossain, M. J. (2009). Transmission of Human Infection with Nipah Virus. *Clinical Infectious Diseases, 49*(11), 1743–1748. doi:10.1086/647951 PMID:19886791

Lundervold, A. (2011). Lecture: Analysis of texture: Practice. *19th Annual Meeting of the International Society for Magnetic Resonance in Medicine(ISMRM).*

Luo, G., & Frey, L. J. (2016). Efficient execution methods of pivoting for bulk extraction of entity-attribute-value-modeled data. *IEEE Journal of Biomedical and Health Informatics, 20*(2), 644–665. doi:10.1109/JBHI.2015.2392553 PMID:25608318

Luz E. J. S., Schwartz W. R., Chavez G. C., Menotti D. (2016). ECG-based heartbeat classification for arrhythmia detection: A survey. *Computer Methods and Programs in Biomedicine, 127,* 144–164.

MacDonald, G. (1957). *The Epidemiology and Control of Malaria.* Oxford University Press.

Mahboob, T., Irfan, R., & Ghaffar, B. (2017, September). Evaluating ensemble prediction of coronary heart disease using receiver operating characteristics. In *2017 Internet Technologies and Applications (ITA)* (pp. 110-115). IEEE.

Mallat, S. G. (1991). Zero-crossing of a wavelet transform. *IEEE Transactions on Information Theory, 37*(4), 1019–1033. doi:10.1109/18.86995

Malthus, T. R. (1970). *An essay on the Principal of Population.* Penguin Books. (Original work published 1798)

Mangai, J. A., Nayak, J., & Kumar, V. S. (2013). A novel approach for classifying medical images using data mining techniques. *International Journal of Computer Science & Electrical Engineering, 1*(2), 188–192.

Mangat, V., & Vig, R. (2014). Dynamic PSO-based associative classifier for medical datasets. *IETE Technical Review (Institution of Electronics and Telecommunication Engineers, India), 31*(4), 258–265. doi:10.1080/02564602.2014.942237

Maraci, M. A., Bridge, C. P., Napolitano, R., Papageorghiou, A., & Noble, J. A. (2017). A framework for analysis of linear ultrasound videos to detect fetal presentation and heartbeat. *J Med Image Anal, 37,* 22–36. doi:10.1016/j.media.2017.01.003 PMID:28104551

Mariam,I. (2017). *UIC Health Informatics Health Data Sciences-blog.* Academic Press.

Marr, D., & Hildreth, E. (1980). Theory of edge detection. *Proceedings of the Royal Society of London. Series B, Biological Sciences, 207*(1167), 187–217. doi:10.1098/rspb.1980.0020 PMID:6102765

Marsanova, L., Ronzhina, M., Smisek, R., Vitek, M., Nemcova, A., Smital, L., & Novakova, M. (2017). ECG features and methods for automatic classification of ventricular premature and ischemic heartbeats: A comprehensive experimental study. *Scientific Reports, 7*(1), 11239. doi:10.103841598-017-10942-6 PMID:28894131

Martis, R.J., Lin, H., Gurupur, V.P., & Fernandes, S. L. (2017). *Frontiers in development of intelligent applications for medical imaging processing and computer vision.* Academic Press.

Materka, A., & Strzelecki, M. (2013). *On the importance of MRI non-uniformity correction for texture analysis. In Signal Processing: Algorithms, Architectures, Arrangements, and Applications.* SPA.

Mathur, S., & Gupta, M. (2014). An Analysis on Color Preservation Using Non-Shannon Entropy Measures for Gray and Color Images. *Fourth International Conference on Advances in Computing and Communications*, 109-112. 10.1109/ICACC.2014.32

Matsumoto, T., Ueda, Y., & Kawaji, S. (2002). A software system for giving clues of medical diagnosis to clinician. *Proceedings of 15th IEEE Symposium on Computer-Based Medical Systems (CBMS 2002)*, 65-70. 10.1109/CBMS.2002.1011356

McCarthy, J., Minsky, M. L., Rochester, N., & Shannon, C. E. (2006). A proposal for the dartmouth summer research project on artificial intelligence, august 31, 1955. *AI Magazine*, *27*(4), 12–12.

McCarty, C. A., Nair, A., Austin, D. M., & Giampietro, P. F. (2007). Informed consent and subject motivation to participate in a large, population-based genomics study: The marshfield clinic personalized medicine research project. *Community Genetics*, *10*(1), 2–9. doi:10.1159/000096274 PMID:17167244

McKhann, G. M., Knopman, D. S., Chertkow, H., Hyman, B. T., Jack, C. R. Jr, Kawas, C. H., Klunk, W. E., Koroshetz, W. J., Manly, J. J., Mayeux, R., Mohs, R. C., Morris, J. C., Rossor, M. N., Scheltens, P., Carrillo, M. C., Thies, B., Weintraub, S., & Phelps, C. H. (2011). The diagnosis of dementia due to Alzheimer's disease: Recommendations from the National Institute on Aging-Alzheimer's Association workgroups on diagnostic guidelines for Alzheimer's disease. *Alzheimer's & Dementia*, *7*(3), 263–269. doi:10.1016/j.jalz.2011.03.005 PMID:21514250

McNeill, M. (1989). ' *Plagues and People.* Anchor Books.

Middleton, D. J., Morrissy, C. J., van der Heide, B. M., Russell, G. M., Braun, M. A., Westbury, H. A., Halpin, K., & Daniels, P. W. (2007). Experimental Nipah virus infection in pteropid bats (*Pteropuspoliocephalus*). *Journal of Comparative Pathology*, *136*(4), 266–272. doi:10.1016/j.jcpa.2007.03.002 PMID:17498518

Minchole, A., Skarp, B., Jager, F., & Laguna, P. (2005). Evaluation of a root mean squared based ischemia detector on the long-term ST database with body position change cancellation. *Computers in Cardiology*, 853–856. doi:10.1109/CIC.2005.1588239

Mining, W. I. D. (2006). Data mining: Concepts and techniques. *Morgan Kaufinann*, *10*, 559–569.

Mir, A., & Dhage, S. N. (2018, August). Diabetes Disease Prediction Using Machine Learning on Big Data of Healthcare. In *2018 Fourth International Conference on Computing Communication Control and Automation (ICCUBEA)* (pp. 1-6). IEEE. 10.1109/ICCUBEA.2018.8697439

Mishra, N. (2018). Internet of Everything Advancement Study in Data Science and Knowledge Analytic Streams. *International Journal of Scientific Research in computer science and Engineering*, *6*(1), 30-36.

Mishra, N., Chang, H. T., & Lin, C. C. (2015). An Iot knowledge reengineering framework for semantic knowledge analytics for BI-services. *Mathematical Problems in Engineering*, *2015*, 2015. doi:10.1155/2015/759428

Mishra, N., Lin, C. C., & Chang, H. T. (2014, December). A cognitive oriented framework for IoT big-data management prospective. In *2014 IEEE International Conference on Communiction Problem-solving* (pp. 124-127). IEEE. 10.1109/ICCPS.2014.7062233

Mishra, N., Thangavel, G., & Samuel, J. M. (2019). A Case Assessment Of Knowledge-Based Fit In Frame For Diagnosis Of Human Eye Diseases. *Journal of Critical Reviews*, *7*(6), 2020.

Mitchell, J. D. (1987). Heavy metals and trace elements in amyotrophic lateral sclerosis. *Neurologic Clinics*, *5*(1), 43–60. doi:10.1016/S0733-8619(18)30934-4 PMID:3550416

Mitchell, J. D., & Borasio, G. D. (2007). Amyotrophic lateral sclerosis. *Lancet, 369*(9578), 2031–2041. doi:10.1016/S0140-6736(07)60944-1 PMID:17574095

Mitra, S., Mitra, M., & Chaudhuri, B. B. (2006). An Approach to a Rough Set Based Disease Inference Engine for ECG Classification. *IEEE Transactions on Instrumentation and Measurement, 55*(6), 2198–2206. doi:10.1109/TIM.2006.884279

Mitrea, D., Nedevschi, S., Socaciu, M., & Badea, R. (2012). The Role of the Superior Order GLCM in the Characterization and Recognition of the Liver Tumors from Ultrasound Images. *Wuxiandian Gongcheng, 21*(1), 79–85.

Moavenian, M., & Khorrami, H. (2010). A qualitative comparison of artificial neural networks and support vector machines in ECG arrhythmias classification. *Expert Systems with Applications, 37*(4), 3088–3093. doi:10.1016/j.eswa.2009.09.021

Mohammad, S., Morris, D. T., & Thacker, N. (2013). Texture Analysis for the Segmentation of Optic Disc in Retinal Images. *IEEE International Conference on Systems, Man, and Cybernetics*, 4265-4270. 10.1109/SMC.2013.727

Moore, P. J., Lyons, T. J., & Gallacher, J. (2019). Random forest prediction of Alzheimer's disease using pairwise selection from time series data. *PLoS One, 14*(2), e0211558. doi:10.1371/journal.pone.0211558 PMID:30763336

Munoz, M., Pong-Wong, R., Canela-Xandri, O., Rawlik, K., Haley, C. S., & Tenesa, A. (2016). Evaluating the contribution of genetics and familial shared environment to common disease using the UK biobank. *Nature Genetics, 48*(9), 980–983. doi:10.1038/ng.3618 PMID:27428752

Murphy, K. P. (2012). *Machine learning: a probabilistic perspective*. MIT Press.

Murthy, H. N., & Meenakshi, M. (2015). ANN, SVM and KNN classifiers for prognosis of cardiac ischemia-a comparison. *Bonfring International Journal of Research in Communication Engineering, 5*(2), 7. doi:10.9756/BIJRCE.8030

Murthy, S. K. (1998). Automatic construction of decision trees from data: A multi-disciplinary survey. *Data Mining and Knowledge Discovery, 2*(4), 345–389. doi:10.1023/A:1009744630224

Muthuchudar, A., & Baboo, S. S. (2013). A Study of the Processes Involved in ECG Signal Analysis. *Int. J. of Scientific and Research Publications, 3*(3), 1–5.

Nabiyev, V. (2003). *Artificial Intelligence: Problems, Methods, Algorithms* (Vol. 724). Seçkin Publishing.

Naik, G. R., & Reddy, K. A. (2016). A new model for ECG signal filtering and feature extraction. *IEEE International Conference on Computer and Communications (ICCC)*, 765-768. 10.1109/CompComm.2016.7924806

Naima, F. A., & Timemy, A. A. (2009). Neural network based classification of myocardial infarction: a comparative study of wavelet and fourier transforms. Academic Press.

Nandhini, M., & Sivanandam, S. N. (2015). An improved predictive association rule based classifier using gain ratio and T-test for health care data diagnosis. *Sadhana - Academy Proceedings in Engineering Sciences, 40*(6), 1683–1699. doi:10.100712046-015-0410-6

Nandhini, M., Rajalakshmi, M., & Sivanandam, S. N. (2017). Experimental and statistical analysis on the performance of firefly based predictive association rule classifier for health care data diagnosis. *Control Engineering and Applied Informatics, 19*(2), 101–110.

Narasingarao, M.R., Manda, R., Sridhar, G.R., Madhu, K., & Rao, A.A. (2009). *A clinical decision support system using multilayer perceptron neural network to assess well being in diabetes*. Academic Press.

Nasiri, J. A., Naghibzadeh, M., Yazdi, H. S., & Naghibzadeh, B. (2009). ECG Arrhythmia Classification with Support Vector Machines and Genetic Algorithm. *Third UKSim European Symposium on Computer Modeling and Simulation.*

Natarajan, P., Krishnan, N., Kenkre, N. S., Nancy, S., & Singh, B. P. (2012). Tumor detection using threshold operation in MRI brain images. *IEEE International Conference on Computational Intelligence and Computing Research*, 1-4. 10.1109/ICCIC.2012.6510299

National Center for Biotechnology Information. (2016). *The Database of Genotypes and Phenotypes (dbGaP)*. Author.

Nidhyananthan, S. S., Saranya, S., & Kumari, R. S. S. (2016). Myocardial infarction detection and heart patient identity verification. *International Conference on Wireless Communications, Signal Processing and Networking (WiSPNET)*, 1107–1111. 10.1109/WiSPNET.2016.7566308

Nikolay, B., Salje, H., Hossain, M.J., Khan, A.K.M.D., & Sazzad, H.M.S. (2019). *Transmission of Nipah Virus - 14 Years of Investigations in Bangladesh*. Doi:10.1056/NEJMoa1805376

Nipah Virus (NiV) CDC. (n.d.). www.cdc.gov

NoSQL - Wikipedia. (n.d.). Retrieved June 22, 2017, from https://en.wikipedia.org/wiki/NoSQL

Nowak, R. (1994). *Walker's bats of the world*. Johns Hopkins University Press.

Ohlhorst, F. (2012). *Big Data Analytics: Turning Big Data into Big Money*. John Wiley & Sons. doi:10.1002/9781119205005

Oluleye, B., Leisa, A., Leng, J., & Dean, D. (2014). A Genetic Algorithm-Based Feature Selection. *International Journal of Electronics Communication and Computer Engineering*, *5*(4), 899–905.

Omran, S. S., Taha, S. M. R., & Awadh, N. A. (2009). ECG Rhythm Analysis by Using Neuro-Genetic Algorithms. *Journal of Basic and Applied Sciences*, *1*(3), 522–530.

Oprea, M. (2006). On the Use of Data-Mining Techniques in Knowledge-Based Systems. *Ecological Informatics*, *6*, 21–24.

Öz, C., Köker, R., & Çakar, S. (2002). *Character-based plate recognition with artificial neural networks*. Paper presented at the Electrical, Electronics and Computer Engineering Symposium (ELECO 2002), Bursa.

Ozbay, Y., Ceylan, R., & Karlik, B. (2006). A fuzzy clustering neural network architecture for classification of ECG arrhythmias. *Computers in Biology and Medicine*, *36*(4), 376–388. doi:10.1016/j.compbiomed.2005.01.006 PMID:15878480

Öztemel, E. (2003). *Artificial neural networks*. Papatya Publishing.

Padhy, S., & Dandapat, S. (2017). Third-order tensor based analysis of multilead ECG for classification of myocardial infarction. *Biomedical Signal Processing and Control*, *31*, 71–78. doi:10.1016/j.bspc.2016.07.007

Padhy, S., Sharma, L., & Dandapat, S. (2016). Multilead ECG data compression using SVD in multiresolution domain. *Biomedical Signal Processing and Control*, *23*, 10–18. doi:10.1016/j.bspc.2015.06.012

Padole, Parekh, & Patel. (2013). Signal Processing Approach for Recognizing Identical Reads From DNA Sequencing of Bacillus Strains. *IOSR Journal of Computer Engineering*, *10*(1), 19-24.

Padole, M. (2014). Distributed approach to pattern matching in genomics. Dept. of Computer Science and Engineering, The M.S University of Baroda. Available http://14.139.121.106/pdf/2014/oct14/1.pdf

Paksoy, S. (2007). A genetic algorithm for project scheduling (PhD). Cukurova University, Adana.

Pal, D., Mandana, K., Pal, S., Sarkar, D., & Chakraborty, C. (2012). Fuzzy expert system approach for coronary artery disease screening using clinical parameters. *Knowledge-Based Systems*, *36*, 162–174. doi:10.1016/j.knosys.2012.06.013

Parashar, U. D., Sunn, L. M., Ong, F., Mounts, A. W., Arif, M. T., Ksiazek, T. G., Kamaluddin, M. A., Mustafa, A. N., Kaur, H., Ding, L. M., Othman, G., Radzi, H. M., Kitsutani, P. T., Stockton, P. C., Arokiasamy, J., Gary, H. E. Jr, & Anderson, L. J. (2000). Case-control study of risk factors for human infection with a new zoonotic Paramyxovirus, Nipah virus, during a 1998–1999 outbreak of severe encephalitis in Malaysia. *The Journal of Infectious Diseases, 181*(5), 1755–1759. doi:10.1086/315457 PMID:10823779

Parsons, S. (2005). Ant Colony Optimization by Marco Dorigo and Thomas Stützle, MIT Press, 305 pp., $40.00, ISBN 0-262-04219-3. *The Knowledge Engineering Review, 20*(1), 92–93. doi:10.1017/S0269888905220386

Pathoumvanh, S., Hamamoto, K., & Indahak, P. (2014). Arrhythmias Detection and Classification base on Single Beeat ECG Analysis. *The 4ᵗʰ International Conference on Information and Communication Technology, Electronics and Electrical Engineering (IJCTEE-2014).*

Patil, P. M. (2016). Review on Prediction of Chronic Kidney Disease using Data Mining Techniques. *International Journal of Computer Science and Mobile Computing, 5*(5), 135.

Patra, D., Das, M. K., & Pradhan, S. (2010). Integration of FCM, PCA and neural networks for classification of ECG arrhythmias. *IAENG Int. J. of Comput. Sci., 36*(3), 24–62.

Paul, R., & Hoque, A. S. M. L. (2009). Optimized entity attribute value model: A search efficient representation of high dimensional and sparse data. *IBC, 3*, 1–6. doi:10.1109/ICCIT.2009.5407131

Paul, R., & Hoque, A. S. M. L. (2010). Optimized column-oriented model: A storage and search efficient representation of medical data. *Information Technology in Bio-and Medical Informatics, ITBAM, 2010*, 118–127. doi:10.1007/978-3-642-15020-3_12

Payan, A., & Montana, G. (2015). *Predicting Alzheimer's disease: a neuroimaging study with 3D convolutional neural networks.* arXiv preprint arXiv:1502.02506

Pereira, C. R., Pereira, D. R., Silva, F. A., Masieiro, J. P., Weber, S. A., Hook, C., & Papa, J. P. (2016). A new computer vision-based approach to aid the diagnosis of Parkinson's disease. *Computer Methods and Programs in Biomedicine, 136*, 79–88. doi:10.1016/j.cmpb.2016.08.005 PMID:27686705

Peter, J., Muller, T., & Freyer, R. (1995). Optimized constraint satisfaction neural network for medical image segmentation. *Neural Networks, Proceedings, IEEE International Conference on, 5*, 2592-2595.

Pham, D. T., & Karaboga, D. (2000). Intelligent Optimisation Techniques. Intelligent Optimisation Techniques. doi:10.1007/978-1-4471-0721-7

Pharwaha, A. P. S., & Singh, B. (2009). Shannon and Non-Shannon Measures of Entropy for Statistical Texture Feature Extraction in Digitized Mammograms. *Proceedings of the World Congress on Engineering and Computer Science, WCECS, 2.*

Phyu, T. N. (2009, March). Survey of classification techniques in data mining. In *Proceedings of the International MultiConference of Engineers and Computer Scientists* (*Vol. 1*, pp. 18-20). Academic Press.

Pohl, K. M., Konukoglu, E., Novellas, S., Ayache, N., Fedorov, A., Talos, I. F., ... & Black, P. M. (2011). A new metric for detecting change in slowly evolving brain tumors: validation in meningioma patients. *Operative Neurosurgery, 68*(suppl_1), ons225-ons233.

Polat, K., Akdemir, B., & Gune, S. (2008). Computer aided diagnosis of ECG data on the least square support vector machine. *Digital Signal Processing, 18*(1), 25–32. doi:10.1016/j.dsp.2007.05.006

Pontryagin, L. S., Boltyanskii, V. G., Gamkrelize, R. V., & Mishchenko, E. F. (1962). *The Mathematical Theory of Optimal Processes*. Wiley.

Poonguzhali, S., & Ravindran, G. (2008). Automatic classification of focal lesions in ultrasound liver images using combined texture features. *Information Technology Journal*, *7*(1), 205–209. doi:10.3923/itj.2008.205.209

Postmus, I., Trompet, S., Deshmukh, H. A., Barnes, M. R., Li, X., Warren, H. R., ... Donnelly, L. A. (2014). Pharmacogenetic meta-analysis of genome-wide association studies of LDL cholesterol response to statins. *Nature Communications*, *5*(1), 5068. doi:10.1038/ncomms6068 PMID:25350695

Powell, J.H. (1993). *Bring Out Your Dead: The Great Plague of Yellow Fever in Philadelphia in 1793*. University of Pennsylvania Press.

Powers, D. M. (2011). Evaluation: From precision, recall and F-measure to ROC, informedness, markedness and correlation. *Journal of Machine Learning Technologies*, 37–63.

Pragna, D. P., Dandu, S., Meenakzshi, M., Jyotsna, C., & Amudha, J. (2017, March). Health alert system to detect oral cancer. In *2017 International Conference on Inventive Communication and Computational Technologies (ICICCT)* (pp. 258-262). IEEE. 10.1109/ICICCT.2017.7975198

Pramanik, M., Gupta, M., & Krishnan, K. B. (2013). Enhancing reproducibility of ultrasonic measurements by new users. *SPIE Medical Imaging International Society for Optics and Photonics*, *8673*, 86730Q. Advance online publication. doi:10.1117/12.2008032

Prasad, T. V. (2012). *Hybrid systems for knowledge representation in artificial intelligence*. arXiv preprint arXiv:1211.2736

Prentzas, J., & Hatzilygeroudis, I. (2007). Categorizing approaches combining rule-based and case-based reasoning. *Expert Systems: International Journal of Knowledge Engineering and Neural Networks*, *24*(2), 97–122. doi:10.1111/j.1468-0394.2007.00423.x

PreprocessingI. (n.d.). https://keras.io/preprocessing/image/

Priyadarshini, R., Dash, N., & Mishra, R. (2014, February). A Novel approach to predict diabetes mellitus using modified Extreme learning machine. In *2014 International Conference on Electronics and Communication Systems (ICECS)* (pp. 1-5). IEEE. 10.1109/ECS.2014.6892740

Priyadharshini, V., & Kumar, S. S. (2015). An Enhanced Approach on ECG Data Analysis using Improvised Genetic Algorithm. *International Research Journal of Engineering and Technology*, *2*(5), 1248–1256.

Priyanka, K. (2014). A Survey on Big Data Analytics in Health Care. *International Journal of Computer Science and Information Technologies*, *5*(4), 5865–5868.

Pryor, T. A. (1988). The HELP medical record system. *MD Computing: Computers in Medical Practice, 5*(5), 22.

Quesnel, P. X., Chan, A. D. C., & Yang, H. (2014). Signal quality and false myocardial ischemia alarms in ambulatory electrocardiograms. *IEEE International Symposium on Medical Measurements and Applications (MeMeA)*, 1–5. 10.1109/MeMeA.2014.6860078

Quinlan, J. R. (1979). Discovering rules by induction from large collections of examples. *Expert systems in the microelectronics age*.

Quinlan, J. R. (1993). *Program for machine learning*. C4. 5.

Quinlan, J. R., & Cameron-Jones, R. M. (1993). FOIL: A midterm report. Lecture Notes in Computer Science, 667, 3–20. doi:10.1007/3-540-56602-3_124

Quinlan, J. R. (2014). *C4. 5: programs for machine learning.* Elsevier.

Ragesh, N. K., Anil, A. R., & Rajesh, R. (2011). Digital image denoising in medical ultrasound images: A Survey. *Proceeding on ICGST AIML-11 Conference,* 67-73.

Raghupathi, W., & Raghupathi, V. (2014). Big data analytics in healthcare: Promise and potential. *Health Information Science and Systems, 2*(1), 3. doi:10.1186/2047-2501-2-3 PMID:25825667

Rahman, S. A., Hassan, S. S., Olival, K. J., Mohamed, M., Chang, L.-Y., Hassan, L., Saad, N. M., Shohaimi, S. A., Mamat, Z. C., Naim, M. S., Epstein, J. H., Suri, A. S., Field, H. E., & Daszak, P. (2010). Characterization of Nipah virus from naturally infected Pteropusvampyrus bats, Malaysia. *Emerging Infectious Diseases, 16*(12), 1990–1993. doi:10.3201/eid1612.091790 PMID:21122240

Rahmatullah, B., Papageorghiou, A. T., & Noble, J. A. (2012). Image analysis using machine learning: anatomical landmarks detection in fetal ultrasound images. Proceeding on Computer Software and Applications, 354-355, doi:10.1109/COMPSAC.2012.52

Rahul, G., & Vijay, K. N. (2012). *Predictive Analytics for Resource Over-commit in IaaS Cloud.* IEEE.

Raihan, M., Mandal, P. K., Islam, M. M., Hossain, T., Ghosh, P., Shaj, S. A., ... More, A. (2019, February). Risk Prediction of Ischemic Heart Disease Using Artificial Neural Network. In *2019 International Conference on Electrical, Computer and Communication Engineering (ECCE)* (pp. 1-5). IEEE. 10.1109/ECACE.2019.8679362

Rajaguru, H., & Prabhakar, S. K. (2017). Performance comparison of oral cancer classification with Gaussian mixture measures and multi layer Perceptron. In *The 16th International Conference on Biomedical Engineering* (pp. 123-129). Springer. 10.1007/978-981-10-4220-1_23

Rajinikanth, V., Satapathy, S. C., Fernandes, S. L., & Nachiappan, S. (2017). Entropy based Segmentation of Tumor from Brain MR Images–A study with Teaching Learning Based Optimization. *Pattern Recognition Letters, 94,* 87–95. doi:10.1016/j.patrec.2017.05.028

Rajliwall, N. S., Davey, R., & Chetty, G. (2018, December). Machine learning based models for Cardiovascular risk prediction. In *2018 International Conference on Machine Learning and Data Engineering (iCMLDE)* (pp. 142-148). IEEE. 10.1109/iCMLDE.2018.00034

Ramya, S., & Radha, N. (2016). Diagnosis of chronic kidney disease using machine learning algorithms. *International Journal of Innovative Research in Computer and Communication Engineering, 4*(1), 812–820.

Rangayyan, R. M., & Reddy, N. P. (2002). Biomedical signal analysis: A case-study approach. *Annals of Biomedical Engineering, 30*(7), 983–983. doi:10.1114/1.1509766

Rasmussen-Torvik, L. J., Stallings, S. C., Gordon, A. S., Almoguera, B., Basford, M. A., Bielinski, S. J., ... Connolly, J. J. (2014). Design and anticipated outcomes of the eMERGE-PGx project: A multicenter pilot for preemptive pharmacogenomics in electronic health record systems. *Clinical Pharmacology and Therapeutics, 96*(4), 482–489. doi:10.1038/clpt.2014.137 PMID:24960519

Ravishankar, H., Prabhu, S. M., Vaidya, V., & Singhal, N. (2016). Hybrid approach for automatic segmentation of fetal abdomen from ultrasound images using deep learning. *IEEE Conference on Global Research,* 779-782, . 2016.7493382.10.1109/ISBI.2016.7493382

Rayavarapu, K., & Krishna, K. K. (2018, March). Prediction of Cervical Cancer using Voting and DNN Classifiers. In *2018 International Conference on Current Trends towards Converging Technologies (ICCTCT)* (pp. 1-5). IEEE. 10.1109/ICCTCT.2018.8551176

Rehm, H. L., Berg, J. S., Brooks, L. D., Bustamante, C. D., Evans, J. P., Landrum, M. J., ... Nussbaum, R. L. (2015). Clingen—The clinical genome resource. *The New England Journal of Medicine, 372*(23), 2235–2242. doi:10.1056/NEJMsr1406261 PMID:26014595

Reiber, G. E., & LaCroix, A. Z. (2016). Older women veterans in the women's health initiative. *The Gerontologist, 56*(Suppl. 1), S1–S5. doi:10.1093/geront/gnv673 PMID:26768382

Riccardo, B., & Blaz, Z. (2009). *Predictive data mining in clinical medicine: Current issues and guidelines*. Elsevier.

Richards, W., & Polit, A. (1974). Texture Matching. *Kybernetic, 16*(3), 155–162. doi:10.1007/BF00271719 PMID:4437126

Rish, I. (2019). An empirical study of the naive Bayes classifier. In Workshop on Empirical Methods in Artificial Intelligence, (pp. 41-46). Academic Press.

Rissanen, J. (1983). A universal prior for integers and estimation by minimum description length. *Annals of Statistics, 11*(2), 416–431. doi:10.1214/aos/1176346150

Robert, F. (2015). Core Concept: Homomorphic encryption. *Proceedings of the National Academy of Sciences of the United States of America, 112*(28), 8515–8516. doi:10.1073/pnas.1507452112 PMID:26174872

Robert, H. M., & Ida, S. (2004). Physicians' Use of Electronic Medical Records: Barriers And Solutions. *Health Affairs*. PMID:15046136

Rodger, L., & Michael, B. (2014). *City Hub: A Cloud-Based IoT Platform for Smart Cities*. IEEE.

Roopa, C. K., & Harish, B. S. (2017). A Survey on various Machine Learning Approaches for ECG Analysis. *International Journal of Computers and Applications, 163*(9).

Rosenblum, S., Samuel, M., Zlotnik, S., Erikh, I., & Schlesinger, I. (2013). Handwriting as an objective tool for Parkinson's disease diagnosis. *Journal of Neurology, 260*(9), 2357–2361. doi:10.100700415-013-6996-x PMID:23771509

Ross, R. (1911). *The Prevention of Malaria*. John Murray.

Ruchika, M. (2015). *A systematic review of machine learning techniques for software fault prediction*. Elsevier.

Ruggieri, S. (2002). Efficient C4. 5 [classification algorithm]. *IEEE Transactions on Knowledge and Data Engineering, 14*(2), 438–444. doi:10.1109/69.991727

Rumelhart, D. E., Hinton, G. E., & Williams, R. J. (1988). Learning representations by back-propagating errors. *Cognitive Modeling, 5*(3), 1.

Russell, S. J., & Norvig, P. (2016). *Artificial intelligence: a modern approach*.

Saal, L. H., Vallon-Christersson, J., Hakkinen, J., Hegardt, C., Grabau, D., Winter, C., ... Schulz, R. (2015). The Sweden Cancerome Analysis Network—Breast (SCAN-B) initiative: A large-scale multicenter infrastructure towards implementation of breast cancer genomic analyses in the clinical routine. *Genome Medicine, 7*(1), 20. doi:10.118613073-015-0131-9 PMID:25722745

Sachdeva, S., & Bhalla, S. (2012). Semantic Interoperability in Standardized Electronic Health Record Databases. *ACM Journal of Data and Information Quality, 3*(1), 1–37. doi:10.1145/2166788.2166789

SadAbadi, H., Ghasemi, M., & Ghaffari, A. (2007). A Mathematical Algorithm for ECG Signal Denoising Using Window Analysis. *Biomedical Papers of the Medical Faculty of the University Palacky, Olomouc, Czechoslovakia, 151*(1), 73–78. doi:10.5507/bp.2007.013 PMID:17690744

Sadiq, A. T., & Shukr, N. H. (2013). Classification of Cardiac Arrhythmia using ID3 Classifier Based on Wavelet Transform. *Iraqi J. of Sci.*, *54*(4), 1167–1175.

Safavian, S. R., & Landgrebe, D. (1991). *A survey of decision tree classifier methodology.* IEEE. doi:10.1109/21.97458

Safdarian, N., Dabanloo, N. J., & Attarodi, G. (2014). A new pattern recog-nition method for detection and localization of myocardial infarction using T-wave integral and total integral as extracted features from one cycle of ECG signal. *Scientific Research Publishing*, *7*, 818.

Sah, R. D., & Sheetalani, J. (2017). Review of Medical Disease Symptoms Prediction Using Data Mining Technique. *Journal of Computational Engineering*, *19*(3), 59–70.

Salchenberger, L. M., Cinar, E. M., & Lash, N. A. (1992). Neural networks: A new tool for predicting thrift failures. *Decision Sciences*, *23*(4), 899–916. doi:10.1111/j.1540-5915.1992.tb00425.x

Sao, P., Hegadi, R., & Karmakar, S. (2015). ECG Signal Analysis Using Artificial Neural Network. *International Journal of Scientific Research (Ahmedabad, India)*, 82–86.

Sarkaleh, M. K., & Shahbahrami, A. (2012). Classification of ECG arrhythmias using Discrete Wavelet Transform and neural networks. *Int. J. of Comput. Sci. Eng. and Applicat.*, *2*(1), 1–13.

Sasikumar, M., Ramani, S., Raman, S. M., Anjaneyulu, K. S. R., & Chandrasekar, R. (2007). *A practical introduction to rule based expert systems.* Narosa Publishing House.

Savitzky–Golay filter. (n.d.). https://en.wikipedia.org/wiki/Savitzky%E2%80%93Golay_filter

Savitzky-Golay Filter. (n.d.b). http://www.statistics4u.com/fundstat_eng/cc_filter_savgolay.html

Savitzky-golay-filter. (n.d.a). https://github.com/swallez/savitzky-golay-filter/blob/master/src/mr/go/sgfilter/SGFilter.java

Schiezaro, M., & Pedrini, H. (2013). Data feature selection based on Artificial Bee Colony algorithm. *EURASIP Journal on Image and Video Processing*, *2013*(1). doi:10.1186/1687-5281-2013-47

Schmidt, M., Baumert, M., Porta, A., Malberg, H., & Zaunseder, S. (2014). Two-dimensional warping for one-dimensional signals–conceptual framework and application to ECG processing. *IEEE Transactions on Signal Processing*, *62*(21), 5577–5588. doi:10.1109/TSP.2014.2354313

Schmoldt, D. L., & Rauscher, H. M. (2012). *Building knowledge-based systems for natural resource management.* Springer Science & Business Media.

Schreiber, G., Wielinga, B., & Breuker, J. (Eds.). (1993). *KADS: A principled approach to knowledge-based system development* (Vol. 11). Academic Press.

Schulman, J., Chen, X., & Abbeel, P. (2017). *Equivalence between policy gradients and soft q-learning.* arXiv preprint arXiv:1704.06440

Seera, M., & Lim, C. P. (2014). A hybrid intelligent system for medical data classification. *Expert Systems with Applications*, *41*(5), 2239–2249. doi:10.1016/j.eswa.2013.09.022

Selvarajah, S., & Kodituwakku, S. R. (2011). Analysis and comparison of texture features for content based image retrieval. *International Journal of Latest Trends in Computing*, *2*(1).

Senthilkumaran, N., & Rajesh, R. (2009). A Study on Rough Set Theory for Medical Image Segmentation. *International Journal of Recent Trends in Engineering*, *2*(2), 236–238.

Serapião, A., & Bannwart, A. C. (2013). Knowledge discovery for classification of three-phase vertical flow patterns of heavy oil from pressure drop and flow rate data. *Journal of Petroleum Engineering.*

Setiawan, N. A., Venkatachalam, P. A., & Fadzil, A. (2009). Rule Selection for Coronary Artery Disease Diagnosis Based on Rough Set. *International Journal of Recent Trends in Engineering, 2*(5), 198–202.

Sexton, R. S., Dorsey, R. E., & Johnson, J. D. (1998). Toward global optimization of neural networks: A comparison of the genetic algorithm and backpropagation. *Decision Support Systems, 22*(2), 171–185. doi:10.1016/S0167-9236(97)00040-7

Shah, N. H., Trivedi, N. D., Thakkar, F. A., & Satia, M. H. (2018). Control Strategies for Nipah Virus. *International Journal of Applied Engineering Research, 13*(21), 15149–15163.

Shahzad, W., & Baig, A. R. (2011). Hybrid associative classification algorithm using ant colony optimization. *International Journal of Innovative Computing, Information, & Control, 7*(12), 6815–6826.

Shamila, M., & Vinuthna, K. (2019). A Review on Several Critical Issues and Challenges in IoT based e-Healthcare System. IEEE.

Shareef, N., Wang, D. L., & Yagel, R. (1999). Segmentation of medical images using LEGION. *IEEE Transactions on Medical Imaging, 18*(1), 74–91. doi:10.1109/42.750259 PMID:10193699

Shareha, A. A. A., Rajeswari, M., & Ramachandram, D. (2008). Textured Renyi Entropy for Image Thresholding. *Fifth International Conference on Computer Graphics, Imaging and Visualisation*, 185-192. 10.1109/CGIV.2008.48

Sharma, K. K., Sharma, N., & Sharma, S. (2012). Comparison of Shannon and Non Shannon Entropy Measures for Threshold Selection in Color Image Segmentation Problems. *International Conference on Electronics Computer Technology*, 533.

Sharma, L. N., & Dandapat, S. (2016). Detecting myocardial infarction by multivariate multiscale covariance analysis of multilead electrocardio-grams. *The International Congress on Information and Communication Technology, Springer Singapore*, 439, pp. 169–179.

Sharma, L. N., Tripathy, R. K., & Dandapat, S. (2015). Multiscale energy and eigenspace approach to detection and localization of myocardial infarction. *IEEE Transactions on Biomedical Engineering, 62*(7), 1827–1837. doi:10.1109/TBME.2015.2405134 PMID:26087076

Sharma, N., Bajpai, A., & Litoriya, R. (2012). Comparison the various clustering algorithms of weka tools. *International Journal of Emerging Technology and Advanced Engineering, 2*(5), 73–80.

Sharmila, S. (2017). *Analysis of Heart Disease Prediction Using Data mining Techniques. International Journal of Advanced Networking & Applications.*

Shawe-Taylor, J., & Cristianini, N. (2004). *Kernel methods for pattern analysis.* Cambridge university press. doi:10.1017/CBO9780511809682

Shepherd, J., Cobbe, S. M., Ford, I., Isles, C. G., Lorimer, A. R., Macfarlane, P. W., McKillop, J. H., & Packard, C. J. (1995). Prevention of coronary heart disease with pravastatin in men with hypercholesterolemia. *The New England Journal of Medicine, 333*(20), 1301–1308. doi:10.1056/NEJM199511163332001 PMID:7566020

Shi, Y., & Eberhart, R. C. (1998). *Parameter selection in particle swarm optimization.* Paper presented at the International conference on evolutionary programming.

Shi, Y., & Eberhart, R. C. (1999). *Empirical study of particle swarm optimization.* Paper presented at the Proceedings of the 1999 Congress on Evolutionary Computation-CEC99 (Cat. No. 99TH8406). 10.1109/CEC.1999.785511

Shiferaw, B., Gelaw, B., Assefa, A., Assefa, Y., & Addis, Z. (2015). Bacterial isolates and their antimicrobial susceptibility pattern among patients with external ocular infections at Borumeda hospital, Northeast Ethiopia. *BMC Ophthalmology, 15*(1), 103. doi:10.118612886-015-0078-z PMID:26268424

Shobitha, S., Amita, P. M., Niranjana, K. B., & Ali, M. A. M. (2018, April). Noninvasive Blood Glucose Prediction from Photoplethysmogram Using Relevance Vector Machine. In *2018 3rd International Conference for Convergence in Technology (I2CT)* (pp. 1-4). IEEE. 10.1109/I2CT.2018.8529481

Signs and Symptoms Nipah Virus (NiV). (n.d.). www.cdc.gov

Silveira, R. M., Agulhari, C. M., Bonatti, I. S., & Peres, P. D. L. (2007). A genetic algorithm to compress the electrocardiograms using parametrized wavelets. *IEEE International Symposium on Signal Processing and Information Technology.* 10.1109/ISSPIT.2007.4458092

SimulatorE. C. G. (n.d.). http://www.mit.edu/~gari/CODE/ECGSYN/JAVA/APPLET2/ecgsyn/ecg-java/source.html

Singh, J., Kamra, A., & Singh, H. (2016, October). Prediction of heart diseases using associative classification. In *2016 5th International Conference on Wireless Networks and Embedded Systems (WECON)* (pp. 1-7). IEEE. 10.1109/WECON.2016.7993480

Singh, A., & Kumar, D. (2017, May). Novel ABC based training algorithm for ovarian cancer detection using neural network. In *2017 International Conference on Trends in Electronics and Informatics (ICEI)* (pp. 594-597). IEEE. 10.1109/ICOEI.2017.8300771

Singh, G., Vadera, M., Samavedham, L., & Lim, E. C. H. (2016). Machine Learning-Based Framework for Multi-Class Diagnosis of Neurodegenerative Diseases: A Study on Parkinson's Disease. *IFAC-PapersOnLine, 49*(7), 990–995. doi:10.1016/j.ifacol.2016.07.331

Singh, M., Singh, S., & Gupta, S. (2014). An information fusion based method for liver classification using texture analysis of ultrasound images. *Information Fusion, 19*, 91–96. doi:10.1016/j.inffus.2013.05.007

Singh, P., Singh, S., & Pandi-Jain, G. S. (2018). Effective heart disease prediction system using data mining techniques. *International Journal of Nanomedicine, 13*, 121–124. doi:10.2147/IJN.S124998 PMID:29593409

Singh, Y. N., Singh, S. K., & Ray, A. K. (2012). Bioelectrical signals as emerging biometrics: Issues and challenges. *ISRN Signal Processing, 2012*, 1–13. doi:10.5402/2012/712032

Sklansky, J. (1978). Image Segmentation and Feature Extraction. *IEEE Transactions on Systems, Man, and Cybernetics, 8*(4), 237–247. doi:10.1109/TSMC.1978.4309944

Soliz, P., Russell, S. R., Abramoff, M. D., Murillo, S., Pattichis, M., & Davis, H. (2008). Independent component analysis for vision-inspired classification of retinal images with age-related macular degeneration. *South authors Symposium on Image Analysis and Interpretation, 65-68.*

Sonawane, J. S., & Patil, D. R. (2014, February). Prediction of heart disease using multilayer perceptron neural network. In *International Conference on Information Communication and Embedded Systems (ICICES2014)* (pp. 1-6). IEEE. 10.1109/ICICES.2014.7033860

Sornmo, L. (1991). *Time-varying filtering for removal of baseline wander in exercise ECGs. Computers in Cardiology, Proceedings.* doi:10.1109/CIC.1991.169066

Specht, D. F. (1990). Probabilistic neural networks. *Neural Networks, 3*(1), 109–118. doi:10.1016/0893-6080(90)90049-Q PMID:18282828

Srimani, P.K., & Koti, M.S. (2014). *Rough set (RS) approach for optimal rule generation in medical datawork*. Academic Press.

Srivastava, V. K., & Prasad, D. (2013). Dwt-Based Feature Extraction from ECG Signal. *American J. of Eng. Research*, *2*(3), 44–50.

Stephanie, C., & Regan, F. (2017). *Risk assessment and decision making in child protective services: Predictive risk modeling in context*. Elsevier.

Storn, R. (1996). Differential evolution design of an IIR-filter. *Proceedings of IEEE international conference on evolutionary computation*. 10.1109/ICEC.1996.542373

Sturm, R. A., & Larsson, M. (2009). Genetics of human iris color and patterns. *Pigment Cell & Melanoma Research*, *22*(5), 544–562. doi:10.1111/j.1755-148X.2009.00606.x PMID:19619260

Suganya, R., & Rajaram, S. (2012). Content based image retrieval of ultrasound liver diseases based on hybrid approach. *American Journal of Applied Sciences*, *9*(6), 938–945. doi:10.3844/ajassp.2012.938.945

Sultana, J., & Podder, C. N. (2016). Mathematical Analysis of Nipah Virus Infections Using Optimal Control Theory. *Zeitschrift für Angewandte Mathematik und Physik*, *4*, 1099–1111. doi:10.4236/jamp.2016.46114

Suman, S. K., & Hooda, N. (2019). Predicting risk of Cervical Cancer: A case study of machine learning. *Journal of Statistics and Management Systems*, *22*(4), 689–696. doi:10.1080/09720510.2019.1611227

Summers, M. J., Madl, T., Vercelli, A. E., Aumayr, G., Bleier, D. M., & Ciferri, L. (2017). Deep machine learning application to the detection of preclinical neurodegenerative diseases of aging. *DigitCult-Scientific Journal on Digital Cultures*, *2*(2), 9–24.

Swain, A., Mohanty, S. N., & Das, A. C. (2016, March). Comparative risk analysis on prediction of Diabetes Mellitus using machine learning approach. In *2016 International Conference on Electrical, Electronics, and Optimization Techniques (ICEEOT)* (pp. 3312-3317). IEEE. 10.1109/ICEEOT.2016.7755319

Syeda-Mahmood, T. F. (2015). *Role of machine learning in clinical decision support (Presentation Recording). In SPIE Medical Imaging*. International Society for Optics and Photonics.

Tafa, Z., Pervetica, N., & Karahoda, B. (2015, June). An intelligent system for diabetes prediction. In *2015 4th Mediterranean Conference on Embedded Computing (MECO)* (pp. 378-382). IEEE. 10.1109/MECO.2015.7181948

Tamura, H., Mori, S., & Yamawaki, Y. (1978). Textural features corresponding to visual perception. *IEEE Transactions on Systems, Man, and Cybernetics*, *8*(6), 460–473. doi:10.1109/TSMC.1978.4309999

Tang, X., & Shu, L. (2014). Classification of Electrocardiogram Signals with RS and Quantum Neural Networks. *Int. J. of Multimedia and Ubiquitous Eng.*, *9*(2), 363–372. doi:10.14257/ijmue.2014.9.2.37

Tao, P. D. (2009, September). Minimum sum-of-squares clustering by DC programming and DCA. In *International Conference on Intelligent Computing* (pp. 327-340). Springer.

Tayel, S., Reif, M., & Dengel, A. (2013). Rule-based Complaint Detection using RapidMiner. In *Conference: RCOMM* (pp. 141-149). Academic Press.

Tereshchenko, L. G., & Josephson, M. E. (2015). Frequency Content and Characteristics of Ventricular Conduction. *Journal of Electrocardiology*, *48*(6), 933–937. doi:10.1016/j.jelectrocard.2015.08.034 PMID:26364232

Thabtah, F. A., Cowling, P., & Peng, Y. (2004). MMAC: A new multi-class, multi-label associative classification approach. *Proceedings - Fourth IEEE International Conference on Data Mining, ICDM 2004*, 217–224. 10.1109/ICDM.2004.10117

The Facts about High Blood Pressure—American Heart Association. (n.d.). Retrieved June 22, 2017, from http://www. heart.org/HEARTORG/Conditions/HighBloodPressure/GettheFactsAboutHighBloodPressure/The-Facts-About-High-Blood-Pressure_UCM_002050_Article.jsp

Tosun, S. (2018). *Software Used in Artificial Neural Networks*. Retrieved from http://www.suleymantosun.com/yapay-sinir-aglari-uygulamasinda-kullanilan-yazilimlar/

Tripathy, B. K., Acharjya, D. P., & Cynthya, V. (2011). A Framework for Intelligent Medical Diagnosis Using Rough Set with Formal Concept Analysis. *International Journal of Artificial Intelligence & Applications*, 2(2), 45–66. doi:10.5121/ijaia.2011.2204

UCI Machine Learning Repository: Liver Disorders Data Set. (n.d.). Retrieved June 22, 2017, from https://archive.ics.uci.edu/ml/datasets/Liver+Disorders

UCI Machine Learning Repository: Thyroid Disease Data Set. (n.d.). Retrieved June 22, 2017, from https:// archive.ics.uci.edu/ml/datasets/Thyroid+Disease

Umer, M., Bhatti, B. A., Tariq, M. H., Zia-ul-Hassan, M., Khan, M. Y., & Zaidi, T. (2014). Electrocardiogram Feature Extraction and Pattern Recognition Using a Novel Windowing Algorithm. *Scientific Research Advances in Bioscience and Biotechnology.*, 5(11), 896–894. doi:10.4236/abb.2014.511103

Understanding Xavier Initialization In Deep Neural Networks. (n.d.). https://prateekvjoshi.com/2016/03/29/understanding-xavier-initialization-in-deep-neural-networks/

Urooj, S., & Singh, S. P. (2016). Geometric invariant feature extraction of medical images using Hu's invariants. *3rd International Conference on Computing for Sustainable Global Development (INDIACom)*, 1560-1562.

Valian, E., Mohanna, S., & Tavakoli, S. (2011). Improved cuckoo search algorithm for feedforward neural network training. *International Journal of Artificial Intelligence & Applications*, 2(3), 36–43. doi:10.5121/ijaia.2011.2304

Vapnik, V. (2013). *The nature of statistical learning theory*. Springer Science & Business Media.

Vardhan, M. H., & Rao, S. V. (2014). GLCM architecture for image extraction. *International Journal of Advanced Research in Electronics and Communication Engineering*, 3(1), 75–82.

Vijayan, V. V., & Anjali, C. (2015, December). Prediction and diagnosis of diabetes mellitus—A machine learning approach. In *2015 IEEE Recent Advances in Intelligent Computational Systems (RAICS)* (pp. 122-127). IEEE.

Vijayarani, S., Dhayanand, S., & Phil, M. (2015). Kidney disease prediction using SVM and ANN algorithms. *International Journal of Computing and Business Research*, 6(2).

Vijayavanan, M., Rathikarani, V., & Dhanalakshmi, P. (2014). Automatic Classification of ECG Signal for Heart Disease Diagnosis using morphological features. *International Journal of Computer Science and Engineering Technology*, 5(4), 449–455.

Vijini, M. (2017). *Towards data science-blog*. Academic Press.

Vimalkumar & Vandra. (2014). Entropy Based Feature Selection For MultiRelational Naïve Bayesian Classifier. *Journal of International Technology and Information Management, 23*(1). https://amethix.com/entropy-in-machine-learning/

Vinken, P. J., & Bruyn, G. W. (Eds(1979*Handbook of clinical neurology*. North-Holland Publishing Company. doi:10.1002/ana.410060526

Vishwa, A., Lal, M. K., Dixit, S., & Vardwaj, P. (2011). Classification of arrhythmic ECG data using machine learning techniques. *Int. J. of Interactive Multimedia and Artificial Intell.*, 1(4), 68–71.

Vishwa, A., Lal, M., Dixit, S., & Vardwaj, P. (2011). Classification of Arrhythmic ECG Data Using Machine Learning Techniques. *International Journal of Interactive Multimedia and Artificial Intelligence*, *1*(4), 67–70. doi:10.9781/ijimai.2011.1411

Vocaturo, E., & Veltri, P. (2017). On the use of Networks in Biomedicine. *FNC/MobiSPC, 2017*, 498-503.

Vocaturo, E., Zumpano, E., & Veltri, P. (2018, July). Features for melanoma lesions characterization in computer vision systems. In *2018 9th International Conference on Information, Intelligence, Systems and Applications (IISA)* (pp. 1-8). IEEE. 10.1109/IISA.2018.8633651

Vocaturo, E., Perna, D., & Zumpano, E. (2019, November). Machine Learning Techniques for Automated Melanoma Detection. In *2019 IEEE International Conference on Bioinformatics and Biomedicine (BIBM)* (pp. 2310-2317). IEEE. 10.1109/BIBM47256.2019.8983165

Vocaturo, E., & Zumpano, E. (2019, November). Dangerousness of dysplastic nevi: a Multiple Instance Learning Solution for Early Diagnosis. In *2019 IEEE International Conference on Bioinformatics and Biomedicine (BIBM)* (pp. 2318-2323). IEEE. 10.1109/BIBM47256.2019.8983056

Vocaturo, E., Zumpano, E., & Veltri, P. (2018, December). Image pre-processing in computer vision systems for melanoma detection. In *2018 IEEE International Conference on Bioinformatics and Biomedicine (BIBM)* (pp. 2117-2124). IEEE. 10.1109/BIBM.2018.8621507

Vyas, V. S., & Rege, P. (2006). Automated texture analysis with Gabor filter. *GVIP Journal*, *6*(1), 35–41.

Wagholikar, K. B., Sundararajan, V., & Deshpande, A. W. (2012). Modeling paradigms for medical diagnostic decision support: A survey and future directions. *Journal of Medical Systems*, *36*(5), 3029–3049. doi:10.100710916-011-9780-4 PMID:21964969

Wagner, R. A., & Fischer, M. J. (1974). The string to string correction problem. *Journal of the Association for Computing Machinery*, *21*(1), 168–173. doi:10.1145/321796.321811

Waldner, J. B. (2007). *Nanocomputers and swarm intelligence*. ISTE.

Wang, J. S., Chiang, W. C., Yang, Y. T., & Hsu, Y. L. (2012). *An effective ECG arrhythmia classification algorithm*. Bio-Inspired Computing and Applications, Springer Berlin Heidelberg. doi:10.1007/978-3-642-24553-4_72

Wang, T. Y., & Chiang, H. M. (2007). Fuzzy support vector machine for multiclass categorization. *Information Processing & Management*, *43*(4), 914–929. doi:10.1016/j.ipm.2006.09.011

Warner, H. R., Olmsted, C. M., & Rutherford, B. D. (1972). HELP—A program for medical decision-making. *Computers and Biomedical Research, an International Journal*, *5*(1), 65–74. doi:10.1016/0010-4809(72)90007-9 PMID:4553324

Weir, B. S. (1990). Genetic data analysis. Methods for discrete population genetic data. Academic Press.

WHA 57.13. (2004). *Genomics and World Health*. Fifty Seventh World Health Assembly Resolution.

What is an intuitive explanation of the Xavier Initialization for Deep Neural Networks? (n.d.). https://www.quora.com/What-is-an-intuitive-explanation-of-the-Xavier-Initialization-for-Deep-Neural-Networks

WHO Nipah Virus (NiV) Infection. (n.d.). www.who.int

WHO. (2002). Genomics and World Health: Report of the Advisory Committee on Health research. Geneva: WHO.

Wong, K. T., Shieh, W. J., Kumar, S., Norain, K., Abdullah, W., Guarner, J., Goldsmith, C. S., Chua, K. B., Lam, S. K., Tan, C. T., Goh, K. J., Chong, H. T., Jusoh, R., Rollin, P. E., Ksiazek, T. G., & Zaki, S. R. (2002). Nipah virus infection: Pathology and pathogenesis of an emerging paramyxoviral zoonosis. *American Journal of Pathology, 161*(6), 2153–2167. doi:10.1016/S0002-9440(10)64493-8 PMID:12466131

Wong, S. Q., Fellowes, A., Doig, K., Ellul, J., Bosma, T. J., Irwin, D., ... Chan, K. S. (2015). Assessing the clinical value of targeted massively parallel sequencing in a longitudinal, prospective population-based study of cancer patients. *British Journal of Cancer, 112*(8), 1411–1420. doi:10.1038/bjc.2015.80 PMID:25742471

World Health Organization. (2006). *Sight test and glasses could dramatically improve the lives of 150 million people with poor vision.* WHO.

Wullianallur, R., & Viju, R. (2013). *An Overview of Health Analytics. J Health Med Informat.*

XiaohuiH. (2006). *PSO Tutorial.* Retrieved from http://www.swarmintelligence.org/tutorials.php

Xu, R., & Wunsch, D. (2008). *Clustering* (Vol. 10). John Wiley & Sons. doi:10.1002/9780470382776

Yang, H. M. (2000). Malaria transmission model for different levels of acquired immunity and temperature-dependent parameters (vector). *Revista de Saude Publica, 34*(3), 223–231. doi:10.1590/S0034-89102000000300003 PMID:10920443

Yang, H. M., & Ferreira, M. U. (2000). Assessing the effects of global warming and local social and economic conditions on the malaria transmission. *Revista de Saude Publica, 34*(3), 214–222. doi:10.1590/S0034-89102000000300002 PMID:10920442

Yanpeng, Q. R. (2019). Li Non-unique decision differential entropy-based feature selection. Elsevier.

Ye, C. Z., Yang, J., Geng, D. Y., Zhou, Y., & Chen, N. Y. (2002). Fuzzy rules to predict degree of malignancy in brain glioma. *Medical & Biological Engineering & Computing, 40*(2), 145–152. doi:10.1007/BF02348118 PMID:12043794

Yekkala, I., Dixit, S., & Jabbar, M. A. (2017, August). Prediction of heart disease using ensemble learning and Particle Swarm Optimization. In *2017 International Conference On Smart Technologies For Smart Nation (SmartTechCon)* (pp. 691-698). IEEE. 10.1109/SmartTechCon.2017.8358460

Yeniay, Ö. (2001). An Overview of Genetic Algorithms. *Anadolu University Journal of Science and Technology, 2*(1), 37–49.

Yeo, M. F., & Agyei, E. O. (1998). Optimising engineering problems using genetic algorithms. *Engineering Computations, 15*(2), 268–280. doi:10.1108/02644409810202684

Yifan& Sharma. (2016). *Diabetes patient Readmission Prediction using Big Data Analytics Tools.* Academic Press.

Yiğit, T., Işık, A. H., & Bilen, M. (2014). Web based educational software for artificial neural networks. *The Eurasia Proceedings of Educational & Social Sciences, 1*, 276–279.

Yin, X., & Han, J. (2003). *CPAR: Classification based on Predictive Association Rules.* doi:10.1137/1.9781611972733.40

Yob, J. M., Field, H., Rashdi, A. M., Morrissy, C., van der Heide, B., Rota, P., bin Adzhar, A., White, J., Daniels, P., Jamaluddin, A., & Ksiazek, T. (2001). Nipah virus infection in bats (order Chiroptera) in peninsular Malaysia. *Emerging Infectious Diseases, 7*(3), 439–441. doi:10.3201/eid0703.017312 PMID:11384522

Yu, L., & Liu, H. (2003). Feature Selection for High-Dimensional Data: A Fast Correlation-Based Filter Solution. *Proceedings, Twentieth International Conference on Machine Learning, 2*, 856–863. https://www.aaai.org/Papers/ICML/2003/ICML03-111.pdf

Yu, S. N., & Chou, K. T. (2008). Integration of independent component analysis and neural networks for ECG beat classification. *Expert Systems with Applications, 34*(4), 2841–2846. doi:10.1016/j.eswa.2007.05.006

Zadeh, L. A. (1965). Fuzzy sets. *Information and Control, 8*(3), 338–353. doi:10.1016/S0019-9958(65)90241-X

Zanella, A., Bui, N., Castellani, A., Vangelista, L., & Zorzi, M. (2014). Internet of things for smart cities. *IEEE Internet of Things Journal, 1*(1), 22-32.

Zare, M. R., Mueen, A., Seng, W. C., & Awedh, M. H. (2011). Combined Feature Extraction on Medical X-ray Images. *Third International Conference on Computational Intelligence, Communication Systems and Networks*, 264-268. 10.1109/CICSyN.2011.63

Žarko, I. P., Pripužić, K., Serrano, M., & Hauswirth, M. (2014, June). Iot data management methods and optimisation algorithms for mobile publish/subscribe services in cloud environments. In *2014 European conference on networks and communications (EuCNC)* (pp. 1-5). IEEE.

Zeraatkar, E., & ... . (2011). Arrhythmia detection based on Morphological and time-frequency Features of t-wave in Electrocardiogram. *Journal of Medical Signals and Sensors, 1*(2), 99–106. doi:10.4103/2228-7477.95293 PMID:22606664

Zhang, Q., & Gao, L. (2010). A Novel Medical Image Feature Extraction Algorithm. *Third International Conference on Intelligent Networks and Intelligent Systems*, 56-59. 10.1109/ICINIS.2010.172

Zhao & Sun. (2019). *Maximum Entropy-Regularized Multi-Goal Reinforcement Learning.* Academic Press.

Zhao, F., Ren, Z., Yu, D., & Yang, Y. (2005). *Application of an improved particle swarm optimization algorithm for neural network training.* Paper presented at the 2005 International Conference on Neural Networks and Brain.

Zheng, X., Shi, J., Zhang, Q., Ying, S., & Li, Y. (2017, April). Improving MRI-based diagnosis of Alzheimer's disease via an ensemble privileged information learning algorithm. In *2017 IEEE 14th International Symposium on Biomedical Imaging (ISBI 2017)* (pp. 456-459). IEEE. https://www.mayoclinic.org/diseases-conditions/alzheimers-disease/symptoms-causes/syc-20350447

Zheng, Y., & Kwoh, C. K. (2011). A Feature Subset Selection Method Based On High-Dimensional Mutual Information. *Entropy (Basel, Switzerland), 13*(4), 2011. doi:10.3390/e13040860

Zhu, X. J. (2005). *Semi-supervised learning literature survey.* University of Wisconsin-Madison Department of Computer Sciences.

Zidelmal, Z., Amirou, A., Abdeslam, D. O., & Merckle, J. (2013). ECG beat classification using a cost sensitive classifier. *Computer Methods and Programs in Biomedicine, 111*(3), 570–577. doi:10.1016/j.cmpb.2013.05.011 PMID:23849928

Ziqing, Z., & Zhou, Y. (2019). *Machine learning guided appraisal and exploration of phase design for high entropy alloys.* Computational Materials, Nature.

Zong, X., Geiser, E. A., Laine, A. F., & Wilson, D. C. (1996). Homomorphic wavelet shrinkage and feature emphasis for speckle reduction and enhancement of echocardiographic images. *Medical Imaging: Image Processing, 2710*, 658–667. doi:10.1117/12.237969

Zucker, S., & Kant, K. (1981). Multiple- level representations for texture discrimination. *Proceedings of the IEEE Conference on pattern Recognition and Image Processing*, 609-614.

Zumpano, E., Iaquinta, P., Caroprese, L., Cascini, G., Dattola, F., Franco, P., ... Vocaturo, E. (2018, December). Simpatico 3d: A medical information system for diagnostic procedures. In *2018 IEEE International Conference on Bioinformatics and Biomedicine (BIBM)* (pp. 2125-2128). IEEE. 10.1109/BIBM.2018.8621090

About the Contributors

Geeta Rani is the Assistant Professor (Senior Grade) at Manipal University Jaipur. She has an enriched experience of ten years in teaching the graduate and post graduate students. She is chief editor of the book "Handbook of Disease Prediction using Machine Learning", to be published by IGI Global. She has published two patents in the applications of Artificial Intelligence. She is awarded with registration of five copyrights for software applications. She has published many articles in the journals of repute, National and International conferences. She also has published four book chapters in the books indexed in SCOPUS and Web of Science. She is working on the funded project recommended by Indian Space Research Organisation. Her one project has been shortlisted in SERB for evaluation. She qualified for the 'Women Scientist-IPR'. She is international trainer for the cloud computing, certified by IBM. She has delivered many invited talks at the national conferences. She is reviewer of many SCI, SCIE and SCOPUS indexed Journals. More than seven IPR are registered in her name.

Pradeep Kumar Tiwari is a research scholar in Computer Science & Engineering Department at Manipal University Jaipur, India. He received the M.Phil degree in Computer Science from the Mahatma Gandhi Chitrakoot Gramodaya Vishwavidyalaya, M.P., India, 2012. The M.C.A degree in Computer Application from the Rajiv Gandhi Proudyogiki Vishwavidyalaya, M.P., India, in 2008. He has held Asst. Professor Positions at The Vindhya Institute of Technology, and the Aditya College of Technology, Satna, M.P, India. His research interests cover the Distributed Computing, Cloud Computing, Virtualization, Grid Computing, Cluster Computing and Network Security. He has published 6 article in refereed international journal and 10 publications in international conferences (i.e. IEEE, Springer). He is reviewer of 5 international conferences and at present, he is reviewer and editorial member of 4 journals.

* * *

Manish Kumar Ahirwar is currently working as an Assistant Professor in Department of Computer Science, University Institute of Technology, RGPV, Bhopal. He has work experience of several years in the field of teaching. His research interests include Data Mining Algorithms, Internet of Things (IoT), Web Development, Machine Learning and Cyber Security. He is a member of IEEE, ACM, IACSIT, IAENG. He has published more than 30 research papers in various International and National Journals and Conferences, including 4 papers in SCIE Journals and more than 10 papers in Scopus Journals. He has also published two Indian patents and two copyrights.

Shiva Shanta Mani B. did her B.Tech in Computer Science and Engineering from Indian Institute of Information Technology Kottayam, India. Currently, she is working as a graduate engineering trainee at L&T Infotech, Bangalore, India. Her area of interest is machine learning and health informatics.

Kerim Kürşat Çevik is the Assistant Professor at the Department of Business Informatics, Akdeniz University. He started to work as a lecturer at Computer Programming Programs Nigde University in 2009. At the end of his PhD studies, he was appointed as an assistant professor in the same program. Recently he has started to work as assistant professor at Akdeniz University. Çevik's research and teaching focus on artificial intelligence, image processing, biomedical, machine learning, computer-aided detection, medical informatics, data mining, mobile programming and computer vision. Çevik studied Electronic and Computer Sciences as an undergraduate and earned a M.Sc. at Selcuk University. He has PhD in Computer Engineering at the Selcuk University.

Ahan Chatterjee is a young and dynamic engineering student at The Neotia University, in the Department of Computer Science and Data Analytics. He has been a part of a research internship at CSIR-CDRI, GoOffer Hyperlocal Pvt. Ltd. as a Research & Development Intern. He also worked as Research Analyst Intern at Research Guruji after his completion of the first year itself. He has 1 accepted and 3 published research articles to his name. He wants to pursue his career in a research-based domain. His field of interest is Data Analytics, Machine Learning, and Artificial Intelligence.

D. K. Chaturvedi is working in Dept. of Elect. Engg, Faculty of Engg, D.E.I., Dayalbagh, Agra since 1989. Presently he is Professor. He did his B.E. from Govt. Engineering College Ujjain, M.P. then he did his M.Tech. and Ph.D. from D.E.I. Dayalbagh. He is gold medalist and received Young Scientists Fellowship from DST, Government of India in 2001-2002 for post doctorial research at Univ. of Calgary, Canada. Also, he had research collaboration with different organizations at national and international level. He is the Fellow - The Institution of Engineers (India), Fellow - Aeronautical Society of India, Fellow - IETE, Sr. Member IEEE, USA and Member of many National and International professional bodies such as IET, U.K., ISTE, Delhi, ISCE, Roorkee, IIIE, Mumbai and SSI etc. The IEE, U.K. recognized his work in the area of Power System Stabilizer and awarded honorary membership to him in 2006. He did many R&D projects of MHRD, UGC, AICTE etc. and consultancy projects of DRDO. He contributed in the national mission of ICT of Govt. of India as Virtual Power Lab Developer. He has guided 10 Ph.Ds., 65 M.Tech. Dissertations and published more than 300 International and National Papers. He has chaired and Co-Chaired many International and National Conferences. He is referee of many International Journals including IEE Proceedings and IEEE Transactions. He is Head of Dept. of Footwear Technology, Convener, Faculty Training and Placement Cell, and Advisor, IEI Students' Chapter (Elect. Engg.), D.E.I. Dayalbagh, Agra.

Arpita Das is an Assistant Professor of Department of Radio Physics and Electronics, University of Calcutta, India. She received her B. Tech, M.Tech and Ph.D. degree in the year 2004, 2006 and 2012 respectively. Her research focuses on Biomedical Image/Signal Analysis, Pattern Recognition, Soft Computing Approaches and FPGA based System Design. She presented many conference papers, published articles in different journals, and contributed chapters in various books.

Poulomi Das is an Assistant Professor of Department of Electronics and Communication Engineering, Omdayal Group of Institutions, MAKAUT, India. She received her M.Tech degree in 2013 from MAKAUT. Presently, she is doing PhD in Department of Radio Physics and Electronics, University of Calcutta. Her research focuses on Medical Image Analysis, Pattern Recognition, Wireless Communication.

Vijaypal Dhaka is an enthusiastic and motivating technocrat with 15 years of industry and academic experience. With his sharp wits, creativity, leading style and passion for students' development, he has created an atmosphere of project development in University. He is strong at technical fixes and impresses by his ability to design solutions. Fostering innovation and providing nurturing eco-system for budding entrepreneurs is his key thrust area. In his able leadership students have won many prizes at National level e.g. Aero India Drone Competition, Pravega at IISc Bengaluru and Innovative Research prize at IIT Bombay are some to mention. He lays strong emphasis on automation projects for University use, developed by students and has been successful in deploying 6 such projects in University. He has served on various key positions including Director-Innovations, Dean-Academics, Chief Editor for International Journal and Head of Department. He has more than 80 publications in Journals of great repute in his name and guided 10 research scholars to earn PhD. His research interests include, Machine Learning, Artificial Intelligence, Image processing and pattern recognition. He has organized 6 International conferences supported by IEEE, ACM, Springer and Elsevier including SIN-2017. He has served as Organizing Secretary and is TPC member for several IEEE Conferences. He has been invited to deliver keynote addresses and plenary talk in various universities and institutions. Dr Dhaka has successfully executed Solar Photo-Voltaic Efficiency Prediction and Enhancement Project funded by SERB (DST, Govt of India). 9 student research projects funded by DST Govt of Rajasthan, India, have been guided by him. He received "World Eminence Awards 2017" for Leading Research Contribution in ICT for the Year 2016, at WS-4 in London on 15th Feb 2017.

Ayushe Gangal is currently pursuing her Bachelor of Technology (B.Tech) degree in the field of Computer Science and Engineering from G.B. Pant Government Engineering College, Delhi, India. She is in the fourth year of her degree's tenure. Her research interests include machine learning, computer vision and neural computing. She has presented a research paper on computer vision in a conference on Advancement in Engineering Sciences in Shri Mata Vaishno Devi University, Katra (J&K). She has published 8 machine learning and computer vision papers in prestigious SCOPUS/SCI-indexed journals along with a patent and she has also co-authored a chapter on disease prediction using machine learning algorithms in IGI Global Publications.

Mayank Gupta is acting as System and IT Analyst in Tata Consultancy services, Noida and expert of Data sciences and Business Analytics. He has skill to visualize the situations from different perspectives and explore the real facts through critical Analysis. He has deep interest in Human health domains.

Pratik Kanani received his Bechelors and Masters Degree from University of Mumbai. Currently he is working as an Assistant Professor in the Department of Computer Engineering at Dwakadas J. Sanghvi College of Engineering. He has more than 25 research contributions in International and National Journals as well as Conferences. He is an active researcher in the field of Network Security, IoT, Machine Learning and Fog Computing. Currently he is pursuing his Doctoral studies from The MS university of Baroda.

Parminder Kaur is working as an Associate Professor in the Department of Computer Science, at Guru Nanak Dev University Amritsar, India. She has done her post-graduation in Mathematics as well as System Software and doctorate in the field of Computer Science. She has more than 60 publications in International/National Journals/Conferences. Her research interests include Component-based Software Engineering, Web Engineering, Software Security, Semantic Web, Digital Image Processing and Service-Oriented Architecture.

Binish Khan is currently pursuing a Dual degree PG Integrated course (B.E. and MTech.) in Computer Science from University Institute of Technology, RGPV, Bhopal. She is eager to work in the field of healthcare in order to improve the prevailing conditions of healthcare system. Her research interests include Classification Algorithms, Web Development, Disease Prediction, Machine Learning and Data Mining. The main idea behind her research is to provide ease to the doctors, various classification techniques can be utilized to predict the liver disease at an early stage so that essential precautions could be undertaken to improve the overall experience of the patients.

Peeyush Kumar is currently pursuing his Bachelor of Technology (B.Tech) degree in the field of Computer Science and Engineering from G.B. Pant Government Engineering College, Delhi, India. He is in the fourth year of his degree's tenure. His research interests include machine learning, computer vision and neural computing. He has published 8 machine learning and computer vision papers in prestigious SCOPUS/SCI indexed journals along with a patent and he has also co-authored a chapter on disease prediction using machine learning algorithms in IGI Global Publications.

Raj Kumar has earned Ph.D. in Electronics Engineering. He has around twenty years of teaching and research. His broad areas of research is Battery Management System, Green Energy, Energy Storage, Smart Instrumentation, Embedded Systems. Now he is involved in capacity building through pedagogy, curriculum and evaluation in higher education.

Upendra Kumar is working as an Assistant Professor in CSE Department in Institute of Engineering & Technology, Lucknow.

Nandhini M. holds an MCA, M.Phil, M.E., Ph.D., in Computer Science. She has been working as an Assistant Professor in Computer Science and Engineering for the last 18 years. She has completed her Ph.D. in the area of data mining. She has more than twelve publications in national and international journals and has presented five papers in international conferences of repute. She has published a book chapter and registered an IPR. She is a reviewer of SCI-indexed journals. She has delivered many invited talks at the national workshops and FDPs. Her research areas include Data mining, Data analytics, and optimization techniques.

Nilamadhab Mishra is currently an Assistant Professor in Post at School of Computing, Debre Berhan University, Ethiopia. He has around 15 years of rich global exposure in Academic Teaching & Research. He publishes numerous peer reviewed researches in SCIE & SCOPUS indexed journals & IEEE conference proceedings, and serves as reviewer and editorial member in peer reviewed Journals and Conferences. Dr. Mishra has received his Doctor of Philosophy (PhD) in Computer Science & Information Engineering from Graduate Institute of Electrical Engineering, College of Engineering, Chang

Gung University (a World Ranking University), Taiwan. He involves in academic research by working, as an Journal Editor, as a SCIE & Scopus indexed Journals Referee, as an ISBN Book Author, and as an IEEE Conference Referee. Dr. Mishra has been pro-actively involved with several professional bodies: CSI, ORCID, IAENG, ISROSET, Senior Member of "ASR" (Hong Kong), Senior Member of "IEDRC" (Hong Kong), and Member of "IEEE ". Dr. Mishra's Research areas incorporate Network Centric Data Management, Data Science: Analytics and Applications, CIoT Big-Data System, and Cognitive Apps Design & Explorations.

Meet Oza is a self-motivated and proficient technocrat. He has won many prizes in the national and international hackathons. He has worked on many projects funded by the national and international agencies. He is pursuing his BTech from Manipal University Jaipur.

Mamta Padole is working as an Associate Professor in the Department of Computer Science and Engineering at The Maharaja Sayajirao University of Baroda. She has more than 20 years of academics and industrial experience. Her research papers are indexed in Web of Science, SCOPUS, DBLP, ACM and IEEE. Her areas of interest are Distributed Computing, Cloud Computing, Fog Computing, IoT, Big Data Analytics and BioInformatics. She is guiding PhD students.

Diviya Prabha is a PhD Research Scholar, Department of Computer Science, Periyar University, Salem, Tamil Nadu, India.

Nidhya R. is presently working as Assistant Professor in the Department of Computer Science & Engineering, Madanapalle Institute of Technology & Science, affiliated to Jawaharlal Nehru Technical University, Anantapuram, India. She received the M.Tech and Ph.D degree from Anna University, Chennai. Her research interests include wireless body area network, network security and data mining. She published many research papers in refereed international journals and IEEE & Springer associated conferences. She is an active member of CSI, ISTE, IAENG, SAISE and ISRD.

Rahul Rajak was a B.Tech student in the Department of Radio Physics and Electronics, University of Calcutta, India. He has completed his B.Tech degree in 2019. Presently, he is doing M.Tech in the Department of Radio Physics and Electronics, University of Calcutta.

Rinkle Rani is working as Associate Professor in Computer Science and Engineering Department, Thapar Institute of Engineering and Technology, Patiala since 2000. She has done her Post graduation from BITS, Pilani and Ph.D. from Punjabi University, Patiala. She has more than 21 years of teaching experience. She has over 120 research papers, out of which 56 are in international journals and 64 are in conferences. She has guided 08 PhD and 46 ME theses. Her areas of interest are Big Data Analytics and Machine Learning. She is a member of professional bodies: ACM, IEEE, and CSI.

Rohit Rastogi received his B.E. degree in Computer Science and Engineering from C.C.S.Univ. Meerut in 2003, the M.E. degree in Computer Science from NITTTR-Chandigarh (National Institute of Technical Teachers Training and Research-affiliated to MHRD, Govt. of India), Punjab Univ. Chandigarh in 2010. Currently he is pursuing his Ph.D. In computer science from Dayalbagh Educational Institute, Agra under renowned professor of Electrical Engineering Dr. D.K. Chaturvedi in area of spiritual consciousness. Dr. Santosh Satya of IIT-Delhi and dr. Navneet Arora of IIT-Roorkee have happily consented him to co supervise. He is also working presently with Dr. Piyush Trivedi of DSVV Hardwar, India in center of Scientific spirituality. He is a Associate Professor of CSE Dept. in ABES Engineering. College, Ghaziabad (U.P.-India), affiliated to Dr. A.P. J. Abdul Kalam Technical Univ. Lucknow (earlier Uttar Pradesh Tech. University). Also, He is preparing some interesting algorithms on Swarm Intelligence approaches like PSO, ACO and BCO etc. Rohit Rastogi is involved actively with Vichaar Krnati Abhiyaan and strongly believe that transformation starts within self.

Swagatam Roy is currently pursuing the second year of engineering at The Neotia University in the Department of Computer Science Engineering with a specialization in Data Analytics. His performance is good in college and the CGPA is increasing in the consecutive semesters. He has good knowledge in C, C++with good application skills in python. Also, 2 papers of him had been published in a renounced journal. His area of interest lies in Data Analytics, machine learning, deep learning, artificial intelligence.

RenugaDevi S. was a M.E student in the Department of Computer Science and Engineering, PSG College of Technology, Coimbatore.

Sivanandam S. N. has a teaching/research experience of more than 52 years. His areas of specialization are Modeling and Simulation, Neural Networks, Fuzzy Systems and Genetic Algorithm, Pattern Recognition, Multidimensional system analysis, Linear and Nonlinear control system, Power System, Numerical methods, Parallel Computing, Data Mining, and Database Security. He is a member of various professional bodies like IE (India), ISTE, CSI, ACS, and SSI. He is a technical advisor for various reputed industries and engineering institutions. He has guided several PhDs successfully in the Modeling and Simulation, Neural Networks, Fuzzy Systems and Genetic Algorithm, Pattern Recognition. He has published more than 100 papers in national and international journals.

Anu Saini received the Bachelor of Technology and Master of Technology degree from the Maharishi Dayanand University Rohtak, Haryana, India in 2004 and 2007 respectively. Ph.D. degree from Jawaharlal Nehru University, New Delhi .She is currently working as a Assistant Professor in the Department of Computer Science and Engineering at G. B. Pant Govt. Engineering College, New Delhi. Her research interests are in Software Engineering, Big Data, and Recommendation Systems. She has published more than 15 papers in the Journals and conferences of repute. She is a lifetime member of the ISTE.

Johny Samuel is a 2 IS research scholar, College of Computing, Debre Berhan University, Ethiopia, Africa.

Sunita Sangwan received the Bachelor of Technology and Master of Technology degree from the Maharishi Dayanand University Rohtak, Haryana, India. She is currently working as a Assistant Professor in the Department of Computer Science and Engineering at G. B. Pant Govt. Engineering College, New Delhi. Her research interests are in Operating systems, Machine Learning, Big data and Data mining. She has published more than 25 papers in the Journals and conferences of repute.

Aman Sharma is currently working as Assistant Professor (Grade-II) in the Department of Computer Science & Engineering at Jaypee University of Information Technology, Waknaghat, Solan, Himachal Pradesh. He has around 5 years of teaching and research experience. He has completed his Ph.D. from the Computer Science & Engineering Department of Thapar Institute of Engineering and Technology, Patiala, Punjab. He obtained his M.E. in Computer Science & Engineering from Thapar Institute of Engineering and Technology, Patiala, Punjab. He has obtained his B.Tech. in Computer Science & Engineering from R.B.I.E.B.T, Mohali, Punjab. He has been a rank holder throughout his studies. He has also obtained A.I.R-1800 in GATE 2013.

Piyush Kumar Shukla received his Bachelor's degree in Electronics & Communication Engineering, LNCT, Bhopal in 2001, MTech. (Computer Science & Engineering) in 2005 from SATI, Vidisha and Ph.D. (Computer Science & Engineering) in 2013 from RGPV, Bhopal, India. He is a member of ISTE (Life Member), IEEE, ACM, IACSIT, IAENG. Currently he is working as an Assistant Professor in Department of Computer Science, University Institute of Technology, RGPV, Bhopal. He has published more than 60 research papers in various International and National Journals and Conferences, including 4 papers in SCIE Journals and more than 10 papers in Scopus Journals. He has also published an Indian patent.

Gurvinder Singh is working as a Professor in the Department of Computer Science, at Guru Nanak Dev University Amritsar, India. He has 23 years of teaching as well as research experience. He has contributed 150 research papers in International / national Journals as well as Conferences. Data Science, Machine Learning and Distributed Processing are his research areas. He is a life member of Punjab Science Congress and Computer Society of India. He is the editorial member of Malaysian as well as Elsevier Journal.

S. Dheva Rajan Srinivasa Varadhan has 13 years of experience in academics and research. His field of research & thrust area is infectious diseases. He was awarded honorary doctorate twice by different Universities abroad for his extensive & dedicated service rendered towards academics and society in the field of Biomathematics. He has authored 6 books and published many research papers in international journals and conferences. His noteworthy contribution and dedicated involvement has led to the achievement of Young Scientist Award. He is a reviewer/editorial board member for many international journals. His area of interest is Bio Mathematics, especially at Infectious Diseases. He has conducted many workshops and seminars in diseases, R programming, and teaching methodologies.

Devesh Kumar Srivastava has been working as a Professor in the Department of Information Technology. He is associated with Manipal University Jaipur since August 2012. His research area is Software Engineering and Data Mining. He has been guiding research scholars in the field of Image Processing, Big Data Analytics and Data Mining He has supervised 8 students for M.Tech Dissertation and 10 B.Tech Students for their final year projects at MUJ. He has organised 2 workshops on open software tools. He has published around many research papers in peer reviewed journals including 2 (SCI and ESCI indexed). Many Scopus index research papers through conferences are published by Springer / ACM/ Elsevier / IEEE conferences. He addressed six Keynote /Invited talks in conferences and chaired many technical sessions at various International Conferences at various locations across India on Communication Technology, Software Engineering and Data Mining.

Amit Kumar Tyagi (GATE, NPwD-JRF, UGC-NET, and ICAR-NET) received his Ph.D degree in 2018 from Pondicherry Central University, Puducherry, India, in area of "Vehicular Ad-hoc Networks". His research interests include Formal Language Theory, Smart and Secure Computing, Privacy (including Genomic Privacy), Machine Learning with Big data, Blockchain Technology, Cyber Physical System etc. He has completed his M.Tech degree from the Pondicherry Central University, Puducherry, India. He joined the Lord Krishna College of Engineering, Ghaziabad (LKCE) for the periods of 2009-2010, and 2012-2013. With more than 08 (Eight) years of teaching and research experience across India, currently he is working as an Assistant Professor in Vellore Institute of Technology, Chennai Campus, Chennai 600127, Tamilnadu, India. Additionally, He is also the recipient/ awarded of the GATE and NPwD-JRF fellowship in 2009, 2016 and 2013. He has been published one major book titled "Know Your Technical (IT) Skills". Also He is a member of various Computer/ Research Communities like IEEE, ISOC, CSI, ISTE, DataScience, MIRLab, etc.

Manikandan V. M. is an Asst. Professor in Computer Science Engineering at SRM University AP, Andhra Pradesh, India. He his Ph.D. from Indian Institute of Information Technology Design and Manufacturing Kancheepuram, Chennai, India after his M.Tech in Software Engineering from Cochin University of Science and Technology, India. His area of research is reversible data hiding, digital image forensics, medical image processing and machine learning. He is a member of The Institution of Engineers (India) and ACM.

Eugenio Vocaturo received a degree in management engineering (2002), a Master in Industrial Engineering Management (2006), a master in Finance issued by SDA Bocconi (2016) and a PhD degree in Information and Communication Technologies at the University of Calabria, Rende, Italy. He has decades of experience as company director, production and logistics manager of business groups. He is currently a contract professor of Computer Science and assistant professor of the Process Mining course at the Department of Computer Science, Modeling, Electronics and Systems Engineering (DIMES) of University of Calabria. His current research interests include machine learning, optimization, issues related to classification problems applied to the medical context, emerging issues related to Cultural Heritage. He is a member of SIBIM (Italian Scientific Society of Biomedical Informatics) and of HL7 Italy (formed in 2003 as part of HL7 International), company responsible for the localization of health standards aiming at promoting the modernization of Italian health IT.

Ashwani Kumar Yadav has done his Ph.D. from Amity University Rajasthan. He did his M. Tech. in VLSI and Embedded System Design and B. Tech. in Electronics & Communication Engineering from MDU Rohtak, Haryana in India. His research interests include image processing, VLSI design and optimization techniques. He has published various research papers in reputed Journals and refereed international conferences. He is also serving as editorial board member and reviewer of reputed journals and conferences.

Shashank Yadav is a research scholar in Department of Computer Science and Engineering at Institute of Engineering & Technology, Lucknow, India.

Index

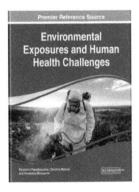
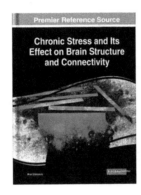
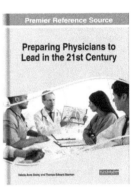
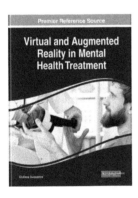
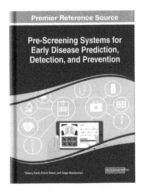
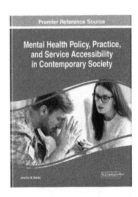
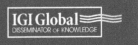

Ensure Quality Research is Introduced to the Academic Community

Become an IGI Global Reviewer for Authored Book Projects

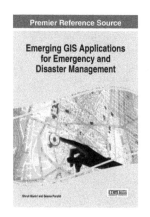
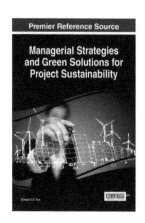
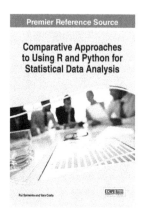
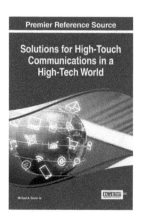

The overall success of an authored book project is dependent on quality and timely reviews.

In this competitive age of scholarly publishing, constructive and timely feedback significantly expedites the turnaround time of manuscripts from submission to acceptance, allowing the publication and discovery of forward-thinking research at a much more expeditious rate. Several IGI Global authored book projects are currently seeking highly-qualified experts in the field to fill vacancies on their respective editorial review boards:

Applications and Inquiries may be sent to:
development@igi-global.com

Applicants must have a doctorate (or an equivalent degree) as well as publishing and reviewing experience. Reviewers are asked to complete the open-ended evaluation questions with as much detail as possible in a timely, collegial, and constructive manner. All reviewers' tenures run for one-year terms on the editorial review boards and are expected to complete at least three reviews per term. Upon successful completion of this term, reviewers can be considered for an additional term.

If you have a colleague that may be interested in this opportunity, we encourage you to share this information with them.

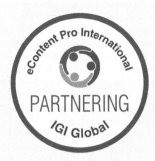

IGI Global Proudly Partners With eContent Pro International

Receive a 25% Discount on all Editorial Services

Editorial Services

IGI Global expects all final manuscripts submitted for publication to be in their final form. This means they must be reviewed, revised, and professionally copy edited prior to their final submission. Not only does this support with accelerating the publication process, but it also ensures that the highest quality scholarly work can be disseminated.

English Language Copy Editing

Let eContent Pro International's expert copy editors perform edits on your manuscript to resolve spelling, punctuaion, grammar, syntax, flow, formatting issues and more.

Scientific and Scholarly Editing

Allow colleagues in your research area to examine the content of your manuscript and provide you with valuable feedback and suggestions before submission.

Figure, Table, Chart & Equation Conversions

Do you have poor quality figures? Do you need visual elements in your manuscript created or converted? A design expert can help!

Translation

Need your documjent translated into English? eContent Pro International's expert translators are fluent in English and more than 40 different languages.

Email: **customerservice@econtentpro.com**   **www.igi-global.com/editorial-service-partners**

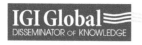

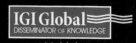

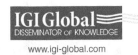
IGI Global's Transformative Open Access (OA) Model:
How to Turn Your University Library's Database Acquisitions Into a Source of OA Funding

In response to the OA movement and well in advance of Plan S, IGI Global, early last year, unveiled their OA Fee Waiver (Offset Model) Initiative.

Under this initiative, librarians who invest in IGI Global's InfoSci-Books (5,300+ reference books) and/or InfoSci-Journals (185+ scholarly journals) databases will be able to subsidize their patron's OA article processing charges (APC) when their work is submitted and accepted (after the peer review process) into an IGI Global journal.*

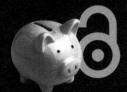

How Does it Work?

1. When a library subscribes or perpetually purchases IGI Global's InfoSci-Databases including InfoSci-Books (5,300+ e-books), InfoSci-Journals (185+ e-journals), and/or their discipline/subject-focused subsets, IGI Global will match the library's investment with a fund of equal value to go toward subsidizing the OA article processing charges (APCs) for their patrons.

   Researchers: Be sure to recommend the InfoSci-Books and InfoSci-Journals to take advantage of this initiative.

2. When a student, faculty, or staff member submits a paper and it is accepted (following the peer review) into one of IGI Global's 185+ scholarly journals, the author will have the option to have their paper published under a traditional publishing model or as OA.

3. When the author chooses to have their paper published under OA, IGI Global will notify them of the OA Fee Waiver (Offset Model) Initiative. If the author decides they would like to take advantage of this initiative, IGI Global will deduct the US$ 1,500 APC from the created fund.

4. This fund will be offered on an annual basis and will renew as the subscription is renewed for each year thereafter. IGI Global will manage the fund and award the APC waivers unless the librarian has a preference as to how the funds should be managed.

Hear From the Experts on This Initiative:

"I'm very happy to have been able to make one of my recent research contributions, 'Visualizing the Social Media Conversations of a National Information Technology Professional Association' featured in the *International Journal of Human Capital and Information Technology Professionals*, freely available along with having access to the valuable resources found within IGI Global's InfoSci-Journals database."

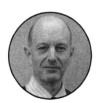

– **Prof. Stuart Palmer**,
Deakin University, Australia

For More Information, Visit: www.igi-global.com/publish/contributor-resources/open-access or contact IGI Global's Database Team at eresources@igi-global.com.

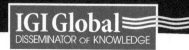
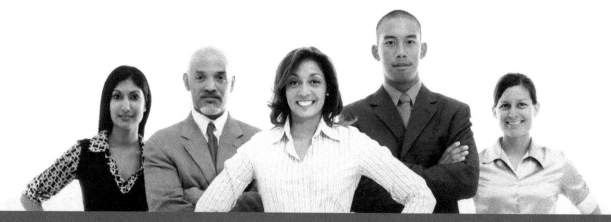

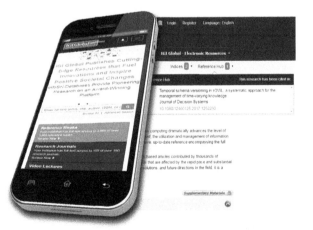
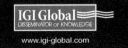

Printed in the USA
CPSIA information can be obtained
at www.ICGtesting.com
LVHW080255151023
761120LV00008B/583